Getting to Good

Arthur L. Caplan • Barbara K. Redman

Editors

Getting to Good

Research Integrity in the Biomedical Sciences

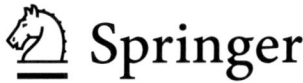 Springer

Editors
Arthur L. Caplan
New York University Langone Medical Center
William F. and Virginia Connolly Mitty
New York, NY, USA

Barbara K. Redman
New York Langone Medical Center
New York, NY, USA

ISBN 978-3-030-09598-7   ISBN 978-3-319-51358-4   (eBook)
https://doi.org/10.1007/978-3-319-51358-4

Preface

A successful scientific career requires a thorough understanding of the various elements of research integrity, also often called the responsible conduct of research (RCR). Many institutions and research funders require an RCR course, especially for PhD students and postdoctoral fellows. Since learning to do science and practicing it will bring you into contact with most of the issues covered in this book, it is important to know what the standards are and how they are evolving. You will follow, enforce, and contribute to them throughout your career.

Renewed developments in meta-science (the science of how to undertake science) are showing how scientific work can reach even higher standards, deemed important because of its societal impact. This examination raises questions of whether changing forms of self-regulation and/or government oversight will support those high standards. A complete record of research leading to a valid body of knowledge requires a literature that reports both positive and negative findings and that checks for their reproducibility as programs of research on important questions accumulate findings. Recently available technologies offer new ways of undermining research integrity (predatory journals, photoshopping images) and of enforcing it (detection of plagiarism and of falsified images).

Research integrity requires scientists, including those who have recently joined the community, to operate ethically in a system that supports ethical practice concurrent with changes in the environment. In the mid-twentieth century, a prominent reformer of science described the essential qualifications of an investigator – "must be well-trained and adequate as a scientist, be unselfish, imaginative, objective and have the ability of generalizing soundly" [1]. While rules and regulations are of key importance, personal virtues are still central for maintaining research integrity. Often it is virtue, the desire to do what is right rather than blindly following a rule, that is key to good conduct. Without a commitment to do what is right by investigators and those who work with them, rules are far less likely to be effective.

This book gives you both rules and the motivation to use them. It will help you reason through an ethical challenge when no rule exists. In addition, each section introduction provides a bit of specific advice about what you need to do or what you should be alert to in facing a potential research integrity issue.

By the way, in the name of research integrity the editors are very grateful to Kelly McBride Folkers and Jessica Wico for all their hard work on this book. It would not exist without them.

Reference

Beecher, H. Experimentation in man. JAMA. 1959;169(5):461–478.

New York, NY, USA   Arthur L. Caplan
                                                                     Barbara K. Redman

Contents

1 Methodology 1
Arthur L. Caplan and Barbara K. Redman

   1.1 Why Most Published Research Findings Are False 2
   John P. A. Ioannidis

   1.2 The Controversy Surrounding Bone Morphogenetic Proteins in the Spine: A Review of Current Research 9
   Joshua W. Hustedt and Daniel J. Blizzard

   1.3 Research Integrity and Everyday Practice of Science 23
   Frederick Grinnell

   1.4 Lessons from the Infuse Trials: Do We Need a Classification of Bias in Scientific Publications and Editorials? 41
   Sohaib Hashmi, Mohamed Noureldin, and Safdar N. Khan

2 Policy 51
Arthur L. Caplan and Barbara K. Redman

   2.1 In Retrospect: Science—The Endless Frontier 52
   Roger Pielke Jr.

   2.2 Publish or Perish Culture Encourages Scientists to Cut Corners 55
   Virginia Barbour

   2.3 "Something of an Adventure": Postwar NIH Research Ethos and the Guatemala STD Experiments 59
   Kayte Spector-Bagdady and Paul A. Lombardo

   2.4 Perverse Incentives 74
   Paula Stephen

   2.5 Flint Water Crisis Yields Hard Lessons in Science and Ethics 78
   Katie L. Burke

3 Reproducibility 95
Arthur L. Caplan and Barbara K. Redman

   3.1 What Does Research Reproducibility Mean? 96
   Steven N. Goodman, Daniele Fanelli, and John P. A. Ioannidis

   3.2 Limited Reproducibility of Research Findings: Implications for the Welfare of Research Participants and Considerations for Institutional Review Boards 103
   Barbara K. Redman and Arthur L. Caplan

   3.3 Quality Time 107
   Monya Baker

4 Human Subjects' Protection 113
Arthur L. Caplan and Barbara K. Redman

**4.1 A Scoping Review of Empirical Research Relating to Quality
and Effectiveness of Research Ethics Review** 114
Stuart G. Nicholls, Tavis P. Hayes, Jamie C. Brehaut,
Michael McDonald, Charles Weijer, Raphael Saginur,
and Dean Fergusson

**4.2 Pharmaceuticalisation and Ethical Review in South
Asia: Issues of Scope and Authority for Practitioners
and Policy Makers** 133
Bob Simpson, Rekha Khatri, Deapica Ravindran,
and Tharindi Udalagama

**4.3 Understanding the Functions and Operations of Data
Monitoring Committees: Survey and Focus Group Findings** 142
Karim A. Calis, Patrick Archdeacon, Raymond Bain, David DeMets,
Miriam Donohue, M. Khair Elzarrad, Annemarie Forrest,
John McEachern, Michael J. Pencina, Jane Perlmutter,
and Roger J. Lewis

**4.4 Women and Fetuses First? An Ethical Case for Giving Priority
in Clinical Research Testing of Zika Vaccines to Pregnant Women** 150
Kelly McBride Folkers and Arthur L. Caplan

4.5 Rethinking the Belmont Report? 162
Phoebe Friesen, Lisa Kearns, Barbara Redman, and Arthur L. Caplan

5 Responsible Authorship 173
Arthur L. Caplan and Barbara K. Redman

5.1 The Problem of Publication-Pollution Denialism 174
Arthur L. Caplan

**5.2 Addressing Research Misconduct and Detrimental
Research Practices: Current Knowledge and Issues** 177
National Academy of Sciences

5.3 Exploring New Approaches 184
National Academy of Sciences

**5.4 A Systematic Review of Research on the Meaning, Ethics
and Practices of Authorship across Scholarly Disciplines** 190
Ana Marusic, Lana Bosnjak, and Ana Jeroncic

**5.5 The Disposable Author: How Pharmaceutical Marketing
is Embraced within Medicine's Scholarly Literature** 208
Alastair Matheson

5.6 Authorship Inflation in Medical Publications 216
Gaurie Tilak, Vinay Prasad, and Annupam B. Jena

6   Mentor-Mentee Responsibilities and Relationships... 223
Arthur L. Caplan and Barbara K. Redman

    **6.1   Closing the Barn Door: Coping with Findings of Research
Misconduct by Trainees in the Biomedical Sciences** 224
Barbara K. Redman and Arthur L. Caplan

    **6.2   Mentoring and Research Misconduct: Analysis of Research
Mentoring in Closed ORI Cases** 234
David E. Wright, Sandra L. Titus, and Jered B. Cornelison

    6.3   Mentorship Matters for the Biomedical Workforce 249
Sally J. Rockey

    6.4   Professional Responsibility 251
C. K. Gunsalus

    6.5   All You Need is Mentorship 256
Robert A. Weinberg, Maya Schuldiner, Hong Wu, Beth Stevens,
Jens Nielsen, P. Robin Hiesinger, and Bassem A. Hassan

7   Plagiarism 261
Arthur L. Caplan and Barbara K. Redman

    7.1   Plagiarism in Research 262
Gert Helgesson and Stefan Eriksson

    **7.2   Text-Based Plagiarism in Scientific Publishing: Issues,
Developments and Education** 274
Yongyan Li

    **7.3   Avoiding Plagiarism, Self-Plagiarism, and Other
Questionable Writing Practices: A Guide to Ethical Writing** 289
Miguel Roig

    7.4   'Dear "Plagiarist': A Scientist Calls Out His Double-Crosser 361
Adam Marcus and Ivan Oransky

    7.5   Defining the Role of Authors and Contributors 366
International Committee of Medical Journal Editors

8   Peer Review 371
Arthur L. Caplan and Barbara K. Redman

    8.1   Let's Make Peer Review Scientific 372
Drummond Rennie

    8.2   A Stronger Post-Publication Culture Is Needed for Better Science........ 376
Hilda Bastian

    8.3   Reviewing Post-Publication Peer Review 380
Paul Knoepfler

9   Research Misconduct 385
Arthur L. Caplan and Barbara K. Redman

   9.1   Shattuck Lecture: Misconduct in Medical Research 387
   John D. Dingell

   **9.2   Ethical Modernization: Research Misconduct and Research
           Ethics Reforms in Korea following the Hwang Affair** 394
   Jongyoung Kim and Kibeom Park

   **9.3   Research Misconduct and Data Fraud in Clinical
           Trials: Prevalence and Causal Factors** 421
   Stephen L. George

   9.4   Repairing Research Integrity 429
   Sandra L. Titus, James A. Wells, and Lawrence J. Rhoades

10   Whistleblowing 435
Arthur L. Caplan and Barbara K. Redman

   10.1   Integrity and Misconduct in Research 436
   Commission on Research Integrity

   10.2   Whistle-Blower Breaks His Silence 453
   David Cyranoski

   10.3   No One Likes a Snitch 456
   Barbara Redman and Arthur Caplan

11   Conflict of Interest 465
Arthur L. Caplan and Barbara K. Redman

   **11.1   Sugar Industry Influence on the Scientific Agenda
           of the National Institute of Dental Research's 1971
           National Caries Program: A Historical Analysis
           of Internal Documents** 467
   Cristin E. Kearns, Stanton A. Glantz, and Laura A. Schmidt

   **11.2   Lessons Learned from the Gene Therapy Trial
           for Ornithine Transcarbamylase Deficiency** 490
   James M. Wilson

   **11.3   Patient Perspectives on Physician Conflict of Interest
           in Industry-Sponsored Clinical Trials for Multiple
           Sclerosis Therapeutics** 498
   Andrew J. Solomon

   **11.4   Industry Support of Medical Research: Important
           Opportunity or Treacherous Pitfall?** 506
   William M. Tierney, Eric M. Meslin, and Kurt Kroenke

12   Data Acquisition, Management and Transparency 515
Arthur L. Caplan and Barbara K. Redman

**12.1   Opentrials: Towards a Collaborative Open Database
         of All Available Information on All Clinical Trials**.................................. 517
Ben Goldacre and Jonathan Gray

**12.2   International Charter of Principles for Sharing
         Bio-specimens and Data**... 530
Deborah Mascalzoni, Edward S. Dove, Yaffa Rubinstein,
Hugh J. S. Dawkins, Anna Kole, Pauline McCormack, Simon Woods,
Olaf Riess, Franz Schaefer, Hanns Lochmüller, Bartha M. Knoppers,
and Mats Hansson

**12.3   Facilitating a Culture of Responsible and Effective
         Sharing of Cancer Genome Data** 539
Lillian L. Siu, Mark Lawler, David Haussler, Bartha Maria Knoppers,
Jeremy Lewin, Daniel J. Vis, Rachel G. Liao, Fabrice Andre, Ian Banks,
J. Carl Barrett, Carlos Caldas, Anamaria Aranha Camargo,
Rebecca C. Fitzgerald, Mao Mao, John E. Mattison,
William Pao, William R. Sellers, Patrick Sullivan,
Bin Tean Teh, Robyn L. Ward, Jean Claude ZenKlusen,
Charles L. Sawyers, and Emile E. Voest

13   International Research Involving Resource-Constrained Countries 549
Arthur L. Caplan and Barbara K. Redman

**13.1   The H3Africa Policy Framework: Negotiating Fairness
         in Genomics**... 550
Jantina de Vries, Paulina Tindana, Katherine Littler, Miche` le Ramsay,
Charles Rotimi, Akin Abayomi, Nicola Mulder, and Bongani M. Mayosi

**13.2   Sponsorship in Non-commercial Clinical Trials: Definitions,
         Challenges and the Role of Good Clinical Practices Guidelines** 554
Raffaella Ravinetto, Katelijne De Nys, Marleen Boelaert, Ermias Diro,
Graeme Meintjes, Yeka Adoke, Harry Tagbor, and Minne Casteels

**13.3   Improving the Informed Consent Process in International
         Collaborative Rare Disease Research: Effective Consent
         for Effective Research** 562
Sabina Gainott, Cathy Turner, Simon Woods, Anna Kole,
Pauline McCormack, Hanns Lochmüller, Olaf Riess, Volker Straub,
Manuel Posada, Domenica Taruscio, and Deborah Mascalzoni

**13.4   The Standard of Care Debate: Can Research in Developing
         Countries Be Both Ethical and Responsive To Those
         Countries' Health Needs?** 570
David Wendler, Ezekiel J. Emanuel, and Reidar K. Lie

**Appendix: Montreal Statement on Research Integrity
in Cross-Boundary Research Collaborations, 2013** 579

Index.. 581

Methodology

Arthur L. Caplan and Barbara K. Redman

Research integrity is now being redefined to require a higher level of methodological quality than has historically been the case. Innovations to reach this new standard fall into several categories: increased use of alternative trial designs with questions about how subject protection can be applied; need to move away from 'P' values and toward effect sizes in statistical analysis and full reporting of research methods including methods of analysis and modified endpoints. Driven by the recognition that the historically dominant standard of the randomized placebo-controlled trial (RCT) is not economically, politically, or scientifically always useful, new trial designs recognize the heterogeneity of disease, the need for timely answers in humanitarian emergencies or for the seriously ill, improvement in trial recruitment and receipt of appropriate treatment, and recognition of the need to synthesize information across trials (Berry 2016). For example, pragmatic trials occur in usual practice settings and raise questions about whether and how patients can opt out and who should review them; basket trials test whether different diseases or subtypes respond to a particular therapy; platform trials test multiple therapies made by different sponsors simultaneously for a particular disease; adaptive trials adjust enrollment during the trial based on accumulating evidence of superiority or inferiority of various arms; cross over designs afford all subjects a chance to experience the active agent in a trial; and cluster randomized trials enroll naturally occurring groups of patients permitting comparisons otherwise not possible in standard trial recruitment. And in many areas of inquiry, integrating qualitative with quantitative findings is becoming standard.

Clinical trial endpoints and surrogates are important for the rapid, accurate accumulation of evidence. Outcomes such as survival, health status, and disease progression may not be evident for a long time. Surrogate endpoints may represent part of the causal chain of disease progression; they must have been validated to be predictive of true endpoints and be sensitive to various ongoing clinical interventions. Surrogate data are now beginning to be accepted by many regulatory agencies for the approval of new drugs and vaccines.

Beyond these methodological innovations, perhaps the most important message for research integrity is that the traditional model of science describes it as a linear process based on logic that is carried out by objective researchers. Grinnell (2013) notes that in reality the scientific practice is much more nuanced, requiring judgments about how to interpret findings or how to diagnose the source of "failed experiments" so as to move forward.

Advice: Read a scientific memoir to get a flavor for how the science was really practiced. Be sure your institution provides full instruction in the methods for your field of research. If you feel it doesn't, ask for more, take relevant courses in an allied discipline, or do an internship with a scientist who is on the cutting edge of innovative methodology. Inadequate methods are a common problem for research integrity; methods well fitted to the research problem support integrity and build your career.

A. L. Caplan · B. K. Redman (✉)
New York University Langone Medical Center,
New York, NY, USA
e-mail: Arthur.Caplan@nyumc.org

© Springer International Publishing AG, part of Springer Nature 2018
A. L. Caplan, B. K. Redman (eds.), *Getting to Good*, https://doi.org/10.1007/978-3-319-51358-4_1

1.1 Why Most Published Research Findings Are False

John P. A. Ioannidis

Ioannidis, J. Why most published research findings are false. *PLoS Medicine* 2(8)e124, 0696–0701 (2005)

Open access, freely available online

Essay

Why Most Published Research Findings Are False

John P. A. Ioannidis

Summary

There is increasing concern that most current published research findings are false. The probability that a research claim is true may depend on study power and bias, the number of other studies on the same question, and, importantly, the ratio of true to no relationships among the relationships probed in each scientific field. In this framework, a research finding is less likely to be true when the studies conducted in a field are smaller; when effect sizes are smaller; when there is a greater number and lesser preselection of tested relationships; where there is greater flexibility in designs, definitions, outcomes, and analytical modes; when there is greater financial and other interest and prejudice; and when more teams are involved in a scientific field in chase of statistical significance. Simulations show that for most study designs and settings, it is more likely for a research claim to be false than true. Moreover, for many current scientific fields, claimed research findings may often be simply accurate measures of the prevailing bias. In this essay, I discuss the implications of these problems for the conduct and interpretation of research.

P ublished research findings are sometimes refuted by subsequent evidence, with ensuing confusion and disappointment. Refutation and controversy is seen across the range of research designs, from clinical trials and traditional epidemiological studies [1–3] to the most modern molecular research [4,5]. There is increasing concern that in modern research, false findings may be the majority or even the vast majority of published research claims [6–8]. However, this should not be surprising. It can be proven that most claimed research findings are false. Here I will examine the key

The Essay section contains opinion pieces on topics of broad interest to a general medical audience.

factors that influence this problem and some corollaries thereof.

Modeling the Framework for False Positive Findings

Several methodologists have pointed out [9–11] that the high rate of nonreplication (lack of confirmation) of research discoveries is a consequence of the convenient, yet ill-founded strategy of claiming conclusive research findings solely on the basis of a single study assessed by formal statistical significance, typically for a *p*-value less than 0.05. Research is not most appropriately represented and summarized by *p*-values, but, unfortunately, there is a widespread notion that medical research articles

> ## It can be proven that most claimed research findings are false.

should be interpreted based only on *p*-values. Research findings are defined here as any relationship reaching formal statistical significance, e.g., effective interventions, informative predictors, risk factors, or associations. "Negative" research is also very useful. "Negative" is actually a misnomer, and the misinterpretation is widespread. However, here we will target relationships that investigators claim exist, rather than null findings.

As has been shown previously, the probability that a research finding is indeed true depends on the prior probability of it being true (before doing the study), the statistical power of the study, and the level of statistical significance [10,11]. Consider a 2×2 table in which research findings are compared against the gold standard of true relationships in a scientific field. In a research field both true and false hypotheses can be made about the presence of relationships. Let R be the ratio of the number of "true relationships" to "no relationships" among those tested in the field. R

is characteristic of the field and can vary a lot depending on whether the field targets highly likely relationships or searches for only one or a few true relationships among thousands and millions of hypotheses that may be postulated. Let us also consider, for computational simplicity, circumscribed fields where either there is only one true relationship (among many that can be hypothesized) or the power is similar to find any of the several existing true relationships. The pre-study probability of a relationship being true is $R/(R + 1)$. The probability of a study finding a true relationship reflects the power $1 - \beta$ (one minus the Type II error rate). The probability of claiming a relationship when none truly exists reflects the Type I error rate, α. Assuming that c relationships are being probed in the field, the expected values of the 2×2 table are given in Table 1. After a research finding has been claimed based on achieving formal statistical significance, the post-study probability that it is true is the positive predictive value, PPV. The PPV is also the complementary probability of what Wacholder et al. have called the false positive report probability [10]. According to the 2×2 table, one gets PPV = $(1 - \beta) R/(R - \beta R + \alpha)$. A research finding is thus

Citation: Ioannidis JPA (2005) Why most published research findings are false. PLoS Med 2(8): e124.

Copyright: © 2005 John P. A. Ioannidis. This is an open-access article distributed under the terms of the Creative Commons Attribution License, which permits unrestricted use, distribution, and reproduction in any medium, provided the original work is properly cited.

Abbreviation: PPV, positive predictive value

John P. A. Ioannidis is in the Department of Hygiene and Epidemiology, University of Ioannina School of Medicine, Ioannina, Greece, and Institute for Clinical Research and Health Policy Studies, Department of Medicine, Tufts-New England Medical Center, Tufts University School of Medicine, Boston, Massachusetts, United States of America. E-mail: jioannid@cc.uoi.gr

Competing Interests: The author has declared that no competing interests exist.

DOI: 10.1371/journal.pmed.0020124

Table 1. Research Findings and True Relationships

Research Finding	True Relationship		
	Yes	**No**	**Total**
Yes	$c(1-\beta)R/(R+1)$	$c\alpha/(R+1)$	$c(R+\alpha-\beta R)/(R+1)$
No	$c\beta R/(R+1)$	$c(1-\alpha)/(R+1)$	$c(1-\alpha+\beta R)/(R+1)$
Total	$cR/(R+1)$	$c/(R+1)$	c

DOI: 10.1371/journal.pmed.0020124.t001

more likely true than false if $(1-\beta)R > \alpha$. Since usually the vast majority of investigators depend on $\alpha = 0.05$, this means that a research finding is more likely true than false if $(1-\beta)R > 0.05$.

What is less well appreciated is that bias and the extent of repeated independent testing by different teams of investigators around the globe may further distort this picture and may lead to even smaller probabilities of the research findings being indeed true. We will try to model these two factors in the context of similar 2 × 2 tables.

Bias

First, let us define bias as the combination of various design, data, analysis, and presentation factors that tend to produce research findings when they should not be produced. Let u be the proportion of probed analyses that would not have been "research findings," but nevertheless end up presented and reported as such, because of bias. Bias should not be confused with chance variability that causes some findings to be false by chance even though the study design, data, analysis, and presentation are perfect. Bias can entail manipulation in the analysis or reporting of findings. Selective or distorted reporting is a typical form of such bias. We may assume that u does not depend on whether a true relationship exists or not. This is not an unreasonable assumption, since typically it is impossible to know which relationships are indeed true. In the presence of bias (Table 2), one gets PPV = $([1-\beta]R + u\beta R)/(R + \alpha - \beta R + u - u\alpha + u\beta R)$, and PPV decreases with increasing u, unless $1-\beta \leq \alpha$, i.e., $1-\beta \leq 0.05$ for most situations. Thus, with increasing bias, the chances that a research finding is true diminish considerably. This is shown for different levels of power and for different pre-study odds in Figure 1.

Conversely, true research findings may occasionally be annulled because of reverse bias. For example, with large measurement errors relationships

are lost in noise [12], or investigators use data inefficiently or fail to notice statistically significant relationships, or there may be conflicts of interest that tend to "bury" significant findings [13]. There is no good large-scale empirical evidence on how frequently such reverse bias may occur across diverse research fields. However, it is probably fair to say that reverse bias is not as common. Moreover measurement errors and inefficient use of data are probably becoming less frequent problems, since measurement error has decreased with technological advances in the molecular era and investigators are becoming increasingly sophisticated about their data. Regardless, reverse bias may be modeled in the same way as bias above. Also reverse bias should not be confused with chance variability that may lead to missing a true relationship because of chance.

Testing by Several Independent Teams

Several independent teams may be addressing the same sets of research questions. As research efforts are globalized, it is practically the rule that several research teams, often dozens of them, may probe the same or similar questions. Unfortunately, in some areas, the prevailing mentality until now has been to focus on isolated discoveries by single teams and interpret research experiments in isolation. An increasing number of questions have at least one study claiming a research finding, and this receives unilateral attention. The probability that at least one study, among several done on the

same question, claims a statistically significant research finding is easy to estimate. For n independent studies of equal power, the 2 × 2 table is shown in Table 3: PPV = $R(1-\beta^n)/(R+1-[1-\alpha]^n - R\beta^n)$ (not considering bias). With increasing number of independent studies, PPV tends to decrease, unless $1-\beta < \alpha$, i.e., typically $1-\beta < 0.05$. This is shown for different levels of power and for different pre-study odds in Figure 2. For n studies of different power, the term β^n is replaced by the product of the terms β_i for $i = 1$ to n, but inferences are similar.

Corollaries

A practical example is shown in Box 1. Based on the above considerations, one may deduce several interesting corollaries about the probability that a research finding is indeed true.

Corollary 1: The smaller the studies conducted in a scientific field, the less likely the research findings are to be true. Small sample size means smaller power and, for all functions above, the PPV for a true research finding decreases as power decreases towards $1-\beta = 0.05$. Thus, other factors being equal, research findings are more likely true in scientific fields that undertake large studies, such as randomized controlled trials in cardiology (several thousand subjects randomized) [14] than in scientific fields with small studies, such as most research of molecular predictors (sample sizes 100-fold smaller) [15].

Corollary 2: The smaller the effect sizes in a scientific field, the less likely the research findings are to be true. Power is also related to the effect size. Thus research findings are more likely true in scientific fields with large effects, such as the impact of smoking on cancer or cardiovascular disease (relative risks 3–20), than in scientific fields where postulated effects are small, such as genetic risk factors for multigenetic diseases (relative risks 1.1–1.5) [7]. Modern epidemiology is increasingly obliged to target smaller

Table 2. Research Findings and True Relationships in the Presence of Bias

Research Finding	True Relationship		
	Yes	**No**	**Total**
Yes	$(c[1-\beta]R + uc\beta R)/(R+1)$	$c\alpha + uc(1-\alpha)/(R+1)$	$c(R+\alpha-\beta R+u-u\alpha+u\beta R)/(R+1)$
No	$(1-u)c\beta R/(R+1)$	$(1-u)c(1-\alpha)/(R+1)$	$c(1-u)(1-\alpha+\beta R)/(R+1)$
Total	$cR/(R+1)$	$c/(R+1)$	c

DOI: 10.1371/journal.pmed.0020124.t002

effect sizes [16]. Consequently, the proportion of true research findings is expected to decrease. In the same line of thinking, if the true effect sizes are very small in a scientific field, this field is likely to be plagued by almost ubiquitous false positive claims. For example, if the majority of true genetic or nutritional determinants of complex diseases confer relative risks less than 1.05, genetic or nutritional epidemiology would be largely utopian endeavors.

Corollary 3: The greater the number and the lesser the selection of tested relationships in a scientific field, the less likely the research findings are to be true. As shown above, the post-study probability that a finding is true (PPV) depends a lot on the pre-study odds (R). Thus, research findings are more likely true in confirmatory designs, such as large phase III randomized controlled trials, or meta-analyses thereof, than in hypothesis-generating experiments. Fields considered highly informative and creative given the wealth of the assembled and tested information, such as microarrays and other high-throughput discovery-oriented research [4,8,17], should have extremely low PPV.

Corollary 4: The greater the flexibility in designs, definitions, outcomes, and analytical modes in a scientific field, the less likely the research findings are to be true. Flexibility increases the potential for transforming what would be "negative" results into "positive" results, i.e., bias, u. For several research designs, e.g., randomized controlled trials [18–20] or meta-analyses [21,22], there have been efforts to standardize their conduct and reporting. Adherence to common standards is likely to increase the proportion of true findings. The same applies to outcomes. True findings may be more common when outcomes are unequivocal and universally agreed (e.g., death) rather than when multifarious outcomes are devised (e.g., scales for schizophrenia

outcomes) [23]. Similarly, fields that use commonly agreed, stereotyped analytical methods (e.g., Kaplan-Meier plots and the log-rank test) [24] may yield a larger proportion of true findings than fields where analytical methods are still under experimentation (e.g., artificial intelligence methods) and only "best" results are reported. Regardless, even in the most stringent research designs, bias seems to be a major problem. For example, there is strong evidence that selective outcome reporting, with manipulation of the outcomes and analyses reported, is a common problem even for randomized trails [25]. Simply abolishing selective publication would not make this problem go away.

Corollary 5: The greater the financial and other interests and prejudices in a scientific field, the less likely the research findings are to be true. Conflicts of interest and prejudice may increase bias, u. Conflicts of interest are very common in biomedical research [26], and typically they are inadequately and sparsely reported [26,27]. Prejudice may not necessarily have financial roots. Scientists in a given field may be prejudiced purely because of their belief in a scientific theory or commitment to their own findings. Many otherwise seemingly independent, university-based studies may be conducted for no other reason than to give physicians and researchers qualifications for promotion or tenure. Such nonfinancial conflicts may also lead to distorted reported results and interpretations. Prestigious investigators may suppress via the peer review process the appearance and dissemination of findings that refute their findings, thus condemning their field to perpetuate false dogma. Empirical evidence on expert opinion shows that it is extremely unreliable [28].

Corollary 6: The hotter a scientific field (with more scientific teams involved), the less likely the research findings are to be true.

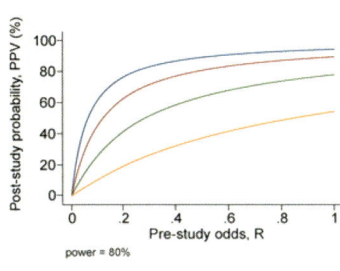

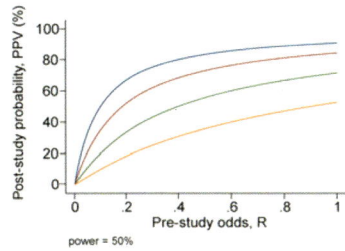

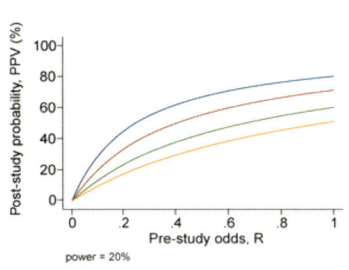

— u=0.05 — u=0.20 — u=0.50 — u=0.80
DOI: 10.1371/journal.pmed.0020124.g001

Figure 1. PPV (Probability That a Research Finding Is True) as a Function of the Pre-Study Odds for Various Levels of Bias, u

Panels correspond to power of 0.20, 0.50, and 0.80.

This seemingly paradoxical corollary follows because, as stated above, the PPV of isolated findings decreases when many teams of investigators are involved in the same field. This may explain why we occasionally see major excitement followed rapidly by severe disappointments in fields that draw wide attention. With many teams working on the same field and with massive experimental data being produced, timing is of the essence in beating competition. Thus, each team may prioritize on pursuing and disseminating its most impressive "positive" results. "Negative" results may become attractive for dissemination only if some other team has found a "positive" association on the same question. In that case, it may be attractive to refute a claim made in some prestigious journal. The term Proteus phenomenon has been coined to describe this phenomenon of rapidly

Table 3. Research Findings and True Relationships in the Presence of Multiple Studies

Research Finding	True Relationship		
	Yes	No	Total
Yes	$cR(1 - \beta^n)/(R + 1)$	$c(1 - [1 - \alpha]^n)/(R + 1)$	$c(R + 1 - [1 - \alpha]^n - R\beta^n)/(R + 1)$
No	$cR\beta^n/(R + 1)$	$c(1 - \alpha)^n/(R + 1)$	$c([1 - \alpha]^n + R\beta^n)/(R + 1)$
Total	$cR/(R + 1)$	$c/(R + 1)$	c

DOI: 10.1371/journal.pmed.0020124.t003

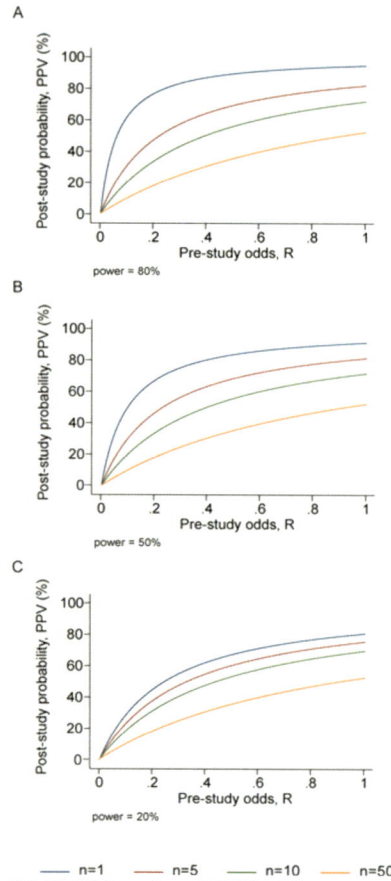

A

B

C

— n=1   — n=5   — n=10   — n=50

DOI: 10.1371/journal.pmed.0020124.g002

Figure 2. PPV (Probability That a Research Finding Is True) as a Function of the Pre-Study Odds for Various Numbers of Conducted Studies, n

Panels correspond to power of 0.20, 0.50, and 0.80.

alternating extreme research claims and extremely opposite refutations [29]. Empirical evidence suggests that this sequence of extreme opposites is very common in molecular genetics [29].

These corollaries consider each factor separately, but these factors often influence each other. For example, investigators working in fields where true effect sizes are perceived to be small may be more likely to perform large studies than investigators working in fields where true effect sizes are perceived to be large. Or prejudice may prevail in a hot scientific field, further undermining the predictive value of its research findings. Highly prejudiced stakeholders may even create a barrier that aborts efforts at obtaining and disseminating opposing results. Conversely, the fact that a field

PLoS Medicine | www.plosmedicine.org   0699   August 2005 | Volume 2 | Issue 8 | e124

Box 1. An Example: Science at Low Pre-Study Odds

Let us assume that a team of investigators performs a whole genome association study to test whether any of 100,000 gene polymorphisms are associated with susceptibility to schizophrenia. Based on what we know about the extent of heritability of the disease, it is reasonable to expect that probably around ten gene polymorphisms among those tested would be truly associated with schizophrenia, with relatively similar odds ratios around 1.3 for the ten or so polymorphisms and with a fairly similar power to identify any of them. Then $R = 10/100,000 = 10^{-4}$, and the pre-study probability for any polymorphism to be associated with schizophrenia is also $R/(R + 1) = 10^{-4}$. Let us also suppose that the study has 60% power to find an association with an odds ratio of 1.3 at $\alpha = 0.05$. Then it can be estimated that if a statistically significant association is found with the p-value barely crossing the 0.05 threshold, the post-study probability that this is true increases about 12-fold compared with the pre-study probability, but it is still only 12×10^{-4}.

Now let us suppose that the investigators manipulate their design, analyses, and reporting so as to make more relationships cross the $p = 0.05$ threshold even though this would not have been crossed with a perfectly adhered to design and analysis and with perfect comprehensive reporting of the results, strictly according to the original study plan. Such manipulation could be done, for example, with serendipitous inclusion or exclusion of certain patients or controls, post hoc subgroup analyses, investigation of genetic contrasts that were not originally specified, changes in the disease or control definitions, and various combinations of selective or distorted reporting of the results. Commercially available "data mining" packages actually are proud of their ability to yield statistically significant results through data dredging. In the presence of bias with $u = 0.10$, the post-study probability that a research finding is true is only 4.4×10^{-4}. Furthermore, even in the absence of any bias, when ten independent research teams perform similar experiments around the world, if one of them finds a formally statistically significant association, the probability that the research finding is true is only 1.5×10^{-4}, hardly any higher than the probability we had before any of this extensive research was undertaken!

---

is hot or has strong invested interests may sometimes promote larger studies and improved standards of research, enhancing the predictive value of its research findings. Or massive discovery-oriented testing may result in such a large yield of significant relationships that investigators have enough to report and search further and thus refrain from data dredging and manipulation.

Most Research Findings Are False for Most Research Designs and for Most Fields

In the described framework, a PPV exceeding 50% is quite difficult to get. Table 4 provides the results of simulations using the formulas developed for the influence of power, ratio of true to non-true relationships, and bias, for various types of situations that may be characteristic of specific study designs and settings. A finding from a well-conducted, adequately powered randomized controlled trial starting with a 50% pre-study chance that the intervention is effective is

eventually true about 85% of the time. A fairly similar performance is expected of a confirmatory meta-analysis of good-quality randomized trials: potential bias probably increases, but power and pre-test chances are higher compared to a single randomized trial. Conversely, a meta-analytic finding from inconclusive studies where pooling is used to "correct" the low power of single studies, is probably false if $R \leq 1:3$. Research findings from underpowered, early-phase clinical trials would be true about one in four times, or even less frequently if bias is present. Epidemiological studies of an exploratory nature perform even worse, especially when underpowered, but even well-powered epidemiological studies may have only a one in five chance being true, if $R = 1:10$. Finally, in discovery-oriented research with massive testing, where tested relationships exceed true ones 1,000-fold (e.g., 30,000 genes tested, of which 30 may be the true culprits) [30,31], PPV for each claimed relationship is extremely low, even with considerable standardization of laboratory and statistical methods, outcomes, and reporting thereof to minimize bias.

Claimed Research Findings May Often Be Simply Accurate Measures of the Prevailing Bias

As shown, the majority of modern biomedical research is operating in areas with very low pre- and post-study probability for true findings. Let us suppose that in a research field there are no true findings at all to be discovered. History of science teaches us that scientific endeavor has often in the past wasted effort in fields with absolutely no yield of true scientific information, at least based on our current understanding. In such a "null field," one would ideally expect all observed effect sizes to vary by chance around the null in the absence of bias. The extent that observed findings deviate from what is expected by chance alone would be simply a pure measure of the prevailing bias.

For example, let us suppose that no nutrients or dietary patterns are actually important determinants for the risk of developing a specific tumor. Let us also suppose that the scientific literature has examined 60 nutrients and claims all of them to be related to the risk of developing this tumor with relative risks in the range of 1.2 to 1.4 for the comparison of the upper to lower intake tertiles. Then the claimed effect sizes are simply measuring nothing else but the net bias that has been involved in the generation of this scientific literature. Claimed effect sizes are in fact the most accurate estimates of the net bias. It even follows that between "null fields," the fields that claim stronger effects (often with accompanying claims of medical or public health importance) are simply those that have sustained the worst biases.

For fields with very low PPV, the few true relationships would not distort this overall picture much. Even if a few relationships are true, the shape of the distribution of the observed effects would still yield a clear measure of the biases involved in the field. This concept totally reverses the way we view scientific results. Traditionally, investigators have viewed large and highly significant effects with excitement, as signs of important discoveries. Too large and too highly significant effects may actually be more likely to be signs of large bias in most fields of modern research. They should lead investigators to careful critical thinking about what might have gone wrong with their data, analyses, and results.

Of course, investigators working in any field are likely to resist accepting that the whole field in which they have spent their careers is a "null field." However, other lines of evidence, or advances in technology and experimentation, may lead eventually to the dismantling of a scientific field. Obtaining measures of the net bias in one field may also be useful for obtaining insight into what might be the range of bias operating in other fields where similar analytical methods, technologies, and conflicts may be operating.

How Can We Improve the Situation?

Is it unavoidable that most research findings are false, or can we improve the situation? A major problem is that it is impossible to know with 100% certainty what the truth is in any research question. In this regard, the pure "gold" standard is unattainable. However, there are several approaches to improve the post-study probability.

Better powered evidence, e.g., large studies or low-bias meta-analyses, may help, as it comes closer to the unknown "gold" standard. However, large studies may still have biases and these should be acknowledged and avoided. Moreover, large-scale evidence is impossible to obtain for all of the millions and trillions of research questions posed in current research. Large-scale evidence should be targeted for research questions where the pre-study probability is already considerably high, so that a significant research finding will lead to a post-test probability that would be considered quite definitive. Large-scale evidence is also particularly indicated when it can test major concepts rather than narrow, specific questions. A negative finding can then refute not only a specific proposed claim, but a whole field or considerable portion thereof. Selecting the performance of large-scale studies based on narrow-minded criteria, such as the marketing promotion of a specific drug, is largely wasted research. Moreover, one should be cautious that extremely large studies may be more likely to find a formally statistical significant difference for a trivial effect that is not really meaningfully different from the null [32–34].

Second, most research questions are addressed by many teams, and it is misleading to emphasize the statistically significant findings of any single team. What matters is the

Table 4. PPV of Research Findings for Various Combinations of Power $(1 - \beta)$, Ratio of True to Not-True Relationships (R), and Bias (u)

$1 - \beta$	R	u	Practical Example	PPV
0.80	1:1	0.10	Adequately powered RCT with little bias and 1:1 pre-study odds	0.85
0.95	2:1	0.30	Confirmatory meta-analysis of good-quality RCTs	0.85
0.80	1:3	0.40	Meta-analysis of small inconclusive studies	0.41
0.20	1:5	0.20	Underpowered, but well-performed phase I/II RCT	0.23
0.20	1:5	0.80	Underpowered, poorly performed phase I/II RCT	0.17
0.80	1:10	0.30	Adequately powered exploratory epidemiological study	0.20
0.20	1:10	0.30	Underpowered exploratory epidemiological study	0.12
0.20	1:1,000	0.80	Discovery-oriented exploratory research with massive testing	0.0010
0.20	1:1,000	0.20	As in previous example, but with more limited bias (more standardized)	0.0015

The estimated PPVs (positive predictive values) are derived assuming $\alpha = 0.05$ for a single study.
RCT, randomized controlled trial.
DOI: 10.1371/journal.pmed.0020124.t004

totality of the evidence. Diminishing bias through enhanced research standards and curtailing of prejudices may also help. However, this may require a change in scientific mentality that might be difficult to achieve. In some research designs, efforts may also be more successful with upfront registration of studies, e.g., randomized trials [35]. Registration would pose a challenge for hypothesis-generating research. Some kind of registration or networking of data collections or investigators within fields may be more feasible than registration of each and every hypothesis-generating experiment. Regardless, even if we do not see a great deal of progress with registration of studies in other fields, the principles of developing and adhering to a protocol could be more widely borrowed from randomized controlled trials.

Finally, instead of chasing statistical significance, we should improve our understanding of the range of R values—the pre-study odds—where research efforts operate [10]. Before running an experiment, investigators should consider what they believe the chances are that they are testing a true rather than a non-true relationship. Speculated high R values may sometimes then be ascertained. As described above, whenever ethically acceptable, large studies with minimal bias should be performed on research findings that are considered relatively established, to see how often they are indeed confirmed. I suspect several established "classics" will fail the test [36].

Nevertheless, most new discoveries will continue to stem from hypothesis-generating research with low or very low pre-study odds. We should then acknowledge that statistical significance testing in the report of a single study gives only a partial picture, without knowing how much testing has been done outside the report and in the relevant field at large. Despite a large statistical literature for multiple testing corrections [37], usually it is impossible to decipher how much data dredging by the reporting authors or other research teams has preceded a reported research finding. Even if determining this were feasible, this would not inform us about the pre-study odds. Thus, it is unavoidable that one should make approximate assumptions on how

many relationships are expected to be true among those probed across the relevant research fields and research designs. The wider field may yield some guidance for estimating this probability for the isolated research project. Experiences from biases detected in other neighboring fields would also be useful to draw upon. Even though these assumptions would be considerably subjective, they would still be very useful in interpreting research claims and putting them in context. ∎

References

1. Ioannidis JP, Haidich AB, Lau J (2001) Any casualties in the clash of randomised and observational evidence? BMJ 322: 879–880.
2. Lawlor DA, Davey Smith G, Kundu D, Bruckdorfer KR, Ebrahim S (2004) Those confounded vitamins: What can we learn from the differences between observational versus randomised trial evidence? Lancet 363: 1724–1727.
3. Vandenbroucke JP (2004) When are observational studies as credible as randomised trials? Lancet 363: 1728–1731.
4. Michiels S, Koscielny S, Hill C (2005) Prediction of cancer outcome with microarrays: A multiple random validation strategy. Lancet 365: 488–492.
5. Ioannidis JPA, Ntzani EE, Trikalinos TA, Contopoulos-Ioannidis DG (2001) Replication validity of genetic association studies. Nat Genet 29: 306–309.
6. Colhoun HM, McKeigue PM, Davey Smith G (2003) Problems of reporting genetic associations with complex outcomes. Lancet 361: 865–872.
7. Ioannidis JP (2003) Genetic associations: False or true? Trends Mol Med 9: 135–138.
8. Ioannidis JPA (2005) Microarrays and molecular research: Noise discovery? Lancet 365: 454–455.
9. Sterne JA, Davey Smith G (2001) Sifting the evidence—What's wrong with significance tests. BMJ 322: 226–231.
10. Wacholder S, Chanock S, Garcia-Closas M, El ghormli L, Rothman N (2004) Assessing the probability that a positive report is false: An approach for molecular epidemiology studies. J Natl Cancer Inst 96: 434–442.
11. Risch NJ (2000) Searching for genetic determinants in the new millennium. Nature 405: 847–856.
12. Kelsey JL, Whittemore AS, Evans AS, Thompson WD (1996) Methods in observational epidemiology, 2nd ed. New York: Oxford U Press. 432 p.
13. Topol EJ (2004) Failing the public health—Rofecoxib, Merck, and the FDA. N Engl J Med 351: 1707–1709.
14. Yusuf S, Collins R, Peto R (1984) Why do we need some large, simple randomized trials? Stat Med 3: 409–422.
15. Altman DG, Royston P (2000) What do we mean by validating a prognostic model? Stat Med 19: 453–473.
16. Taubes G (1995) Epidemiology faces its limits. Science 269: 164–169.
17. Golub TR, Slonim DK, Tamayo P, Huard C, Gaasenbeek M, et al. (1999) Molecular classification of cancer: Class discovery and class prediction by gene expression monitoring. Science 286: 531–537.
18. Moher D, Schulz KF, Altman DG (2001) The CONSORT statement: Revised recommendations for improving the quality of reports of parallel-group randomised trials. Lancet 357: 1191–1194.
19. Ioannidis JP, Evans SJ, Gotzsche PC, O'Neill RT, Altman DG, et al. (2004) Better reporting of harms in randomized trials: An extension of the CONSORT statement. Ann Intern Med 141: 781–788.
20. International Conference on Harmonisation E9 Expert Working Group (1999) ICH Harmonised Tripartite Guideline. Statistical principles for clinical trials. Stat Med 18: 1905–1942.
21. Moher D, Cook DJ, Eastwood S, Olkin I, Rennie D, et al. (1999) Improving the quality of reports of meta-analyses of randomised controlled trials: The QUOROM statement. Quality of Reporting of Meta-analyses. Lancet 354: 1896–1900.
22. Stroup DF, Berlin JA, Morton SC, Olkin I, Williamson GD, et al. (2000) Meta-analysis of observational studies in epidemiology: A proposal for reporting. Meta-analysis of Observational Studies in Epidemiology (MOOSE) group. JAMA 283: 2008–2012.
23. Marshall M, Lockwood A, Bradley C, Adams C, Joy C, et al. (2000) Unpublished rating scales: A major source of bias in randomised controlled trials of treatments for schizophrenia. Br J Psychiatry 176: 249–252.
24. Altman DG, Goodman SN (1994) Transfer of technology from statistical journals to the biomedical literature. Past trends and future predictions. JAMA 272: 129–132.
25. Chan AW, Hrobjartsson A, Haahr MT, Gotzsche PC, Altman DG (2004) Empirical evidence for selective reporting of outcomes in randomized trials: Comparison of protocols to published articles. JAMA 291: 2457–2465.
26. Krimsky S, Rothenberg LS, Stott P, Kyle G (1998) Scientific journals and their authors' financial interests: A pilot study. Psychother Psychosom 67: 194–201.
27. Papanikolaou GN, Baltogianni MS, Contopoulos-Ioannidis DG, Haidich AB, Giannakakis IA, et al. (2001) Reporting of conflicts of interest in guidelines of preventive and therapeutic interventions. BMC Med Res Methodol 1: 3.
28. Antman EM, Lau J, Kupelnick B, Mosteller F, Chalmers TC (1992) A comparison of results of meta-analyses of randomized control trials and recommendations of clinical experts. Treatments for myocardial infarction. JAMA 268: 240–248.
29. Ioannidis JP, Trikalinos TA (2005) Early extreme contradictory estimates may appear in published research: The Proteus phenomenon in molecular genetics research and randomized trials. J Clin Epidemiol 58: 543–549.
30. Ntzani EE, Ioannidis JP (2003) Predictive ability of DNA microarrays for cancer outcomes and correlates: An empirical assessment. Lancet 362: 1439–1444.
31. Ransohoff DF (2004) Rules of evidence for cancer molecular-marker discovery and validation. Nat Rev Cancer 4: 309–314.
32. Lindley DV (1957) A statistical paradox. Biometrika 44: 187–192.
33. Bartlett MS (1957) A comment on D.V. Lindley's statistical paradox. Biometrika 44: 533–534.
34. Senn SJ (2001) Two cheers for P-values. J Epidemiol Biostat 6: 193–204.
35. De Angelis C, Drazen JM, Frizelle FA, Haug C, Hoey J, et al. (2004) Clinical trial registration: A statement from the International Committee of Medical Journal Editors. N Engl J Med 351: 1250–1251.
36. Ioannidis JPA (2005) Contradicted and initially stronger effects in highly cited clinical research. JAMA 294: 218–228.
37. Hsueh HM, Chen JJ, Kodell RL (2003) Comparison of methods for estimating the number of true null hypotheses in multiplicity testing. J Biopharm Stat 13: 675–689.

1.2   The Controversy Surrounding Bone Morphogenetic Proteins in the Spine: A Review of Current Research

Joshua W. Hustedt and Daniel J. Blizzard

Hustedt, J, Blizzard, D. The controversy surrounding bone morphogenetic proteins in the spine: A review of current research. *Yale Journal of Biology and Medicine* 87(4), 549–561 (2014)

YALE JOURNAL OF BIOLOGY AND MEDICINE 87 (2014), pp.549-561.
Copyright © 2014.

REVIEW

The Controversy Surrounding Bone Morphogenetic Proteins in the Spine: A Review of Current Research

Joshua W. Hustedt, MD, MHS*, and Daniel J. Blizzard, MD, MHS

Department of Orthopaedics and Rehabilitation, Yale School of Medicine, New Haven, Connecticut

Bone morphogenetic proteins have been in use in spinal surgery since 2002. These proteins are members of the TGF-beta superfamily and guide mesenchymal stem cells to differentiate into osteoblasts to form bone in targeted tissues. Since the first commercial BMP became available in 2002, a host of research has supported BMPs and they have been rapidly incorporated in spinal surgeries in the United States. However, recent controversy has arisen surrounding the ethical conduct of the research supporting the use of BMPs. Yale University Open Data Access (YODA†) recently teamed up with Medtronic to offer a meta-analysis of the effectiveness of BMPs in spinal surgery. This review focuses on the history of BMPs and examines the YODA research to guide spine surgeons in their use of BMP in spinal surgery.

INTRODUCTION

The frequency of spinal fusion procedures has significantly increased over the last 15 years, concurrent with the increasing popularity and use of osteobiologics to improve fusion. Lumbar and cervical fusion are the most common spine surgeries performed in the United States, with a combined annual rate of approximately 450,000 operations [1]. Although there have been numerous advances in surgical fixation techniques, nonunion still occurs in 10 percent to 15 percent of patients [2]. Despite advancements in materials and constructs, instrumentation remains only a temporizing measure — biologic processes are re-

*To whom all correspondence should be addressed: Joshua W. Hustedt, Department of Orthopaedics and Rehabilitation, Yale School of Medicine, PO Box 208071, New Haven, CT 06511; Tel: 203-737-7463; Fax: 203-785-7132; Email: joshua.hustedt@gmail.com.

†Abbreviations: BMP, bone morphogenetic protein; BMA, bone marrow aspirate; TGF-β, transforming growth factor beta; rhBMP, recombinant human bone morphogenetic protein; GDF-5, growth differentiation factor 5; IDE, investigational device exemption; ACS, absorbable collagen sponge; ALIF, anterior lumbar interbody fusion; PLF, posterolateral fusion; PLIF, posterior lumbar interbody fusion; TLIF, transforaminal lumbar interbody fusion; OSI, Oswestry Disability Index; ICBG, iliac crest bone graft; FRA, femoral ring allografts; RE, retrograde ejaculation; YODA, Yale University Open Data Access; FDA, Food and Drug Administration.

Keywords: spinal fusion, spine, postoperative complications, bone morphogenetic proteins

quired to solidify an arthrodesis for long-term fusion success.

Successful fusion is contingent upon multiple host and graft characteristics. Low bone density, alcohol abuse, cigarette smoking, and long fusions are known risk factors for nonunion. To augment spinal fusion, bone graft is often used, and bone graft material must have sufficient osteoconductive and osteoinductive activities to promote healing. For healing to occur, osteogenic cells lay down new bone on an acceptable scaffolding (osteoconductivity) and stimulate differentiation of stem cells or osteoprogenitor cells into osteoblasts (osteoinduction). Given the critical role graft materials play in driving successful fusion, substantial research efforts have focused upon methods to augment this biologic process in order to achieve stable fusion in circumstances which otherwise would be unfeasible.

Autograft, most commonly taken from the iliac crest, remains the gold-standard graft material as it naturally possess both osteoinductive and osteoconductive properties and is associated with a low risk of infection and rejection. However, autograft is associated with several disadvantages, including increased procedure time, limited donor site availability, and donor site pain — with rates that vary significantly in the literature [3-7]. Allograft circumvents donor site morbidity but has been associated with increased rates of infection and rejection and has poor osteoconductive properties [8,9]. These limitations, combined with a nontrivial incidence of nonunion, have stimulated research into potential alternatives or improvements, including bone morphogenetic proteins (BMPs) and bone marrow aspirate (BMA). BMPs have traditionally been preferred over BMA as head-to-head studies have shown the superiority of BMPs in animal models [10].

BMPs are a unique group of cytokines with osteoinductive activity that belong to the transforming growth factor beta (TGF-β) super-family [11]. In 1965, Urist demonstrated the ability of BMPs to induce ectopic differentiation of cartilage and bone in rodents [12]. New bone production required

for a solid fusion occurs as a result of a series of complex cascades involving osteoprogenitor cells and numerous osteogenic growth factors and competing effects of osteoclasic and osteoblastic cells. BMPs function through a variety of pathways that include the initiation of an increase in alkaline phosphatase and parathyroid hormone levels, as well as an increase in expression of osteocalcin (a marker for differentiated osteoblasts). When bound to transmembrane receptors on mesenchymal stem cells, BMPs induce differentiation into osteoprogenitor cells and form new bone.

Following the sequencing and cloning of BMP genes in the early 1990s, mass production of different BMPs became feasible. In the past decade, 20 individual human recombinant BMPs (rhBMPs) possessing various bone and cartilage stimulation characteristics have been identified [13]. Numerous trials and case series have since evaluated the use of these biologics as adjuvants or alternatives to autograft in spinal fusion. The results and complications of these studies have varied with regard to the specific subtype of rhBMP used, anatomic location of fusion, surgical approach, and the specific authors conducting the studies [4].

Early positive results subsequently led to the Food and Drug Administration (FDA) approval of rhBMPs for use in human surgery [3]. Although the FDA approved usage in the spine is limited to a specific carrier, approach, and range of levels, clinical off-label use of these compounds is rampant. In their 2009 study, Cahill et al. reported that by 2006, rhBMP was used in 25 percent of all fusion procedures in the United States and 40 percent of lumbar fusions [14]. While the liberal usage of rhBMPs has led to improved success rates for many procedures, serious, unforeseen complications have been encountered. Given that much of the off-label use of rhBMPs occurs outside the context of a clinical trial, the true incidence of bad outcomes is unknown. Furthermore, a majority of early studies were industry sponsored and performed by surgeons with high levels of investment in the success of BMP. As more independent research has become available, it has been clear that the early studies were flawed in their research design and biased in their outcomes.

Much remains unknown about these powerful compounds. The risk of uncontrolled bone formation, BMP antibody formation, bone resorprtion, immunogenicity, urethrogenital complications, and malignancies have yet to be fully characterized. All of this on the recent backdrop of research controversy makes it difficult for clinicians to understand the proper use of BMP in a clinical setting. Therefore, we have undertaken to provide a review that examines the evidence for and against BMP, chronicles the controversy surrounding BMP, and provides insight into new research in a better effort to provide clinicians with a working framework in which to apply BMP in their clinical practices.

CONTROVERSY IN COMPLICATION RATES WITH rhBMP-2 USE

Despite BMPs' widespread use, controversy about its effectiveness remains. Controversy surrounds conflicting studies on the success and failure of rhBMP-2 and whether it is superior to autograft from the iliac crest as well as underreporting of adverse side effects in early clinical trials of rhBMP-2 [15,16]. Starting in 2006, independent research groups started to report serious side effects of rhBMP-2 use, with complication rates ranging from 20 to 70 percent [4]. The most notable complications included retrograde ejaculation, seroma formation, bone overgrowth, osteolysis, and an increased risk of cancer. Serious side effects began arising in BMP usage in the cervical spine with large seroma formations placing pressure on airways and causing major postoperative morbidity and mortality complications. In June 2008, the FDA placed a warning on BMP use in the cervical spine due to severe dysphagia postoperatively [17].

Soon after the FDA warning, additional concerns arose with the *Wall Street Journal* reporting that Medtronic was under investi-

gation by the federal government for off-label use of INFUSE (rhBMP-2) [18]. Additional lawsuits were also reported, claiming damages on behalf of the federal government with evidence from former Medtronic employees alleging illegal marketing, including "indictments paid to doctors to use INFUSE" [4]. Even worse, an early study showing the effective use of rhBMP-2 was retracted by the *Journal of Bone and Joint Surgery* after allegations of research misconduct and fraud by the author [19]. It was later reported that the author had significant financial ties to the manufacturer of rhBMP-2 [20]. To say the least, the reputation of rhBMP-2 was tarnished, and the clinical use of BMP was questioned.

In an effort to sort out the madness and provide true evidence-based medicine for the use of rhBMP-2, Medtronic agreed to team up with the Yale University Open Data Access Project (YODA). In this collaboration, Medtronic offered to provide all of its clinical data to the Yale investigators who would independently analyze and interpret the data of all known clinical trials of rhBMP-2. In June 2013, the first two systematic reviews and meta-analyses from this collaboration were reported in the *Annals of Internal Medicine* [15,16].

The reports had four important findings. First, the reports found that in aggregate, the current data does not show a significant improvement in fusion rates with rhBMP-2 as compared to autograft iliac crest bone graft. Second, both BMP-2 and iliac crest bone graft are associated with similar rates of retrograde ejaculation and neurological complications when used in anterior interbody lumbar fusion or posterolateral fusion. This seems to not be associated with the graft material but inherent to the patient population. Third, there is clear evidence that BMP-2 usage leads to high rates of complication in anterior cervical procedures and high rates of ectopic bone formation in posterior lumbar interbody procedures. And fourth, although there is a slight risk of cancer with the use of BMP-2, the absolute risk remains very small and therefore most likely clinically insignificant (Table 1).

Table 1. Summary of Yale Open Access Study.

1. No difference in fusion rates between rhBMP-2 and autograft iliac crest bone graft

2. Both rhBMP-2 and iliac crest bone graft are associated with similar rates of retrograde ejaculation and neurological complications when used in anterior interbody lumbar fusion or posterolateral fusion

3. There is clear evidence that rhBMP-2 usage leads to high rates of complication in anterior cervical procedures and high rates of ectopic bone formation in posterior lumbar interbody procedures

4. Although there is a slight increased relative risk of cancer with the use of BMP-2, the absolute risk remains very small and therefore most likely clinically insignificant

The findings of the Yale University Open Data Access project mark an important new milestone in clinical research by combining the resources of an invested company with the independent review of an academic institution. In light of these findings, we have undertaken to offer both the history of BMPs' development alongside recent YODA evidence to offer clinical practice guidelines for five major spinal surgery applications in the following sections.

TYPES OF BMPs

Although 20 different BMPs have been discovered, only BMP-2 is currently FDA approved and available in recombinant form for use in human spine surgery. BMP-7, or OP-1, was previously given a Humanitarian Device Exemption and ultimately was not approved by the FDA. Additionally, growth differentiation factor 5 (GDF-5), a member of the TGF-β superfamily and closely related to BMPs, has also been preliminarily tested in humans.

rhBMP-2

In 1997, a prospective randomized control trial evaluating the use of rhBMP-2 was conducted under an FDA-approved investigational device exemption (IDE) [21]. In this pilot study, the rhBMP-2 (Genetics Institute, Cambridge, MA) was delivered on an absorbable collagen sponge (ACS) carrier (Integra Life Sciences, Plainsboro, NJ) and placed into a titanium interbody fusion device (LT-Cage; Medtronic Sofamor Danek).

The authors concluded that fusion not only occurred, but occurred more reliably in the patients who received rhBMP-2 [21]. In a multicenter follow-up study, InFUSE Bone Graft/LT-CAGE Lumbar Tapered Fusion Device (Medtronic Sofamor Danek, Memphis, TN) and autograft were compared for clinical and radiographic fusion following anterior lumbar interbody fusion (ALIF). Successful radiographic fusion was achieved in 94.5 percent of the experimental group versus 88.7 percent in the control group at 2-year follow-up. In the control group, 32 percent of patients reported graft site discomfort and 16 percent were bothered by its appearance at 2-year follow-up [3]. Citing this work as a pivotal study, Medtronic was granted FDA approval in 2003 for the use of rhBMP-2 in conjunction with the LT-CAGE™ Lumbar Tapered Fusion Device for ALIF. Contraindications included pregnancy, material allergy, infection, and previous tumor near the site of implantation.

Although only specifically tested and FDA approved for ALIF, off-label, or "physician-directed application," of IN-FUSE is widespread. Publication of initial clinical results indicating superior fusion rates compared to autograft and no complications encouraged many surgeons to begin using rhBMP-2 off-label — initially restricted to patients with known risk factors for nonunion and later with more generalized use. It is easy to see why as patients with diabetes, hypothyroidism, or a history of smoking have been shown to have reduced fusion rates [22]. The attractiveness of augmenting these risk factors brought many surgeons onboard with BMP use. In the United States alone, BMP use in spinal fusions increased from 0.7 percent in 2002 to 25 percent in 2006, with Medtronic reporting nearly $400 million dollars in sales in 2012 [4,17].

Anterior Lumbar Interbody Fusion

In their 2002 landmark study, Burkus et al. showed that patients treated with rhBMP-2 with an LT-CAGE Lumbar Tapered Fusion Device (Medtronic Sofamor Danek, Memphis, TN, USA) had statistically superior outcomes with regard to length of surgery, blood loss, hospital stay, reoperation rate, median time to return to work, and fusion rates at 6, 12, and 24 months, as well as Oswestry Disability Index (OSI) scores and Physical Component and Pain Index scores at 3, 6, 12, and 42 months compared to patients treated with iliac crest bone graft (ICBG) [3]. Although this study was able to prove non-inferiority, it lacked sufficient statistical power to prove fusion superiority of rhBMP-2 versus autograft. In a follow-up study, combining datasets from two additional clinical trials, a 24-month fusion success rate of 94.4 percent (201/213) for rhBMP-2 and 89.4 percent (252/282) for autograft was found, showing statistical superiority of rhBMP-2 with respect to fusion [23]. At 6 years, 98 percent of the study group showed radiographic fusion and 79 percent had an improvement in the OSI score of > 15 points [24].

In two related, prospective FDA-approved Investigation Device Exemption (IDE) studies, Burkus et al. also evaluated the use of rhBMP-2 in ALIF with structural cortical allografts and the INTER FIX Threaded Fusion Device (Medtronic Sofamor Danek, Memphis, TN, USA) versus ICBG [23,25]. Patients treated with rhBMP-2 had superior clinical and radiographic outcomes compared with patients who had received ICBG. The study group was found to have significantly higher rates of radiographic fusion than the control group at all time-points with a difference of 99 percent and 76 percent, (p < 0.001) respectively at 2 years. Similarly, the authors also found that

the INTER FIX device packed with rhBMP-2 led to improved ODI outcomes, improved radiographic fusion rate, and improved rate of return to work compared to ICBG controls.

In a non-industry sponsored, prospective cohort study in 2006, investigators evaluated the outcomes for patients undergoing ALIF with femoral ring allografts (FRAs) with ICBG and rhBMP-2. In contrast to Burkus et al. [25], the study found that rhBMP-2 paradoxically caused a trend toward higher rates of nonunion (56 percent) compared to ICBG (36 percent) as well as aggressive resorption of the FRAs [26]. One year later, an industry-sponsored trial using FRAs with pedicle screw fixation reported statistically superior clinical outcomes and fusion rates at all follow-up time points for patients with rhBMP-2 added to the FRAs (but no comparison to FRAs with ICBG) [27].

Although rhBMP-2 has been shown to significantly improve fusion rates in ALIF and early studies revealed no increased rate of rhBMP-2 related complications, more recent studies have revealed an array of complications. Multiple reports and trials have reported significant endplate resorption, osteolysis, and graft subsidence with rhBMP-2 used in ALIF [28-30]. Although many reports denied resultant clinical symptoms or effect of fusion, Carragee et al. reported a higher reoperation rate in patients treated with rhBMP-2, principally attributed to graft subsidence complications [4]. rhBMP-2 has also been implicated in increased rates of retrograde ejaculation (RE) following ALIF. Baseline rates of RE in ALIF without rhBMP-2 have been established to be less than 1 percent [31-33], but rates of RE with rhBMP-2 have been shown to be statistically significantly higher at 6 to 7 percent [34,35].

In spite of varying evidence, ALIF is the only FDA-approved application of rhBMP-2. Findings from YODA suggest no difference between rhBMP-2 and autograft iliac crest. However, iliac crest bone graft requires an additional surgical site operation. When autograft is not available or an additional procedure is not desired, rhBMP-2 is

Table 2. Recommendations for use of rhBMP-2.

Anterior Lumbar Interbody Fusion (ALIF)	No difference between rhBMP-2 and ICBG. However, iliac crest bone graft requires additional surgical site operation. When autograft is not available or procedure is not desired, rhBMP-2 is a reliable alternate. Retrograde ejaculation and neurological complications are equal with both rhBMP-2 and ICBG.
Anterior Cervical Fusion	An FDA warning has been issued to not use rhBMP-2 in the anterior cervical spine due to inflammation causing severe dysphagia and airway compromise.
Posterolateral Fusion (PLF)	No difference between rhBMP-2 and ICBG. However, iliac crest bone graft requires additional surgical site operation. When autograft is not available or procedure is not desired, rhBMP-2 is a reliable alternate.
Posterior Interbody Lumbar Fusion (PLIF)	Use of rhBMP-2 has been associated with high rates of ectopic bone formation leading to neurological compromise. ICBG is preferred.
Transforaminal Interbody Fusion (TLIF)	Use of rhBMP-2 has been associated with seroma formation and neurological compromise. Further evidence is needed, but judicious use of rhBMP-2 is recommended due to complications.

a reliable alternate. YODA found retrograde ejaculation and neurological complications to be equal in both autograft and BMP augmented ALIF surgeries (Table 2) [16].

Posterolateral Lumbar Fusion

Two large, prospective randomized multicenter trials have evaluated the use of rhBMP-2 in posterolateral lumbar fusion (PLF). The first, conducted in 2002, compared three groups of patients with single-level degenerative disc disease undergoing PLF: autograft with pedical screw fixation, rhBMP-2 with pedical screw fixation, and rhBMP-2 without pedical screw fixation [36]. At 17 months follow-up, the fusion rate in the autograft group was 40 percent compared to a 100 percent fusion rate in the patients who received rhBMP-2 (with or without internal fixation). These authors demonstrated that rhBMP-2 at a dose of 20 mg per side can achieve PLF at a higher rate than iliac crest autograft alone.

The second study in 2009 compared the use of autograft and higher dose rhBMP-2 (AMPLIFY rhBMP-2 Matrix; Medtronic So-famor Danek) in single-level, instrumented PLF. This study reported an 89 percent fusion rate in the autograft group (n = 224) and a 96 percent fusion rate in the rhBMP-2/CRM group (n = 239) at 2 years follow-up (p = 0.014). Clinical outcome measures were similar between the two groups, and the re-operation rate was significantly higher in the autograft group (16 percent vs. 8 percent, P = 0.015). Of the patients in the autograft group, 60 percent reported donor site iliac crest pain at 2 years follow-up [37]. Several smaller studies have found similar results of superior fusion rates with the use of rhBMP-2 in PLF compared to ICBG with minimal complications [22,38-41].

Concerns with the use of rhBMP-2 in PLF include risk for complications from heterotopic ossification and post-surgical edema and seroma formation. A study in 2008 reported a case of post-operative psoas ossification with subsequent development of pain along the iliac wing, groin, and greater trochanter 3 months after surgery [42]. In a 2010 retrospective review of 130 patients undergoing PLF with rhBMP-2, authors reported a 4.6 percent incidence of sterile seromas requiring surgical exploration (no data for seroma incidence in ICBG group for comparison) [43].

In accordance with the large body of positive study results and limited published reports of serious complications, Medtronic applied for FDA approval of higher dose rhBMP-2, AMPLIFY, for application in posterolateral spine fusion. In March 2011, the application for FDA was rejected due to concerns about potential increased risk of malignancy [4].

Recent YODA evidence shows that while there may be a small increased relative risk of malignancy with the use of rhBMP-2 in PLF, the absolute risk remains very low and therefore clinically insignificant. Findings show no difference between rhBMP-2 and ICBG in PLF and also show higher rates of ectopic bone formation in PLF procedures. Therefore, rhBMP-2 may be useful when autograft is not available in PLF surgery, and the benefits outweigh the risks of ectopic bone formation (Tables 1 and 2) [16].

Posterior Lumbar Interbody Fusion

Multiple clinical studies have shown positive fusion results using rhBMP-2 in posterior lumbar interbody fusion (PLIF), but have also identified a high propensity for the development of heterotopic bone formation. When comparing PLIF with rhBMP-2 in two INTER FIX cages (Medtronic Sofamor Danek, Memphis, TN) versus autograft, fusion rates were 92.3 percent for the rhBMP-2 group versus 77.8 percent for the control group, with no significant difference in clinical improvement between the two groups [5]. Although the findings show favorable results, ectopic bone formation away from the PLIF cages in preliminary CT imaging caused the investigators to suspend recruitment in the study. There was statistically significantly more extradiscal bone formation in the BMP group (75 percent; 24 of 32 patients) compared with the control group (13 percent; 4 of 31 patients). Despite the statistical significance, there was no relationship found between this bone formation and clinical symptoms.

Follow-up studies found a similar higher incidence of asymptomatic hetero-topic bone formation in patients treated with rhBMP-2 [44,45]. A case report also showed the formation of ectopic bone following PLIF with rhBMP-2 that led to neurologic impairment and subsequent revision surgery [46]. However, some authors have shown high fusion rates with no incidence of heterotopic bone formation [46,47]. In addition to heterotopic bone formation, cage migration following PLIF with rhBMP-2 has been described [29]. Meta-analysis data from YODA suggests clinicians should avoid rhBMP-2 use in PLIF procedures due to concern about ectopic bone formation and neurological compromise (Table 2) [16].

Transforaminal Lumbar Interbody Fusion

The off-label use of rhBMP-2 in transforaminal lumbar interbody fusion (TLIF) is becoming increasingly common. Although there are no prospective, randomized studies evaluating the use of rhBMP-2 in TLIF, results from several retrospective studies support its clinical efficacy. In a series of 74 patients who underwent single and multiple-level TLIF with rhBMP-2 applied on an ACS and combined with allograft or autograft, all patients had developed radiographic fusion at 10 months follow-up [48]. No complications or adverse reactions attributed specifically to the rhBMP-2 were reported, although two patients had persistent postoperative radiculitis. A similar study retrospectively reviewed clinical and radiographic outcomes in 48 patients who underwent single-level TLIF using rhBMP-2 [49]. Radiographic fusion was achieved in 95.8 percent of patients, improvement in symptoms was reported in 83 percent of patients, and satisfaction with surgical outcome was reported in 84 percent of patients. However, 27.1 percent of patients had one or more complications, including transient postoperative radiculitis (8/48), vertebral osteolysis (3/48), nonunion (2/48), and symptomatic ectopic bone formation (1/48).

Complications with rhBMP-2 used in TLIF have been reported in several case series and reports. Postoperative radiculitis has been a complication of TLIF surgery with rhBMP-2, with rates as high as 20 percent being reported [50]. Also, ectopic bone formation following TLIF using rhBMP-2 has been reported in many case reports, with cases of symptomatic, delayed neural compression in patients following TLIF using rhBMP-2 [51]. Finally, vertebral osteolysis has been reported to occur in 5.8 to 7.4 percent [50,52]. Although the osteolytic defects filled spontaneously in most of these patients, a small subset of these patients were later found to have osteomyelitis that required revision debridement and reconstruction.

Given the variety and frequency of complications associated with rhBMP-2 use in TLIF, additional caution should be exercised in implementing BMP use in TLIF procedures. Further evidence is needed in order to make practice guidelines, and in the meantime, judicious use of rhBMP-2 in TLIF procedures is recommended due to complications (Table 2) [16].

Anterior Cervical Fusion

The efficacy of rhBMP-2 to promote fusion in the cervical spine has been well documented in numerous clinical studies. In their prospective, randomized, FDA-approved pilot trial, Baskin showed a 100 percent fusion rate and no increase in complications when using rhBMP-2 versus autograft within an allograft ring [53]. In subsequent studies with larger sample sizes and less contained doses of rhBMP-2, the efficacy of achieving solid fusion was further supported with 100 percent fusion rates when rhBMP-2 was added to absorbable collagen sponges, PEEK cages, bioabsorbable spacers, and allograft rings. Despite the common finding that rhBMP-2 was equivalent or superior to autograft in promoting fusion, there emerged a clear increase in the incidence of soft-tissue related complications.

In 2006, authors reported high complication rates in 151 patients who underwent anterior cervical fusion using high-dose rhBMP-2 (2.1mg/level) [54]. Overall, 23.2 percent (35/151) experienced complications, including 15 patients diagnosed with a hematoma (of whom eight were surgically

evacuated) and 13 patients with either a prolonged hospital stay or hospital readmission because of swallowing/breathing difficulties or dramatic swelling without hematoma. Although there was no study group for comparison, the authors concluded that rate of complications differed from their significant surgical experience in anterior cervical fusion without rhBMP-2. Two years later, another report of soft tissue swelling emerged in a series of 200 patients who underwent single- or multilevel anterior cervical fusion with PEEK spacers filled with an ACS impregnated with varying doses of rhBMP-2 [55]. During the study, they decreased the dose of rhBMP-2 twice. The first reduction from 2.1mg to 1.05mg/level was due to an observation of asymptomatic excess bony formation. The second reduction from 1.05mg to 0.7mg/level was due to the authors noting anecdotal reports of dysphagia with higher concentration. The authors did not find a significant difference in dysphagia or swelling between the study group and historical controls, and there were not a sufficient number of patients to compare complications between patients receiving the different doses of rhBMP-2. However, the authors of this study agreed with the conclusions of other studies suggesting a relationship between complication rates and increased rhBMP-2 concentration.

Although there is a breadth of literature documenting high complication rates with rhBMP-2 usage in anterior cervical surgery, it is difficult to assess true risk given the design of most of the published studies. Specifically, surgical technique, instrumentation, concentration of rhBMP-2, and number of levels fused are not controlled between studies. Furthermore, in multiple instances, authors cite that their use of rhBMP-2 was due to their patients having known risk factors for pseudarthrosis. Most importantly, the only prospective, randomized trial evaluating rhBMP-2 in anterior cervical fusion found that that there was no increased rate of complication. However, in light of the serious adverse events reported in the literature, the FDA released a public health notification warning of the life-threatening risks associated with rhBMP-2 in anterior cervical fusion and recommended that "practitioners either use approved treatments or consider enrolling as investigators in approved clinical studies" [17]. Currently, clinical recommendations are to avoid the use of rhBMP-2 in anterior cervical fusion (Table 2) [16].

OP-1

OP-1, also known as BMP-7, is another member of the TGF-β family that has received significant investigation for clinical use in the spine. Initial animal studies of spinal fusion rates suggested OP-1 was a promising new BMP. In 2000, a study in a New Zealand White Rabbit model showed a 100 percent intertransverse process lumbar fusion rate with OP-1 versus a 63 percent fusion rate for autograft alone [56]. Two years later, additional authors showed a superior bone formation rate with OP-1 versus autograft alone in a Canine model of posterolateral arthrodesis [57].

These early animal studies led Vaccaro et al. to perform safety and efficacy trials of OP-1 in patients with grade I or II spondylolisthesis. The safety and efficacy of OP-1 was first assessed in 2003 in a 12-patient study in which the authors showed a 70 percent rate of bridging bone formation and an 89 percent clinical success rate at 1-year follow-up when OP-1 was used in conjunction with autograft [58,59]. The authors then examined the efficacy of OP-1 versus autograft alone in a study examining 36 patients with neurogenic claudication and spondylolisthesis who underwent decompression laminectomy and one-level uninstrumented PLF [60]. Successful radiographical fusion was found in 74 percent of OP-1 patients versus 60 percent of patients with autograft alone. These two studies led to an FDA Humanitarian Device Exemption approval in 2004 to allow up to 4,000 patients a year to receive OP-1 for revision PLF in patients who suffer from factors that complicate healing or for whom autograft harvest is not feasible.

Based on the success of the early pilot studies, Vaccaro et al. undertook a large,

prospective, randomized, controlled multicenter clinical trial of 295 patients to demonstrate the noninferiority of OP-1 versus autograft in patients with spondylolisthesis undergoing one-level posterior decompression and uninstrumented posterolateral intratransverse process arthrodesis [61]. The investigators hypothesized that OP-1 would prove as efficacious as autograft alone, and therefore serve as a potential replacement, circumventing the morbidity of an autograft procedure. However, the study results showed superior results for autograft versus OP-1, with bone formation in 51.9 percent of OP-1 patients compared to 73.5 percent of autograft patients on plain films at 2-year follow-up. The authors questioned if the result was due to the insensitivity of plain films to assess for bridging bone formation and decided to add an additional 3-year follow-up with a CT scan for 257 of the original 295 patients. CT results at 3 years again suggested the superiority of autograft, with 36 percent of autograft patients showing evidence of bridging bone formation versus 26 percent of OP-1 patients [62].

The findings of the large Vaccaro et al. study ultimately lead to the FDA rejection of Pre-Market Approval of OP-1 in April 2009. While this has been a significant setback in the clinical use of OP-1, studies are ongoing to find an optimal dosage and delivery system for OP-1 in the future.

GDF-5

GDF-5, also known as cartilage-derived morphogenetic protein-1or BMP-14, is under development in combination with a specific collagen carrier called Healos (DePuy Spine, Inc., Raynham, MA), a cross-linked type I collagen with hydroxyapatite coating that serves as a vehicle for cellular attachment and vascular ingrowth. The collagen carrier is further soaked in bone marrow aspirate during preparation to provide adequate stem cells for bone growth. When used together with bone marrow aspirate, Healos has shown promising results in terms of fusion in both animal and human studies.

Animal studies have shown that Healos has strong potential for clinical benefit. A pre-clinical study using GDF-5 0.5 and 1.0 mg/cc Healos doses showed abundant bone formation and 100 percent fusion in a New Zealand Rabbit model [63]. A similar study compared Healos and autograft in a posterolateral instrumented spinal fusion in sheep and found 100 percent fusion in both the Healos and autograft groups [64]. These early animal study results, combined with many others, propelled Healos into clinical testing.

Clinical testing of Healos and bone marrow aspirate are ongoing. However, a few successful clinical studies have been promising. A trial of Healos was conducted in 2006, in which the authors compared 50 spinal fusion operations using Healos to 50 matched controls using autograft alone [65]. For posterolateral lumbar fusions, there were equivalent radiologic fusion rates for the two groups with no significant difference in the subjective and objective clinical outcomes. There were no lasting complications associated with Healos use compared with a 14 percent persisting donor site complication rate in the autograft patients. Similar positive results have been shown with Healos in ACDF [62], TLIF [63], and PLF [64] procedures [19,66,67].

These early clinical trials suggest Healos has potential to have great clinical benefit in spinal fusion procedures. However, it remains to be seen if Healos will have the same effect as other BMPs. In a study comparing Healos and INFUSE (BMP-2), Kraiwattanapong et al. showed that INFUSE was far superior to Healos in their posterolateral lumbar spine fusion model in New Zealand White Rabbits [10]. In the study, 100 percent (12/12) of rabbits had successful fusion with INFUSE, while 0 percent (0/12) had successful fusion with Healos. The data on Healos should be questioned, as the fusion rates for Healos are not similar to other reported fusion rates in rabbits, but the study highlights the need to compare Healos with other BMPs.

The animal and clinical studies on Healos suggest it has great clinical potential in spinal fusion; however, the data is limited and more research must be undertaken to identify the risks and benefits of using Healos in spinal fusion techniques. Additionally, studies have not been undertaken to compare Healos to other BMPs, which will be essential in determining the clinical efficacy of Healos.

SUMMARY AND FUTURE DIRECTIONS

Recent research calls into question the ultimate fate of rhBMP-2 in its superiority to autograft from the iliac crest. The Yale University Open Access Project's published studies offer important insight for clinicians in their determination to use BMPs in spinal surgery. The authors of this study suggest judicious use of rhBMP-2 in spinal surgery. rhBMP-2 will likely hold an important role in future spinal surgery, as it offers augmentation options when autograft from the iliac crest is either unavailable or the side effects of the procedure are unwanted by the patients (Table 2). However, it is most likely that recent findings will temper the widespread use of BMP in a majority of spinal fusions where iliac bone graft is a reliable option.

In addition, ongoing research in spinal fusion augmentation offers many alternates to BMP-2 usage. Most promising is the ever-increasing use of bone marrow aspirate to augment spinal fusion. Recent studies have described the use of bone marrow aspirate derived from the vertebral body, which is already accessed during spinal fusion procedures with instrumentation, resulting in augmented fusion rates and no donor site morbidity [68-70]. Additionally, further studies with GDF-5 may provide safer, more efficacious osteobiologics for certain spinal surgeries.

In conclusion, surgeons should be aware that aggregate data analysis from the Yale University Open Access Project does not suggest that rhBMP-2 is superior to autograft iliac bone graft. Additionally, surgeons should be wary of use of rhBMP-2 in the cervical spine, aware of complications of ectopic bone growth in posterolateral fusion, and judicious when using BMP in transforaminal interbody fusion due to seroma formation. Overall, rhBMP-2 remains a viable option for complex cases when autograft iliac bone graft is not desirable or available. Further research and evaluation of the clinical data is ongoing and will likely further provide evidence for the use of BMPs in spinal fusion. Spinal surgeons should remain aware of current research in order to practice current evidence-based medicine.

REFERENCES

1. Resnick DK. Evidence-based spine surgery. Spine (Phila Pa 1976). 2007;32(11):S15-9.
2. Hsu WK, Wang JC. The use of bone morphogenetic protein in spine fusion. Spine J. 2008;8(3):419-25.
3. Burkus JK, Gornet MF, Dickman CA, Zdeblick TA. Anterior lumbar interbody fusion using rhBMP-2 with tapered interbody cages. J Spinal Disord Tech. 2002;15(5):337-49.
4. Carragee EJ, Hurwitz EL, Weiner BK. A critical review of recombinant human bone morphogenetic protein-2 trials in spinal surgery: emerging safety concerns and lessons learned. Spine J. 2011;11(6):471-91.
5. Haid RW Jr, Branch CL Jr, Alexander JT, Burkus JK. Posterior lumbar interbody fusion using recombinant human bone morphogenetic protein type 2 with cylindrical interbody cages. Spine J. 2004;4(5):527-38; discussion 38-9.
6. Mroz TE, Wang JC, Hashimoto R, Norvell DC. Complications Related to Osteobiologics Use in Spine Surgery A Systematic Review. Spine. 2010;35(9):S86-104.
7. Smoljanovic T, Bojanic I, Pecina M. The Use of Bone Morphogenetic Protein in Lumbar Spine Surgery. J Bone Joint Surg Am. 2009;91A(8):2045-6.
8. Agarwal R, Williams K, Umscheid CA, Welch WC. Osteoinductive bone graft substitutes for lumbar fusion: a systematic review Clinical article. J Neurosurg Spine. 2009;11(6):729-40.
9. Resnick DK, Choudhri TF, Dailey AT, Groff MW, Khoo L, Matz PG, et al. Guidelines for the performance of fusion procedures for degenerative disease of the lumbar spine. Part 16: bone graft extenders and substitutes. J Neurosurg Spine. 2005;2(6):733-6.
10. Kraiwattanapong C, Boden SD, Louis-Ugbo J, Attallah E, Barnes B, Hutton WC. Comparison of Healos/bone marrow to INFUSE(rhBMP-2/ACS) with a collagen-ceramic sponge bulking agent as graft substitutes for lumbar spine fusion. Spine. 2005;30(9):1001-7.
11. Zlotolow DA, Vaccaro AR, Salamon ML, Albert TJ. The role of human bone morphogenetic proteins in spinal fusion. J Am Acad Orthop Surg. 2000;8(1):3-9.
12. Carlisle E, Fischgrund JS. Bone morphogenetic proteins for spinal fusion. Spine J. 2005;5(6 Suppl):240S-9S.
13. Axelrad TW, Einhorn TA. Bone morphogenetic proteins in orthopaedic surgery. Cytokine Growth Factor Rev. 2009;20(5-6):481-8.
14. Cahill KS, Chi JH, Day A, Claus EB. Prevalence, Complications, and Hospital Charges Associated With Use of Bone-Morphogenetic Proteins in Spinal Fusion Procedures. JAMA. 2009;302(1):58-66.
15. Fu R, Selph S, McDonagh M, Peterson K, Tiwari A, Chou R, et al. Effectiveness and harms of recombinant human bone morphogenetic protein-2 in spine fusion: a systematic review and meta-analysis. Ann Intern Med. 2013;158(12):890-902.
16. Simmonds MC, Brown JV, Heirs MK, Higgins JP, Mannion RJ, Rodgers MA, et al. Safety and effectiveness of recombinant human bone morphogenetic protein-2 for spinal fusion: a meta-analysis of individual-participant data. Ann Intern Med. 2013;158(12):877-89.
17. Life-threatening complications associated with recombinant human bone morphogenetic protein in cervical spine fusion. US Food and Drug Administration [Internet]. 2008. [cited 25 Jul 2013]. Available from: http://www.fda.gov/MedicalDevices/Safety/AlertsandNotices/PublicHealthNotifications/ucm062000.htm.
18. Carrey-Rou J, McGinty T. Medtronic Surgeons Held Back, Study Says. Wall Street Journal. June 29, 2011.
19. Carter JD, Swearingen AB, Chaput CD, Rahm MD. Clinical and radiographic assessment of transforaminal lumbar interbody fusion using HEALOS collagen-hydroxyapatite sponge with autologous bone marrow aspirate. Spine J. 2009;9(6):434-8.
20. Armstrong D. Medtronic paid the surgeon accused of falsifying study nearly $800,000. Wall Street Journal. June 18, 2009.
21. Boden SD, Zdeblick TA, Sandhu HS, Heim SE. The use of rhBMP-2 in interbody fusion cages - Definitive evidence of osteoinduction in humans: A preliminary report. Spine. 2000;25(3):376-81.
22. Glassman SD, Dimar JR, Burkus K, Hardacker JW, Pryor PW, Boden SD, et al. The efficacy of rhBMP-2 for posterolateral lumbar fusion in smokers. Spine. 2007;32(15):1693-8.
23. Burkus JK, Heim TE, Gornet MF, Zdeblick TA. Is INFUSE bone graft superior to autograft bone? An integrated analysis of clinical trials using the LT-CAGE lumbar tapered fusion device. J Spinal Disord Tech. 2003;16(2):113-22.
24. Burkus JK, Gornet MF, Shuler TC, Kleeman TJ, Zdeblick TA. Six-Year Outcomes of Anterior Lumbar Interbody Arthrodesis with Use of Interbody Fusion Cages and Recombinant Human Bone Morphogenetic Protein-2. J Bone Joint Surg Am. 2009;91(5):1181-9.

25. Burkus JK, Sandhu HS, Gornet MF, Longley MC. Use of rhBMP-2 in combination with structural cortical allografts: Clinical and radiographic outcomes in anterior lumbar spinal surgery. J Bone Joint Surg Am. 2005;87(6):1205-12.

26. Pradhan BB, Bae HW, Dawson EG, Patel VV, Delamarter RB. Graft resorption with the use of bone morphogenetic protein: Lessons from anterior lumbar interbody fusion using femoral ring allografts and recombinant human bone morphogenetic protein-2. Spine. 2006;31(10):E277-84.

27. Slosar PJ, Josey R, Reynolds J. Accelerating lumbar fusions by combining rhBMP-2 with allograft bone: a prospective analysis of interbody fusion rates and clinical outcomes. Spine J. 2007;7(3):301-7.

28. Hansen SM, Sasso RC. Resorptive response of rhBMP2 simulating infection in an anterior lumbar interbody fusion with a femoral ring. J Spinal Disord Tech. 2006;19(2):130-4.

29. Vaidya R, Sethi A, Bartol S, Jacobson M, Coe C, Craig JG. Complications in the Use of rhBMP-2 in PEEK Cages for Interbody Spinal Fusions. J Spinal Disord Tech. 2008;21(8):557-62.

30. Vaidya R, Weir R, Sethi A, Meisterling S, Hakeos W, Wybo CD. Interbody fusion with allograft and rhBMP-2 leads to consistent fusion but early subsidence. J Bone Joint Surg Br. 2007;89(3):342-5.

31. Kang B-U, Choi W-C, Lee S-H, Jeon SH, Park JD, Maeng DH, et al. An analysis of general surgery-related complications in a series of 412 minilaparotomic anterior lumbosacral procedure. J Neurosurg Spine. 2009;10(1):60-5.

32. Sasso RC, Best NM, Mummaneni PV, Reilly TM, Hussain SM. Analysis of operative complications in a series of 471 anterior lumbar interbody fusion procedures. Spine. 2005;30(6):670-4.

33. Sasso RC, Kitchel SH, Dawson EG. A prospective, randomized controlled clinical trial of anterior lumbar interbody fusion using a titanium cylindrical threaded fusion device. Spine. 2004;29(2):113-21.

34. Carragee EJ, Mitsunaga KA, Hurwitz EL, Scuderi GJ. Retrograde ejaculation after anterior lumbar interbody fusion using rhBMP-2: a cohort controlled study. Spine J. 2011;11(6):511-6.

35. Jarrett CD, Heller JG, Tsai L. Anterior Exposure of the Lumbar Spine With and Without an "Access Surgeon" Morbidity Analysis of 265 Consecutive Cases. J Spinal Disord Tech. 2009;22(8):559-64.

36. Boden SD, Kang J, Sandhu H, Heller JG. Use of recombinant human bone morphogenetic protein-2 to achieve posterolateral lumbar spine fusion in humans - A prospective, randomized clinical pilot trial - 2002 Volvo Award in clinical studies. Spine. 2002;27(23):2662-73.

37. Carreon LY, Glassman SD, Djurasovic M, Campbell MJ, Puno RM, Johnson JR, et al. RhBMP-2 Versus Iliac Crest Bone Graft for Lumbar Spine Fusion in Patients Over 60 Years of Age A Cost-Utility Study. Spine. 2009;34(3):238-43.

38. Dawson E, Bae HW, Burkus JK, Stambough JL, Glassman SD. Recombinant Human Bone Morphogenetic Protein-2 on an Absorbable Collagen Sponge with an Osteoconductive Bulking Agent in Posterolateral Arthrodesis with Instrumentation A Prospective Randomized Trial. J Bone Joint Surg Am. 2009;91(7):1604-13.

39. Glassman SD, Carreon LY, Djurasovic M, Campbell MJ, Puno RM, Johnson JR, et al. RhBMP-2 Versus Iliac Crest Bone Graft for Lumbar Spine Fusion. Spine. 2008;33(26):2843-9.

40. Hamilton DK, Smith JS, Reames DL, Williams BJ, Shaffrey CI. Use of recombinant human bone morphogenetic protein-2 as an adjunct for instrumented posterior arthrodesis in the occipital cervical region: An analysis of safety, efficacy, and dosing. J Craniovertebr Junction Spine. 2010;1(2):107-12.

41. Lee KB, Taghavi CE, Hsu MS, Song KJ, Yoo JH, Keorochana G, et al. The efficacy of rhBMP-2 versus autograft for posterolateral lumbar spine fusion in elderly patients. Eur Spine J. 2010;19(6):924-30.

42. Brower RS, Vickroy NM. A case of psoas ossification from the use of BMP-2 for posterolateral fusion at L4-L5. Spine. 2008;33(18):E653-5.

43. Garrett MP, Kakarla UK, Porter RW, Sonntag VKH. Formation of Painful Seroma and Edema After the Use of Recombinant Human Bone Morphogenetic Protein-2 in Posterolateral Lumbar Spine Fusions. Neurosurgery. 2010;66(6):1044-9.

44. Joseph V, Rampersaud YR. Heterotopic bone formation with the use of rhBMP2 in posterior minimal access interbody fusion - A CT analysis. Spine. 2007;32(25):2885-90.

45. Meisel HJ, Schnoring M, Hohaus C, Minkus Y, Beier A, Ganey T, et al. Posterior lumbar interbody fusion using rhBMP-2. Eur Spine J. 2008;17(12):1735-44.

46. Wong DA, Kumar A, Jatana S, Ghiselli G, Wong K. Neurologic impairment from ectopic bone in the lumbar canal: a potential complication of off-label PLIF/TLIF use of bone morphogenetic protein-2 (BMP-2). Spine J. 2008;8(6):1011-8.

47. Geibel PT, Boyd DL, Slabisak V. The Use of Recombinant Human Bone Morphogenic Protein in Posterior Interbody Fusions of the Lumbar Spine A Clinical Series. J Spinal Disord Tech. 2009;22(5):315-20.

48. Villavicencio AT, Burneikiene S, Nelson EL, Bulsara KR, Favors M, Thramann J. Safety of transforaminal lumbar interbody fusion and intervertebral recombinant human bone

morphogenetic protein-2. J Neurosurg Spine. 2005;3(6):436-43.

49. Rihn JA, Makda J, Hong J, Patel R, Hilibrand AS, Anderson DG, et al. The use of RhBMP-2 in single-level transforaminal lumbar interbody fusion: a clinical and radiographic analysis. Eur Spine J. 2009;18(11):1629-36.

50. Rihn JA, Patel R, Makda J, Hong J, Anderson DG, Vaccaro AR, et al. Complications associated with single-level transforaminal lumbar interbody fusion. Spine J. 2009;9(8):623-9.

51. Chen NF, Smith ZA, Stiner E, Armin S, Sheikh H, Khoo LT. Symptomatic ectopic bone formation after off-label use of recombinant human bone morphogenetic protein-2 in transforaminal lumbar interbody fusion Report of 4 cases. J Neurosurg Spine. 2010;12(1):40-6.

52. Balseiro S, Nottmeier EW. Vertebral osteolysis originating from subchondral cyst end plate defects in transforaminal lumbar interbody fusion using rhBMP-2. Report of two cases. Spine J. 2010;10(7):e6-e10.

53. Baskin DS, Ryan P, Sonntag V, Westmark R, Widmayer MA. A prospective, randomized, controlled cervical fusion study using recombinant human bone morphogenetic protein-2 with the CORNERSTONE-SR (TM) allograft ring and the ATLANTIS (TM) anterior cervical plate. Spine. 2003;28(12):1219-24.

54. Shields LBE, Raque GH, Glassman SD, Campbell M, Vitaz T, Harpring J, et al. Adverse effects associated with high-dose recombinant human bone morphogenetic protein-2 use in anterior cervical spine fusion. Spine. 2006;31(5):542-7.

55. Tumialan LM, Pan J, Rodts GE, Mummaneni PV. The safety and efficacy of anterior cervical discectomy and fusion with polyetheretherketone spacer and recombinant human bone morphogenetic protein-2: a review of 200 patients. J Neurosurg Spine. 2008;8(6):529-35.

56. Grauer J, Patel T, Erulkar J, Troiano N, Panjabi M, Friedlaender G. 2000 Young Investigator Research Award winner. Evaluation of OP-1 as a graft substitute for intertransverse process lumbar fusion. Spine (Phila Pa.). 2001;26(2):127-33.

57. Cunningham BW, Shimamoto N, Sefter JC, Dmitriev AE, Orbegoso CM, McCarthy EF, et al. Osseointegration of autograft versus osteogenic protein-1 in posterolateral spinal arthrodesis: emphasis on the comparative mechanisms of bone induction. Spine J. 2002;2(1):11-24.

58. Vaccaro AR, Patel T, Fischgrund J, Anderson DG, Truumees E, Herkowitz H, et al. A pilot safety and efficacy study of OP-1 putty (rhBMP-7) as an adjunct to iliac crest autograft in posterolateral lumbar fusions. Eur Spine J. 2003;12(5):495-500.

59. Vaccaro AR, Anderson DG, Patel T, Fischgrund J, Truumees E, Herkowitz HN, et al.

Comparison of OP-1 Putty (rhBMP-7) to iliac crest autograft for posterolateral lumbar arthrodesis: a minimum 2-year follow-up pilot study. Spine. 2005;30(24):2709-16.

60. Vaccaro AR, Patel T, Fischgrund J, Anderson DG, Truumees E, Herkowitz HN, et al. A pilot study evaluating the safety and efficacy of OP-1 putty (rhBMP-7) as a replacement for iliac crest autograft in posterolateral lumbar arthrodesis for degenerative spondylolisthesis. Spine. 2004;29(17):1885-92.

61. Vaccaro AR, Whang PG, Patel T, Phillips FM, Anderson DG, Albert TJ, et al. The safety and efficacy of OP-1 (rhBMP-7) as a replacement for iliac crest autograft for posterolateral lumbar arthrodesis: minimum 4-year follow-up of a pilot study. Spine J. 2008;8(3):457-65.

62. Munns J, Park D, Singh K. Role of osteogenic protein-1/bone morphogenetic protein-7 in spinal fusion. Orthopedic Research and Reviews. 2009;1:11-21.

63. Magit DP, Maak T, Trioano N, Raphael B, Hamouria Q, Polzhofer G, et al. Healos/recombinant human growth and differentiation factor-5 induces posterolateral lumbar fusion in a New Zealand white rabbit model. Spine. 2006;31(19):2180-8.

64. Kim DH, Jahng TA, Fu TS, Zhang HY, Novak SA. Evaluation of HealosMP52 osteoinductive bone graft for instrumented lumbar intertransverse process fusion in sheep. Spine. 2004;29(24):2800-8.

65. Neen D, Noyes D, Shaw M, Gwilym S, Fairlie N, Birch N. Healos and bone marrow aspirate used for lumbar spine fusion - A case controlled study comparing healos with autograft. Spine. 2006;31(18):E636-40.

66. Khoueir P, Oh BC, DiRisio DJ, Wang MY. Multilevel anterior cervical fusion using a collagen-hydroxyapatite matrix with iliac crest bone marrow aspirate: An 18-month follow-up study. Neurosurgery. 2007;61(5):963-70.

67. Ploumis A, Albert TJ, Brown Z, Mehbod AA, Transfeldt EE. Healos graft carrier with bone marrow aspirate instead of allograft as adjunct to local autograft for posterolateral fusion in degenerative lumbar scoliosis: a minimum 2-year follow-up study. J Neurosurg Spine. 2010;13(2):211-5.

68. Badrinath R, Bohl DD, Hustedt JW, Webb ML, Grauer JN. Only prolonged time from abstraction found to affect viable nucleated cell concentrations in vertebral body bone marrow aspirate. Spine J. 2014;14(6):990-5.

69. Hustedt JW, Jegede KA, Badrinath R, Bohl DD, Blizzard DJ, Grauer JN. Optimal aspiration volume of vertebral bone marrow for use in spinal fusion. Spine J. 2013;13(10):1217-22.

70. Risbud MV, Shapiro IM, Guttapalli A, Di Martino A, Danielson KG, Beiner JM, et al. Osteogenic potential of adult human stem cells of the lumbar vertebral body and the iliac crest. Spine (Phila Pa 1976). 2006;31(1):83-9.

1.3 Research Integrity and Everyday Practice of Science

Frederick Grinnell

Grinnell, F. Research integrity and everyday practice of science. *Science and Engineering Ethics* 19(3), 193–199 (2013). © Springer Science+Business Media B.V. 2012. Imprint of SpringerNature

Sci Eng Ethics (2013) 19:685–701
DOI 10.1007/s11948-012-9376-5

ORIGINAL PAPER

Research Integrity and Everyday Practice of Science

Frederick Grinnell

Received: 21 April 2012 / Accepted: 14 June 2012 / Published online: 28 June 2012
© Springer Science+Business Media B.V. 2012

Abstract   Science traditionally is taught as a linear process based on logic and carried out by objective researchers following the scientific method. Practice of science is a far more nuanced enterprise, one in which intuition and passion become just as important as objectivity and logic. Whether the activity is committing to study a particular research problem, drawing conclusions about a hypothesis under investigation, choosing whether to count results as data or experimental noise, or deciding what information to present in a research paper, ethical challenges inevitably will arise because of the ambiguities inherent in practice. Unless these ambiguities are acknowledged and their sources understood explicitly, responsible conduct of science education will not adequately prepare the individuals receiving the training for the kinds of decisions essential to research integrity that they will have to make as scientists.

Keywords   Responsible conduct of research · Science education ·
Science policy · Philosophy of science

Introduction

In 2002, the National Academies Institute of Medicine (IOM) published a report called *Integrity in Scientific Research* (National Academies—Institute of Medicine 2002). The IOM committee wrote that "Integrity in research embraces the aspirational standards of scientific conduct rather than simply the avoidance of questionable practices." More than mere compliance, understanding and commitment to research integrity should be an institutional output along with the research

F. Grinnell (✉)
Department of Cell Biology, Program in Ethics in Science and Medicine,
UT Southwestern Medical Center, Dallas, TX 75390, USA
e-mail: frederick.grinnell@utsouthwestern.edu

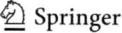 Springer

itself (Figure 3.1 in the IOM report). Education in responsible conduct of research (RCR) was viewed by the IOM committee as the essential means to encourage research integrity.

RCR training in the United States began in 1989 when the National Institutes of Health (NIH) announced that NIH training programs should teach the principles of scientific integrity as an integral part of training efforts (U.S. Department of Health and Human Services 1989). For many years, most details regarding how to conduct RCR education and what subjects to cover were left to the institutions providing the instruction. Beginning in 2011, NIH provided expanded guidance concerning format, overall subject matter, faculty participation, duration and frequency of RCR instruction (National Institutes of Health 2011). Beginning in 2010, the National Science Foundation (NSF) also introduced an RCR training requirement for undergraduates, graduate students, and postdoctoral fellows receiving NSF support (National Science Foundation 2010). The new NIH and NSF requirements strongly encourage institutions to make RCR instruction part of the core educational curriculum rather than an ancillary component.

This essay concerns the fundamental orientation of RCR education. The perspective presented is that research integrity should be taught in the context of everyday practice of science (Grinnell 1992, 2009). Consider the following example that will be discussed later in detail. Research papers frequently contain only a small portion of the data collected. Moreover, the data presented often are arranged to tell the best story even though doing so is historically inaccurate. What are students to think—what do they learn—when they realize these features? Is the research paper honest? In an intellectual sense, yes, and consistent with the conventions of everyday practice. But it an absolute sense, the paper is false.

The 2010 *Singapore Statement on Research Integrity* begins with the principle *Honesty in all aspects of research* (2nd World Conference on Research Integrity 2010). Such aspirational documents about research integrity as well as RCR courses based on theory of science will not by themselves adequately prepare the individuals receiving RCR training for the kinds of decisions essential to research integrity that they will have to make as scientists. Because of ambiguities inherent in everyday practice such as the example of research papers mentioned above, ethical challenges will arise in every aspect of research. RCR education that fails to acknowledge these ambiguities and make explicit their sources loses its relevance for the students receiving the training.

In what follows, I begin by contrasting everyday practice with the textbook and linear models of science. Then, I discuss the problem of objectivity in science given the influence of personal biography on what one does and how one does it. Subsequent sections will focus on the two central practices of science, discovery and credibility, Discovery means learning new things about the world. Credibility means convincing others of the correctness of what one has learned. Final sections will deal with the sociopolitical environment in which research is conducted and with the question whether RCR education should begin earlier in the science curriculum.

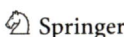 Springer

Everyday Practice of Science

Towards the beginning of his classic work *Against Method*, Paul Feyerabend wrote,

> The history of science will be as complex, chaotic, full of mistakes, and entertaining as the ideas it contains, and these ideas will be as complex, full of mistakes, and entertaining as are the minds of those who invented them. Conversely, a little brainwashing will go a long way in making the history of science duller, simpler, more uniform, more 'objective' and more easily accessible to treat by strict and unchangeable rules… Science education as we know it today has precisely this aim. (Feyerabend 1975)

Science comes in three versions: textbook, linear model, and everyday practice. From the first two versions, one can learn a lot about the theory of science but not so much about what actually happens in the laboratory or the field. Textbooks offer facts with little possibility to understand their origins. As Harvard University president James Conant commented in *Science and Common Sense*.

> The stumbling way in which even the ablest of the scientists of every generation have had to fight through thickets of erroneous observations, misleading generalizations, inadequate formulations, and unconscious prejudice is rarely appreciated by those who obtain their scientific knowledge from textbooks. (Conant 1951)

The linear model offers a description of science in which the path from hypothesis to discovery follows a direct line guided by objectivity and logic as if the facts were waiting to be observed and collected by dispassionate researchers. The linear model exemplifies how scientists communicate with each other when they make their research findings public in papers and lectures. Formulated as *the scientific method*, the linear model provides the traditional focus of science education.

"It is commonly believed," wrote Harold Schilling—introducing the image of science as cranking out discoveries,

> that science is a sort of intellectual machine, which, when one turns a crank called 'the scientific method,' inevitably grinds out ultimate truth in a series of predictably sequential steps, with complete accuracy and certainty (Schilling 1958).

Shilling's description exactly fits the expectation that arises from science education based on the linear model.

Everyday practice focuses on what actually happens in the conduct of research. Rather than textbooks and research papers, the best place to find this version of science is in scientific memoirs and other historical accounts. When Sir Peter Medawar reviewed Jim Watson's memoir *The Double Helix*, Medawar commented about how the book offered key insights about practice of science,

> No layman who reads this book with any kind of understanding will every again think of the scientist as a man who cranks a machine of discovery. No beginner in science will henceforward believe that discovery is bound to come

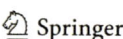 Springer

his way if only he practices a certain method, goes through a certain well-defined performance of hand and mind. (Medawar 1968)

Reading *The Double Helix* one quickly leans that the path to discovery is anything but linear, and that the researchers involved are anything but disinterested.

Biography and Personality

Research programs vary in focus from highly descriptive to mathematical and theoretical. They range in size from one or several individuals working in a single laboratory to hundreds of collaborators interacting world-wide. Whatever the focus and size of the research program, responsible conduct of research begins with the individual investigator.

Thomas Kuhn is best known for his book *The Structure of Scientific Revolutions* in which he makes a distinction between normal and revolutionary science and describes *paradigms* as community-shared sets of beliefs and acceptable ways of problem solving that guide practice during periods of normal science (Kuhn 1962). Although less well appreciated, Kuhn also emphasized that beyond values shared by the community, scientific judgment by individuals depends on biography and personality (Kuhn 1979). The interface between prevailing beliefs of the community and individual biography and personality always will be the starting point for subsequent work. Others have reached similar conclusions and offered operational terms for the influence of biography and personality, e.g., *schemata* (Piaget 1970), *thematic presuppositions* (Holton 1973), and *thought styles* (Fleck 1979).

The term *thought style* comes from Ludwik Fleck's book *Genesis and Development of a Scientific Fact* (Fleck 1979), which traces the transformation of beliefs about syphilis from the 15th to 20th century. Fleck described a researcher's thought style as the cluster of education, experience, temperament, and life situation that establishes the particular standpoint from which the person approaches the work at hand. Here, intuition blends with logic; conviction blends with skepticism.

At every step of the discovery and credibility process, the thought style will influence what the person experiences, how experience is interpreted, and what actions are taken in response. These actions include making decisions about what research problems to study; how to design experiments; and how to distinguish between data and noise.

Decisions produce commitments. For instance, deciding to study a particular research question takes for granted:

- That prior research was somehow incomplete or incorrect leaving behind an unanswered question to be investigated.
- That adequate methodological, infrastructure, personnel, and financial resources are available to answer the question.
- That finding the answer will be worth the effort.

Because resources of time, money and personnel are limiting, carrying out one project almost always means that something else will not be accomplished. What if

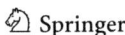

the investigator's starting assumptions are wrong, i.e., the problem already has been solved by others; or finding a solution is beyond the abilities of the research group; or even if the problem is solved successfully, the community thinks it is unimportant? Being wrong ultimately can result in failure to achieve the accomplishments that advance one's career as a scientist. Recognizing the influence of biography and personality makes it clear why researchers can never be objective and dispassionate in the way imagined by the linear model of science. Indeed, given the context of biography and personality, one wonders—what is the source of objectivity in science?

Discovery

Creativity, originality, novelty—these words reflect the gold standard of science. The goal of discovery is to be first to know something new about the world—to go where no one has gone before. By contrast, researchers usually find little reward (and therefore little incentive) to simply replicate and confirm what others already have done. Achieving recognition and fame are symbols of success in carrying out *new-search* not *re-search*. But achieving new-search is not easy. Indeed, creative thinking is hard to teach and rarely part of the science education curriculum (DeHaan 2011).

In everyday practice, the path to discovery frequently is convoluted with lots of dead ends. Failure is frequent. The pressure to produce is great. Why is discovery so hard? The Greek philosopher Plato argued that discovery is not just difficult, but impossible! In the *Dialogues*, Meno asks Socrates:

> How will you look for it, Socrates, when you do not know at all what it is? How will you aim to search for something you do not know at all? If you should meet with it, how will you know that this is the thing that you did not know?

Socrates answers:

> I know what you want to say, Meno…that a man cannot search either for what he knows or for what he does not know. He cannot search for what he knows – since he knows it, there is no need to search – nor for what he does not know, for he does not know what to look for. (Plato 380 B.C.E.)

The exchange between Meno and Socrates points to the paradox of discovery. If an investigator searches for and finds what he already knows and can recognize, then nothing new has been discovered. Discovery requires searching for what is beforehand unknown and not yet recognizable, but how is that possible?

Plato's paradox captures the problem that every researcher encounters. The already known and expected can act as an impediment to discovery by constraining investigators from seeing and thinking anything more. Claude Bernard, one of the first experimental physiologists, emphasized the foregoing difficulty in his classic 1865 work, *An Introduction to the Study of Experimental Medicine.*

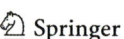 Springer

Men who have excessive faith in their theories or ideas are not only ill prepared for making discoveries; they also make very poor observations. Of necessity, they observe with a preconceived idea, and when they devise an experiment, they can see, in its results, only a confirmation of their theory. In this way they distort observations and often neglect very important facts because they do not further their aim. (Bernard 1957)

For Plato, discovery is an event with two outcomes. *It's one of them*, or *I didn't see anything*. In practice, discovery occurs as a process. Through this process, new things can be noticed even if they are not understood at the moment. *It looks like one of them, but I'm not sure*, or *I don't know what it is, I've never seen one before*. Noticing what does not fit into one's expectations becomes the starting point. Learning to see how after all it does fit becomes the discovery.

Sometimes, one notices and learns something new without being explicitly aware of having done so. We know more than we can tell, said Michael Polanyi, describing the tacit dimension of knowledge (Polanyi 1983). Discovery results from getting in touch with that tacit knowledge. Commenting on the 50th anniversary of the discovery of the Operon in gene regulation, Nobel Laureate François Jacob wrote that a moment occurred when he sensed "in a flash" the relationship between the research going on at the two ends of corridor where he worked at the Pasteur Institute in Paris (Jacob 2011).

> Our breakthrough was the result of "night science": a stumbling, wandering exploration of the natural world that relies on intuition as much as it does on the cold, orderly logic of "day science."

Frequently, it is not the individual alone, but the individual engaged with others that leads to recognition of what has been learned. Fleck describes these interactions in terms of an expanding community of thought styles.

> Thoughts pass from one individual to another, each time a little transformed, for each individual can attach to them somewhat different associations. Strictly speaking, the receiver never understands the thought exactly in the way the transmitter intended it to be understood. After a series of such encounters, practically nothing is left of the original content. Whose thought is it that continues to circulate? (Fleck 1979)

Disagreements about "whose thought is it" can easily lead to disputes regarding priority of discovery and authorship.

Not only do we know more than we can tell, but also we do more than we intend. In this case, noticing new things is made possible by unintended experiments. Nobel Laureate Max Delbrück facetiously called doing more than we intend the *principle of limited sloppiness* (Hayes 1982). By sloppiness, Delbrück did not mean technical error, although the history of science shows that important discoveries sometimes occur through technical error. Rather Delbrück was commenting on the openness of experimental design. Because knowledge is limiting and researchers do not know exactly what they are looking for, experimental design can result in unexpected outcomes. The decision to study old problems with new technologies is a useful

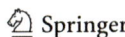

strategy to increase opportunities to notice something new (de Solla Price 1983). Once noticed, unanticipated outcomes can become the first step towards important new discoveries.

Charles Peirce gave the name *abduction*, in contrast to *deduction* or *induction*, to the logic of discovery by unintended experiments. Neither of the latter, he argued, could result in any new ideas (Peirce 1958). Peirce formulated the logic of abduction as follows.

> The surprising fact C is observed.
> But if A were true, C would be self-evident.
> Consequently, there is ground to suspect that A is true.

According to Peirce's analysis, experimental results can be thought of as pieces of a jigsaw puzzle. An unexpected result (C)—noticed because it is "surprising"—can be seen as fitting into a puzzle (A) that had not been under investigation at the time the experiment was planned and carried out. Noticing the new piece (C) opens the possibility of focusing on the new puzzle (A) in which the new piece appears to fit.

Experiments

As experiments proceed, they divide into three categories: heuristic, demonstrative, and—most common—failed. Heuristic experiments offer researchers new insights into the problem under investigation including evidence that disproves a new hypothesis. Demonstrative experiments re-work heuristic findings, if necessary, into a form suitable for making discovery claims public. Failed experiments arise when results are inconclusive or uninterpretable, which may occur for many reasons including technical errors, uncertain methods, or poor study design. Success in science frequently depends on turning failed experiments into new starts.

Carrying out any experiment requires guessing what will be the outcome. The guess becomes the basis for study design. Because the answer is not known in advance (otherwise why do the experiment—Plato's paradox revisited), every experiment tests both the investigator's explicit hypothesis about how things are and implicit hypothesis about the type of methodology and design adequate to answer the question under investigation. Finding the "right" answer always will be a work in progress.

In his memoir *The Statue Within*, François Jacob describes the failures that he and his colleagues encountered as they tried to demonstrate the existence of mRNA.

> We were to do very long, very arduous experiments… But nothing worked. We had tremendous technical problems… Full of energy and excitement, sure of the correctness of our hypothesis, we started our experiment over and over again. Modifying it slightly. Changing some technical detail.
> Our confidence crumbled. We found ourselves lying limply on a beach, vacantly gazing at the huge waves of the Pacific crashing onto the sand. Only a few days were left before the inevitable end. But should we keep on? What

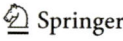 Springer

was the use? Suddenly, Sydney gives a shout. He leaps up, yelling, "The magnesium! It's the magnesium!" Immediately we get in Hildegaard's car and race to the lab to run the experiment one last time…Sydney had been right. It was indeed the magnesium that gave the ribosomes their cohesion. But the usual quantities were insufficient…This time we added plenty of magnesium. (Jacob 1988)

The hypothesis had been correct; the method used to test the hypothesis had been incorrect.

Karl Popper suggested that research advances by falsification of hypotheses (Popper 1959). Because every experiment tests both the hypothesis and the adequacy of the experiment to test the hypothesis, conclusions always will be open to interpretation and debate. One does not give up a good hypothesis just because the data do not fit, at least not at first. Popper's notion of falsification might work for linear science, but in everyday practice, the significance of falsification is aspirational. Researchers should be open to the possibility of being wrong.

Besides the uncertainty of experimental methodology and design, a second aspect of "don't give up the hypothesis just because of the data don't fit" concerns anomalous research findings. In *The Structure of Scientific Revolutions* (Kuhn 1962), Kuhn describes how anomalous findings accompany research during normal science and accumulate until their presence becomes so overwhelming that a crises occurs, which is the point at which revolutionary science begins. However, during normal science, the natural tendency for researchers will be to overlook anomalous findings. Here is what Nobel Laureate Rita Levi-Montalcini wrote regarding her research that ultimately led to discovery of nerve growth factor, a key regulator of cell growth and development.

> Even though I possessed no proof in favor of the hypothesis, in my secret heart of hearts, I was certain that the [cancerous] tumors that had been transplanted into the embryos would in fact stimulate [nerve] fiber growth.

The tumors stimulated fiber growth but, unexpectedly, Levi-Montalcini found a similar effect with normal tissue fragments. She described this observation as "the most severe blow to my enthusiasm that I could ever have suffered."

> After suffering the brunt of the initial shock at these results, in a partially unconscious way I began to apply what Alexander Luria, the Russian neuropsychologist has called 'the law of disregard of negative information'… facts that fit into a preconceived hypothesis attract attention, are singled out and remembered. Facts that are contrary to it are disregarded, treated as exception, and forgotten. (Levi-Montalcini 1988)

If Levi-Montalcini had focused on the anomalous result, she might have abandoned the research project. Instead, she continued to believe in the unique importance of the factor in tumor biology. Years later, she returned to study the importance of nerve growth factor with normal tissues.

The foregoing examples turned out to be success stories for the researchers involved. However, sticking to one's hypothesis in the face of contrary data or

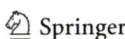

ignoring anomalous data is risky business. The challenge is to be aware of the choices that one is making and to know when to give up a hypothesis even though it is a good one. Error is common. Failure is frequent.

Research Papers

The adage *publish or perish* concerns both researchers and the discoveries that they make. When researchers do not publish, they put their careers a risk. When discoveries are not made public, it is as if the work was never performed.

Research papers provide the formal mechanism by which investigators make public the details of their discovery claims. Papers typically describe the small collection of demonstrative experiments carried out with the much larger set of failures omitted. It would not be unusual for ten research notebooks worth of experiments to become a ten page research paper.

As the research proceeds, investigators and co-workers make judgments about experimental outcomes and decide what results count as data versus experimental noise. Unlike high school and college science experiments, no one knows the right answer in advance. Heuristic principles can help distinguish data from noise but rarely are sufficient. Given the uncertainty, experience and intuition (biography and personality) become equally important.

In any particular case, the way that results are selected and used by one investigator might appear self-serving and inappropriate to another. As the National Academies 1992 report *Responsible Science* comments, "The selective use of research data is another area where the boundary between fabrication and creative insight may not be obvious." (National Academies Panel on Scientific Responsibility and the Conduct of Research 1992)

In his work describing the charge on the electron, Nobel laureate Robert A. Millikan based his calculations on 58 out of 140 oil drop experiments, which he called the "golden events" (Holton 1973). In reporting his findings, Millikan said that he included "all" the data in making his calculation. The discrepancy (58 vs. 140) led the Sigma Xi Research Society in its pamphlet *Honor in Science* to describe Millikan's published work as "one of the best known cases of cooking" (i.e., falsifying data by unrepresentative selection; Jackson 1984).

Several years after *Honor in Science* was published, Sigma Xi awarded its annual McGovern Science and Society Award to physicist David Goodstein. Goodstein entitled his award lecture "In the case of Robert Andrews Millikan." He argued that the 58 drops selected by Millikan were all of the drops that fit the criteria Millikan had used to distinguish which results counted as data. The other drops did not count for one reason or another (Goodstein 2001).

In addition to presenting only a selected set of data, research papers also typically rewrite history to present a logical and internally consistent account of the studies. Just as failed experiments are omitted, so will be failed hypotheses that have been discarded and older experiments at one time believed to be demonstrative but reinterpreted or discarded in light of later findings.

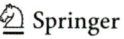 Springer

The paper published in *Nature* in which Jacob and co-workers describe the evidence for mRNA (Jacob 1988) offers a much different account from that found in Jacob's memoir. Instead of "sure of the correctness of our hypothesis," one reads early on, "A priori, three types of hypothesis may be considered to account for the known facts of phage protein synthesis…" Then comes a logical discussion of how these three types of hypotheses might be distinguished. When the subject turns to magnesium,

> The bulk of the RNA synthesized after infection is found in the ribosome fraction, provided that the extraction is carried out in 0.01 M magnesium ions[12]. Lowering of the magnesium concentration in the gradient, or dialyzing the particles against low magnesium, produces a decrease of the B band and an increase of the A band. At the same time, the radioactive RNA leaves the B band to appear at the bottom of the gradient.

The beach and Sydney's shout are gone. The citation to reference 12 makes it appear as if the experiments had been carried out from the beginning with high (0.01 M) magnesium as recommended previously by others. The summer of "But nothing worked. We had tremendous technical problems." becomes an intentional control experiment showing the result of lowering the magnesium concentration.

"Writing a paper" writes Jacob,

> is to substitute order for the disorder and agitation that animate life in the laboratory… To replace the real order of events and discoveries by what appears as the logical order, the one that should have been followed if the conclusions were known from the start. (Jacob 1988)

The paper converts the process of discovery into an announcement of a discovery claim, a scientific short story whose plot is none other than the scientific method.

In an essay called *Is the scientific paper a fraud?* Sir Peter Medawar complained that research publications distort science—"a totally mistaken conception, even a travesty, of the nature of scientific thought." One cannot not learn from the publications the "adventures of the mind" leading researchers to make their discoveries (Medawar 1963). While RCR education would benefit from teaching about the adventures of the mind leading to discoveries, the function of research papers is not to teach about the nature of scientific thought but rather to make it as easy as possible for new discovery claims to be understood and used.

Notwithstanding his essay, Medawar was no different from everyone else when it came to his own practice. Rupert Billingham, Medawar's younger collaborator in the work establishing the field of transplantation immunology for which Medawar won the Nobel Prize, published an autobiographical essay containing a section called "The most important lecture I've ever attended."

> In 1947 Medawar gave a joint paper on our work… It was obvious to me that in this lecture the only items that were sacrosanct or inviolable were actual factual observations. Hypotheses could be invented or rejected at will, and the chronology of the experiments conducted and the reasons for embarking upon them could be altered to make the best possible story.

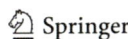 Springer

In a subsequent session of this symposium Dr. J. H. Woodger gave what amounted to a lecture on scientific method. I was amused when he cited Medawar's contribution as a model of its kind, exemplifying how an investigation should be tackled. Obviously, it had never occurred to Woodger that Medawar's narrative represented a gross travesty of the true history of the project. (Billingham 1974)

If one is looking for a historically accurate picture a particular piece of research, then research notebooks would be the only potential source of information. Because research publications contain only a representative selection of data and present the findings in a logical rather than historically accurate fashion, keeping and preserving a historical record in essential for research integrity. Existence of the detailed notebook historical record allows researchers potentially to share all of their data with others and to explain and justify their choices if asked to do so.

Trust

Discussions of research integrity frequently emphasize the importance of trust. For instance, the aspirational code of ethics of the American Society of Biochemistry and Molecular Biology begins,

Members … are engaged in the quest for knowledge … with the ultimate goal of advancing human welfare. Underlying this quest is the fundamental principle of trust. The [society] encourages its members to engage in the responsible practice of research required for such trust by fulfilling the following obligations. (American Society of Biochemistry and Molecular Biology 1998)

Trust between investigators plays a central role in the discovery and credibility processes. It begins in each research group where a necessary feature for normal functioning is that investigators trust each other to do what they say and to get the results that they describe. When multiple groups are involved in a collaborative research project, then the degree of trust required increases with the physical and disciplinary distances in between.

When investigators make their work public in the form of scientific manuscripts or submitted grant applications, reviewers trust that the completed work or preliminary studies were carried out as described and led to the results reported. Researchers, on the other hand, trust that reviewers of their submitted manuscripts and research grant proposals will not misuse the information that they learn. Here the situation becomes tricky. The contents of submitted manuscripts and grant applications are privileged and confidential, but reviewers will be not be able to unlearn what they have learned during the review process. Moreover, the best peer-reviewers often are those most knowledgeable about a subject, and who have the most to gain by advance knowledge of the others' work and ideas. Scientific peer-review resembles a bizarre version of poker in which competitors show each other their cards for analysis and comment but expect that everyone will continue to play their own cards unaffected by what has been seen.

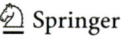 Springer

The National Academies' defines conflict of interest as:

> any financial or other interest which conflicts with the service of the
> individual because it (i) could significantly impair the individual's objectivity
> or (ii) could create an unfair competitive advantage for any person or
> organization. (The National Academies 2003)

According to part (ii), scientific peer-review system is inherently conflicted. Yet the
rigor of peer-review generally is credited with the success of contemporary science.

Credibility

Once a discovery claim is made public, the credibility process can begin. Because
scientists bring biography and personality to their work, discovery claims can be no
more than *protoscience*, inseparable from the subjectivity and ownership associated
with the investigator or research group that makes the claim. For a discovery claim
to become a scientific discovery, the researcher must turn towards the larger
community.

Making a discovery claim public allows individual researchers to transcend their
own subjectivity through intersubjectivity. Intersubjectivity is at the base of all
social interactions. People live in a shared world and experience the world in similar
ways. If two individuals interchange places, then they will (sort of) see, hear, think
similar things—*reciprocity of perspectives* (Schutz 1967). In science, intersubjectivity means that researchers will be able to verify and validate each others work if
it is correct. Through the credibility process, the individual researcher's existential
me/here/now becomes the scientific community's anyone/anywhere/anytime.
Objective knowledge is the goal, not the starting point. The community rather
than the individual provides the source of objectivity in science. Paraphrasing
William James' pragmatic conception of truth (James 1975),

> Credible discoveries are those that we can assimilate, validate, corroborate,
> and verify… The credibility of a discovery is not a stagnant property inherent
> in it. Credibility happens to a discovery. It becomes credible, is made credible
> by events … Its verity is the process of verification. Its validity is the process
> of validation. (paraphrased)

That the credibility process goes on and on and on is the self-correcting feature of
science. As a consequence, what was believed at first to be correct and important,
frequently turns out later to be wrong or overstated (Ioannidis 2005).

At the beginning of the credibility process, the attitude of the community towards
discovery claims can be summed up by the inscription on the coat of arms of the
Royal Society—*Nullius in verba*—which Sir Peter Medawar translated as *Don't
take anybody's word for it!* Because of the novelty associated with discovery,
intersubjectivity can act as a double-edged sword. Nobel Laureate Albert Szent-
Györgyi's characterized discovery as *seeing what everybody else has seen and
thinking what nobody else has thought*. Szent-Györgyi's idea is captured in René
Magritte's 1936 oil painting *Perspicacity*, which shows a seated artist staring at a

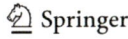

solitary egg on a draped table but painting a bird in full flight on the canvas. The more novel a discovery claim, the more likely it will challenge prevailing scientific beliefs with the outcome of *non*-reciprocity of perspectives, which can lead, at least at first, to skepticism if not outright rejection.

The history of Nobel Prizes includes many examples of novel discoveries that were either ignored or disputed for years, e.g., tumor viruses (Nobel Prize in 1966), chemiosmotic theory (Nobel Prize in 1978), transposable elements (Nobel Prize in 1983), catalytic ribonucleic acid (Nobel Prize in 1989), and prions (Nobel Prize in 1997).

Nobel Laureate Barbara McClintock explicitly commented in her Nobel banquet speech about why her research went unaccepted for so long,

> I have been asked, notably by young investigators, just how I felt during the long period when my work was ignored, dismissed, or aroused frustration.... My understanding of the phenomenon responsible for rapid changes in gene action... was much too radical for the time. A person would need to have my experiences, or ones similar to them, to penetrate this barrier. (McClintock 1983)

Ralph Steinman shared (posthumously) in the 2011 Nobel Prize in Physiology and Medicine. After he won the 2007 Lasker Prize for his work, the chair of the Lasker Committee wrote,

> Why were Steinman's early studies ignored, neglected and often denigrated by the immunological community? Longstanding dogma... made it easy for immunologists to brush aside Steinman's experiments and ideas on dendritic cells, and to view them as some type of Victorian curiosity with little or no relevance to the mainstream of immunology. Fortunately, Steinman's passionate belief in his data and his unshakable self-confidence propelled him forward despite the criticisms of his colleagues. (Goldstein 2007)

Ironically, when skepticism about the novel discoveries leads one's research findings to be ignored, neglected and denigrated, success sometimes requires the individual to become an advocate—a passionate advocate—for the work. How to become a passionate advocate for one's work and yet remain intellectually honest becomes the challenge. Of course, in the end the community might be right.

The Research Environment

While responsible conduct of research begins with the individual investigator, the overall research environment can exert a profound influence (National Academies—Institute of Medicine 2002). The complex intersection of society, government and research institution (academic, independent, industrial) creates the moral climate in which the individual does the work. In general, attitudes towards one's surrounding moral climate influence individual behavior. Science is no different. Empirical

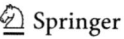 Springer

evidence suggests that scientists' perceptions of the research environment impacts their commitment to research integrity (Martinson et al. 2006).

Political, economic and cultural factors exert an important influence on what science will be done, who will do it, and how the work will be financed. For instance, soft money support of US academic researcher salaries began in 1960, when the President's Science Advisory Committee (PSAC) recommended that federal agencies provide support for basic research and graduate education. However, PSAC envisioned a block grant support mechanism and commented about "the need for avoiding situations in which a professor becomes partly or wholly responsible for raising his own salary" (President's Science Advisory Committee 1960). Contrary to PSAC's recommendation, what has evolved is a system in which it is precisely the professors who are now responsible for raising their own salaries. Success in doing so can influence getting a job, keeping a job, and keeping one's salary even if one's job is tenured.

Linking a researcher's position and salary to the ability to win external research funding creates potential conflicts of interest and commitment. Satisfying the demands of one's external funding review panel can become more important than satisfying the internal demands of the university or research center such as teaching, clinical practice and service. Because graduate students and postdoctoral fellows frequently also are supported by research grants, they straddle the line between employee and trainee. What is in the best interests of a trainee's education may not be in the best interests of research productivity.

In today's environment, the grant-supported research group increasingly resembles a small business. The principle investigator (owner/operator) generates grants and contracts (income) to support students, postdoctoral fellows and other staff (employees) who produce papers and patents (products) described in seminars and scientific conferences (advertising) to the scientific community (potential buyers). Acting as small business owners, scientists take on new roles beyond research directors. They become personnel and business managers, activities that come with their own ethical challenges. And when principle investigators transition from science to business entrepreneurs, *patent and prosper* replaces the traditional goal of *publish or perish* (Schachman 2006).

Should RCR Education Should Begin Earlier in the Science Curriculum?

The overarching aim of this essay has been to show the importance of orienting RCR education towards everyday practice rather than theory of science. The examples presented demonstrate that in every aspect of research, ethical challenges inevitably will arise because of the ambiguities of practice. One way to help teach about these ambiguities would be to incorporate scientific memoirs and other historical accounts of science into RCR education. A separate issue to be raised in this final section is the question whether RCR education should begin earlier in the science curriculum in connection with activities such as science laboratory experiments and science fair.

In chemistry laboratory with an unknown to investigate, getting anything close to the predicted result sometimes is impossible regardless how carefully the student

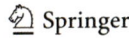
Springer

works given time constraints and quality of reagents. Yet getting the "right" result often determines the grade. As a result, writing a lab report based on the calculated amount of end product—not the amount actually determined—sometimes becomes the path to success (B. Fisher, Survival skills and ethics program, University of Pittsburgh, Personal communication, 2011). Does this sort of chemistry lab experience encourage students to falsify data?

In physics laboratory, pendulum experiments exemplify the potential for ambiguity. A National Academies study *America's Lab Report: Investigations in High School Science* describes the problem as follows,

> [W]hen discussing a pendulum in class, a physics teacher may ignore without discussion a host of variables that may affect its operation. However, when a student starts doing a simple experiment with a pendulum, these variables suddenly become relevant… The student may feel betrayed by the apparent mismatch between the neatness of a phenomenon as presented in a textbook and the inherent messiness and ambiguity of the same phenomenon encountered in the laboratory. (National Academies National Research Council 2006)

So how are these difficulties managed?

> To reduce the potential confusion and to help students attain one goal—mastery of subject matter—a typical high school pendulum activity is "cleaned up." This activity is designed to guide students toward making observations that will verify the accepted scientific principle that the period of a pendulum (the time it takes to swing out and back) depends on the length of the string and the force of gravity. It focuses only on science content. (National Academies National Research Council 2006)

Similar to chemistry laboratory, the emphasis is on the right answer not the right practice. Ironically, some research suggests that the inherent openness and ambiguity of science laboratory experiments, including opportunities to design one's own messy experiments, has the potential to promote critical thinking skills and collaborative problem solving similar to that which takes place in everyday practice of science, e.g., (Roth 1994; Etkina et al. 2010).

Science fair has a different set of problems. Studies in the education literature, albeit not many in number, have demonstrated that outright scientific misconduct occurs in science fair, especially when student participation is compulsory. Out of time, having difficulty choosing a topic, lacking resources that they feel they need, about one in five students makes up their data (Shore et al. 2007). A recent student conducted survey of science fair research integrity at duPont Manual High School in Louisville, KY, reported that 65 % of the respondents admitting to falsifying their data. The survey also concluded that 20 % of the students had "abused the scientific method" by altering their hypothesis after finishing their study (Manoharan 2011). Altering one's hypothesis in response to the data may be an abuse of the linear scientific method, but it is not an abuse of what researchers do in practice. Lumping together falsification of data with changing a hypothesis to fit the data reflects a

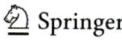 Springer

mistaken impression of what doing science entails, just the sort of misunderstanding that RCR education carried out in connection with science fair might correct.

Earlier introduction of RCR education into the science curriculum should be considered for science laboratory experiments and science fair. Doing so could provide unique opportunities to clarify misimpressions on the part of students (and their teachers) about the nature and practice of science.

Conclusion

If science really were a linear process based on logic and carried out by objective observers following the scientific method, then aspirational documents about research integrity along with courses based on theory of science would be sufficient for RCR training. However, because practice of science is a more ambiguous enterprise, a more nuanced approach to research integrity education is required, one that acknowledges and makes explicit the ambiguities inherent in practice and the ethical challenges to which they give rise. Achieving research integrity requires creating a research environment that openly recognizes and engages these ethical challenges and makes explicit their sources.

Acknowledgments Thanks to Mark Frankel, Kenneth Pimple, William Snell and Thomas Mayo for their helpful comments and suggestions regarding this essay.

References

2nd World Conference on Research Integrity. (2010). Singapore statement on research integrity, from http://www.singaporestatement.org/statement.html.

American Society of Biochemistry and Molecular Biology. (1998). Code of ethics, from http://ethics.iit.edu/ecodes/node/3898.

Bernard, C. (1957). *An introduction to the study of experimental medicine (1865)*. New York, NY: Dover Publications, Inc.

Billingham, R. E. (1974). Reminiscences of a "transplanter". *Transplantation Proceedings, 6*, 5–17.

Conant, J. B. (1951). *Science and common sense*. New Haven, CT: Yale University Press.

de Solla Price, D. (1983). The science/technology relationship, the craft of experimental science, and policy for the improvement of high technology innovation. In National Science Foundation (Ed.), *Role of basic research in science and technology*. Washington, DC: U.S. Government Printing Office.

DeHaan, R. L. (2011). Science education. Teaching creative science thinking. *Science, 334*, 1499–1500.

Etkina, E., Karelina, A., Ruibal-Villasenor, M., Rosengrant, D., Jordan, R., & Hmelo-Silver, C. E. (2010). Design and reflection help students develop scientific abilities: Learning in introductory physics laboratories. *Journal of the Learning Sciences, 19*, 54–98.

Feyerabend, P. (1975). *Against method*. New York: Verso.

Fleck, L. (1979). *Genesis and development of a scientific fact (1935)*. Chicago, IL: University of Chicago Press.

Goldstein, J. L. (2007). Creation and revelation: Two different routes to advancement in the biomedical sciences. *Nature Medicine, 13*, 1151–1154.

Goodstein, D. (2001). In the case of Robert Andrews Millikan. *American Scientist, 89*, 54–60.

Grinnell, F. (1992). *The scientific attitude* (2nd ed.). New York, NY: Guilford Press.

Grinnell, F. (2009). *Everyday practice of science: Where intuition and passion meet objectivity and logic*. New York: Oxford University Press.

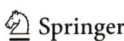

Hayes, W. (1982). Max Ludwig Henning Delbruck. *Biographical Memoirs of the Fellows of the Royal Society, 28*, 58–90.

Holton, G. (1973). *Thematic origins of scientific thought: Kepler to Einstein.* Cambridge, MA: Harvard University Press.

Ioannidis, J. P. (2005). Why most published research findings are false. *PLoS Medicine, 2*, e124.

Jackson, C. I. (1984). *Honor in science.* New Haven, CT: Sigma Xi, The Scientific Research Society.

Jacob, F. (1988). *The statue within.* New York, NY: Basic Books Inc.

Jacob, F. (2011). The birth of the operon. *Science, 332*, 767.

James, W. (1975). Pragmatism's conception of truth (1907). In *Pragmatism and the meaning of truth* (pp. 95–113). Cambridge, MA: Harvard University Press.

Kuhn, T. S. (1962). *The structure of scientific revolutions.* Chicago, IL: University of Chicago Press.

Kuhn, T. S. (1979). Objectivity, value judgement, and theory choice. In T. S. Kuhn (Ed.), *The essential tension.* Chicago, IL: University of Chicago Press.

Levi-Montalcini, R. (1988). *In praise of imperfection.* New York, NY: Basic Books Inc.

Manoharan, J. (2011, 04/22/2011). Scientific misconduct starts early, from http://www.biotechniques. com/news/Scientific-misconduct-starts-early/biotechniques-314589.html.

Martinson, B. C., Anderson, M. S., Crain, A. L., & de Vries, R. (2006). Scientists' perceptions of organizational justice and self-reported misbehaviors. *Journal of Empirical Research on Human Research Ethics, 1*, 51–66.

McClintock, B. (1983). Nobel banquet speech—December 10, 1983. In T. Frängsmyr (Ed.), *Les Prix Nobel.* Stockholm: Almqvist & Wiksell International.

Medawar, P. B. (1963). Is the scientific paper a fraud? The Listener (September 12), pp. 377–378.

Medawar, P. B. (1968). Lucky Jim. The New York Review of Books, March 28, 1968.

National Academies National Research Council. (2006). *America's lab report: Investigations in high school science.* Washington, DC: National Academies Press.

National Academies Panel on Scientific Responsibility and the Conduct of Research. (1992). *Responsible science: Ensuring the integrity of the research process.* Washington, DC: National Academies Press.

National Academies—Institute of Medicine. (2002). *Integrity in scientific research: Creating an environment that promotes responsible conduct.* Washington, DC: National Academy Press.

National Institutes of Health. (2011). Update on the requirement for instruction in the responsible conduct of research, from http://grants.nih.gov/grants/guide/notice-files/NOT-OD-10-019.html.

National Science Foundation. (2010). Chapter IV—grantee standards; Part B. Responsible Conduct of Research (RCR), from http://www.nsf.gov/pubs/policydocs/pappguide/nsf10_1/aag_4.jsp.

Peirce, C. P. (1958). Harvard lectures on pragmatism (1903). In C. Hartshorne, P. Weiss & A. Burks (Eds.), *Collected papers of Charles sanders Peirce* (Vols. 1–6, 5, pp. 188–189). Cambridge, MA: Harvard University Press.

Piaget, J. (1970). *Genetic epistemology* (E. Duckworth, Trans.). New York, NY: W.W. Norton & Co.

Plato. (380 B.C.E.). Meno 80 d-e, from http://classics.mit.edu/Plato/meno.html.

Polanyi, M. (1983). *The tacit dimension (1966).* Gloucester, MA: Peter Smith Publishers.

Popper, K. R. (1959). *The logic of scientific discovery.* New York, NY: Basic Books Inc.

President's Science Advisory Committee. (1960). *Scientific progress, the universities, and the federal government (President's Science Advisory Committee).* Washington, DC: U.S. Government Printing Office.

Roth, W.-M. (1994). Experimenting in the constructivist high school physics laboratory. *Journal of Research in Science Teaching, 31*, 197–223.

Schachman, H. K. (2006). From "publish or perish" to "patent and prosper". *Journal of Biological Chemistry, 281*, 6889–6903.

Schilling, H. K. (1958). A human enterprise. *Science, 127*, 1324–1327.

Schutz, A. (1967). *The phenomenology of the social world* (G. Walsh & F. Lehnert, Trans.). Evanston, IL: Northwestern Univ. Press.

Shore, B. M., Delcourt, M. A. B., Syer, C. A., & Schapiro, M. (2007). The phantom of the science fair. In B. M. Shore, M. W. Aulis, & M. A. B. Delcourt (Eds.), *Inquiry in education, volume II: Overcoming barriers to successful implementation.* New York, NY: Routledge.

The National Academies. (2003). Policy on committee composition and balance and conflicts of interest for committees used in the development of reports (May 12, 2003), from http://www.national academies.org/coi/bi-coi_form-0.pdf.

U.S. Department of Health and Human Services. (1989). Requirement for programs on the responsible conduct of research in national research service award institutional training programs, from http:// grants.nih.gov/grants/guide/historical/1989_12_22_Vol_18_No_45.pdf.

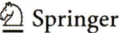 Springer

1.4 Lessons from the Infuse Trials: Do We Need a Classification of Bias in Scientific Publications and Editorials?

Sohaib Hashmi, Mohamed Noureldin, and Safdar N. Khan

Hashmi, S, Noureldin, M, Khan, S. Lessons from the infuse trials: do we need a classification of bias in scientific publications and editorials? *Current Review of Musculoskeletal Medicine* 7(3), 193–199 (2014). © Springer Science+Business Media New York 2014. Imprint of SpringerNature.

Table 1 reprinted from Schulz KF, Altman DG, Moher D. CONSORT 2010 statement:updated guidelines for reporting parallel group randomised trials. BMJ. 2010;340:c332. doi:https://doi.org/10.1136/bmj.c332. With permission from BMJ Publishing Group Ltd.

Table 2 reprinted from Boutron I, Moher D, Tugwell P, Giraudeau B, Poiraudeau S, Nizard R, et al. A checklist to evaluate a report of a nonpharmacologicaltrial (CLEAR NPT) was developed using consensus. J ClinEpidemiol. 2005;58:123340. doi:https://doi.org/10.1016/j.jclinepi.2005.05.004. With automatic permission from Elsevier via STM Permissions Guidelines

Curr Rev Musculoskelet Med (2014) 7:193–199
DOI 10.1007/s12178-014-9223-1

SPINE: BMP (K SINGH, SECTION EDITOR)

Lessons from the infuse trials: do we need a classification of bias in scientific publications and editorials?

Sohaib Hashmi · Mohamed Noureldin · Safdar N. Khan

Published online: 31 May 2014
© Springer Science+Business Media New York 2014

Abstract The original 13 Food and Drug Administration industry-sponsored recombinant human bone morphogenetic protein-2 (rhBMP-2) trials investigating its use in spinal fusion all reported no associated adverse events. However, subsequent series of studies began reporting complication rates that were much higher than those that were initially published. Critical analysis of the original rhBMP-2 industry-associated data found systematic alignment favoring positive outcomes with no proven clinical advantage over bone graft. The sources of potential bias leading to inaccurate reporting of original rhBMP-2 efficacy and safety profile include flawed study design, methodological technique, data reporting and analysis, and significant financial conflict of interest. As such, to ensure the integrity of the scientific literature, further measures should be taken by researchers, surgeons, authors, journal editors and reviewers to assess for potential sources of bias.

Keywords Infuse trials · BMP · Bias · Adverse events · Bias classification system

Introduction

The original discovery of bone morphogenetic protein (BMP) in 1965 by Urist [1] was followed by extensive preclinical and translational research in the application of these growth factors in spine fusion surgery. There was a need in selected patients to investigate alternatives and adjuncts to autologous iliac crest bone graft (ICBG) that would prove to be effective and safe. ICBG is considered the gold standard in spinal fusion with inherent osteoinductive, osteoconductive, and neovascularization properties, fusion rates varying from 40 % to 100 % [2].

The Food and Drug Administration (FDA) initially approved rhBMP-2 (Infuse; Medtronic Sofamor Danek, Memphis, TN) in the use of anterior lumbar interbody fusions (ALIF) with the LT-CAGE (Medtronic Sofamor Danek, Memphis, TN) in patients with degenerative disc disease at 1 level from L4–S1. The authors of the original industry-sponsored or industry-associated studies of rhBMP-2 all reported the efficacy in applications including both anterior and posterior cervical and lumbar fusion surgery [3–14]. Additionally, the authors of these studies stated similar safety profiles with no adverse effects or complications attributable to rhBMP-2 in any study. Favorable research findings regarding the use of rhBMP-2 in spinal fusion surgery has undoubtedly contributed to its increased utilization from 0.7 % in 2002 to 25 % in 2006, as the off-label use of rhBMP-2 expanded to nearly 73 % of the total use by 2007 [15•].

With the complexity of mechanisms and interactions of growth factors, the nature and time course of adverse events would prove to be difficult to predict. However, clear concerns in the clinical application of rhBMP-2 were cited including bony overgrowth, interaction with nearby neural structures, local and systemic toxicity, osteoclastic activation, and potential for cancer risk [16]. A divergence from the previously reported safety profile surfaced as the literature reported a greater frequency of complications associated with the use of rhBMP-2 in spinal fusion.

This disparity in the findings resulted in scrutiny by the scientific community, press, and government regarding the safety of BMP and the overarching peer review and editorial process. In a systematic review, Carragee et al concluded that the original industry-sponsored publications were systematically aligned in favor of BMP use for spinal fusion surgery, in

S. Hashmi · M. Noureldin · S. N. Khan (✉)
Division of Spine Surgery, Department of Orthopaedic Surgery,
Wexner Medical Center at The Ohio State University, 456 W 10th
Ave, Columbus, OH 43210, USA
e-mail: Safdar.Khan@osumc.edu

turn contributing to the widespread off-label use and associated the complications [17••].

The reporting and publication of the inaccurate safety profile and results of original industry-sponsored rhBMP-2 trials occurred as a result of clear bias. Bias has been defined as any process at any stage of inference that tends to produce results or conclusions that differ systematically from the truth [18]. Substantial methodological, operational, reporting, editorial, and financial bias leads one to question the efficacy of rhBMP-2 in both on-label and off-label uses. The critique of the original rhBMP-2 trials varied from the scientific community to the government including Consumer Reports, The Wall Street Journal, the Milwaukee Journal Sentinel, US Senate, the New York Times, and the Department of Justice all chiming in on this controversial topic [19••]. Following this investigation, Medtronic commissioned the Yale University Open Data Access (YODA) project to report the safety and efficacy of rhBMP-2. Using data from the original 13 trials and 31 cohort studies, these authors concluded that rhBMP-2 has no proven clinical advantage over bone graft and may be associated with significant sequelae, thereby making it difficult to identify clear indications for rhBMP-2 [20••]. In light of the subsequent conflicting assessments of rhBMP-2 with regards to efficacy and safety, it is crucial to clarify the systematic flaws of the original trials in order to improve understanding and reporting of bias in the scientific literature.

Lessons from systematic failures of the infuse trials

Systematic review of the original rhBMP-2 by Carragee et al [17••] fostered awareness of the current shortcomings in the peer review process, specifically as is it pertains to reporting of novel biological technologies for clinical application. The authors' analysis of the complete data presented by the 13 industry-sponsored studies shed light upon several areas of bias, whether intentional or unintentional, from the level of the author to publication editors. The importance of maintaining a high degree of scientific integrity relies on professionalism from the investigators and peer review for clinicians and the public to understand the published literature [21•]. Appraisal in limitations of the formative publications provides understanding of potential sources of bias in the peer review process and guidance of direction in how to face these challenges.

The FDA's premarket approval (PMA) investigations were open label investigations in which researchers, surgeons, and patients knew treatment allocation of the involved subjects. Nonblinded assessment is a significant source for potential conscious or unconscious bias. A recent meta-analysis of 16 trials with subjective outcomes demonstrated that nonblinded assessors exaggerated the effectiveness of treatment with a pooled effect size of 68 % (95 % CI, 14 %–230 %). The authors concluded that the significant evidence of observer

bias in randomized clinical trials with subjective scale outcomes and failure to blind the assessors of outcomes resulted in a high risk of substantial bias [22]. In a review of randomized clinical trials published from 2002-2004 in the Journal of Bone and Joint Surgery (American Volume) and Spine, approximately half did not report attempts to reduce bias in the Materials or Methods sections [23]. While surgical studies may be more difficult to blind compared with nonsurgical trials, efforts must be made in order to minimize potential bias.

All of the original BMP studies employed noninferiority trial designs rather than superiority trial designs. This model is intended to show that a new treatment is "not acceptably worse" than the current standard treatment. Debate regarding the use of such trials began in the mid-1900s as some authors have argued that the complexity of the study design and difficulty in verification as reasons against the utilization of noninferiority models [24]. Furthermore, noninferiority trials often carry "substantial methodological flaws" and subsequent risk for type II errors [25]. A review including 162 randomized controlled trials of noninferiority and equivalence hypotheses reported that only 20 % of articles fulfilled reporting requirements specific to this study type, in addition to 12 % of trials with misleading conclusions [26]. It has been suggested that BMP use would be better proven through superiority trials [21•].

Carragee et al [17••] included analysis of control group techniques in the assessment of the industry-sponsored BMP trials. The authors reported several discrepancies from the established literature of ICBG and local bone autograft use in spine fusion. The posterolateral fusion trials comparing rhBMP-2 with ICBG did not incorporate facet preparation, thus, fusion at facet joints was not radiographically assessed. The quantity of ICBG used was also disproportionately lower with as little as 7 cc. In addition, local bone autograft harvested from the decompression was discarded rather than being applied to augment the ICBG volumes. The control group of the posterior lumbar interbody fusion (PLIF) trial may have had unnecessary ICBG harvest, as local bone autograft alone has been shown to be sufficient for fusion, thereby contributing to preventable handicap. In addition, Carragee et al noted that the reporting of ICBG harvest-site morbidity was higher (50 %–95 %) than previous estimates. The methodological techniques used in the original BMP studies place the control ICBG groups at higher risk for poorer quality fusion, nonunion, and potential failure when compared with the standard surgical method for lumbar spinal fusion [17••].

Each of the 13 original BMP trials under-reported complications and adverse events related to BMP use when compared with additional data available through the FDA and unsponsored trials. As a result, a near-perfect safety profile of BMP was established. However, Carragee et al reported that the complication rates associated with BMP were 5 %– 15 % in anterior procedures and included implant displacement, subsidence, infection, urogenital events, and retrograde ejaculation. The authors also cited complication rates associated with posterior fusion procedures ranging from 25 %– 50 % including radiculitis, ectopic bone formation, osteolysis, and poorer global outcomes [17••]. Of serious concern, Carragee et al demonstrated a greater apparent risk of a new malignancy with groups treated with the 40 mg dose of rhBMP-2 per level. However, even more alarming was the lack of reporting on this issue in the original publication even though it was significantly discussed in the FDA Executive Summary [14]. Carragee et al attributed "fundamental error in the statistical analysis of uncommon and serious adverse events within each of the original studies" behind the low rates of complications. In addition, the authors cited the need for sensitivity in the detection of adverse events in noninferiority trials [17••].

As all of the original BMP trials were industry-sponsored, the authors had significant financial conflict of interests. Since the authors involved in these trials received payments during and after the study periods, a strong conflict of interest was present. Carragee et al estimated the magnitude of the financial gain, with a median payment of $12 million for 12 of the 13 studies with no information available for 1 study [17••]. Conflict of interest statements reported in these trials were marred with vague and inconsistent statements. In combination with an absence of standardized methodology and ascertainment protocol, including successful fusion outcome, the authors were prone to bias in favor of BMP use [21•].

Recommendations of bias classification in scientific publication

Critical assessment of the original industry-sponsored rhBMP-2 trials has provided insight into the potential sources of bias that must be carefully be addressed to maintain a high degree of scientific validity. The systematic bias leading toward reporting and publication of favorable outcomes for BMP use in respected orthopedic journals brings into question the current state of the editorial review process. In addition to the use of current guidelines to ensure quality reporting, including Consolidated Standards of Reporting Trials (CONSORT) [27, 28], checklist to evaluate a report of a nonpharmacologic trial (CLEAR NPT) [29]; Preferred reporting items for systematic reviews and meta-analyses (PRISMA) [30]; Strengthening the Reporting of Observational studies in Epidemiology (STROBE) [31]; Meta-analysis Of Observational Studies in Epidemiology (MOOSE) [32], a scientific classification system of bias is necessary to further appraise the quality of the published literature.

The Levels of Evidence rating system [33] was introduced in 2003 to categorize literature based upon the study quality

and design. This 5-level rating system, with Level I evidence being randomized control trials with least bias, allowed for critical appraisal for researchers, editorial reviewers, clinicians, and the public at large regarding the quality rating of scientific articles. Obremskey et al reviewed clinical scientific articles published from January to June 2013 in 9 different orthopedic journals and reported that 11.3 % were Level I, 20.7 % were Level II, 9.9 % were Level III, and 58.1 % were Level IV [34]. The scarcity of higher level of evidence literature is further compounded by a variability of quality between the level I evidence articles. In a review of level I evidence from January 2003 to December 2004, Poolman et al demonstrated low Cochrane reporting quality scores among the individual methodological safeguards with further that scores that did not significantly differ between Level I and Level II studies [35].

The CONSORT statement checklist was established to improve the reporting of randomized control trial design, conduct, analysis, interpretation, and assessment of the validity of results (Table 1) [27, 28]. CONSORT does not deem the use of arbitrarily determined and set statistical significance ($P<0.05$) as a criterion to identify possible associations with infrequent but serious adverse events, as those under-reported in the original rhBMP-2 trials during the pharmacologically active period [17••]. Divergence from the recommended COSNORT guidelines is not exclusive to the rhBMP-2 FDA trials. In an evaluation of the adherence to CONSORT guidelines of 196 randomized control trials in the orthopedic trauma literature, Bhandari et al reported an adherence rate of 36 % of the critical CONSORT items and 32 % of the total CONSORT items [36]. Recognizing the differences between medical and surgical trials and the limited applicability of CONSORT in surgical trials, a more applicable 10-item CLEAR NPT checklist was developed (Table 2) [29]. Chan and Bhandhari evaluated the methodological quality of 87 randomized control trials in 8 orthopedic journals from 2004 to 2008 [37]. The authors demonstrated that 84 % of studies did not clearly report the concealment of the treatment allocation while only 20 % described the experience of the surgeon. Furthermore, blinding was unclear in 55 % of patients, 72 % of ward staff, 74 % of rehabilitation staff, 46 % of clinical outcome assessors, and 38 % of nonclinical outcome assessors. A recent review of the randomized control trials in spine surgery from 2005 to 2010 reported that only 10 % report surgical experience, which is usually a description of the learning curve [38]. Equally as alarming, 77 % of studies were unclear about the concealment of treatment allocation, 68 % were unclear regarding the blinding of participants, 77 % were unclear regarding the blinding of outcome assessors, and 67 % were unclear of adhering to the intention-to-treat principle [38]. The implementation of guidelines such as CONSORT and CLEAR NPT aim to minimize methodological bias and improve the quality of reporting among the randomize control

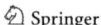

Table 1 CONSORT 2010 updated checklist

Title and abstract	
	Identification as a randomized trial in the title
	Structured summary of trial design, methods, results, and conclusions (for specific guidance see CONSORT for abstracts 21 31)
Introduction	
Background	Scientific background and explanation of rationale
Objectives	Specific objectives or hypotheses
Methods	
Trial design	Description of trial design (such as parallel, factorial) including allocation ratio
	Important changes to methods after trial commencement (such as eligibility criteria), with reasons
Participants	Eligibility criteria for participants
	Settings and locations where the data were collected
Interventions	The interventions for each group with sufficient details to allow replication, including how and when they were actually administered
Outcomes	Completely defined pre-specified primary and secondary outcome measures, including how and when they were assessed
	Any changes to trial outcomes after the trial commenced, with reasons
Sample size	How sample size was determined
	When applicable, explanation of any interim analyses and stopping guidelines
Randomization	
Sequence	Method used to generate the random allocation sequence
Generation	Type of randomization; details of any restriction (such as blocking and block size)
Allocation concealment mechanism	Mechanism used to implement the random allocation sequence (such as sequentially numbered containers), describing any steps taken to conceal the sequence until interventions were assigned
Implementation	Who generated the random allocation sequence, who enrolled participants, and who assigned participants to interventions
Blinding	If done, who was blinded after assignment to interventions (for example, participants, care providers, those assessing outcomes) and how
	If relevant, description of the similarity of interventions
Statistical methods	Statistical methods used to compare groups for primary and secondary outcomes
	Methods for additional analyses, such as subgroup analyses and adjusted analyses
Results	
Participant flow	For each group, the numbers of participants who were randomly assigned, received intended treatment, and were analyzed for the primary outcome
	For each group, losses and exclusions after randomization, together with reasons
Recruitment	Dates defining the periods of recruitment and follow-up
	Why the trial ended or was stopped
Baseline data	A table showing baseline demographic and clinical characteristics for each group
Numbers analyzed	For each group, number of participants (denominator) included in each analysis and whether the analysis was by original assigned groups
Outcomes and estimation	For each primary and secondary outcome, results for each group, and the estimated effect size and its precision (such as 95 % CI)
	For binary outcomes, presentation of both absolute and relative effect sizes is recommended
Ancillary analyses	Results of any other analyses performed, including subgroup analyses and adjusted analyses, distinguishing pre-specified from exploratory
Harms	All important harms or unintended effects in each group (for specific guidance see CONSORT for harms 28)
Discussion	
Limitations	Trial limitations, addressing sources of potential bias, imprecision, and, if relevant, multiplicity of analyses
Generalizability	Generalizability (external validity, applicability) of the trial findings
Interpretation	Interpretation consistent with results, balancing benefits and harms, and considering other relevant evidence
Other information	
Registration	Registration number and name of trial registry
Protocol	Where the full trial protocol can be accessed, if available
Funding	Sources of funding and other support (such as supply of drugs), role of funders

From [28], with permission

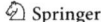

Table 2 Final checklist of items to assess quality of randomized controlled trials of nonpharmacologic treatment

	Possible answers
1. Was the generation of allocation sequences adequate?	Yes; No; Unclear
2. Was the treatment allocation concealed?	Yes; No; Unclear
3. Were details of the intervention administered to each group made available?	Yes; No; Unclear
4. Were care providers' experience or skill in each arm appropriate?	Yes; No; Unclear
5. Was participant (ie, patients) adherence assessed quantitatively?	Yes; No; Unclear
6. Were participants adequately blinded?	Yes; No, because blinding is not feasible; No, although blinding is feasible; Unclear
6.1. If participants were not adequately blinded	
6.1.1. Were all other treatments and care (ie, co-interventions) the same in each randomized group?	Yes; No; Unclear
6.1.2. Were withdrawals and lost to follow-up the same in each randomized group?	Yes; No; Unclear
7. Were care providers or persons caring for the participants adequately blinded?	Yes; No, because blinding is not feasible; No, although blinding is feasible; Unclear
7.1. If care providers were not adequately blinded	
7.1.1. Were all other treatments and care (ie, co-interventions) the same in each randomized group?	Yes; No; Unclear
7.1.2. Were withdrawals and lost to follow-up the same in each randomized group?	Yes; No; Unclear
8. Were outcome assessors adequately blinded to assess the primary outcomes?	Yes; No, because blinding is not feasible; No, although blinding is feasible; Unclear
8.1. If outcome assessors were not adequately blinded, were specific methods used to avoid ascertainment bias (systematic differences in outcome assessment)?	Yes; No; Unclear
9. Was the follow-up schedule the same in each group?	Yes; No; Unclear
10. Were the main outcomes analyzed according to the intention-to-treat principle?	Yes; No; Unclear

From [29], with permission

trials, especially in the current time of reliance upon comparative effectiveness research. Tangible progress, however, may only be realized with more standardized and strict adherence to the established guidelines.

With the strong relationship between the medical device industry and the orthopedic surgery specialty, conflicts of interest are simply unavoidable. Favorable outcomes like those seen in device-sponsored rhBMP-2 trials are not unique. Results are favorable to the implant manufacturer in 73 % of industry-sponsored studies compared with 44 % of independent studies (odds ratio, 3.3; 95 % CI, 2.4–4.5) for spine implants; 93 % and 37 %, respectively, for hip implants; and 75 % and 20 % for knee implants [39]. With the Food and Drug Administration and Public Health Service guidelines suggesting that $5000 to $25,000 of financial relationships with a study sponsor pose a risk of systematic bias, Carragee et al argue that it is impossible to estimate the potential bias from the multimillion-dollar financial industry dealings that involved the original rhBMP-2 trials [40•].

In an effort to increase transparency and potential bias, required disclosures of industry relationships been implemented by many journals. Yet, there is substantial variability of reported financial disclosure between journals. One industry-sponsored study investigating rhBMP-2 use with posterior spinal instrumentation disclosed that "The manuscript submitted does not contain information about medical device(s)/

drug(s). Institutional funds were received in support of this work. No benefits in any form have been or will be received from a commercial party related directly or indirectly to the subject of this manuscript" [12]. Furthermore, the accuracy of industry payment disclosure has significant incongruity. In an evaluation of inconsistencies between physician disclosures and payments reported by industry, authors found that Medtronic and Depuy Spine payments were disclosed by 12.1 % and 8.75 % of physicians attending the 2011 North American Spine Society annual meeting, respectively [41•]. This physician reporting discrepancy is especially concerning, as The Physician Payment Sunshine Act (PPSA) will require the industry to disclose anything of value that has been given to physicians by 2014. It is clear that more standardized practices must be adopted to decrease disclosure discrepancy and increase transparency.

The role for greater transparency may extend to editorial staff of journals in addition to authors and researchers. Journal publication of industry-sponsored studies with inherent systematic alignment for favorable results contributes to a significant source of potential bias in spine literature. In a retrospective review of articles published in the journal Spine from January 2002 to July 2003, the authors reported that industry support was noted for 15.9 %, foundation support for 12.7 %, government support for 10.2 %, and institution support for 3.2 % [42]. The odds ratio regarding the association between

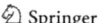

industry funded reporting of positive results was 3.3 times that of studies with other funding sources ($P<0.001$). The authors suggest that study design bias, experimental technique bias, result interpretation bias, or publication bias as potential sources of bias. One author with significant financial conflicts of interest in the original rhBMP-2 trials also served as the Editor-in-Chief of a journal that published these articles [5, 8]. Editorial conflicts of interest have played a role in the systematic failure surrounding the original rhBMP-2 papers reporting favorable outcomes [19••]. To further minimize financial conflicts of interest, editorial disclosures may address the increasingly industry-sponsored landscape of the scientific literature.

Conclusions

The original 13 rhBMP-2 industry-sponsored trials significantly under-reported adverse events and complications associated with rhBMP-2 use in spinal fusion surgery, thereby contributing to widespread promotion of on- and off-label use. The subsequent literature review, however, found serious complications ranging from 20 % to 70 % in all settings, which were 10–50 times the original estimates from the industry-associated trials [17••]. The YODA Project, commissioned to report on the safety and efficacy of rhBMP-2, concluded that "rhBMP-2 has no proven clinical advantage over bone graft and may be associated with important harms, making it difficult to identify clear indications for rhBMP-2. Earlier disclosure of all relevant data would have better informed clinicians and the public than the initial published trial reports did" [20••]. A significant degree of systematic bias undoubtedly contributed to the alignment of favorable outcomes reported in earlier industry-sponsored rhBMP-2 trials, while later independent investigations of the same data from FDA randomized control trials led to differing conclusions. In an effort to better assess the extent of the present and potential bias in the scientific literature, standardized classification and reporting of study design, methodology, data analysis and reporting, and financial conflicts of interests must be advocated. This responsibility must be shared between the scientific community including researchers, surgeons, authors, editors, and reviewers to ensure sufficient integrity of the published literature, which guides clinical decision-making and patient treatment.

Compliance with Ethics Guidelines

Conflict of Interest Sohaib Hashmi, Mohamed Noureldin, and Safdar N. Khan declare that they have no conflict of interest.

Human and Animal Rights and Informed Consent This article does not contain any studies with human or animal subjects performed by any of the authors.

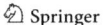 Springer

References

Papers of particular interest, published recently, have been highlighted as:
- Of importance
- • Of major importance

1. Urist MR. Bone: formation by autoinduction. Science. 1965;150: 893–9.
2. Grabowski G, Cornett CA. Bone graft and bone graft substitutes in spine surgery: current concepts and controversies. J Am Acad Orthop Surg. 2013;21:51–60. doi:10.5435/jaaos-21-01-51.
3. Boden SD, Zdeblick TA, Sandhu HS, Heim SE. The use of rhBMP-2 in interbody fusion cages. Definitive evidence of osteoinduction in humans: a preliminary report. Spine. 2000;25:376–81.
4. Boden SD, Kang J, Sandhu H, Heller JG. Use of recombinant human bone morphogenetic protein-2 to achieve posterolateral lumbar spine fusion in humans: a prospective, randomized clinical pilot trial: 2002 Volvo Award in clinical studies. Spine. 2002;27: 2662–73. doi:10.1097/01.brs.0000035320.82533.06.
5. Burkus JK, Gornet MF, Dickman CA, Zdeblick TA. Anterior lumbar interbody fusion using rhBMP-2 with tapered interbody cages. J Spinal Disord Tech. 2002;15:337–49.
6. Burkus JK, Transfeldt EE, Kitchel SH, Watkins RG, Balderston RA. Clinical and radiographic outcomes of anterior lumbar interbody fusion using recombinant human bone morphogenetic protein-2. Spine. 2002;27:2396–408. doi:10.1097/01.brs.0000193.26290.dd.
7. Baskin DS, Ryan P, Sonntag V, Westmark R, Widmayer MA. A prospective, randomized, controlled cervical fusion study using recombinant human bone morphogenetic protein-2 with the CORNERSTONE-SR allograft ring and the ATLANTIS anterior cervical plate. Spine. 2003;28:1219–24. doi:10.1097/01.brs. 0000065486.22141.ca. discussion 25.
8. Burkus JK, Heim SE, Gornet MF, Zdeblick TA. Is INFUSE bone graft superior to autograft bone? An integrated analysis of clinical trials using the LT-CAGE lumbar tapered fusion device. J Spinal Disord Tech. 2003;16:113–22.
9. Haid Jr RW, Branch Jr CL, Alexander JT, Burkus JK. Posterior lumbar interbody fusion using recombinant human bone morphogenetic protein type 2 with cylindrical interbody cages. Spine J. 2004;4: 527–38. doi:10.1016/j.spinee.2004.03.025. discussion 38–9.
10. Boakye M, Mummaneni PV, Garrett M, Rodts G, Haid R. Anterior cervical discectomy and fusion involving a polyetheretherketone spacer and bone morphogenetic protein. J Neurosurg Spine. 2005;2:521–5. doi:10.3171/spi.2005.2.5.0521.
11. Burkus JK, Sandhu HS, Gornet MF, Longley MC. Use of rhBMP-2 in combination with structural cortical allografts: clinical and radiographic outcomes in anterior lumbar spinal surgery. J Bone Joint Surg Am. 2005;87:1205–12. doi:10.2106/jbjs.d.02532.
12. Glassman SD, Dimar III JR, Burkus K, Hardacker JW, Pryor PW, Boden SD, et al. The efficacy of rhBMP-2 for posterolateral lumbar fusion in smokers. Spine. 2007;32:1693–8. doi:10.1097/BRS. 0b013e318074c366.
13. Dawson E, Bae HW, Burkus JK, Stambough JL, Glassman SD. Recombinant human bone morphogenetic protein-2 on an absorbable collagen sponge with an osteoconductive bulking agent in posterolateral arthrodesis with instrumentation. A prospective randomized trial. J Bone Joint Surg Am. 2009;91:1604–13. doi:10. 2106/jbjs.g.01157.
14. Dimar II JR, Glassman SD, Burkus JK, Pryor PW, Hardacker JW, Carreon LY. Clinical and radiographic analysis of an optimized rhBMP-2 formulation as an autograft replacement in posterolateral lumbar spine arthrodesis. J Bone Joint Surg Am. 2009;91:1377–86. doi:10.2106/jbjs.h.00200.

Curr Rev Musculoskelet Med (2014) 7:193–199   199

15.• Spengler DM. Resetting standards for sponsored research: do conflicts influence results? Spine J. 2011;11:492–4. doi:10.1016/j.spinee.2011.05.001. *Commentary on Carragee et al "A critical review of recombinant human bone morphogenetic protein-2 trials in spinal surgery: emerging safety concerns and lessons learned" raises questions regarding state of peer-review process, conflicts of interest, and regulation and use of rhBMP-2.*

16. Poynton AR, Lane JM. Safety profile for the clinical use of bone morphogenetic proteins in the spine. Spine. 2002;27(16 Suppl 1): S40–8.

17.•• Carragee EJ, Hurwitz EL, Weiner BK. A critical review of recombinant human bone morphogenetic protein-2 trials in spinal surgery: emerging safety concerns and lessons learned. Spine J. 2011;11: 471–91. doi:10.1016/j.spinee.2011.04.023. *This article compared data published in the original 13 industry-sponsored rhBMP-2 studies with data provided in the FDA website and spinal literature investigating BMP use concluding that the original industry-sponsored articles systemically aligned to report positive results of BMP use in spinal fusion.*

18. Owen R. Reader bias. JAMA. 1982;247:2533–4. doi:10.1001/jama.1982.03320430037027.

19.•• Carragee EJ, Ghanayem AJ, Weiner BK, Rothman DJ, Bono CM. A challenge to integrity in spine publications: years of living dangerously with the promotion of bone growth factors. Spine J. 2011;11: 463–8. doi:10.1016/j.spinee.2011.06.001. *This editorial states the precedence for critical review and cause of discrepancy between the original industry-sponsored BMP studies compared with later studies reporting higher rate of adverse events with use of BMP.*

20.•• Fu R, Selph S, McDonagh M, Peterson K, Tiwari A, Chou R, et al. Effectiveness and harms of recombinant human bone morphogenetic protein-2 in spine fusion: a systematic review and meta-analysis. Ann Intern Med. 2013;158:890–902. doi:10.7326/0003-4819-158-12-201306180-00006. *This independent systematic review and meta-analysis of 17 industry-sponsored studies and subsequent publications regarding rhBMP-2 use in spine fusion surgery concluded rhBMP-2 has no proven clinical advantage over bone graft and may be associated with important harms, unclear indications for proper use of rhBMP-2, and earlier disclosure of original BMP studies would have better informed clinicians and the public.*

21.• Mirza SK. Folly of FDA-approval studies for bone morphogenetic protein. Spine J. 2011;11:495–9. doi:10.1016/j.spinee.2011.05.009. *This commentary on Carragee et al "A critical review of recombinant human bone morphogenetic protein-2 trials in spinal surgery: emerging safety concerns and lessons learned" discusses the systematic bias leading to the reporting of highly favorable results in the original industry-sponsored spinal fusion studies with rhBMP-2.*

22. Hrobjartsson A, Thomsen AS, Emanuelsson F, Tendal B, Hilden J, Boutron I, et al. Observer bias in randomized clinical trials with measurement scale outcomes: a systematic review of trials with both blinded and nonblinded assessors. CMAJ. 2013;185:E201–11. doi:10.1503/cmaj.120744.

23. Khan SN, Mermer MJ, Myers E, Sandhu HS. The roles of funding source, clinical trial outcome, and quality of reporting in orthopedic surgery literature. Am J Orthop. 2008;37:E205–12. discussion E12.

24. Garattini S, Bertele V. Non-inferiority trials are unethical because they disregard patients' interests. Lancet. 2007;370:1875–7. doi:10.1016/s0140-6736(07)61604-3.

25. Kaul S, Diamond GA. Good enough: a primer on the analysis and interpretation of noninferiority trials. Ann Intern Med. 2006;145:62–9.

26. Le Henanff A, Giraudeau B, Baron G, Ravaud P. Quality of reporting of noninferiority and equivalence randomized trials. JAMA. 2006;295:1147–51. doi:10.1001/jama.295.10.1147.

27. Begg C, Cho M, Eastwood S, Horton R, Moher D, Olkin I, et al. Improving the quality of reporting of randomized controlled trials. The CONSORT statement. JAMA. 1996;276:637–9.

28. Schulz KF, Altman DG, Moher D. CONSORT 2010 statement: updated guidelines for reporting parallel group randomised trials. BMJ. 2010;340:c332. doi:10.1136/bmj.c332.

29. Boutron I, Moher D, Tugwell P, Giraudeau B, Poiraudeau S, Nizard R, et al. A checklist to evaluate a report of a nonpharmacological trial (CLEAR NPT) was developed using consensus. J Clin Epidemiol. 2005;58:1233–40. doi:10.1016/j.jclinepi.2005.05.004.

30. Moher D, Liberati A, Tetzlaff J, Altman DG. Preferred reporting items for systematic reviews and meta-analyses: the PRISMA statement. J Clin Epidemiol. 2009;62:1006–12. doi:10.1016/j.jclinepi.2009.06.005.

31. Elm EV, Altman DG, Egger M, Pocock SJ, Gøtzsche PC, Vandenbroucke JP. Strengthening the reporting of observational studies in epidemiology (STROBE) statement: guidelines for reporting observational studies. BMJ. 2007;335:806–8. doi:10.1136/bmj.39335.541782.AD.

32. Stroup DF, Berlin JA, Morton SC, Olkin I, Williamson GD, Rennie D, et al. Meta-analysis of observational studies in epidemiology: a proposal for reporting. Meta-analysis Of Observational Studies in Epidemiology (MOOSE) group. JAMA. 2000;283:2008–12.

33. Wright JG, Swiontkowski MF, Heckman JD. Introducing levels of evidence to the journal. J Bone Joint Surg Am. 2003;85-A:1–3.

34. Obremskey WT, Pappas N, Attallah-Wasif E, Tornetta III P, Bhandari M. Level of evidence in orthopaedic journals. J Bone Joint Surg Am. 2005;87:2632–8. doi:10.2106/jbjs.e.00370.

35. Poolman R, Struijs P, Krips R, Sierevelt I, Lutz K, Bhandari M. Does a "Level I Evidence" rating imply high quality of reporting in orthopaedic randomised controlled trials? BMC Med Res Meth. 2006;6:44.

36. Bhandari M, Guyatt GH, Lochner H, Sprague S, Tornetta III P. Application of the Consolidated Standards of Reporting Trials (CONSORT) in the fracture care literature. J Bone Joint Surg Am. 2002;84-A:485–9.

37. Chan S, Bhandari M. The quality of reporting of orthopaedic randomized trials with use of a checklist for nonpharmacological therapies. J Bone Joint Surg Am. 2007;89:1970–8. doi:10.2106/jbjs.f.01591.

38. van Oldenrijk J, van Berkel Y, Kerkhoffs GM, Bhandari M, Poolman RW. Do authors report surgical expertise in open spine surgery related randomized controlled trials? A systematic review on quality of reporting. Spine. 2013;38:857–64. doi:10.1097/BRS.0b013e31827ecb1c.

39. Gelberman RH, Samson D, Mirza SK, Callaghan JJ, Pellegrini Jr VD. Orthopaedic surgeons and the medical device industry: the threat to scientific integrity and the public trust. J Bone Joint Surg Am. 2010;92:765–77. doi:10.2106/jbjs.i.01164.

40.• Carragee EJ, Baker RM, Benzel EC, Bigos SJ, Cheng I, Corbin TP, et al. A biologic without guidelines: the YODA project and the future of bone morphogenetic protein-2 research. Spine J. 2012;12:877–80. doi:10.1016/j.spinee.2012.11.002. *This editorial comments on fundamental flaws in existing studies investigating the efficacy and safety involving BMP-2 in spine surgery, including limitations in methodological, operational, and reporting issues.*

41.• Buerba RA, Fu MC, Grauer JN. Discrepancies in spine surgeon conflict of interest disclosures between a national meeting and physician payment listings on device manufacturer web sites. Spine J. 2013;13:1780–8. doi:10.1016/j.spinee.2013.05.032. *In this comparison of publically available disclosure/payment data, authors concluded discrepancy rates between what spine surgeons disclosed at NASS 2011 and what companies reported for their consultants were high demanding need for more standardized practice in reporting of financial conflict of interests.*

42. Shah RV, Albert TJ, Bruegel-Sanchez V, Vaccaro AR, Hilibrand AS, Grauer JN. Industry support and correlation to study outcome for papers published in Spine. Spine. 2005;30:1099–104. discussion 105.

References

Berry D. Emerging innovations in clinical trial design. Clin Pharmacol Ther. 2016;99(1):82–91.

Grinnell F. Research integrity and everyday practice of science. Sci Eng Ethics. 2013;19(3):193–9.

Additional Suggested Reading

Berry D. Emerging innovations in clinical trial design. Clin Pharmacol Ther. 2016;99(1):82–91. (*Provides a review of emerging clinical trial designs driven by increasing recognition that diseases and patients are heterogeneous.*)

Grinnell F. Research integrity and everyday practice of science. Sci Eng Ethics. 2013;19(3):685–701. (*Notes that "science is traditionally taught as a linear process based on logic and carried out by objective researchers following the scientific method" is not accurate. Research integrity should be taught as it is carried out in the everyday practice of science.*)

Weintraub W, Luscher T, Pocock S. The perils of surrogate endpoints. Eur Heart J. 2015;36(33):2212–8. (*Describes the difficult but necessary steps in validating surrogate endpoints.*)

Policy

Arthur L. Caplan and Barbara K. Redman

Science policy creates a de facto contract between science and society involving the provision of public resources to pay for research, while requiring honoring a regulatory system and creating the institutions to perform research. All of these policy elements have an effect on research integrity, and as those effects become known, they suggest how the policy elements are performing to support valid science while also protecting research subjects and insuring that public money is being used responsibly.

The notion of a contract flows from the post World War II era, building on the considerable helpfulness of science in the Allied war effort. The post-war period emphasized that the integrity and independence of the investigator was essential and that science would self-regulate with its own moral standards (Pielke 2010). But a series of scandals such as the Tuskegee sexually transmitted syphilis disease experiments (1932–1972) showed that lack of government oversight including attention to bias and conflict of interest was inadequate (Spector-Bagdady and Lombardo 2013). A more modern scandal, the Flint, Michigan, water crisis in which residents were exposed for years to harmful levels of lead in their drinking water (Burke 2016), seemed to rest on loyalty to state and federal regulatory agencies, both of which ignored evidence with serious consequences to public health. In this case, the research standards were well established, but their implementation ensnared in politics, was ignored.

By the last quarter of the 20th century, restraints on science self-governance yielded regulations in human subjects protection (1970s) and animal subjects protection (1980s) (Krimsky 1995) and, in the late 1990s, conflict of interest and research misconduct. The scope of public accountability has been widening. Most recently, in the face of large increases in the number of scientists worldwide but stable public financial resources, scientific leaders have diagnosed an unsustainable hypercompetitive environment (Alberts et al. 2014).

An evolving form of research integrity involves calls from within science for scientists to engage in political debate and become accountable, as well as to influence decisions about funding (Sarewitz 2016). Sound science policy demands not just input from scientists but also early engagement with public and political discourse. Researchers can make real contributions by educating the public about their work and demonstrating that they follow the highest standards of integrity.

Advice: Your professional organization will be up-to-date on research policies that affect your field. Join as a student member and participate in policy-influencing activities. And don't be afraid to give a presentation on your work and the ethics that guide you to a public audience.

A. L. Caplan · B. K. Redman (✉)
New York University Langone Medical Center,
New York, NY, USA
e-mail: Arthur.Caplan@nyumc.org

© Springer International Publishing AG, part of Springer Nature 2018
A. L. Caplan, B. K. Redman (eds.), *Getting to Good*, https://doi.org/10.1007/978-3-319-51358-4_2

2.1   In Retrospect: Science—The Endless Frontier

Roger Pielke Jr.

Pielke R. In retrospect: Science—The Endless Frontier. *Nature* 2010 August 19; 466:922–923. © 2010 Macmillan Publishers Limited. All rights reserved. Imprint of SpringerNature.

Figure 1 reprinted with permission from Getty Images.

Figure 2 reprinted with permission from Roger Pielke Jr.

OPINION

NATURE|Vol 466|19 August 2010

for example, how physicians will use genetic data for diagnosis and treatment, and whether individuals will welcome or fear knowledge of what their genomes hold for the future.

Such social change will follow, I believe, when useful applications of genomic information become available. They might tell us how to alter our lifestyles to improve our health, or distinguish which drugs will be of benefit or have serious side effects, or may guide the development of new drugs. But this will take time. We are only at the beginning of interpreting the sequence and understanding

what variants mean for the individual.

Drawing the Map of Life is one of many books that have been written about the HGP. The volume does not add much to earlier descriptions of the project's genesis, such as *Genome* by Jerry Bishop and Michael Waldholz (Simon and Schuster, 1990) and *The Gene Wars* by Robert Cook-Deegan (W. W. Norton, 1994). In *Cracking the Genome* (Free Press, 2001), Kevin Davies brought us up to the completion of the draft sequences. More recently, protagonists John Sulston and Venter have told their contrasting personal stories, while

James Shreeve has written a detailed study of Venter's contributions.

All of these books are valuable; what is now needed is a scholarly history of the HGP. *Drawing the Map of Life* is not that book, but it offers an enjoyable account of the project from origin to conclusion and beyond. ■

Jan Witkowski is executive director of the Banbury Center and a professor in the Watson School of Biological Sciences, Cold Spring Harbor Laboratory, New York 11724, USA. He is co-author of *Recombinant DNA: Genes and Genomes*.
e-mail: witkowsk@cshl.edu

In Retrospect: *Science — The Endless Frontier*

Vannevar Bush's pivotal report that marked the beginning of modern science policy catapulted the phrase 'basic research' into popular usage, explains **Roger Pielke Jr**.

**Science — The Endless Frontier.
A Report to the President on a Program for Postwar Scientific Research**
by Vannevar Bush
National Science Foundation: 1960 (reprint).
First published 1945.

The US government's landmark report *Science — The Endless Frontier* was published 65 years ago last month. Commissioned by President Franklin D. Roosevelt and prepared by electrical engineer Vannevar Bush, who directed US government research during the Second World War, the document distilled the lessons of wartime into proposals for subsequent federal support of science. Although its bold recommendations were only partly implemented, the document is ripe for reappraisal today: it marked the beginning of modern science policy.

Bush's report called for a centralized approach to government-sponsored science, largely shielded from political accountability. The creation of the National Science Foundation in 1950, a small agency with a limited mandate, was far from the sweeping reform set out in the 30-page report and its appendices. However, its publication ushered in a new era in which science was viewed as vital for progress towards national goals in health, defence and the economy. Government funding for research and development consequently increased by more than a factor of ten from the 1940s to the 1960s.

The influence of *Science — The Endless Frontier* stems largely from its timing, coming at the tail end of a war in which science-based technology had been crucial. The development

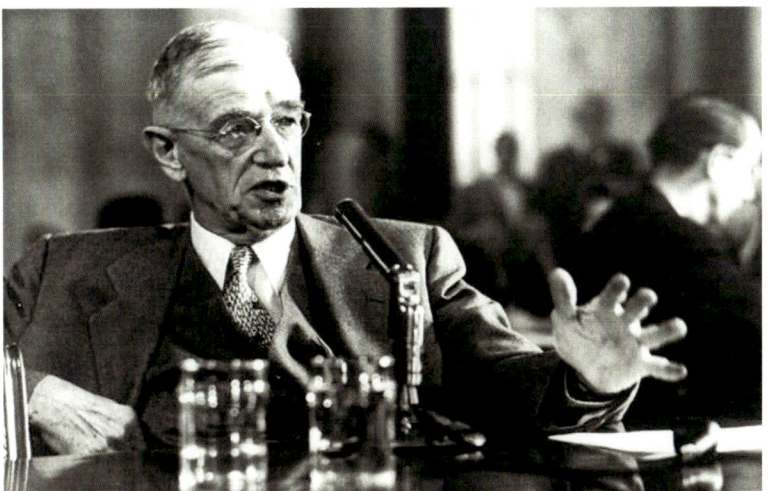

Engineer Vannevar Bush's proposals led to the creation of the National Science Foundation in 1950.

of the atomic bomb, radar and penicillin meant that Bush's declaration that "scientific progress is essential" to public welfare found a receptive audience. Bush also adopted innovative language that capitalized on this new-found government credulity.

In particular, he broadened the meaning of the phrase 'basic research'. In using it to refer simultaneously to the demands of policymakers for practical innovation and to the interests of scientists in curiosity-driven enquiry, he satisfied both sectors.

Before the report, pleas by scientists to expand government support for research had met with only limited success. Prominent calls

along similar lines were made to no avail in 1924 by the UK National Union of Scientific Workers (NUSW) and in 1929 by US agriculture secretary Arthur Hyde. The poor response might have been due to the confused messages offered to protect the integrity of pure research. In a 1921 essay, for example, the NUSW president declared that scientific research has "no industrial bearing at all" but later stated that it is "the foundation of progress in industry". Not surprisingly, most policy-makers shrugged.

Some political leaders did champion government support for basic research before 1945. Prior to Hyde's appointment, US agriculture secretary Henry C. Wallace had argued in

NATURE|Vol 466|19 August 2010

OPINION

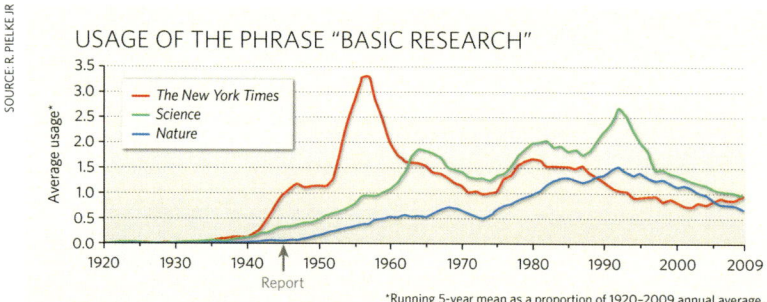

USAGE OF THE PHRASE "BASIC RESEARCH"

The New York Times
Science
Nature

Report

*Running 5-year mean as a proportion of 1920–2009 annual average.

SOURCE: R. PIELKE JR

The fluid meaning of "basic research" galvanized science-policy discussions in the mid-twentieth century.

the early 1920s (one of the first narrow uses of the phrase) that the agency should fund more "basic research" to enhance agricultural productivity. At the time, Wallace's call for investment was counter-intuitive because US agriculture was suffering from being too efficient; a surfeit of production depressed prices and caused hardship for farmers. But he reasoned presciently that consumption would catch up in the longer term. Wallace did not live to see his vision realized, but his son, Henry A. Wallace, picked up the baton, first as agriculture secretary under Roosevelt (1933–40) and then as Roosevelt's vice-president (1941–45). During the war, the younger Wallace served as liaison between Roosevelt and Bush.

Bush was selected by his friend and neighbour Vice-President Wallace to draft *Science — The Endless Frontier*. As director of the Office of Scientific Research and Development, Bush had credibility and good connections within both the science and policy camps. This meant that when the report was released — less than two weeks before the Hiroshima atomic bomb was detonated — it was well positioned to influence. When Wallace's political fortunes fell, leadership in science policy completed its switch from the agriculturists to the physicists, and the language of science policy changed too.

With its inherent inscrutability, Bush's 'basic' research descriptor helped to secure a pragmatic compromise between scientists and politicians. The concepts of 'pure' and 'fundamental' research had long presented a narrow view of science in terms of benefits only to scientists. By contrast, basic research could be carried out for curiosity's sake — satisfying scientists — and could meet national needs, pleasing the politicians. Bush later recalled how the phrase made it easy to convey that "work that had been regarded by many as interesting but hardly of real impact on a practical existence, had been basic to the production of a bomb that had ended a war."

The publication of *Science — The Endless Frontier* entrenched the concept of government patronage of scientific research in policy discourse. The setting up of the National Science Foundation and countless other policy reports cemented it. "Institutions and statistics are what gave stability to the fuzzy concept of basic research," wrote science-policy scholar Benoît Godin in 2000. The speed with which science and society discussions were reframed is demonstrated by usage of the phrase in *The New York Times*, which rose rapidly from 4 mentions in 1944 to a peak of 159 mentions in 1957 (see 'Usage of the phrase "basic research"').

In recent decades, science policy has shifted its focus towards conferring measurable benefits to society. The fuzzy concept of basic research no longer seems to fit — nebulous descriptions of benefit are insufficient in today's competitive environment for public funds. Consequently, use of the phrase has declined since the early 1990s, as indicated by mentions in *Science* and *Nature* (see 'Usage of the phrase "basic research"'). Other terms, such as 'transformative research', have sprung up to fill the gap; even 'fundamental research' has made an ironic return. And science policy itself has been renamed by scholars of science studies: as collaborative assurance, socially robust science, use-inspired basic research and other monikers that have meanings largely known only to that community.

Words alone cannot bridge the gap between the different interests of scientists and politicians in pursuing research: governments demand relevance; scientists desire freedom. The so-far futile search for a language that is relevant today both reflects and reinforces the unsettled nature of science policy. In the six decades since *Science — The Endless Frontier* was written, research and policy have been transformed. Our framework for discussing both needs to catch up. ∎

Roger Pielke Jr is at the Center for Science and Technology Policy Research, University of Colorado, Boulder, Colorado 80309, USA.
e-mail: pielke@colorado.edu

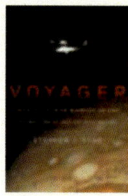

Launched in 1977, the twin Voyager probes are true explorers. Among the earliest spacecraft to visit the neighbourhoods of Jupiter and Saturn, they will soon exit the Solar System and witness interstellar space. Environmental historian Stephen Pyne sets these missions within the wider arc of human exploration in *Voyager* (Viking, 2010). He examines the origins of the planetary exploration programme in cold war politics, and looks to modern frontiers of discovery, such as journeys to the ocean floor or beneath Antarctica's ice sheets.

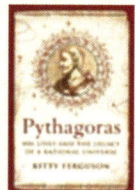

Pythagoras held that the Universe is rational, and that there is order and unity to all things. In *Pythagoras* (Icon, 2010), science writer Kitty Ferguson pieces together the life story of the ancient Greek philosopher and his followers. She asks how his interest in mathematics arose and how his convictions developed. She unravels how Pythagoras's influence has spread across the ages, to underpin the work of great scientists such as Nicolaus Copernicus, Johannes Kepler and Isaac Newton, together with modern figures such as Stephen Hawking.

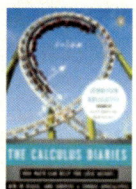

Mathematics fills some people with fear. In *The Calculus Diaries* (Penguin, 2010), science writer Jennifer Ouellette makes maths palatable using a mix of humour, anecdote and enticing facts. She describes how she overcame her own phobia of numbers and how maths forms the basis of modern life. Using everyday examples, such as petrol mileage and fairground rides, Ouellette makes even complex ideas such as calculus and probability appealing.

BOOKS IN BRIEF

2.2 Publish or Perish Culture Encourages Scientists to Cut Corners

Virginia Barbour

The Conversation, September 22, 2015. Author: Viginia Barbour, Executive Officer, Australasian Open Access Support Group, Australian National University. https://the-conversation.com/publish-or-perish-culture-encourages-scientists-to-cut-corners-47692.

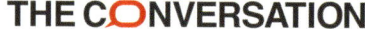

THE CONVERSATION

Academic rigor, journalistic flair

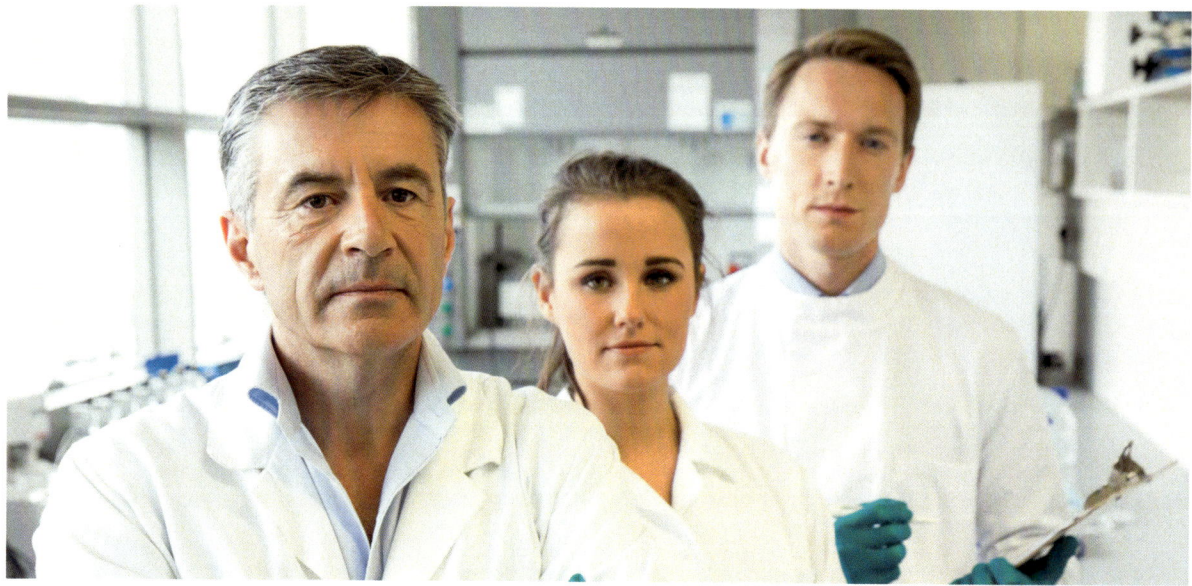

Publish or perish culture encourages scientists to cut corners

September 22, 2015 4.14pm EDT

Which of these researchers has fudged their results to get ahead? wavebreakmedia

Last week there was another very public case of a journal article being retracted as a result of academic misconduct. This time it was in the Journal of the American Medical Association (JAMA), with the lead author – Dr Anna Ahimastos, working at Melbourne's Baker IDI – reportedly admitting she fabricated data.

Sadly, the story is all-too familiar. But this is not to say that science is imperiled, only that we need to ensure the reward and support structures in academia promote the best practices rather than corner cutting.

We have only recently begun looking closely at how the scientific literature could function better, and what can go wrong. And there are conflicting opinions on how to handle underlying problems.

Peer review is currently the primary tool we have for assessing papers prior to publication. Although it has its strengths, especially when overseen by skilled editors, it can't pick up all instances of fraud or sloppy scientific practices.

Author

Virginia Barbour

Executive Officer, Australasian Open Access Support Group, Australian National University

In the past these errors may have lain hidden for many years, or never come to light. Now, post publication scrutiny is picking up more and more papers with questionable data. This is leading to corrections, or even **retractions**. Websites such as **Retraction Watch** have sprung up to document these retractions.

Peerless research

To non-academics, this might all seem rather surprising. Isn't science governed by strict protocols for performing and reporting research?

Well, no. Unlike industrial processes, for example, which have standard operating procedures and oversight, science is usually organised locally. Expert laboratory heads typically have the responsibility for the oversight of their laboratories' work.

Many laboratories work as part of larger collaborations, which may have their own checks and balances in place, as do the academic institutions to which they belong. Even so, ultimately the researchers and individual laboratories are responsible for their own work.

The medical sciences have developed their own standards of **reporting studies**, including **clinical trials**. But even these standards are not employed universally.

The system of rewards within science is possibly even more perplexing. Academia is a highly competitive profession. The basic training in science is a PhD, with more than 6,000 awarded each year in Australia alone, which is many more than can ever end up as career researchers, even at the lowest level.

The situation gets worse the more senior a researcher gets. According to a 2013 discussion document **less than 5%** of those who were originally awarded PhDs find permanent academic positions. Even these senior researchers rarely have permanent positions, but are instead expected to compete for funding every few years.

And the primary way academics compete is in the number of papers they publish in peer reviewed journals, especially the handful of what are considered to be top journals, such as **Science**, http://www.nature.com/**link text** and **The Lancet**.

Under pressure

Why does this all matter? Doesn't this competition lead to selection of the best of the best in research and a faster pace of advancement of science? In fact, the reverse may be the case.

In a seminal paper published in 2005, provocatively titled **Why Most Published Research Findings are False**, John Ioannidis discussed a number of reasons why research may be unreliable. One finding was that papers in highly competitive areas were more likely to be false than papers in less competitive fields.

In 2014, the Nuffield Council on Bioethics probed these issues among UK researchers in a year long study. What they found was alarming.

Researchers stated that there was strong pressure on them to publish in a limited number of top journals, "resulting in important research not being published, disincentives for multidisciplinary research, authorship issues, and a lack of recognition for non-article research outputs". Even worse was that the need to get into these top journals led to "scientists feeling tempted or under pressure to compromise on research integrity and standards".

What can be done? Increasingly, groups of scientists are coming together to develop standards in reporting, conduct and reproducibility. Organisations such as the Committee on Publication Ethics (COPE), which I chair, advise editors on how to handle problem papers.

Perhaps most interestingly, a number of technological innovations have arisen that could lead to more reliable science, if adopted widely. Probably the most important innovation is that of Open Science, i.e. open access to research publications, and open access to the data and methodology that underpins those publications.

But we also need to develop ways to reward scientists who do make their publications, data and methodology open for scrutiny, and don't just pursue publication in top journals.

Research data organisations, such as the Australian National Data Service (ANDS), are developing the infrastructure for systematic and standardised ways of linking to data, but as yet funders and institutions do not routinely reward such behaviour.

In the end, science is a human endeavour. And like humans everywhere, those who work in it will do what they are rewarded for, for better or for worse. So we need to make sure those reward structures are encouraging good quality research, not the opposite.

   Peer Review   Academic publishing   Science fraud   Retractions

2.3 "Something of an Adventure": Postwar NIH Research Ethos and the Guatemala STD Experiments

Kayte Spector-Bagdady and Paul A. Lombardo

Spector-Bagdady, K, Lombardo, P. "Something of an adventure": postwar NIH research ethos and the Guatemala STD experiments. *Journal of Law Medicine and Ethics* 41, 697–710 (2013).

"Something of an Adventure":
Postwar NIH Research Ethos and the Guatemala STD Experiments

Kayte Spector-Bagdady and Paul A. Lombardo

Introduction

Since their revelation to the public, the sexually transmitted disease (STD) experiments in Guatemala from 1946 to 1948 have earned a place of infamy in the history of medical ethics. During these experiments, Public Health Service (PHS) researchers intentionally exposed over 1,300 non-consenting Guatemalan soldiers, prisoners, psychiatric patients, and commercial sex workers to gonorrhea, syphilis, and/or chancroid under conditions that have shocked the medical community and public alike.[1] Expert analysis has found little scientific value to the experiments as measured by current or contemporaneous research standards.[2]

Such an obvious case of research malfeasance, which violated research norms in place both in the past and now, has been uniformly repudiated. The Guatemala STD experiments were labeled "clearly unethical" by President Barack Obama and "reprehensible" by the Secretaries of State and Health and Human Services.[3] The Presidential Commission for the Study of Bioethical Issues, charged by the President to undertake a "thorough fact-finding investigation" into the Guatemala STD experiments,[4] described the studies as "clearly and grievously wrong."[5] The public now knows what happened in Guatemala, and those actions have been universally condemned, but the question remains: if the Guatemala STD experiments were so "ethically impossible," how did the U.S. government approve their funding in the first place? Much of the blame for the STD experiments in the

media reports has been directed at Dr. John C. Cutler, a senior surgeon at the PHS and the lead investigator in Guatemala.[6] His records, although inconsistent and incomplete, provide the most thorough documentation of what took place in Guatemala. They also provide clear evidence that Dr. Cutler knew some would conclude that this work was unethical. In the absence of his records, we would still not know about the Guatemala STD experiments — with their revelation, Dr. Cutler's name has become synonymous with unethical research.

Public health research, however, is rarely an individual activity. The events in Guatemala did not just happen because a rogue scientist exploited a loophole in an underdeveloped administrative scheme. Making Dr. Cutler the focus of blame in the Guatemala STD scandal limits our understanding of the scope of responsibility for the experiments. Many others were complicit in planning, approving, advising, and participating in the STD research. Such a focus diminishes the lessons we can apply to ethical analysis of current human participant research. If Dr. Cutler had not joined the PHS, the Guatemala STD experiments might still have occurred. They were not merely the product of a malevolent individual; they were generated and supported by a structured grant system and a defined research environment.

This structured research grant system was the new National Institutes of Health (NIH) system. The World War II contract process of directed research

Kayte Spector-Bagdady, J.D., M. Bioethics, *is an Associate Director at the Presidential Commission for the Study of Bioethical Issues (Washington, DC). She received her J.D. from the school of law and M. Bioethics from the Perlman School of Medicine of the University of Pennsylvania (Philadelphia, PA).* **Paul A. Lombardo, Ph.D., J.D.,** *is a Senior Advisor at the Presidential Commission for the Study of Bioethical Issues (Washington, DC) and the Bobby Lee Cook Professor of Law at Georgia State University (Atlanta, GA).*

gave way in 1946 to an NIH grant process encouraging scientific freedom under the Division of Research Grants (DRG). We argue in this article that tension existed at the time between the need for a system of governmental oversight and the desire to foster free scientific inquiry. The push towards scientific freedom coupled with a lack of attention to serious conflicts of interest at the grant review level did not offer sufficient protection to the subjects of federally funded research.

to prevent the abuses perpetrated on the subjects of the Guatemala STD experiments, it is critical for researchers to understand the impetus behind these regulations and be able to apply such ethical lessons to their daily interactions. Regulations and ethics are not coextensive — there will inevitably be times where a participant must rely on the ethical responsibility of an investigator. Ethics training is a critical element in a researcher's education to inform compliance with

Such an obvious case of research malfeasance, which violated research norms in place both in the past and now, has been uniformly repudiated. The Guatemala STD experiments were labeled "clearly unethical" by President Barack Obama and "reprehensible" by the Secretaries of State and Health and Human Services.

The failure to address these tensions adequately was a major element leading to the eventual corruption of the Guatemala experiments. In the Guatemala STD study context, respect for scientific freedom trumped administrative accountability, and the desire to engage the most preeminent experts for funding review overwhelmed attention to the conflicts and biases those experts faced. Without the detailed regulatory structure in place now for both grant review and treatment of research participants, this initial NIH process left protection of research subjects to the virtue of individual researchers, and the approval of their close colleagues and superiors.[7]

In this article we document the system of research review in place at the time of the Guatemala experiments and the ethos of scientific freedom for investigators that it promised. The NIH launched these experiments as part of a transition from the wartime contract process to a "new horizon" of postwar research grants. The inaugural NIH study section recommended approval of the Guatemala STD experiments at its first meeting. While the DRG required annual reports from its grantees, the Guatemala researchers were able to time their more questionable experiments so as to evade detailed reporting. We also look at the web of relationships that generated the experiments and provided a support system for them over time.

The needs to reconcile governmental oversight of research with scientific freedom and to mitigate conflicts of interest in areas requiring specialized expertise are issues that continue to challenge participant research today.[8] While current grant review and human subjects research regulations are designed

the spirit of even the most well-tailored regulatory structure. Comprehensive understanding of what could happen when "high ethical purposes and completely good morals"[9] of researchers are assumed and not cultivated is crucial to understanding the requisite value of ethics education and building the responsible investigator.

Science in Wartime: The Federal Medical Research Funding Process

At the turn of the 20th century in the United States, Congress allotted minimal funding for research grants related to the investigation of disease. The agencies created to fund research focused on matters relating to war. Congress created the National Academy of Sciences in 1863 to identify and employ scientific talent that could advance national objectives during the Civil War.[10] The National Research Council began to carry out studies for the National Academy of Sciences, and in 1916 the Council of National Defense was established to coordinate resources and industry preparation for the U.S. effort in World War I.[11]

In 1935, President Franklin Roosevelt established the National Resources Committee to provide recommendations, plans, data, and information about the development of national resources.[12] The Committee went on to release a report entitled "Research — a National Resource" that argued that government agencies should be granted more latitude for the use of research funds so that scientists could tangentially build upon research as they were conducting it "following the unforeseen leads which research itself reveals." The National Resources Committee saw research as "something of an adventure; and the more freedom it enjoys, the more likely it is to achieve important results."[13]

On the brink of the American involvement in World War II, the Roosevelt Administration established the Office of Scientific Research and Development (OSRD) to assume research contracts "issued for the purpose of assuring adequate provision for research on scientific and medical problems relating to national defense."[14] The Committee on Medical Research was also inaugurated to "advise and assist the Director in the performance of his medical research duties with special reference to the mobilization of medical and scientific personnel of the nation [and]...to recommend to the Director the need for and character of contracts to be entered into with universities, hospitals, and other agencies conducting medical research activities for research and development in the field of medical science."[15] (See Figure I).

Although the National Resources Committee had advised broad latitude for investigators, under the OSRD contract process, those who wished to receive funding had to complete a proposal including the: 1) "subject of investigation with its background, present state of knowledge, significance in national defense and plan of attack;" 2) "personnel, materials, and financial requirements;" 3) "investigative facilities available;" and 4) estimated duration of research. If an investigator received funding, he was required to conduct the research as defined in the contract, submit bi-monthly progress reports, and file a final report.[16]

Dr. Joseph Earle Moore was the Director of the Venereal Disease Division at Johns Hopkins University and Chair of the Subcommittee on Venereal Disease under the National Research Council (the

research arm of the National Academies).[17] Although Dr. Moore was excited by medical advancements during World War II, he warned that "[t]he success or failure of a National Research Foundation depends, not on money alone, but even more largely on the administration of it. Politics, bureaucracy, red tape, incompetent leadership – these can render sterile and futile the expenditure of any sum."[18] In an early draft of *Organizing Scientific Research for War: The Administrative History of the Office of Scientific Research and Development*, Irvin Stewart conceded that a level of bureaucratic research oversight was appropriate in a time of war, when scientific "[c]oordination...could not be sustained through publication of results for that was either impossibly slow or, in classified fields, altogether absent." In contrast, once hostilities ceased he argued that "supervision of research is unnecessary and coordination is gradually sustained by ordinary channels of publication and scientific meetings."[19]

In four years OSRD administered some 2,515 contracts worth about $454 million.[20] By 1944 and the impending defeat of Germany, however, OSRD Director Vannevar Bush decided that some of its contracts could be transferred to "a permanent civilian organization which might in peacetime supplement the work of the Army and the Navy...."[21] PHS Surgeon General Thomas Parran and the NIH Director Rolla Dyer advocated for assigning this ongoing work to the NIH[22] — the biomedical research laboratory of the PHS.[23] With the passage of the Public Health Service Act in July that same year, Surgeon General Parran and his Advisory Council assumed responsibility for the research grant system, the duty of recommending project funding, and any "additional means as [the Surgeon General] deems necessary or appropriate" to administer such grants.[24] Upon dissolution of the OSRD in December 1945, 42 projects previously administered by that agency were taken over by the PHS.[25]

During World War II, OSRD directed research funding primarily toward topics of interest to the armed services. As many considered syphilis "one of the most pressing problems of military medicine,"[26] and an anticipated 7,000,000 work days a year were lost to gonorrheal infection,[27] contracts that supported research into

Figure I

Structure of OSRD in 1941

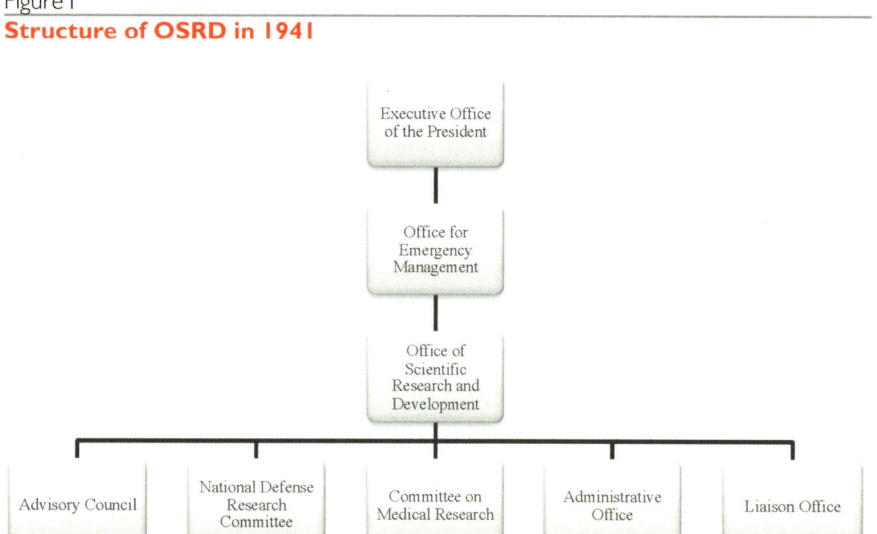

the prevention and treatment of STDs took priority. When the war ended, "the lion's share of research appropriations" remained tied up in military research and a major portion of that research — almost half of the contracts transferred from OSRD — involved penicillin therapy trials for syphilis.[28]

Studies of penicillin and other "miracle drugs" had heightened popular expectations for rapid scientific advancement during the war.[29] To the average citizen at the time, there was a "new optimism about the power of science."[30] Government medical officials worked to channel this optimism into enthusiasm for federally-funded research. At a lecture at Dartmouth College in December of 1945, Surgeon General Parran identified the government as the most realistic source of support for medical research. He argued that such a program "must assure complete freedom for the institutions and the individual scientists in developing and conducting their research work."[31] The financial significance of grant funding for researchers was obvious. Grant applications surged as the total expenditure for medical research rose from $18,000,000 in 1941 to $115,000,000 in 1946.[32] Congress also put aside a special appropriation of $800,000 to produce antibiotics.[33] Under Dr. Parran's leadership, the NIH presented plans for the federal expansion of public health initiatives when "[t]he time was ripe and the postwar budget could stand the cost."[34]

"New Horizons in Medical Research": Scientific Freedom under the Division of Research Grants

Surgeon General Parran preferred a research grant structure over OSRD's contractual requirements.[35] Contracts were for specific directed research on behalf of the government,[36] but a research grants structure lessened government control and encouraged investigator independence.[37] The PHS's acceptance of OSRD's contracts as grants, however, called for a new administrative structure. The NIH Director Dr. Dyer appointed Dr. Cassius Van Slyke, Assistant Chief of the PHS Venereal Disease Division, as the Chief of the new DRG in January of 1946.[38] With so much funding already devoted to penicillin and STD research, it made sense to place a physician with related experience in a leadership role in the new office under the NIH.

Dr. Van Slyke was committed to eliminating many of the burdens posed by the administrative oversight of contract research. One thing that had "especially bothered" him about the wartime contract process was that it "required a lot of paperwork...."[39] He shared his vision for the future of research grants in his article "New Horizons in Medical Research," where he

declared that the establishment of the DRG signaled the "complete acceptance of a basic tenet of the philosophy upon which the scientific method rests: The integrity and independence of the research worker and his freedom from control, direction, regimentation, and outside interference."[40] Dr. Van Slyke agreed with the National Resources Committee regarding the benefits of scientific latitude and endorsed maximum flexibility for researchers to change the direction of funded research as "bypaths quite often lead to more important findings than do the roads from which they branch."[41] Dr. Van Slyke distributed the article to many academic scientists for their endorsement before publishing it in *Science*.[42]

Dr. Van Slyke structured his division so that "[r]esearch under the Research Grants programs is conducted with the full independence and autonomy of the research investigator."[43] In contrast to the biweekly reporting requirement of the contract structure, he believed that only brief annual scientific progress reports should be required from grantees:

> In order not to divert the time of the researcher unnecessarily from the actual conduct of the research investigation, only annual scientific progress reports are requested. It is not desired that the preparation of these reports present any long, tedious burden to the investigator, and it is therefore requested that they contain only such data in a brief, clear, and concise manner as will permit the appropriate Study Section and National Advisory Council to be adequately informed as to the conduct of the research investigations since the submission of the previous progress report.[44]

He later reported that under his system "wide latitude is allowed [for] the responsible scientific investigator in the use of research grants funds. Recipients of awards are given complete freedom to conduct projects in whatever ways they choose."[45] In Dr. Van Slyke's new "medical research program of scientists and by scientists,"[46] scientific freedom promised scientific progress, and governmental oversight required under the contract process had stifled that freedom. Dr. Van Slyke's mantra of scientific freedom permeated the PHS research grants program. Dr. Ernest Allen, appointed from the PHS Venereal Disease Division by Dr. Van Slyke as Assistant Chief of the DRG,[47] noted that "[t]hose who established the [DRG] believed that maximum progress can be achieved only if the scientist enjoys freedom to experiment without direction or interference, and they drew up policies and procedures accordingly."[48] Under Dr. Van Slyke's program "[t]he investigator works on problems of his own choosing and is not obliged to adhere to a preconceived plan. He is free to publish as he sees fit and to change his research without clearance if he finds new and more promising leads. He has almost complete budget freedom as long as he uses the funds for research purposes and expends them in accordance with local institutional rules."[49] Dr. Van Slyke believed his was a system dealing with men of "high ethical purposes and completely good morals."[50] He later observed that "[w]e didn't have to worry about legalities, or a legalistic approach to this thing at all. We were just dealing with the kind of folks that wouldn't cheat a penny."[51] Dr. Van Slyke, and those who helped him create the grant review process, were "completely in favor of trusting the scientist and we set up such a program that trusted him. If [the scientist] let us down — well, that was the exception. It was far and away the exception."[52]

This vision was the foundation of the NIH grant review process. Dr. James A. Shannon,[53] the Director of the NIH, testified before a committee of the House of Representatives in 1962 that investigators with research grants "are not conducting research for NIH. They are exploring ideas of their own choosing..." and are "free to plan and conduct their investigations as they see fit."[54] This had been "true from the beginnings of the program...[and was] in response to a fundamental philosophy." Dr. Shannon argued that "science will advance most rapidly, and that as a consequence, practical findings will emerge most rapidly and in the greatest profusion, if science is unfettered by restrictions – if scientists are given freedom to follow their ideas.... Selection of good men and good ideas — and rejection of the inferior — is the key."[55]

The funding process under the DRG involved dual review of both a specialized study section and an appropriate Advisory Council. The goal of the study sections was to distance the grant review system from the government-driven research decisions of World War II and create a structure of "peer review" under which DRG placed advisory power in the hands of preeminent members of the relevant scientific community.[56] Dr. Van Slyke envisioned "the scientific community of America," as opposed to the government, deciding who would receive grant funds because he believed that "if we couldn't trust the scientists of this country to do a job properly, we couldn't trust anybody."[57]

The study sections had two responsibilities: (1) to be aware of the status of research generally in their field to identify areas to be expanded upon and encouraged, and (2) to review applications for grant money in that field and forward a recommendation to the appropri-

ate Advisory Council.[58] The study section reviewed the science; the Advisory Council approved the funding. The standard application reviewed by the study section was a four-page form with a 200-word summary of the project.[59] The form included information on objectives, methods, and the budget.[60] After the study section finished a review of "scientific merit and confidence in the principal investigator," they formulated an official recommendation. Advisory Councils took DRG policy goals into consideration,[61] but study section recommendations were the primary factor in determining which grants to approve and send to the Surgeon General for final endorsement.[62]

"Good Men and Good Ideas": Approval and Scientific Freedom in the Guatemala STD Studies

Necessary Review Expertise and Conflicts of Interest
Because of the influx of wartime penicillin contracts, the Syphilis Study Section was the first to begin its work. It held its inaugural meeting on February 7-8, 1946.[63] Dr. Moore, who had earlier voiced his concerns on "politics, bureaucracy, red tape, and incompetent leadership" as barriers to the success of national research efforts,[64] moved from his prior appointment as Chair of the Venereal Disease Subcommittee of the National Research Council to become the Chair of the Syphilis Study Section. Drs. John Mahoney, of the PHS, Venereal Disease Research Laboratory (VDRL), and John Stokes, of the Institute for the Control of Syphilis, University of Pennsylvania, also relocated from the National Research Council's Subcommittee to the Syphilis Study Section.[65]

Other members of the Syphilis Study Section included PHS officers Drs. Harry Eagle and John Heller, along with Dr. Thomas Turner, of the Johns Hopkins School of Hygiene and Public Health.[66] At their inaugural meeting, the Syphilis Study Section approved the Guatemala STD experiments, which they later described as "dealing with the experimental transmission of syphilis to human volunteers and improved methods of prophylaxis,"[67] for recommendation to the National Advisory Health Council.[68]

On March 8-9th, 1946 the Advisory Council met to discuss the new grant approval process and to review the recommendations of the study sections. At this meeting, the Advisory Council approved Research Grant (RG)-65 for the "[p]rophylaxis and treatment of gonorrhea and syphilis."[69] The Advisory Council named "Guatemala" as the "Grantee" of the funds and the "Pan American Union" as the "Investigator."[70] Dr. Cutler explained that while the grant was made from the DRG to the Pan American Sanitary Bureau, the VDRL "assumed responsibility for scientific and technical direction of the project and provided necessary personnel," including himself.[71] Dr. John Mahoney was listed as the principal investigator of the grant.[72]

The primary goal of study sections was to evaluate grant applications using the best available expertise, and a small number of preeminent researchers, whose interests and allegiances overlapped, dominated the field of STD research. Conflicts of interest were a concern. As a later historian noted: "[d]espite the fact that individual members of these review groups are required to absent themselves whenever a grant application from their own institution is under consideration, there is unavoidably some conflict of interest built into this system. No man can be completely objective about a grant application from an esteemed colleague who has just stepped out of the room, or even from one of the colleagues' close associated."[73]

Dr. Mahoney was a member of the Syphilis Study Section and also the Director of the VDRL. All of the U.S. investigators were from his laboratory and Dr. Mahoney himself was later confirmed as the principal investigator.[74] However, there is no evidence to suggest whether or not he abstained from the Study Section discussion regarding the Guatemala STD experiments.[75]

In 1943, Drs. Mahoney and Richard Arnold of the VDRL discovered that penicillin could cure syphilis quickly and effectively.[76] (Dr. Mahoney also published with Dr. Van Slyke in 1943 concerning the use of penicillin for gonorrhea).[77] While Drs. Mahoney and Arnold continued refining their research on the administration and dosing of penicillin, they also turned to exploring the *prevention* of infection through a post-exposure prophylaxis wash called "orvus-mapharsen" that they had found to be effective in rabbits.[78] Small-scale studies of their orvus-mapharsen wash had been conducted, but "while the results were suggestive they were inconclusive."[79] Therefore, "[i]t was felt that carefully controlled studies on relatively small groups of individuals exposed to a high risk of infection were required before the preparation could be prepared for wide spread use, particularly in the Armed Services."[80] Indeed, the stated objectives of the Guatemala STD experiments were to continue testing the effectiveness of penicillin as well as research the efficacy of orvus-mapharsen in humans.[81] Dr. Cutler, who worked for Drs. Mahoney and Arnold at the VDRL, was selected to manage these studies in Guatemala. Both physicians acted as Dr. Cutler's supervisors.[82]

Due to his strong personal interest in the success of his prophylaxis and oversight of the study, Dr. Mahoney's involvement in the study section that recommended the Guatemala STD experiments for approval raises serious concerns. When the grant for the study of "[p]rophylaxis and treatment of gonorrhea and syphilis" in Guatemala came before the Syphilis Study Section, not only was the principal investigator a member, the main therapies under investigation were a continuation of his work.

The personal interest of the Syphilis Study Section in the Guatemala STD experiments did not end there. Dr. Van Slyke was an STD physician himself. He received his initial training in the PHS Venereal Disease Division, rising to Assistant Chief of that unit. He had just completed his service as Associate Director of the VDRL under Dr. Mahoney.[83] Dr. Van Slyke served as the Syphilis Study Section Executive Secretary, responsible for coordinating the review of the applications.[84]

Dr. Heller of the Syphilis Study Section was the Chief of the Division of Venereal Disease at the PHS, where he worked with Dr. Mahoney and recruited Dr. Van Slyke (before his move to DRG).[85] After the renewal of the Guatemala STD experiments in 1947, Dr. Heller accompanied Drs. Van Slyke and Mahoney to visit the Guatemala City study site.[86] He asked Dr. Cutler to take "photographic records" of the experiments for him to use later for teaching.[87] Above and beyond the annual reporting requirements of grantees to study sections, Dr. Heller also received copies of Dr. Cutler's monthly reports from Guatemala, which Dr. Mahoney requested he keep confidential.[88] At the time Dr. Heller was approving the Guatemala STD experiments on the Syphilis Study Section, he was also overseeing his own syphilis experiments in Tuskegee, Alabama — experiments that Dr. Cutler would later join. (See Figure II).

Study Section Chair Dr. Joseph Moore also considered a site visit to Guatemala.[89] When Dr. Moore was the Chair of the National Research Committee's Venereal Disease Subcommittee, he was instrumental in the approval of gonorrhea prophylaxis experiments in Terre Haute, Indiana where researchers intentionally exposed prisoners to gonorrhea through many of the same intentional exposure methods used in Guatemala. His colleagues on the Terre Haute study included Drs. Van Slyke, Mahoney, and Cutler.[90]

Dr. Eagle of the Syphilis Study Section was doing his own work on penicillin and syphilis, using doses of the antibiotic as a prophylactic. When Waldemar Kaempffert, science editor for the *New York Times*, reported on Dr. Eagle's research in rabbits, Kaempffert noted that while Dr. Eagle's "case holds good for rabbits...no tests on human beings have yet been made. To settle the human issue quickly it would be necessary to shoot living syphilis germs into human bodies, just as Dr. Eagle shot them

Figure II

Involvement in the Syphilis Study Section in the Terre Haute and Guatemala Experiments

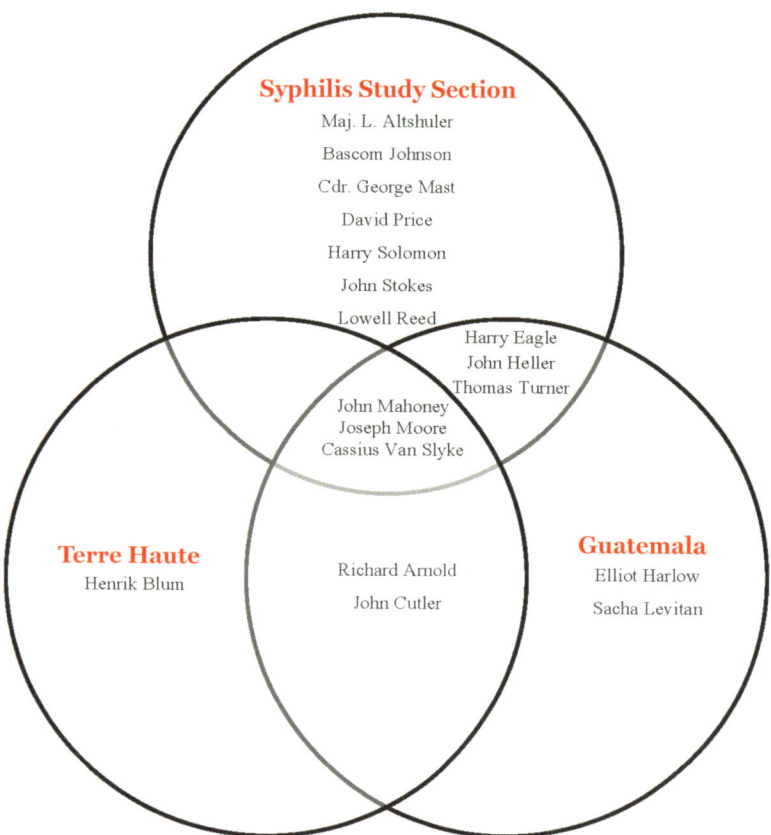

all the arrangements" of the experiments and was "very much interested in the project." After a debriefing on Guatemala, "a merry twinkle came into his eye when he said, 'You know, we couldn't do such an experiment in this country.'"[94] When Dr. Parran left the Surgeon General's office in late 1948, Dr. Mahoney noted his exit to Dr. Cutler: "we have lost a very good friend and that it appears to be advisable to get our ducks in line. In this regard we feel that the Guatemala project should be brought to the innocuous stage as rapidly as possible."[95]

In sum, when the Guatemala STD experiments were recommended for funding by the Syphilis Study Section, one member of the study section was the principal investigator of the protocol; two members had worked with the principal investigator previously on the Venereal Disease Subcommittee; two members had been involved in the Terre Haute gonorrhea experiments with the Executive Secretary and the investigator on the ground in Guatemala; and two members and the Executive Secretary worked or had worked together at the PHS Venereal Disease Division — the laboratory which "assumed responsibility for scientific and technical direction" of the protocol at issue. Out of the twelve members of the Syphilis Study Section, five members and the Executive Secretary either visited the experiments in Guatemala and/or tried to join in on the work.

Governmental Oversight and Free Scientific Inquiry
REPORTING REQUIREMENTS

Although the wartime research contract process required bi-weekly progress reports from federal grantees,[96] Dr. Van Slyke avoided placing this burden on the investigators funded by grants — he requested only brief annual reports for the study section and Advisory Council.[97] Dr. Cutler did send monthly progress reports from Guatemala to Dr. Mahoney[98] and sent edited versions to the Pan American Sanitary Bureau.[99] However, the Pan American Sanitary Bureau closely aligned itself with the PHS at the time, which assigned "practically all of [the Pan American

into rabbits. Since this is ethically impossible, it may take years to gather the information needed."[91] Dr. Eagle did not heed Kaempffert's warning. In fact, he asked to travel to Guatemala to conduct human experiments on Dr. Cutler's subjects *after* Kaempffert's comment. Dr. Mahoney objected to Dr. Eagle joining the work, and warned Dr. Cutler that "Doctor Van Slyke made a hurried trip from Washington recently to tell us that Harry Eagle is about to complain to the Surgeon General [Parran] that I have not been extremely enthusiastic about allowing him to enter the Guatemala study."[92]

Dr. Eagle was not the only Syphilis Study Section member who wanted to do his own research in Guatemala. Dr. Turner of Johns Hopkins asked Dr. Mahoney to have the Guatemala researchers "check on the pathogenicity in man of the rabbit spirochete" that he had been working on.[93] Even Surgeon General Parran, who had final approval authority for all grants before the DRG, was reportedly "familiar with

Sanitary Bureau's] professional staff...." Dr. Hugh S. Cumming Sr. led both organizations as the U.S. Surgeon General until 1936, at which point he retired from the PHS but remained the Director of the Pan American Sanitary Bureau until 1947.[100]

Intentional exposure experiments began in the Guatemalan Army in February 1947 and followed in the penitentiary and psychiatric hospital in May.[101] The following month, Dr. Cutler wrote to Dr. Mahoney with concerns about even the limited reporting they were doing:

> First, as you know, it is imperative that the least possible be known and said about this project, for a few words to the wrong person here, or even at home, might wreck it or parts of it. We have found that there has been more talk here than we like with knowledge of the work turning up in queer places.... The four of us in our project have carefully discussed the matter and all felt that we should do all possible to keep knowledge of our project restricted. Thus I should like to ask your permission to send the detailed reports and discussions of our work directly to you and not through any other person here. In order to conform to the [Pan American Sanitary Bureau] requirement for monthly reports we can continue to send the barest summaries of our progress.[102]

Dr. Mahoney agreed with Dr. Cutler in his response the following week and assured him that he would reiterate the secretive nature of his forwarded reports to Dr. Heller:

> In regard to the amount of gossip which the work in Guatemala has engendered, we are doing our utmost here to restrict our own conversations and those of others bearing upon the matter. We have also been aware of considerable conversation and discussion being carried out in rather high places, much of which has not helped the work greatly. We are forwarding all of your reports to Doctor Heller in a way which we hope will prevent their being read by unauthorized persons. I will write him again in the matter.[103]

The National Advisory Council approved Guatemala funding in March 1946.[104] When the PHS researchers arrived in Guatemala, they began by conducting serology studies that compared the accuracy of different syphilis diagnostic blood tests in the Guatemalan population and by treating already-infected military patients with penicillin. In February 1947, they also conducted an experiment in the Army in which 15 soldiers had intercourse with two commercial sex workers who were infected with gonorrhea.[105]

In March the brief annual report to the Syphilis Study Section and Advisory Council was due, and the Advisory Council renewed RG-65.[106] Within weeks of filing this report the PHS researchers began intentional exposure experiments in the penitentiary and the psychiatric hospital. They abandoned their initial experiment design of "normal exposure" to commercial sex workers and injected syphilis spirochetes directly into their subjects.[107] As the RG-65(c) funding drew to a close in June 1948, Dr. Cutler urged Dr. Mahoney that he should request further funding to continue the STD experiments.[108] Dr. Mahoney disagreed, saying "a new grant has some drawback in that it will require a progress report dealing with the work which has been accomplished. This we might not care to do at the present time."[109] Dr. Van Slyke, however, gave his approval to the researchers to continue to use any remaining grant funds in Guatemala for up to 6 months after the expiration of the grant.[110]

When the Guatemala researchers completed their first annual reporting requirement to the Division of Research Grants in March 1946, the major work they had completed was on serological testing; only one sexual intercourse prophylaxis experiment had been conducted. The next month, the PHS researchers moved into the Guatemala City Penitentiary as well as the Psychiatric Hospital and began exposing subjects to STDs via "artificial inoculation." Over the next year their research expanded to include injection of syphilis spirochetes into the blood stream and spinal column, abrading genitals to apply a syphilitic emulsion, and applying gonorrheal pus to subjects' mucus membranes. In 21 months of intentional exposure experiments, involving 1,300 subjects, the PHS investigators would have only filed one annual report to the Division of Research Grants describing only serological testing, penicillin treatment, and one sexual intercourse experiment of 15 subjects.[111]

SCIENTIFIC FREEDOM
Dr. Van Slyke's new research grants system adopted the perspective of the National Resources Committee that "[a] further advantage to research which would result from latitude in the use of funds is the possibility of following the unforeseen leads which research itself reveals."[112] Dr. Van Slyke later explained "we never did hold [the scientists] to their stated purpose. They were free to turn any way they wanted to."[113]

In the Guatemala STD experiments the original plan had been to test Drs. Mahoney and Arnold's orvus-mapharsen prophylaxis wash in prisoners who were having sexual intercourse with commercial sex workers infected with syphilis. Sex work was legal in prisons in Guatemala, thereby allowing for "normal exposure" to STDs. The hope was to test the prophylaxis through as natural a method as possible to establish a "rapid and unequivocal answer as to the value of various prophylactic techniques."[114]

The original PHS protocol immediately posed challenges. The subjects could not be infected with STDs dependably (the same problem that forced the abandonment of the Terre Haute prison gonorrhea study), which prevented the reliable testing of the post-exposure prophylaxis.[115] Dr. Cutler decided that the solution was more aggressive exposure techniques and

"unforeseen leads" and moved on to exposing subjects in the Psychiatric Hospital to syphilis through oral ingestion[122] and injecting syphilitic material "directly into the central nervous system" in the base of subjects' skulls.[123] He also performed transmission experiments in which he applied gonorrheal pus to subjects' urethras, rectums, and eyes.[124] After Dr. Mahoney refused to apply for more funding or to submit a new report to DRG, Dr. Cutler tested the orvus-mapharsen prophylaxis for a third STD, exposing the abraded skin of 131 soldiers and psychiatric patients to chancroid in October of 1948.[125] Dr. Van Slyke's extension of the renewed RG-65 ended in December of 1948, after which Dr. Cutler left Guatemala.[126]

Although much of the public commentary on the Guatemalan STD experiments has targeted the failings of Dr. Cutler, we offer a different critique by focusing on the institutional context and research ethos that shaped the outcome of the PHS STD research in Guatemala. Dr. Cutler had daily responsibility for the conduct of the experiments, but a "new horizon" of grant-based scientific review allowed this work to proceed.

began abrading subjects' penises by hand and rubbing in syphilitic material.[116] Around the same time, Dr. Mahoney wrote to Dr. Cutler that "Dr. Heller [of the Syphilis Study Section] would feel considerably more secure if we were to set up an advisory group of leading figures in the world of science to serve as a background for the study." He went on to confide that "[t]here are several men whom I would not mind being associated with the work. There are several other leading figures who, I think, would be a distinct detriment."[117] Dr. Mahoney also disapproved of Dr. Cutler's more aggressive approach and argued that the scarification and abrasion techniques were "drastic...beyond the range of natural transmission and will not serve as a basis for the study of a locally applied prophylactic agent."[118] Dr. Mahoney warned Dr. Cutler that if he was not able to resolve the prophylactic experiments, they would only have their serology and penicillin treatment work and "would surely have difficulty in selling an expensive project of this kind to the [Public Health] Service."[119]

Dr. Cutler believed, however, that the more aggressive the exposure technique, the more vigorously he could prove the prophylaxis' value in preventing both syphilis and gonorrhea.[120] Even though scarification and abrasion methods proved effective at infecting subjects,[121] Dr. Cutler decided to continue to follow his

Conclusions and Implications

Although much of the public commentary on the Guatemalan STD experiments has targeted the failings of Dr. Cutler, we offer a different critique by focusing on the institutional context and research ethos that shaped the outcome of the PHS STD research in Guatemala. Dr. Cutler had daily responsibility for the conduct of the experiments, but a "new horizon" of grant-based scientific review allowed this work to proceed. The freedom that Dr. Cutler was able to exercise allowed him to ignore the heightened concern for the welfare of research participants that characterized planning for the Terre Haute experiments, as well as the general movement at the end of World War II. Dr. Van Slyke later emphasized that under his new structure federally funded researchers were supposed to "make sure that in treating [a research subject] we weren't subjecting him to any unusual danger." He insisted that if "untoward effects" occurred, treatment would be stopped "so that [the subject] wouldn't be hurt."[127] But with a new grant system based on the discretion of the investigator, no one held Dr. Cutler accountable to such considerations. Serious professional conflicts marked the review of RG-65. Many of the members of the Syphilis Study Section were close colleagues and had worked together and with the principal investigator before as researchers and reviewers. Dr. Mahoney stood to benefit from the success of his new prophylactic treatment that Dr. Cutler was studying in Guatemala, and several other study section members attempted to advance their own work as part of the grant they had already approved.

The researchers in Guatemala abandoned their original ineffective exposure methodology in favor of much more invasive techniques. The flexible grant process allowed this change with federal funding. Dr. Cutler's correspondence affirms that he was aware that some colleagues might consider his new methods a violation of the norms of research ethics.[128] However, the investigators' efforts to keep the work secret and the lack of formal reporting under the grant structure allowed these violations to continue. While many of the Syphilis Study Section members had a detailed awareness of the work going on in Guatemala, it is clear from the researchers' emphasis on secrecy and discretion that if others found out about the STD work they believed it would have meant an end to the experimentation.

Twenty years after the Guatemala STD experiments, Dr. Henry K. Beecher argued in his seminal article on "Ethics and Clinical Research" that examples of unethical experimentation on humans had been growing since World War II. Dr. Beecher found that "[t]he data are suggestive of widespread problems" and that it was "evident...that unethical or questionably ethical procedures are not uncommon."[129] Dr. Beecher placed the onus of ethical behavior on "the more reliable safeguard provided by the presence of an intelligent, informed, conscientious, compassionate, responsible investigator."[130] The Guatemala STD experiments, however, demonstrate that reliance on such an investigator is not enough to protect all research participants all of the time. The new NIH peer review system, put in place just as the Guatemala studies were about to begin, and stressing "scientific merit and confidence in the principal investigator,"[131] revealed critical flaws in its first implementation.

Peer review still forms the basis of the NIH's dual review grant process. As late as 1996, the Director of DRG described the leadership style reflected in his agency as having been "inherited from Ernest Allen and Cassius Van Slyke, whose guiding precept was that no procedural obstacle should be allowed to stand in the way of scientific opportunity."[132] A plethora of infamous research scandals however led to modern scientific peer review and research participant regulations to combat just the types of problems present in Guatemala.[133] The NIH has reformed its policies on conflicts of interest in the peer review process. Regulations now prohibit those with real or apparent conflicts of interest from reviewing the applica-

tion at issue, conflicts including the possibility of financial benefit or any other interest likely to bias the reviewer's evaluation.[134] The perception that peer review groups "are biased toward one of their own" is "long-standing" and assumed[135] by the regulations and another qualified group must review a member's research proposal.[136] The NIH continues to refine its review process today, most recently considering a pilot program for anonymous grant review.[137] Institutional review board approval is also necessary for federally-funded human research, requiring protections such as minimization of risk, equitable subject selection, informed consent, and additional safeguards for vulnerable populations such as prisoners and people with mental disabilities.[138] These regulations support the grant review process so that participant protections do not solely rely on the discretion of an investigator.

Making Dr. Cutler the sole culpable party for what happened in Guatemala limits the breadth of the import of this case. There will always be immoral individuals. Critical for participant protection is a regulatory system that mandates, to the extent possible, correct behavior. Today, conflict of interest regulations, along with other layers of protections, make the funding of unethical research much less likely in the first place. Human subjects regulations and institutional review boards provide another layer of protection against unethical research once it is funded. But what is legal and what is ethical do not always have the same scope – sometimes regulations permit an action that is unethical, and sometimes the ethically optimal choice may fall outside regulatory boundaries. Ethics training is essential to encourage compliance with the spirit, as well as letter, of the law and inform actions in the space in which something may be legal but unethical. A comprehensive understanding of professional ethics also allows researchers to identify times where lawmakers should recalibrate regulations to reinforce ethical action. It is impossible to prevent a researcher from ever having to make an ethical assessment. The responsible investigator remains an important ideal.

Comprehensive ethics education can help build and support this responsible investigator. Scandals like the Guatemala STD studies give students stark examples of why "completely good morals" cannot be assumed, but must be taught, learned, and embodied. Ethical researchers do not self-select, they must be cultivated. A system built on the ethos of "good men and good ideas" alone is not enough to guarantee federal funding is used to advance good science. It takes regulatory research participant protections in addition to professional ethics education to achieve the longstanding ideal of the responsible investigator and ensure ethical research.

Acknowledgements

The findings and conclusions in this paper are those of the authors and do not necessarily represent the official position of the Department of Health and Human Services or the Presidential Commission for the Study of Bioethical Issues. The authors would like to thank Lisa M. Lee, Ph.D., M.S. and Jonathan Moreno, Ph.D., for their insightful comments and review.

References

1. H. F. Lynch, "Ethical Evasion or Happenstance and Hubris? The U.S. Public Health Service STD Inoculation Study," *The Hastings Center Report* 42, no. 2 (2012): 30 ("There is a new entry in the long catalog of historic research abuses."). Soldiers and prisoners had sexual intercourse with infected sex workers, and soldiers and psychiatric patients were injected with infected material in many parts of their bodies including genitals, eyes, and spinal columns. See generally, S. Reverby, 'Normal Exposure' and Inoculation Syphilis: A PHS 'Tuskegee' Doctor in Guatemala, 1946-48," *Journal of Policy History* 23, no. 1 (2011): 6-28; see also, Presidential Commission for the Study of Bioethical Issues (Bioethics Commission 118), "'Ethically Impossible:' STD Research in Guatemala from 1946-1948," (2011). Both Dr. Reverby and the Bioethics Commission describe this research in detail. In this article, the authors have chosen to cite directly to primary documents, rather than repeating citations to secondary sources, so that readers can easily verify the sources cited in this article and to encourage future scholarship on original sources. Many of the PCSBI Human Subjects Protection (HSP) I Archives sources are available online at <http://bioethics.gov/node/654> (last visited July 26, 2013). All of the PCSBI I Archives sources are available at the National Archives in Morrow, GA under Research Group 22, PCSBI, Record of the Guatemala Study. All of the documents archived by John C. Cutler are available at the National Archives online collection at <http://www.archives.gov/research/health/cdc-cutler-records/> (last visited August 13, 2013).
2. Faulty scientific design plagued the studies. Investigators altered or omitted data and information in final reports. See Bioethics Commission, *supra* note 1, at 95.
3. Secretary of State H. R. Clinton and Secretary of Health and Human Services K. Sebelius, "Joint Statement by Secretaries Clinton and Sebelius on a 1946-1948 Study" (2010), *available at* <http://www.state.gov/secretary/rm/2010/10/148464.htm> (last visited July 26, 2013); President B. Obama, "Memorandum re: Review of Human Subjects Protection (2010)," *available at* <http://bioethics.gov/cms/sites/default/files/news/Human-Subjects-Protection-Letter-from-President-Obama-11.24.10.pdf> (last visited July 26, 2013).
4. See Obama, *supra* note 3.
5. See Bioethics Commission, *supra* note 1, at 6.
6. See K. Minogue, "U.S. Officials Apologize for 'Appalling' 1940s Syphilis Study," ScienceInsider, October 1, 2010, *available at* <http://news.sciencemag.org/scienceinsider/2010/10/usofficials-apologize-forappalling.html> (last visited July 26, 2013). While media accounts have generally focused on the role of Dr. Cutler, accounts in the scholarly literature, e.g. Reverby and the Bioethics Commission, *supra* note 1, as well as other more recent publications cited in this paper, have provided a broader analysis of the Guatemala episode.
7. There has been a movement in the rhetoric of human research away from humans being "subjects of" research towards "participants in" research. See P. M. Boynton, "Letters: People should participate in, not be subjects of, research," *British Medical Journal* 317 (Nov. 28, 1998): 1521. The vulnerable populations involved in the Guatemala research, however, were clearly *subjects of* unethical research. In addition, 45 C.F.R. 46 currently uses the term "subject." Therefore, for the purposes of this paper, we used the term "subject" for the Guatemalans involved in the STD research and when referencing current federal regulation, but "participant" when discussing the current research environment. Also, the increasing importance of statistical argument in designing clinical trials, and the infrastructure that grew to support them is described in detail in H. M. Marks, *The Progress of Experiment: Science and Therapeutic Reform in the United States, 1900-1990* (New York: Cambridge University Press, 1997). Marks also discusses the early work on penicillin by scientists like Joseph Earle Moore on the National Research Council, and the transition of funding from the National Research Council to the NIH in detail, see *id.*, at 98-128. Victoria Harden also provides a history of the legislative and administrative initiatives that led to establishment of the NIH in V. Harden, *Inventing the NIH: Federal Biomedical Research Policy, 1887-1937* (Baltimore: Johns Hopkins University Press, 1986).
8. See, e.g., the recent Advanced Notice of Proposed Rulemaking on "Human Subjects Research Protections" which still grapples with ensuring that government regulated participant protections are "commensurate with the level of risk of the research study" in order to protect participants in high risk studies, while allowing lower risk studies to proceed more efficiently. Human Subjects Research Protections, Department of Health and Human Services, "Enhancing Protections for Research Subjects and Reducing Burden, Delay, and Ambiguity for Investigators," 76 *Fed. Reg.* 44512, 44514-44521. See also, P. Basken, "NIH Considered Anonymity for Grant Applications," *The Chronicle of Higher Education*, December 10, 2012, *available at* <http://chronicle.com/article/NIHConsiders- Anonymity-for/136227/> (last visited July 29, 2013); and S. Wessely, "Peer Review of Grant Applications: What Do We Know?" *The Lancet* 352, no. 9124 (1998): 301-302. For a look at the continued challenges of conflict of interest disclosure generally see G. Loewenstein et al, "The Unintended Consequences of Conflict of Interest Disclosure," *JAMA* 307, no. 7 (2012): 669-670.
9. C.J. Van Slyke, "Health Sciences," Oral History Research Office, Columbia University (1976): at 29.
10. I. Stewart, *Organizing Scientific Research for War: The Administrative History of the Office of the Scientific Research and Development* (Boston: Little, Brown and Company, 1948): at 4.
11. *Id.*, at 5, 7.
12. F. D. Roosevelt, Executive Order 7065, The National Resources Committee is Created, *available at* <http://www.presidency.ucsb.edu/ws/index.php?pid=15075> (last visited July 29, 2013).
13. National Resources Committee, *Research – A National Resource* (Washington, D.C.: United States Government Printing Office, 1938): 16.
14. An Advisory Council was also established "to advise and assist the Director with respect to the co-ordination of research activities carried on by private and governmental research groups...." See Stewart (1948), *supra* note 10, at 36-37. These contracts were originally that of the National Defense Research Committee, which was charged with coordinating, supervising, and conducting scientific research on problems underlying the development, production, and use of mechanisms and devices of warfare. The National Defense Research Committee later became advisory to the Office of Scientific Research and Development. *Id.*, at 7-8, 37-38.
15. *Id.*, at 39.
16. *Id.*, at 103.
17. See Stewart (1948), *supra* note 10, at 5. In June of 1940, the National Research Council decided to create a Subcommittee on Venereal Disease to make "general recommendations to The Surgeons General of the Army and Navy concerning the prevention and treatment of the venereal diseases and with acting in a consultative capacity on questions in its special field that might originate from the armed services." P. Padget, "Diagnosis and Treatment of the Venereal Diseases: Historical Note," *International Medicine in World War II, Vol. II: Infectious Diseases* (Washington D.C.: Office of the Surgeon General, Department of the Army, 1963): at 409.

18. Letter from J. E. Moore, Chairman, Subcommittee on Venereal Diseases to A. N. Richards, Chairman, Committee on Medical Research (Oct. 9, 1945) in PCSBI HSP I Archives, NARA-II_0000117.
19. I. Stewart, First Draft of Proposed C.M.R. Chapter for Irvin Stewart's Administrative History of OSRD (1945): 20-21 in PCSBI HSPI Archives, NARA-II_0000373-74.
20. R. Mandel, *A Half Century of Peer Review 1946-1996* (Bethesda, MD: Division of Research Grants, National Institutes of Health, 1996): at 8.
21. *Id.*, at 11.
22. *Id.*, at 12.
23. R. E. Miles, Jr., *The Department of Health, Education, and Welfare* (New York: University Press of America, 1974): at 169.
24. Mandel, *supra* note 20, at 11-12.
25. *Id.*, at 20.
26. J. F. Mahoney, "An Experimental Resurvey of the Basic Factors Concerned in Prophylaxis in Syphilis," *The Military Surgeon* (1936): 351-363, at 351.
27. Letter from J. E. Moore, Chairman, Subcommittee on Venereal Diseases, National Research Council to A. N. Richards, Chairman, Committee on Medical Research, National Research Council (Feb. 1, 1943) in PCSBI HSPI Archives, NARA-II_0000176.
28. See Mandel, *supra* note 20, at 15-16, 23. Three physicians including Drs. John Mahoney and R.C. Arnold (both later involved in the Guatemala STD experiments) discovered in 1943 that penicillin cured syphilis. J. F. Mahoney, R. C. Arnold, and A. Harris, "Penicillin Treatment of Early Syphilis: A Preliminary Report," *American Journal of Public Health and the Nation's Health* 33, no. 12 (1943): 1387-91.
29. See Miles, *supra* note 23, at 169; see, e.g., "Medicine: New Magic Bullet," *Time Magazine*, October 25, 1943.
30. "The practical experience and specific progress from 1942 through 1945 brought about a new philosophical attitude toward government's role in science and health and new optimism about the power of science, particularly organized science." S. P. Strickland, *The Story of the NIH Grants Program* (New York: University Press of America, 1989): at 17.
31. "By carefully nurturing the peer review process and by cultivating rapport with Congress, Surgeon General Parran and NIH Director Dyer won the allegiance of a substantial majority of academic scientists and laid the institutional foundations for the nationwide extramural structure that would emerge in the following decade." Mandel, *supra* note 20, at 15-16.
32. K. M. Endicott and E. M. Allen, "The Growth of Medical Research 1941-1953 and the Role of Public Health Service Research Grants," *Science* 118, no. 3065 (1953): 337-43, at 337.
33. See Mandel, *supra* note 20, at 22.
34. See Miles, *supra* note 23, at 169.
35. See Mandel, *supra* note 20, at 19.
36. See Stewart (1948), *supra* note 10, at 103.
37. See C. J. Van Slyke, "New Horizons in Medical Research," *Science* 104, no. 2711 (1946): 559-67, at 559.
38. See Mandel, *supra* note 20, at 20, 22; C. J. Van Slyke, "Standard Form 61: Appointment Affidavits" (n.d.) in PCSBI HSPI Archives, NPRC_0002846.
39. See Strickland, *supra* note 30, at 31.
40. See Van Slyke, *supra* note 37, at 559.
41. *Id.*
42. See Mandel, *supra* note 20, at 30. This article was a major policy statement about the direction that government funding grants would take and the role of scientific independence in that program.
43. See Van Slyke, *supra* note 37, at 563.
44. *Id.*
45. C. J. Van Slyke, 'Research Grants Awarded by National Institute of Health,' (Sept. 23, 1947) 1, in PCSBI HSPI Archives, MISC_0000037.
46. See Strickland, *supra* note 30, at 32.
47. See Mandel, *supra* note 20, at 22. As Assistant Chief of the DRG during the Guatemala experiments, Dr. Allen was also

the one to convey to the researchers that they could use the remaining grant money to continue their work in Guatemala for up to 6 months after the grant's expiration. Letter from E. M. Allen to J. R. Murdock (June 28, 1948) in PCSBI HSPI Archives, CTLR_0001182.
48. See Endicott and Allen, *supra* note 32, at 341.
49. *Id.*
50. See Van Slyke, *supra* note 9, at 29.
51. *Id.*
52. *Id.*, at 42-43.
53. Dr. Shannon was the chair of the Malaria Study Section in 1947 and became the Associate Director of Research under Dr. Van Slyke at the National Heart Institute in 1948. See Van Slyke (1976), *supra* note 9, at 50. E. M. Allen, "Historical View: Early Years of NIH Research Grants," *NIH Alumni Association Newsletter* (II)(1980): 6-8, also in PCSBI HSPI Archives, MISC_0000064.
54. This Committee was investigating NIH expenditures. J.A. Shannon, "The Administration of Grants by the National Institutes of Health," *Hearings Before the Subcommittee on Intergovernmental Relations of the Committee on Government Operations of the House of Representatives 87th Cong.* (March 28-30, 1962): at 14. Lawmakers had challenged the NIH budget, and other questions had been raised in light of the seeming avalanche of new funding that NIH had disbursed. L. Stark, *Behind Closed Doors: IRBs and the Making of Ethical Research* (Chicago: University of Chicago Press, 2012): at147-48.
55. See Shannon, *supra* note 54, at 14.
56. See Mandel, *supra* note 20, at 1; Miles, *supra* note 23, at 177.
57. Van Slyke, *supra* note 9, at 28-29. Dr. Van Slyke later elaborated that setting up the Division this way was 'the easiest way to run it...It just puts your responsibilities on somebody else's shoulders. But those shoulders are a devil lot more competent to carry it than any single federal bureaucrat I know of.' *Id.*, at 64.
58. See Van Slyke, *supra* note 37, at 561.
59. See Mandel, *supra* note 20, at 46.
60. See Van Slyke, *supra* note 37, at 562.
61. See Miles, *supra* note 23, at 180.
62. See Van Slyke, *supra* note 37, at 562.
63. See Mandel, *supra* note 20, at 23; *see also* Memorandum from E.M. Allen to R.E. Dyer, (Mar. 8, 1946) in PCSBI HSPI Archives, NARA-II_0000129.
64. Letter from J.E. Moore, Chairman, Subcommittee on Venereal Diseases to A.N. Richards, Chairman, Committee on Medical Research (Oct. 9, 1945) in PCSBI HSPI Archives, NARAII_0000117.
65. See Padget, *supra* note 17, at 409; Van Slyke, *supra* note 37, at 567. Prior to the Subcommittee on Venereal Disease's recommendations, the diagnosis and treatment of syphilis in the Army followed the protocol outlined by Dr. Stokes in *Modern Clinical Syphilology*. J. H. Stokes, *Modern Clinical Syphilology* (Philadelphia: W.B. Saunders Co., 19236).
66. Other members included: David E. Price (NIH), Lowell J. Reed (Johns Hopkins School of Hygiene and Public Health), Harry C. Solomon (Boston Psychopathic Hospital), Maj. L. N. Altshuler (Army), Cdr. George W. Mast (Navy), and Bascom Johnson (Veterans Administration). Van Slyke, *supra* note 37, at 567.
67. [Draft] letter from J. E. Moore, Chairman, Syphilis Study Section to C.J. Van Slyke (May 1947), found in letter from J.E. Moore, Chairman, Syphilis Study Section to Members of the Syphilis Study Section, National Institute of Health (May 26, 1947), in PCSBI HSPI Archives, NARA-II_0000033.
68. National Advisory Health Council Meeting, U.S. Public Health Service (Mar. 8-9, 1946): at 13, in PCSBI HSPI Archives, NARA-II_0000547. Even though a later memo by Dr. Allen states that '[c]opies of the minutes of the meeting and of papers presented are on file in the Research Grants office...' the protocol for the Guatemala STD research or minutes of this meeting have not been located. Memorandum from E.M.

Allen to R.E. Dyer (Mar. 8, 1946), in PCSBI HSPI Archives, NARA-II_0000129.

69. See National Advisory Health Council, *supra* note 68 at 10, 13.

70. *Id.*

71. J. C. Cutler, Final Syphilis Report (Feb. 24, 1955): at 9, in PCSBI HSPI Archives, CTLR_0000641.

72. Supplemental Information Submitted in Connection with 1948 Amendment to Budget: Status of Grants, State of Illinois; Grants Paid, Fiscal Yr 1946 & 1947: at 5, in PCSBI HSPI Archives, NARA-II_0000076. When the grant was renewed in 1947, Dr. Fred Soper, the Director of the Pan American Sanitary Bureau, was listed as the Principal Investigator. National Advisory Health Council, U.S. Public Health Service, Minutes of Meeting (Mar. 14-15, 1947), in PCSBI HSPI Archives, NARA-II_0000047. While it appears from correspondence that Dr. Soper did visit the Guatemala experiments, it is not clear how much he knew about what they entailed. See, e.g., Letter from J. F. Mahoney to J. C. Cutler (June 30, 1947), in PCSBI HSPI Archives, CTLR_0001077.

73. "Organizational expert Harold Seidman has characterized scientific research as 'the only pork barrel for which the pigs determine who gets the pork.'" See Miles, *supra* note 23, at 179.

74. Supplemental Information Submitted in Connection with 1948 Amendment to Budget, *supra* note 72, at 5.

75. The minutes of this meeting have not been located, see *supra* note 68. However, the listing of "Guatemala" as the grantee and the "Pan American Union" as the investigator may have allowed Dr. Mahoney to recommend the grant. See National Advisory Health Council (1946), *supra* note 68 at 13.

76. See Mahoney, *supra* note 28.

77. J. F. Mahoney, C. Ferguson, M. Buchholtz, and C. J. Van Slyke, "The Use of Penicillin Sodium in the Treatment of Sulfonamide-Resistant Gonorrhea in Man," *The American Journal of Syphilis, Gonorrhea, and Venereal Disease* 27, no. 5 (1943): 525-528.

78. See Cutler, *supra* note 71, at 7, in PCSBI HSPI Archives, CTLR_0000639. Orvusmapharsen was a 10-percent argyrol (i.e., silver) intra-urethral instillation.

79. *Id.*

80. *Id.*

81. *Id.*, at 22, PCSBI HSPI Archives, CTLR_0000654. J. C. Cutler, Experimental Studies in Gonorrhea (Oct. 29, 1952): at 1, in PCSBI HSPI Archives, CTLR_0001278.

82. See Cutler, *supra* note 71, in PCSBI HSPI Archives, CTLR_0000629.

83. See Van Slyke, *supra* note 37.

84. See Mandel, *supra* note 20, at 25. By December, however, it appears Dr. Van Slyke was replaced with Dr. Price. See Van Slyke, *supra* note 37, at 567.

85. See Allen, *supra* note 53, at 1, in PCSBI HSPI Archives MISC_0000063; Van Slyke, *supra* note 9, at 23.

86. Letter from J. C. Cutler to J. F. Mahoney (Mar. 12, 1947), in PCSBI HSPI Archives, CTLR_0001054.

87. J. C. Cutler to R. C. Arnold (Aug. 21, 1946) in PCSBI HSPI Archives CTLR_0001216. Almost 600 photographs in Guatemala were taken of the subjects, prophylactic procedures, and symptomatic results of the STD exposures. Bioethics Commission, *supra* note 1, at 110.

88. Letter from J. F. Mahoney to J. C. Cutler (June 30, 1947) in PCSBI HSPI Archives CTLR_0001077. Those reports otherwise went to Drs. Mahoney and Arnold – not Syphilis Study Section members.

89. Letter from J. F. Mahoney to J. C. Cutler. (Oct. 15, 1946) in PCSBI HSPI Archives, CTLR_0001200. It is unclear if Dr. Moore actually visited the Guatemala study site.

90. J. F. Mahoney, C. J. Van Slyke, J. C. Cutler, and H. L. Blum, "Experimental Gonococcic Urethritis in Human Volunteers," *American Journal of Syphilis, Gonorrhea, and Venereal Disease* 30, no. 1 (1946): 1-39.

91. W. Kaempffert, "Notes on Science: Syphilis Prevention," *New York Times*, April 27, 1947, at E9.

92. Letter from J. F. Mahoney to J. C. Cutler (May 5, 1947) in PCSBI HSPI Archives, CTLR_0001243.

93. See Mahoney, *supra* note 89.

94. Letter from G. R. Coatney to J. C. Cutler (Feb. 17, 1947) in PCSBI HSPI Archives CTLR_0001051. See Lynch, *supra* note 1, for further debate regarding the Parran comment. In addition, as this article was under review, the American Sexually Transmitted Diseases Association decided to remove the name of Dr. Thomas Parran from its lifetime achievement award, in large part because of his role in the Guatemala research described in this article. See L. K. Altman, "Of Medical Giants, Accolades and Feet of Clay," *New York Times*, April 1, 2013, at D3. For a series of essays discussing Dr. Parran's legacy, see also *Sexually Transmitted Diseases* 40, no. 4 (2013): 275-284.

95. Letter from J. F. Mahoney to J.C. Cutler (Feb. 19, 1948) in PCSBI HSPI Archives, CTLR_0001223.

96. See Stewart, *supra* note 10, at 103.

97. See Van Slyke, *supra* note 37, at 563.

98. Letter from J. C. Cutler to J. F. Mahoney (Oct. 31, 1946) in PCSBI HSPI Archives CTLR_0001199.

99. Letter from J. C. Cutler to J. F. Mahoney (June 22, 1947) in PCSBI HSPI Archives CTLR_0001241. See, e.g., Letter from J. R. Murdock to J. C. Cutler, forwarded by W. J. McAnally, Jr. (Dec. 26, 1947) in PCSBI HSPI Archives, CTLR_0001102.

100. F. L. Soper, *Report of the Director of the Pan-American Sanitary Bureau to the Member Governments of the Pan American Sanitary Organization: January 1947-April 1950* (n.d.): at 30, in PCSBI HSPI Archives, PAHO_0000486. The Pan American Sanitary Bureau later became part of the Pan American Sanitary Organization, which then was renamed the Pan American Health Organization. M. Cueto, *The Value of Health: A History of the Pan American Health Organization* (Rochester: University of Rochester Press, 2007): 63-108.

101. See Bioethics Commission, *supra* note 1, at 116.

102. Letter from J. C. Cutler to J. F. Mahoney (June 22, 1947) in PCSBI HSPI Archives CTLR_0001241.

103. Letter from J. F. Mahoney to J.C. Cutler (June 30, 1947) in PCSBI HSPI Archives CTLR_0001077.

104. National Advisory Health Council, *supra* note 68, at 10, 13, PCSBI HSPI Archives, NARA-II_0000544, NARA-II_0000547.

105. J. C. Cutler, Gonorrheal experiment #1 (1947) in PCSBI HSPI Archives, CTLR_0001736-79.

106. National Advisory Health Council, U.S. Public Health Service, "Minutes of Meeting March 14-15" (1947): at 58, in PCSBI HSPI Archives, NARA-II_0000473, NARA-II_0000530.

107. See Cutler, *supra* note 71, PCSBI HSPI Archives, CTLR_0000694.

108. The funding was authorized through June 1948. Letter from J. C. Cutler to J. F. Mahoney, forwarded by W. J. McAnally, Jr., (Aug. 26, 1948) in PCSBI HSPI Archives, CTLR_0001163.

109. Letter from J. F. Mahoney to J. C. Cutler, forwarded by F. L. Soper, Director, Pan-American Sanitary Bureau (Sept. 3, 1948) in PCSBI HSPI Archives, CTLR_0001161.

110. Letter from E. M. Allen to J. R. Murdock (June 28, 1948) in PCSBI HSPI Archives, CTLR_0001182.

111. This annual report has not been located, but would have described the "scientific progress" up to that point.

112. See National Resources Committee, *supra* note 13, at 16.

113. See Van Slyke, *supra* note 9, at 35.

114. See Cutler, *supra* note 81, at 2, PCSBI HSPI Archives, CTLR_0001279; Cutler, *supra* note 71, at 8, PCSBI HSPI Archives, CTLR_0000640.

115. If the researchers could not establish what percentage of subjects became infected after exposure to an STD naturally, they could not establish the preventative effect of the prophylactic wash.

116. See Cutler, *supra* note 71, at 8, PCSBI HSPI Archives, CTLR_0000766.

117. Letter from J. F. Mahoney to J. C. Cutler (May 5, 1947) in PCSBI HSPI Archives, CTLR_0001243.

118. Letter from J. F. Mahoney to J. C. Cutler (Sept. 8, 1947) in PCSBI HSPI Archives, CTLR_0001234.
119. Letter from J. F. Mahoney to J. C. Cutler (Sept. 8, 1947) in PCSBI HSPI Archives, CTLR_0001233.
120. See Cutler, *supra* note 81, at 12, PCSBI HSPI Archives, CTLR_0001290; Cutler, *supra* note 71, PCSBI HSPI Archives, CTLR_0000701.
121. See Cutler, *supra* note 71, at 5, PCSBI HSPI Archives, CTLR_0000763.
122. *Id.*, PCSBI HSPI Archives, CTLR_0000728.
123. *Id.*, at 13, PCSBI HSPI Archives, CTLR_0000836.
124. See Insane Asylum (Asilo de Alienados) and Prison Patient Records (Various dates), in PCSBI HSPI Archives, CTLR_0004157.
125. J. C. Cutler, Chancroid Experiment (n.d.) in PCSBI HSPI Archives, CTLR_0000951, CTLR_0000969.
126. See Bioethics Commission, *supra* note 1, at 117.
127. See Van Slyke, *supra* note 9, at 22-23.
128. See Bioethics Commission, *supra* note 1, at 97-101.
129. H. K. Beecher, "Ethics and Clinical Research," *New England Journal of Medicine* 274, no. 24 (1966): 1354-60, at 1354-55.
130. *Id.*, at 1360.
131. See Allen, *supra* note 53, at 6-8, in PCSBI HSPI Archives MISC_0000064.
132. See Mandel, *supra* note 20, at vii.
133. Examples include the Tuskegee syphilis experiments, the Jewish Chronic Disease Hospital cancer experiments, and the Willowbrook State School Hepatitis A experiments. See J. D. Arras, "The Jewish Chronic Disease Hospital Case," J. H. Jones, "The Tuskegee Syphilis Experiment," and W.M. Robinson and B.T. Unruh, "The Hepatitis Experiments at Willowbrook State School," in E. J. Emanuel et al., eds., *The Oxford Textbook of Clinical Research Ethics* (New York: Oxford University Press, 2008): at 73-96. 13442 C.F.R. 52h.2, 52h.5 (2004).
134. 42 C.F.R. 52h.5 (2004).
135. "Scientific Peer Review of Research Grant Applications and Research and Development Contract Projects," 69 *Fed. Reg.* 272, 275 (Jan. 5, 2004).
136. 42 C.F.R. Part 52h.5(d) (2004).
137. P. Basken, "NIH Considered Anonymity for Grant Applications," *The Chronicle of Higher Education*, December 10, 2012, available online at <http://chronicle.com/article/NIH-Considers-Anonymity-for/136227/> (last visited August 13, 2013).
138. 45 C.F.R. §46.111 (2009).

2.4   Perverse Incentives

Paula Stephen

Stephan, P. Perverse incentives. *Nature* 484(7392), 29–31 (2012). © 2010 Macmillan Publishers Limited. All rights reserved. Imprint of SpringerNature.

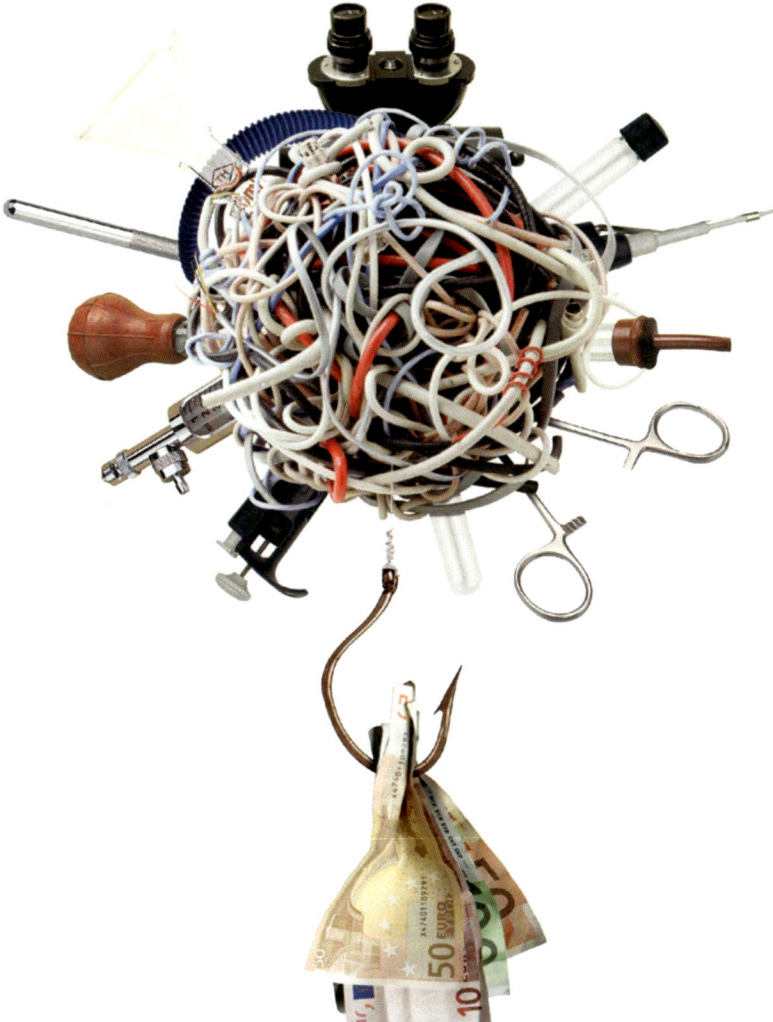

ILLUSTRATION BY VIKTOR KOEN

Perverse incentives

Counterproductive financial incentives divert time and resources from the scientific enterprise. We should spend the money more wisely, says **Paula Stephan**.

Scientists may portray themselves as not being motivated by money, but they and the institutions where they work respond in spades to financial opportunities. Incentives that encourage people to make one decision instead of another for monetary reasons play an important part in science. This is good news if the incentives are right. But if they are not, they can cause considerable damage to the scientific enterprise.

For instance, cash incentives adopted by countries such as China, South Korea and Turkey encourage local scientists to submit papers to high-end journals despite the low probability of success. These payments have achieved little more than overloading reviewers, taking them away from their work, and have increased submissions by the three countries to the journal *Science* by 46% in recent years, with no corresponding increase in the number of publications[1].

Sadly, science is full of incentives gone awry. Look no further than expanding PhD programmes that produce graduates with almost no career prospects, or the growth of lab space with no apparent increase in productivity.

The economic rules behind science were written without much consideration for unintended consequences, but such consequences abound because people and institutions are so responsive to incentives. And in the current economic climate, no one can afford to waste time or resources. In a world of tight budgets, getting the incentives right is more important than ever.

BAD DIRECTIONS

Consider the financial calculations that encourage universities to hire a series of postdocs rather than staff scientists. Postdocs earn around half to two-thirds of a staff scientist's salary. They are young, have fresh perspectives and new ideas and are temporary, so can be let go when budgets decline[2]. But, in reality, postdocs are not cheap: substantial resources — both their own and society's — have been invested in training them.

If a postdoc doesn't get a research job, taxpayers do not get a return on their investment. Neither does the postdoc: someone who did not go to graduate school and entered the labour market in 2001 was earning about US$58,000 in 2008; a first-year postdoc who started graduate school in the United States in 2001 was making around $37,000 in 2008 on graduation[3]. During a three-year postdoc position, a scientist gives up more than $60,000 on average in return for highly uncertain job prospects. And many postdocs will not get a research job. There are few faculty openings, and limited numbers of research positions in government and industry. So even if individual postdocs cost less, from a societal perspective they can be expensive.

Equally harmful are rules that encourage scientists to support graduate students on a research assistantship (RA) rather than on a training grant, despite evidence that the ▶

SUMMARY

● Science is full of incentives that encourage bad financial choices, such as expanding labs and hiring too many temporary scientists.

● These incentives hurt both individual scientists and society as a whole, which gets minimal return on its investment when someone is trained for a field with no career prospects.

● The way forward is to fix incentives that are damaging the system, by considering their true social and personal cost.

▶ latter produces better outcomes. Part of the reason is that RA funding comes with an additional amount to cover the university's overhead, or indirect rate, which may be as high as 50%. For those on training grants from the US National Institutes of Health (NIH) in Bethesda, Maryland, that amount is capped at 8%. This difference easily translates into an institution getting at least $12,000 more for every RA-supported student. Other considerations affect the choice of RAs over training grants, too — RAs are under the direct control of principal investigators, whereas graduate students on training grants are less so.

However, training grants are arguably better for scientists in the long term. Importantly, they give departments the incentive to provide a high-quality training experience, because renewals for training-grant awards are evaluated on the quality of the PhD experience and placement outcomes. By contrast, scientists who support students on research grants are not required on renewal to disclose where graduates end up being placed. Some principal investigators collect this information, but departments typically do not — my informal survey of 45 science departments found only two that were able to report where their students had been placed. Without this knowledge, prospective students will not be able to judge whether a lab is a good place to begin a successful science career.

The growth of labs is another result of incentives. Bigger is seen as better: more funding, more papers, more citations and more trainees — regardless of whether the market can sustain their employment. Some institutions pay bonuses to faculty members on the basis of the amount of external funding they receive[4]. But, again, too many trainees creates a glut of people who will not find suitable jobs. It would have been more efficient for both the students and society to steer them in a different direction. And big labs can be wasteful — an analysis by the US National Institute of General Medical Sciences in Bethesda, Maryland, found that an increase in funding is not associated with a substantial increase in output when measured by the number of grant-linked publications[5].

Other economic incentives indirectly render the scientific process less efficient — such as the tendency of scientists to avoid risk by submitting to funding organizations only those proposals that they consider 'sure bets'. This tendency comes from the need for faculty members to obtain grants to support their salary, the emphasis on preliminary data in grant applications and the difficulty of obtaining funding in today's climate.

> *"The building boom is now costing the scientific enterprise by creating space that cannot be paid for."*

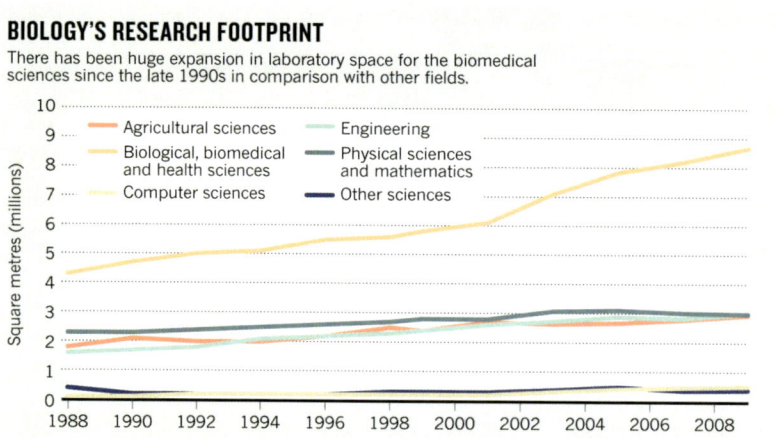

BIOLOGY'S RESEARCH FOOTPRINT
There has been huge expansion in laboratory space for the biomedical sciences since the late 1990s in comparison with other fields.

SOURCE: US NATL. SCI. FOUND.

If most scientists are risk-averse, there is little chance that transformative research will occur, leading to significant returns from investments in research and development. Funding bodies sometimes give money specifically for field-changing research, but not nearly enough — Pioneer grants from the NIH fund fewer than 1% of applicants.

In the European Union, there are strong incentives for researchers to team up with colleagues in other countries. This is because most funding opportunities under the various research Framework programmes require consortia to be made up of at least three entities in three different European countries. No collaboration, no grant. Is this a good use of resources? Although there is evidence that collaboration leads to better research, I do not know of any that supports the idea that those collaborators should come from different countries. The extra costs of coordination — organizing the work, travel, meetings and so on— can be large relative to the money being invested in research.

Universities are also driven by incentives. By hiring faculty members on 'soft' money, with grants providing the salary, the institutions bear almost none of the risks. Furthermore, universities prefer to put up a new building or invest millions in remodelling existing lab space rather than house scientists in older buildings that they already own. Why? One reason is that debt can be an accounting asset. A US government accounting rule called A21 means that the more debt universities have from construction, the more they can add to grants for overhead costs. If a university borrows $100 million to build a new facility and pays 4% interest, it can increase its indirect rate by including the $4-million interest payment in the calculation. The building binge is further fuelled by competition among universities: recruiting senior faculty members requires space, and lots of it.

What is so bad about institutions putting up new research facilities? The answer lies in what economists call 'incidence' — who eventually pays. Before the global financial crisis, universities had hoped to recoup the money through increased indirect costs and through the 'buy-out' money they receive from funding agencies to cover the salaries of permanent faculty members working on grants. But now that grants are harder to get, that money isn't coming in. Unless states and private institutions default, someone will have to pay the bonds. The money is likely to come from the physical sciences, the humanities and social sciences, as well as cutbacks in hiring across departments. In short, the building boom is now costing the scientific enterprise by creating excess space that cannot be paid for.

FIX WHAT'S BROKEN
The way forward is to alter these damaging incentives. The scientific enterprise should cut back on the demand for graduate research assistants by establishing more research institutes that are not focused on the production of PhDs, such as the Howard Hughes Medical Institute's Janelia Farm campus in Ashburn, Virginia. Research institutes, by producing fewer PhDs, lead to a better balance between supply and the limited number of research jobs. Abstinence, after all, is the most effective form of birth control.

In addition, we should consider ways of making graduate students and postdocs more costly to universities, to discourage their overuse and reflect their social cost. One possibility is to 'tax' the two positions, making them more expensive relative to other staff types, thereby providing an incentive to employ permanent rather than temporary staff. Principal investigators and their departments should also be required to report placement data online as part of all research-grant applications. This would allow society to monitor the return on its investment, and students to assess job outcomes.

Training grants should be made more

economically attractive. And rules should be altered to limit the amount of interest payments universities can include when calculating indirect rates, and the amount of faculty members' salaries that can be charged to grants, thereby dulling the incentive to hire people for soft-money positions. Shifting evaluations from projects to people, and de-emphasizing the importance of metrics in hiring and promotion, could encourage scientists to work on riskier projects[6].

Many of the problems now faced by science accelerated when biomedical funding started to increase steeply. For instance, the doubling of the NIH budget from 1998 to 2003 triggered universities to hire more people and build more buildings, while scientists increased the number of grants they submitted and the size of their labs (see 'Biology's research footprint'). Now, this biomedical machine needs increasing amounts of money to sustain itself — larger labs need more grants, which leads to lower success rates, with calls for more funding.

Biomedical research has done much to contribute to increased life expectancy. But it seems likely that diminishing returns have set in. New drugs are slower in coming to market and there was a less than stellar increase in US publications associated with the NIH doubling[7]. Moreover, many of the breakthroughs that have contributed to better health outcomes have come from other fields of science — such as the laser and magnetic resonance imaging. Funds for the physical sciences in the United States (in terms of the percentage of federal research funding) are close to a 35-year low. Perhaps it is time for deans in the biomedical sciences to rent some of that excess space to their colleagues in chemistry and physics. ∎

Paula Stephan *is professor of economics at Georgia State University in Atlanta, Georgia 30303, USA, and a research associate at the National Bureau of Economic Research in Cambridge, Massachusetts. She is author of* How Economics Shapes Science *(Harvard Univ. Press, 2012).*
e-mail: pstephan@gsu.edu

1. Franzoni, C., Scellato, G. & Stephan, P. *Science* **333,** 702–703 (2011).
2. Stephan, P. *How Economics Shapes Science* (Harvard University Press, 2012).
3. Current Population Survey, Table P-28 (United States Census Bureau, 2010); available at http://go.nature.com/neix5i
4. Mallon, W. T. & Korn, D. *Science* **303,** 476–477 (2004).
5. Berg, J. 'Another Look at Measuring the Scientific Output and Impact of NIGMS Grants' (22 November 2010); available at http://go.nature.com/dae21z
6. Azoulay, P., Graff Zivin, J. S. & Manso, G. *Incentives and Creativity: Evidence from the Academic Life Sciences* (2010); available at http://go.nature.com/biey9d
7. Sacks, F. *The Scientist* (11 September 2007), available at http://go.nature.com/bpa3xr

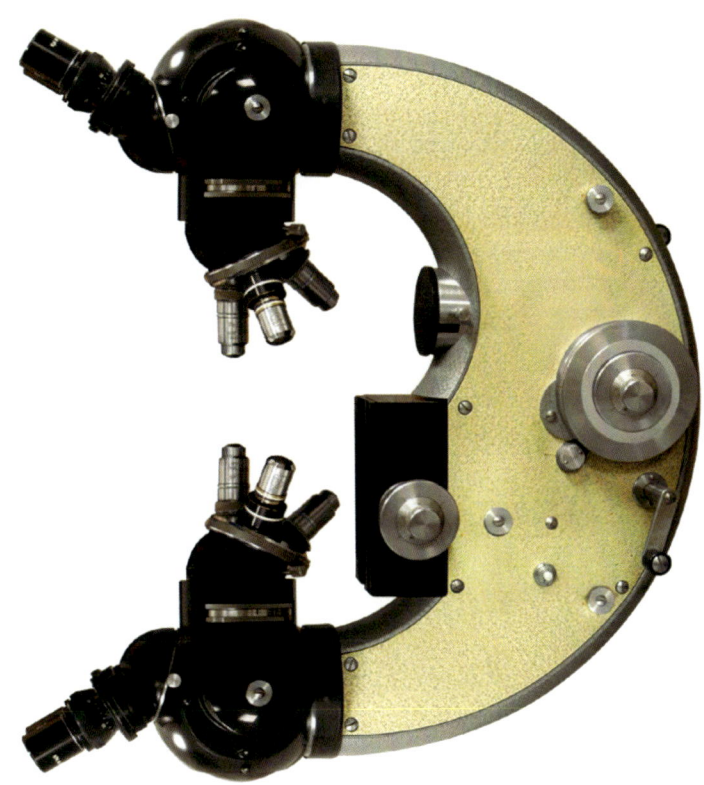

ILLUSTRATION BY VIKTOR KOEN

Turn the scientific method on ourselves

How can we know whether funding models for research work? By relentlessly testing them using randomized controlled trials, says **Pierre Azoulay**.

In times of tight budget constraints, scientists' wranglings about the real and perceived sins of public funding agencies become particularly acute. Complaints usually lead to the creation of a panel of respected, thoughtful and well-meaning scientists who come up with a plan of reform based on their intuition and experience. Funding agencies, who are genuinely concerned about improving the productivity of the scientific enterprise, often adopt these recommendations, at least in part. In one example of this process, the US National Institutes of Health (NIH) in Bethesda, Maryland, has created a large array of funding mechanisms, each one targeted to a particular problem — including the K99/R00 or 'kangaroo' grants, which pair postdoctoral scientists with mentors to help them to prepare for tenure-track faculty positions and funding independence. Not only is this range of mechanisms confusing and costly to administer, but the effectiveness of such reforms is never seriously evaluated.

It is time to turn the scientific method on ourselves. In our attempts to reform the institutions of science, we should adhere to the same empirical standards that we insist on when evaluating research results. We already know how: by subjecting proposed reforms to a prospective, randomized ▶

2.5   Flint Water Crisis Yields Hard Lessons
          in Science and Ethics

Katie L. Burke

Burke, K. Flint water crisis yields hard lessons in science and ethics. *American Scientist* 104(3), 134–136 (2016). https://www.americanscientist.org/article/flint-water-crisis-yields-hard-lessons-in-science-and-ethics.

Flint Water Crisis Yields Hard Lessons In Science And Ethics

BY KATIE L. BURKE (/AUTHOR/KATIE_L._BURKE)

Q&A with Virginia Tech civil engineer Marc Edwards on uncovering the water crises in Flint, Michigan and Washington, DC and his efforts to keep it from happening again.

ETHICS (/TOPICS-NAMES/ETHICS) · POLICY (/TOPICS-NAMES/POLICY) · SOCIOLOGY (/TOPICS-NAMES/SOCIOLOGY)

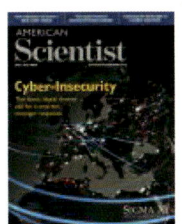

THIS ARTICLE FROM ISSUE

MAY-JUNE 2016

VOLUME 104, NUMBER 3

PAGE 134

DOI: **10.1511/2016.120.134**

(/)

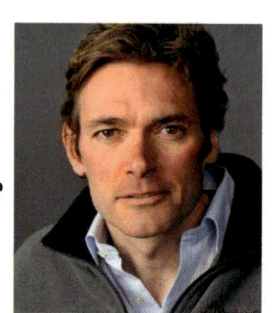

Like many scientists, *Virginia Tech civil engineer Marc Edwards chose his career to serve the public good. But his experience uncovering the Flint, Michigan, water crisis, where citizens were exposed to high levels of lead because of government and scientific negligence, has been a stark reminder of what can happen when science is misused or ignored. To make matters worse, the Flint water crisis is a repeat of very recent history. About a decade ago, Edwards revealed high lead levels in public water in Washington, DC, exposing misconduct at the U.S. Centers for Disease Control and Prevention (CDC), U.S. Environmental Protection Agency (EPA), and District of Columbia Water and Sewer Authority (WASA). At the time, in 2003, Edwards was conducting WASA-funded research investigating an unprecedented number of small leaks in copper water pipes in the DC area as well as EPA-subcontracted research on water lead levels. He found some lead concentrations in the thousands of parts per billion and realized that WASA had given out misinformed advice about drinking water. But after he notified the agency, WASA refused to issue a new memo to alert people. Soon after, WASA threatened to withhold the results from his sampling program as well as $110,000 of funding he had recently proposed, unless he stopped the studies*

(/)

of water in local homes. Edwards refused, and the EPA terminated his

subcontract. Edwards continued his research, paying his team out of his own

pocket when he had to. In March 2004, the CDC published a report that

concluded that the lead levels from blood tests of DC children were not high

enough for concern. After congressional hearings, the EPA ruled later in 2004

that WASA violated federal regulation. In 2009 congressional hearings, the CDC

report was found to be flawed, because it left out samples, a fact that had

come to light after Edwards reanalyzed the full data set. Digital features editor

Katie L. Burke interviewed Edwards about his experiences and how he is

working to prevent another incident like the ones in Flint and DC.

Studies by you and others have now shown that tens of thousands of

homes in Washington, DC, had elevated levels of lead in their water. Lead

levels in some water samples you tested were so high that they could be

classified as hazardous waste. How could scientists and regulatory

agencies let that happen?

The DC water crisis was the most fundamental betrayal of the public trust and

scientific integrity in black and white that I have ever seen or even heard of,

having reviewed case study after case study. With no profit motive whatsoever,

these people [those in leadership positions at WASA, EPA, and CDC] poisoned

an entire city, covered it up completely, and made sure that these kids and

their families never even got a penny to help with the extra educational needs

that they have [as a result of the poisoning]. It took me working as a volunteer

crazy person for six years to prove that kids were hurt.

(/) Five people [Seema Bhat, Jim Bobreski, Sue Kanen, Jerome Krough, and Ralph Scott] put their professional lives on the line in DC. They were fired. Two won whistleblower lawsuits, but no one really ever thanked these people. The perpetrators and the federal government who caused the DC lead crisis covered it up every step of the way.

If it comes down to a decision between their reputation and the truth, the truth will lose every single time with these agencies, because they are not rewarded for being loyal to the human race. They're rewarded for being loyal to their agency. That's the kind of people we have, unfortunately, in positions of power.

How can the agencies prevent another DC or Flint water crisis?

If you ever want to know why something like Flint happens, you only have to look at how we destroy good people and promote weak, unethical cowards. At that point, it's just what you expect. We should expect more Flints in the future unless we get the system fixed.

What have you found to be the most effective way to reach people when you talk about failing public infrastructure that is underfunded?

If you look at every projection of the federal budget, due to mismanagement and entitlement, discretionary spending is going down. That's happening at the federal, state, and local level. We are in an era where the pie is getting smaller. That is going to create unprecedented pressure on all aspects of science and

(/)   engineering. It's going to pressure us to be unethical in some situations to make sure we get our positions taken care of. We have to prioritize like we never have before.

What do we value as a society? From my perspective, critical infrastructure, you have to advocate for that, because without it, civilization is lost. That's what happened in Flint. They lost their ability to get clean water. People left town. This happened in Rome roughly two millennia ago. When the aqueducts no longer functioned, Rome lost 95 percent of its population. A civilization can literally end if you don't invest in these priorities.

I think we also have to be aware that this is a prioritization process. We have to engage in these debates and fully realize that there are other priorities for the shrinking pie. Education is getting the short end of the stick as well. You have to have some humility about that, look at the economic realities, and try to do more with less. It's the ultimate science and engineering challenge to still serve mankind, even though the fiscal reality is that we're not going to get increased funding and in all likelihood we're going to get less.

You now have a reputation as a whistleblower. Have you always had a skeptical attitude toward the research establishment?

Before my experiences in DC, I was incredibly naive. I was about 40 years old, and I didn't know anything about the history of scientific misconduct. I hadn't even accepted the idea that scientists at federal agencies with no profit motive

(/)

whatsoever would behave unethically. I think a lot of America is just waking up to that possibility based on what we exposed in Flint.

It was very difficult for me to accept, because I was to some extent willfully blind, in retrospect. I was a danger to myself and others, because I didn't really understand the dark side of science, which is the dark side of humans. We're all imperfect, and humans can screw up anything. Growing up worshipping at the altar of science, if you will, and thinking of science just as a good, and thinking that if I'm a scientist or engineer then I'm by definition doing good. The idea that science might be used for bad in a Western democracy hadn't really entered into my mind-set.

What went through your head as you began to realize that government scientists were lying?

It was an extremely traumatic experience for me to learn this the hard way, to see that corrupt officials couldn't care less about facts and scientific truths if it meant protecting their reputation or advancing their agency's agenda. At one point I'd lost about 30 pounds when I realized what the EPA was up to. My heart started racing, and I told my wife, "I'm going to die." I told her goodbye. Thankfully, I didn't die. I'm sure some people out there wish I had.

Do you think you would have been better off in your early career if you'd been more aware of the likelihood of encountering scientific misconduct?

(/)   You can really mess yourself up, I think, just from being that naive and uninformed. It's a real problem that we as scientists aren't aware of our history. We're not taught about how everything human about us can push us to do unethical things. We face those pressures day in and day out, and it's only by properly using the scientific method and honoring it that we can stop ourselves from reaching the wrong conclusions that hurt people. Science really is this amazing tool that if it's done properly you will more often than not reach the correct conclusion, which is important, I hope we would all agree. But to the extent that you let down your guard and lack moral humility, you will wake up some day having done something horrible, even though you started down this path with the best of intentions.

Why and how do these scientists end up hurting rather than helping the public with their flawed research?

I believe that the vast majority of scientists entering the profession from high school, based on my personal observation, view science as a public good and a force to create a better world. Gradually, if you look at our educational institutions and the workplace, what happens is we are taught to become willfully blind. We're taught to become cynical. We're taught that we can't do better than the status quo, and that if this agency's corrupt, there's nothing we can do about that. We feel powerless. We become part of the problem.

This all happens naturally, to the point that a lot of people end up becoming something that they once abhorred. They become people who practice science and engineering and end up harming people.

(/)

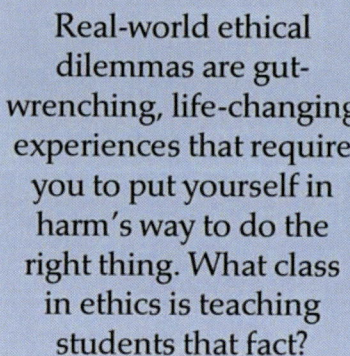
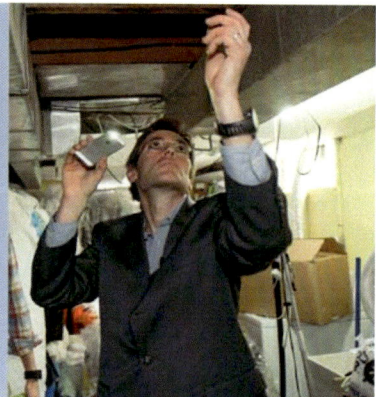

You now co-teach with anthropologist Yanna Lambrinidou an ethics class at Virginia Tech called Engineering Ethics and the Public. How do you approach mentoring future scientists in this class to help them avoid these pitfalls?

We have to tell people that heroism is difficult. Otherwise, everyone would be doing it, and it wouldn't be heroism. It's our experience and our hypothesis in the class, Dr. Lambrinidou's and mine, that ethics instruction in this country is 100 percent wrong in how it's approached. It is presented as if "you know the rules, and we're going to teach you them. Then, if you follow them, everything will turn out just fine." It's like a chess game, and if you know the rules, you'll win. That's not the real world. Real-world ethical dilemmas are gut-wrenching, life-changing experiences that require you to put yourself in harm's way to do the right thing. What class in ethics is teaching students that fact? We try to instill ethical street-smarts in students.

(/)   What we do in the class is make sure people understand who they are, what they stand for, where they will draw the line, and to write that down at this early point in their career. We put them in real-world situations where everything is pushing them to do the wrong thing. They see how strong a person you have to be to uphold scientific integrity. They come away realizing, "Wow, this is not easy to remain ethical in a perverse incentive structure." We go through case studies that show how heroic actors do the right thing, put their career on the line to protect the public, and are fired.

One of our best examples is what we call the press conference. We have each student role-play that they're one of the agencies that was involved in perpetrating and covering up the Washington, DC, lead crisis. We give them briefing materials that tell each agency what they know at that moment in time and how their agency owns a little piece of this problem because of their past mistakes. We then let them know the public is angry. In a few days they're going to give a press conference and answer questions.

When we do that, nine times out of ten the students find themselves lying. It's fascinating. We then play the videotape from the actual people at the press conferences telling the exact same lies. They very quickly learn that telling the truth is not necessarily your first inclination. Throughout the semester they get to see how a half lie turns into a bigger lie, which turns into a bigger lie, until eventually you create the epic examples of scientific misconduct.

The Washington, DC, lead crisis goes on to this day. Kids that were hurt might get their day in court next summer, at which point they're out of high school.

(/) Once you've lived through those kinds of experiences, you realize that you have

to work very hard to be ethical. You gain moral humility, which is necessary in

science and engineering. You're only one bad mistake from becoming someone

that you once would've been disgusted by.

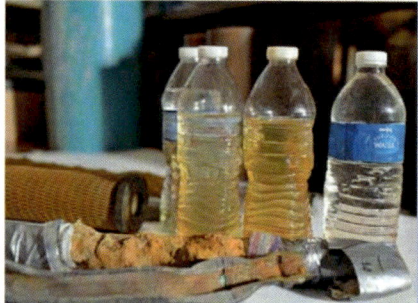

Who do we point to for students to emulate? Well, it's the person who's got the big multimillion-dollar center and is getting all the money. Is that the modern hero of science?

Do we need to change the stories we tell ourselves and others about what it takes to be a good scientist?

It's interesting who we glorify in science and how divorced from reality it is. If

you consider the typical stereotype of heroism in science, it's about a path

where someone makes a discovery through hard work, creates something of

tremendous value for the world, and they bestow this gift on the world and

receive rewards. It feeds the virtuous cycle between science and the public.

Who are we putting forward as heroes for students to follow? I believe that

currently who we make the role models in our field, it's very narrow. It is the

people who've achieved the goals of the perverse incentive structure. Who do

we point to for students to emulate? Well, it's the person who's got the big

multimillion-dollar center and is getting all the money, getting all the

publications, is at the top of this pyramid supporting all these researchers. Is

that the modern hero of science? I guess so, but not to me.

(/)   My heroes are people whose story you might not even know. For example,

Peter Buxtun exposed the Tuskegee experiment (*Buxtun was an*

epidemiologist once employed by the U.S. Public Health Service (PHS), who

acted as a whistleblower in 1972 to expose an experiment that studied the

natural progression of syphilis, which became treatable during the course of

the 40-year experiment, in hundreds of poor African-American men under the

auspices of free health care). He fought for five years to get the PHS to stop

this horrific human experiment. He went through two review panels, fighting,

and those panels each time told him to go do something else because they felt

there was nothing wrong with the Tuskegee experiment. He didn't give up. It

wasn't until it got into the press and there was a congressional hearing that

folks in positions of power at PHS realized, "Wow, this really looks bad. People

are mad at us." As a result, we now have institutional review boards and

human subjects training. To me, he went the true hero's journey.

Researchers speaking out about science's dark side are often warned that

doing so can be dangerous, because it feeds anti-science rhetoric. How do

you respond?

Well, the same logic applied in the Catholic Church when pedophilia was

rampant, we now know, and people were stopped from calling it out. Folks in

positions of power were saying, "This is going to hurt the church. This is going

to hurt our reputation." I understand where they're coming from. I don't get

any pleasure from talking about this. The people in the Catholic Church who

were whistleblowers did not get pleasure from pointing out that their

(/) colleagues were pedophiles. But what is the cost of not speaking out? The cost is people get hurt. The cost is you end up damaging the institution you love even more. It wasn't until the public learned about it that they finally had no choice but to get this fixed.

Who loves science more: the people who are willfully blind and are fearful of talking honestly about our problems, or someone who loves it so much that they're willing to try to fix it? No one loves science and engineering more than me. No one loses more sleep over what I've had to do than me. It kills me to speak out, but I am not going to sit by and let more people get hurt. I'm not going to let the institution of science and engineering go down this path if I have a word to say about it, because all humanity, all civilization, rests on scientists and engineers doing their jobs, and we cannot do our job if we are not trustworthy. I'm frankly more fearful about what will happen if I don't speak out than if I lose my career.

(/)

0 Comments   **American Scientist**   🔴 **Login** ▾

♡ Recommend 8   ⬆ **Share**   Sort by Newest ▾

👤   ┌──┐
       │ Start the discussion…   │
       └──┘

        LOG IN WITH

                            OR SIGN UP WITH DISQUS (?)

                            ┌──┐
                            │ Name   │
                            └──┘

                            Be the first to comment.

ALSO ON **AMERICAN SCIENTIST**

Science in the Post-Truth Era

6 comments • 7 months ago●

   Jamie Vernon — Thank you for your
   comment. You may want to read Matt
   Nisbet's article that was mentioned in …

Photoshopping the Universe

1 comment • 7 months ago●

   Rob Pettengill — It's good to see the
   misconception that an un-manipulated
   image is a truer representation of reality …

An Updated Prehistory of the Human Pelvis

2 comments • 9 months ago●

   RichW9090 — There is no functional reason
   why that should be so.

An Illness Observed: A Conversation with Julie Rehmeyer

20 comments • 3 months ago●

   AndyPR — Thank you, American Scientist,
   for covering this subject accurately. Us
   patients have been so used to …

(/)

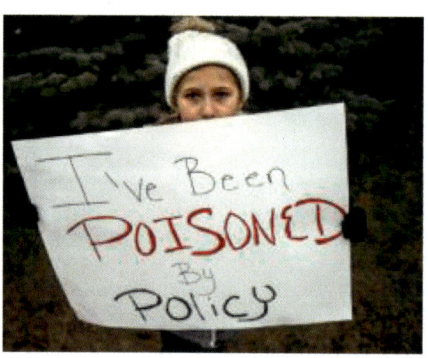

READ MORE IN THIS ISSUE

Moving Forward After Flint (/Article/Moving-Forward-After-Flint)

ALL TOPICS (/TOPICS-NAMES/ALL)

MORE IN ETHICS

- TOPICS (/TOPICS-NAMES/ALL)

- FEATURES (/TOPICS-NAMES/ALL?FIELD_MEDIA_TID=338)

- BLOGS (/BLOGS/ALL)

- (✔) VIDEO (/TOPICS-NAMES/ALL?FIELD_MEDIA_TID=103

- PODCASTS (/TOPICS-NAMES/ALL?FIELD_MEDIA_TID

- MAGAZINE (/MAGAZINE/ISSUES/ALL)

- ARCHIVE (HTTP://WWW.JSTOR.ORG/JOURNAL/AMER

- SUBSCRIBE (HTTPS://ECOMMERCE.SIGMAXI.ORG/EC

- NEWSLETTER (/USER?DESTINATION=NODE/3796)

- ABOUT US (/CONTENT/ABOUT-US)

- ADVERTISE (/CONTENT/ADVERTISE)

- LOGIN (/USER/LOGIN)

- REGISTER (/USER/REGISTER)

- SEARCH (/SEARCH/NODE)

- HELP

(/magazine/issues/2017/july-august)

The past decade has seen an explosion of...

SUBSCRIBE (HTTPS://ECOMMERCE.SIGMAXI.ORG/ECOM/#S

GIVE A GIFT (HTTPS://ECOMMERCE.SIGMAXI.ORG/ECOM/#S

DONATE (HTTPS://WWW.SIGMAXI.ORG/ABOUT/DONATE

A Publication of

(https://www.sigmaxi.org/)

References

Alberts B, Kirschner M, Tilghman S, Varmus H. Rescuing US biomedical research from its systemic flaws. PNAS. 2014;111(16):5773–7.

Burke K. Flint water crisis yields hard lessons in science and ethics. Am Sci. 2016;104(3):134–6.

Krimsky S. Science, society, and the expanding boundaries of moral discourse. In: Gavroglu K, Stachel J, Wartofsky M, editors. Science, politics and social practice. Boston: Kluwer Academic Publishers; 1995.

Pielke R. In retrospect: Science—The endless frontier. Nature. 2010;466:922–3.

Sarewitz D. Saving science. New Atlantis. 2016;49:5–40.

Spector-Bagdady K, Lombardo P. "Something of an adventure": postwar NIH research ethos and the Guatemala STD experiments. J Law Med Ethics. 2013;41:697–710.

Additional Suggested Reading

Alberts B, Kirschner M, Tilghman S, Varmus H. Rescuing US biomedical research from its systemic flaws. PNAS. 2014;111(16):5773–7. (*Suggests immediate changes needed to reverse the unsustainable path of the biomedical research enterprise in the United States.*)

Kaiser D, Moreno J. Self-censorship is not enough. Nature. 2012;492:345–7. (*Describes 1975 history of self-censorship around recombinant DNA until scientists could develop safety protocols, and 2012 voluntary moratorium on flu-virus research but concludes that self-censorship is insufficient.*)

Kretser A, Murphy D, Dwyer J. Scientific integrity resource guide: Efforts by federal agencies, foundations, nonprofit organizations, professional societies, and academia in the United States. Crit Rev. Food Sci Nutr. 2017;57(1):163–80. (*Provides a resource on scientific integrity standards.*)

Reproducibility

3

Arthur L. Caplan and Barbara K. Redman

While reproducibility has long been a cornerstone of the scientific method, it is currently an active area for reaffirming scientific standards. Medicine, psychology, neuroscience, genetics, and economics are examples of fields actively working to assess the quality of their science.

Some irreproducibility is an inevitable part of cutting edge science and of the variability of biological systems, but rigorous scientific practice that permits replication is also essential. Such practices include blinding of outcome assessment, power calculation to determine sample size, use of positive and negative controls, random allocation of subjects (where appropriate), validation of cell lines, reagents and antibodies, computer code documented and tested for accuracy, and auditing to insure methodological compliance at all sites. Systematic reviews have also been found to need more reproducible search strategies (Koffel and Rethlefsen 2016).

Replication has usually meant obtaining same results by using precisely the same methods and materials. In an effort to establish consistent definitions, Goodman and colleagues suggest: methods reproducibility, results reproducibility (akin to replication), and inferential reproducibility. It should be noted that the level of detail needed to describe a study methodologically is not typically found in publications. Open data allows validation of published findings as well as supporting novel analyses. Inferential reproducibility calls attention to the fact that not all investigators will draw the same conclusions from the same results and may use different analytical strategies, but their findings should still correlate if valid (Goodman et al. 2016).

Some of the most vigorous and organized work on reproducibility by independent investigators is being done in psychology. These efforts have shown that underpowered studies and publication bias can be corrected (Etz and Vanderkerckhove 2016) and that this field also has to be sensitive to contextual differences (Van Bavel et al. 2016) . In all fields, literature linked with subsequent correcting or corroborating literature can be helpful in tracking consistency or inconsistency of results from similar experiments (Pulverer 2015).

Reliability of the scientific record and integrity of scientific inquiry require high levels of quality and documented reproducibility where possible.

Advice: Check the quality of scientific practices in your field, especially that of the particular line of research on which your own work is building. See if there are any prior problems or scandals. Try to be aware of retracted work. Gather evidence of reproducibility for the problem you are studying to be sure it is solid enough that you are not wasting your time or that of others.

As a reviewer of manuscripts or grant applications or in service on editorial boards, help to adopt policies that support quality science and assure its publication no matter whether the findings are negative or positive.

A. L. Caplan · B. K. Redman (✉)
New York University Langone Medical Center,
New York, NY, USA
e-mail: Arthur.Caplan@nyumc.org

© Springer International Publishing AG, part of Springer Nature 2018
A. L. Caplan, B. K. Redman (eds.), *Getting to Good*, https://doi.org/10.1007/978-3-319-51358-4_3

3.1 What Does Research Reproducibility Mean?

Steven N. Goodman, Daniele Fanelli, and John P. A. Ioannidis

Goodman SN, Fanelli D, Ioannidis JPA. What does research reproducibility mean? Science Translational Medicine 2016 June 1;341:1–6.

PERSPECTIVE

SCIENTIFIC INTEGRITY

What does research reproducibility mean?

Steven N. Goodman,* Daniele Fanelli, John P. A. Ioannidis

The language and conceptual framework of "research reproducibility" are nonstandard and unsettled across the sciences. In this Perspective, we review an array of explicit and implicit definitions of reproducibility and related terminology, and discuss how to avoid potential misunderstandings when these terms are used as a surrogate for "truth."

Concern about the reproducibility of scientific research has been steadily rising recently with reports that the results of experiments in numerous domains of science could not be replicated (1, 2). Whereas problems in biomedical research have garnered most of the attention, concerns have touched almost every field in the biological and social sciences and beyond (3) (Fig. 1). As the movement to examine and enhance the reliability of research expands, it is important to note that some of its basic terms—reproducibility, replicability, reliability, robustness, and generalizability—are not standardized. This diverse nomenclature has led to confusion, both conceptual and operational, about what kind of confirmation is needed to trust a given scientific result. Here, we dissect this vocabulary, explore the reasons for the confusion, and offer a framework to improve both communication and understanding.

DEFINING THE TERMS
Although the importance of multiple studies corroborating a given result is acknowledged in virtually all of the sciences (Fig. 1), the modern use of "reproducible research" was originally applied not to corroboration, but to transparency, with application in the computational sciences. Computer scientist Jon Claerbout coined the term and associated it with a software platform and set of procedures that permit the reader of a paper to see the entire processing trail from the raw data and code to figures and tables (4). This concept has been carried forward into many data-intensive domains, including epidemiology (5), computational biology (6), economics (7), and clinical trials (8). According to a U.S. National Science Foundation (NSF) subcommittee on replicability in science (9), "*reproducibility* refers to the ability of a researcher to duplicate

the results of a prior study using the same materials as were used by the original investigator. That is, a second researcher might use the same raw data to build the same analysis files and implement the same statistical analysis in an attempt to yield the same results…. Reproducibility is a minimum necessary condition for a finding to be believable and informative."

Documenting this kind of reproducibility thus requires, at minimum, the sharing of analytical data sets (original raw or processed data), relevant metadata, analytical code, and related software. Reproducibility defined in this way mainly addresses issues of trust that data and analyses are as represented. The definition does not specify to what extent deviations are acceptable. Such reproducibility does not add new evidential weight, although greater subjective weight is often accorded to evidence that is more highly trusted. New evidence is provided by new experimentation, defined in the NSF report as "replicability," which refers to "the ability of a researcher to duplicate the results of a prior study if the same procedures are followed but new data are collected."

Although the preceding conceptual distinctions might seem clear, the definitions do not provide clear operational criteria for what constitutes successful replication or reproduction. Furthermore, the terminology is not universally used, and sometimes the meanings above are reversed. Consider the language of Francis Collins, director of the U.S. National Institutes of Health (NIH), in his commentary on plans to enhance research reproducibility (10):

"… a complex array of other factors seems to have contributed to the lack of reproducibility. Factors include poor training of researchers in experimental design, increased emphasis on making provocative statements rather than presenting technical details, and publications that do not report basic elements of ex-

perimental design. Some irreproducible reports are probably the result of coincidental findings that happen to reach statistical significance, coupled with publication bias. Another pitfall is overinterpretation of creative 'hypothesis-generating' experiments, which are designed to uncover new avenues of inquiry rather than to provide definitive proof for any single question. Still, there remains a troubling frequency of published reports that claim a significant result, but fail to be reproducible."

This short passage covers a wide range of issues subsumed under the rubric of reproducibility: design, reporting, analysis, interpretation, and corroborating studies (that is, replication, as previously defined). If one looks at the terminology being used across the scientific literature, one finds similar variation and intermingling of concepts. For example, the largest-scale attempt to replicate experiments in psychology was published with the title "Estimating the reproducibility of psychological science," (2) clearly allying the term "reproducibility" with the conduct of new studies.

One notable absence from this diverse lexicon is the word "truth." The fundamental concern of Collins and others is, in fact, not reproducibility per se, but whether scientific claims based on scientific results are true. Below, we discuss how treating reproducibility as an end in itself—rather than as an imperfect surrogate for scientific truth—is partly responsible for the current terminological and operational morass, and suggest how we can benefit by refocusing on cumulative evidence and truth.

A NEW LEXICON FOR RESEARCH REPRODUCIBILITY
We start the process of clarification by proposing a new terminology to distinguish between the various interpretations of reproducibility. Rather than offer new technical meanings for words whose common language interpretations are nearly identical (such as reproducibility, replicability, and repeatability), we propose to ally the word reproducibility—currently the most widely used single term in this domain—with descriptors for the underlying construct. This yields three terms: methods reproducibility, results reproducibility, and inferential reproducibility. Although we apply these terms mainly to the biomedical field, they have utility across many domains of science, each of which has different conventions and cultures about how

Meta-Research Innovation Center at Stanford (METRICS), Stanford University, Stanford, CA 94305, USA.
*Corresponding author. Email: steve.goodman@stanford.edu

PERSPECTIVE

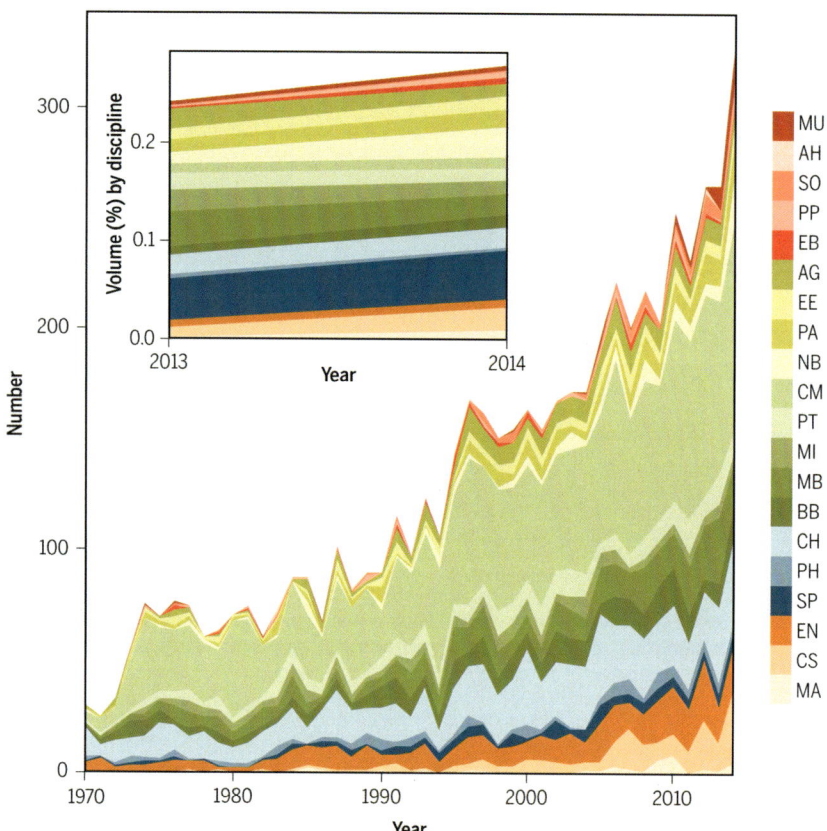

Fig. 1. Reports rising. Number of publications recorded in Scopus that have, in the title or abstract, at least one of the following expressions: research reproducibility, reproducibility of research, reproducibility of results, results reproducibility, reproducibility of study, study reproducibility, reproducible research, reproducible finding, or reproducible result. Papers are classified by discipline on the basis of the journal, following an adaptation and expansion of Thomson Reuters' Essential Science Indicators classification system. Journals not included in the latter database were hand-classified on the basis of their name. The subplot reports the percentage over the total number of records for each discipline, in the last 2 years of the series. Disciplines legend: MA, mathematics; CS, computer sciences; EN, engineering; SP, space science; PH, physics; CH, chemistry; BB, biology and biochemistry; MB, molecular biology; MI, microbiology; PT, pharmacology and toxicology; CM, clinical medicine; NB, neurobiology and behavior; PA, plant and animal sciences; EE, environment and ecology; AG, agricultural sciences; EB, economics and business; PP, psychology and psychiatry; SO, social sciences, general; AH, arts and humanities; MU, multidisciplinary. The time series was truncated at 2014.

to handle the role of chance, the level of certainty required for making published claims, and the adopted criteria for "proof" (Table 1) (*11*).

Methods reproducibility is meant to capture the original meaning of reproducibility, that is, the ability to implement, as exactly as possible, the experimental and computational procedures, with the same data and tools, to obtain the same results. Results reproducibility refers to what was previously described as "replication," that is, the production of corroborating results in a new study, having followed

the same experimental methods. Inferential reproducibility, not often recognized as a separate concept, is the making of knowledge claims of similar strength from a study replication or reanalysis. This is not identical to results reproducibility, because not all investigators will draw the same conclusions from the same results, or they might make different analytical choices that lead to different inferences from the same data. Here, we explore the definitions and operational complexities of each of these concepts.

Methods reproducibility

Methods reproducibility refers to the provision of enough detail about study procedures and data so the same procedures could, in theory or in actuality, be exactly repeated. Operationally, this can mean different things in different sciences. In the biomedical sciences, this means, at minimum, a detailed study protocol, a description of measurement procedures, the data gathered, the data used for analysis with descriptive metadata, the analysis software and code, and the final analytical results. In laboratory science, how key reagents and biological materials were created or obtained can be critical. In theory, these requirements are clear, but in practice, the level of procedural detail needed to describe a study as "methodologically reproducible" does not have consensus. For example, the detection of batch effects, which have been responsible for a number of high-visibility claims and retractions, can require information on exactly which samples were tested on which machine in what order and on what day, together with calibration data. This level of detail is typically not provided in publications and is not always retained by the investigator.

In the clinical sciences, the definition of which data need to be examined to ensure reproducibility can be contentious. The relevant data could be anywhere along the continuum from the initial raw measurement (such as a pathology slide or image), to the interpretation of those data (the pathologic diagnosis), to the coded data in the computer analytic file. Many judgments and choices are made along this path and in the processes of data cleaning and transformation that can be critical in determining analytical results. Last, even if there is consensus on the appropriate analytical data set, methodologic reproducibility requires an understanding of which and how many analyses were performed and how the particular analyses reported in a published paper were chosen. So, whether a particular study is to be considered methodologically reproducible is contingent on whether there is general agreement about the level of detail needed in the description of the measurement process, the degree of processing of the raw data, and the completeness of the analytic reporting.

Results reproducibility

Results reproducibility (previously described as replicability) refers to obtaining the same results from the conduct of an independent study whose procedures are as closely matched

PERSPECTIVE

Table 1. Examples of differences that affect the approach to reproducibility in distinct scientific domains.

Degree of determinism

Signal to measurement-error ratio

Complexity of designs and measurement tools

Closeness of fit between hypothesis and experimental design or data

Statistical or analytic methods to test hypotheses

Typical heterogeneity of experimental results

Culture of replication, transparency, and cumulating knowledge

Statistical criteria for truth claims

Purposes to which findings will be put and consequences of false conclusions

to the original experiment as possible. As with methods reproducibility, this might be clear in principle but is operationally elusive. The problem arises in settings where there is substantial random error in any result, making unclear the criteria for considering results to be "the same." The intuition and logic of results reproducibility are derived from systems that are deterministic or for which the signal-to-error ratio is exceedingly high. But, when the same intuition and logic are applied to studies with substantive stochastic components, the paradigm of accumulating evidence might be more appropriate than any binary criteria for successful or unsuccessful replication.

In a deterministic system (for example, computational research), the outcome is determined by the initial conditions. Methods reproducibility is often demonstrated through results reproducibility because the two are linked by determinacy—the signal-to-noise ratio is effectively infinite. A single failure to reproduce the original results with identical inputs casts doubt on the methodology and on any predictions (*12*).

Closely related is a proof-of-principle study, which demonstrates a new phenomenon not previously observed; for example, delivery of the first normal, live-born infant derived from in vitro fertilization or a first case of human limb regeneration would be sufficient to show that such phenomena are possible. That said, a first demonstration will not be accepted without intensive, independent scrutiny of the methods employed and the outcomes claimed, in order to rule out the possibility of misconduct, selective reporting, or procedural compromise. Failure to replicate the phenome-

non under circumstances that preclude ancillary causes (for example, mistaken diagnosis, faulty procedures, measurement error, biased design, or fraud) constitutes effective disproof of the original claim. This type of scrutiny helped debunk claims of cold fusion (*13*) and pluripotent stem cell creation (*14*).

The bright-line logic of deterministic and proof-of-principle studies is superficially mimicked through statistical significance testing; findings that are statistically significant are often regarded either as literally true or, at least, as justifying a knowledge claim, and those that aren't are regarded as either confirming the null hypothesis or inconclusive. However, it is inappropriate to combine null hypothesis–significance testing with intuition from fields of science with determinacy or very high signal-to-noise ratios. Statistical significance by itself tells very little about whether one study has "replicated" the results of another. For example, two studies that show identical 10% survival differences between the treatment and control arms would have very different degrees of statistical significance if their sample sizes were substantially different. If one was highly significant and the other far from significance, the two studies might be reported individually as supporting opposite conclusions, in spite of the fact that they are mutually corroborative.

An interpretive error complementary to the one described above involves the assumption that multiple studies that fail to demonstrate statistical significance necessarily confirm the absence of an effect. This fallacy was demonstrated, for example, in a well-known early meta-analysis of the effect of tamoxifen on breast cancer survival (*15*). (Meta-analysis is the mathematical pooling of results of multiple independent studies that investigate the same research question.) In this pooled analysis, 25 of 26 individual studies of tamoxifen's effect were not statistically significant. Naïvely, these nonsignificant findings could be described as having been replicated 25 times. Yet, when properly pooled, they cumulatively added up to a definitive rejection of the null hypothesis with a highly statistically significant 20% reduction in mortality. So the proper approach to interpreting the evidential meaning of independent studies is not to assess whether or not statistical significance has been observed in each, but rather to assess their cumulative evidential weight.

The above example involved randomized experiments without major bias. If major biases are at play, having multiple statistically

significant studies and even a statistically significant summary result for a meta-analysis does not guarantee that a genuine effect exists. For example, many studies on single nutrients and even their meta-analyses show significant associations with cancer or death risk, but most reflect confounding and reporting biases (*16*). What matters in such scientific fields is not replication defined by the presence or absence of statistical significance, but the evaluation of the cumulative evidence and assessment of whether it is susceptible to major biases, due to either the study design or the self-selection of subjects in ways that are unknown or not measurable.

It is easier to statistically define nonreplication than replication, through statistical tests of heterogeneity, which can evaluate whether the difference between two or more experimental results might be due to the play of chance. Two or more studies are judged to be statistically heterogeneous when the between-study variance in reported effects is substantially greater than what is expected from sampling error. Such tests, however, are greatly underpowered and therefore unreliable when comparing several studies, particularly when they are small or imprecise (*17*). Conversely, when there are many large studies, tests for heterogeneity might demonstrate statistical heterogeneity (and, therefore, lack of results reproducibility) even if the effect sizes of different studies are close (*17*) and regarded as scientifically equivalent. Therefore, a preferred way to assess the evidential meaning of two or more results with substantive stochastic variability is to evaluate the cumulative evidence they provide vis-á-vis a hypothesis of interest and not whether one contradicts or discredits the other through the lens of statistical significance.

Whether experiments can be pooled to provide cumulative evidence depends further on which features of a study or results are considered scientifically equivalent enough to pool. For example, in a recent replication effort of the anti-Leishmania activity of tested peptides, it was difficult to tell whether replication had been achieved or not; the peptides were found to have anti-Leishmania activity, but at concentrations 10 to 50 higher than in the original experiments and close to the toxicity range of eukaryotic human cells (*18*). Rejection of the null hypothesis in the two sets of experiments was insufficient to garner consensus about results reproducibility when consensus was missing about the operational scientific question, that is, whether the peptides had activity at low (and clinically relevant) con-

PERSPECTIVE

centrations or at any concentration. These experiments could be regarded as conflicting on the first question and mutually supportive on the second, so the question of results reproducibility is always dependent on the specificity of the underlying scientific question.

In the absence of a consensus on what constitutes successful results reproduction, investigators employ a range of operational definitions, as occurred in the case of the evaluation of the (results) reproducibility of 100 psychology studies conducted by the Open Science Collaboration (2). They acknowledged the lack of an accepted definition and so examined the studies from a variety of perspectives: significance levels, effect sizes, the number of studies whose effect size was within the confidence interval of another selected study, whether the combined estimate of the original and replication studies was statistically significant and finally, a "subjective assessment" of reproducibility. The lack of a single accepted definition opened the door to controversy about their methodological approach and conclusions (19).

Robustness and generalizability

We briefly introduce these terms because they are sometimes used in lieu of the term reproducibility. Robustness refers to the stability of experimental conclusions to variations in either baseline assumptions or experimental procedures. It is somewhat related to the concept of generalizability (also known as transportability), which refers to the persistence of an effect in settings different from and outside of an experimental framework. The issue of generalizability arises in clinical trials and other types of studies in which the context of how an intervention is delivered and the types of subjects tested are highly relevant. When a universal property of nature or biology is being explored, generalizability is often assumed, and the concept of robustness of a finding to minor variations in experimental procedures is more frequently invoked. Whether a study design is similar enough to the original to be considered a replication, a "robustness test," or some of many variations of pure replication that have been identified, particularly in the social sciences (for example, conceptual replication, pseudoreplication), is an unsettled question (12).

Inferential reproducibility

This dimension of reproducibility, while underrecognized, might be the most important one. It refers to the drawing of qualitatively similar conclusions from either an independent replication of a study or a reanalysis of the original study. Inferential reproducibility is not identical to results reproducibility or to methods reproducibility, because scientists might draw the same conclusions from different sets of studies and data or could draw different conclusions from the same original data, sometimes even if they agree on the analytical results. The aforementioned debate about the interpretation of the psychology reproducibility results could be seen as an example of this (19). There are many contributors to these differences, including different assessments of the prior probability of the hypotheses being explored—which can only be examined through a Bayesian lens—and different choices about how to analyze and report data, which we will discuss under the general rubric of "multiplicity."

Bayesian perspectives. What scientists and science users are really concerned about when they debate research reproducibility is the truth of research claims. Research reproducibility and other related concepts can be regarded as ways to operationalize truth. To express this informally, if a finding can be reliably repeated, it is likely to be true, and if it cannot be, its truth is in question (20). Unfortunately, the standard frequentist approach to statistics does not allow the assigning of a probability of truth to a hypothesis or claim (21). However, the philosophy underlying Bayesian statistics does: The probability that a claim is true after an experiment is a function of the strength of the new experimental evidence combined with how likely it was to be true before the experiment. Viewed through this lens, the aim of repeated experimentation is to increase the amount of evidence, measured on a continuous scale, either for or against the original claim.

How much evidence needs to be gathered for effective proof depends on the prior probability of the original hypothesis, which itself depends on prior evidence. If a hypothesis is highly unlikely a priori, such as the presence of extrasensory perception or the therapeutic effect of homeopathy, a large amount of high-quality evidence would have to be gathered to outweigh the very strong prior reasons to view such claims skeptically (22, 23). Conversely, for a hypothesis based on a plausible, coherent, and robust body of prior work, such as the research that preceded the development of imatinib for leukemia (24), a claim is more likely to be true both before and after an experiment that supports it. Under the

Bayesian paradigm, every study contributes evidence that adds to the prior evidence, represented by the a priori probability of truth of a given claim. Reproducibility plays no formal role except that repeated experiments with similar findings will generate strong cumulative evidence, which can confirm or refute an initial finding.

A hybrid Bayesian-frequentist index that captures the traditional notion of results reproducibility is predictive power: the probability that, given a result in one experiment, the next experiment of specified design will be statistically significant. This probability has been dubbed the replication (25) or reproducibility probability (26). After a significant result, this probability is typically far lower than most scientists suspect, due to the random variation of the P value. This phenomenon shows that the failure to observe a significant result in a second experiment of similar design is to be expected and cannot be used as a criterion to undermine the credibility of the first experiment (25–28).

Multiplicity. Multiplicity, combined with incomplete reporting, might be the single largest contributor to the phenomenon of nonreproducibility, or falsity, of published claims. Multiplicity can arise in many ways, including testing many hypotheses in one experiment, testing one hypothesis many times or in multiple ways in one or more studies, and other maneuvers that virtually guarantee a chance observation that will appear to strongly support some hypotheses. A diverse vocabulary has developed in various fields for the biases or practices that can mislead because of multiplicity (Table 2). These range from the conduct of multiple experiments (and reporting only "good" ones) to the use of multiple endpoints, multiple predictors, and, perhaps most invisibly, the fitting of many mathematical or statistical models. Coupled with incomplete or selective reporting, these practices are a formula for generating findings unlikely to be supported by further experimentation. However, the adverse effects of multiplicity can be greatly ameliorated through complete reporting of analytical procedures and choices (for example, reporting the total number of associations tested or models considered).

These practices are likely to thrive when there is low consensus on the correct methodology and what is considered sufficiently complete reporting. Many scientific fields have seen an increasing burden of multiplicity,

PERSPECTIVE

Table 2. Terminology to describe practices that introduce or hide multiplicity.

Multiple comparisons (many statisticians)

File-drawer problem (29)

Pseudoreplication (32)

Significance questing (33)

Data mining, dredging, torturing (34)

Hypothesizing after the results are known (HARKing) (30)

Data snooping (35)

Selective outcome reporting (36)

Silent multiplicity (37)

Specification searching (38)

P-hacking (31)

because they have expanded their capacity to measure more variables and to fit increasingly complex models. Scientific fields that routinely work with multiple hypotheses without correcting for or reporting the occurrence of multiplicity run a higher risk of non-reproducibility of results or inferences.

A variety of old and new practices that are described as specific forms of bias actually result from multiplicity. The classic file-drawer publication bias problem (wherein non-significant or "uninteresting" results are not published) (29) results in bias under the assumption that multiple studies are being produced independently but a biased sample is published. The acronym "HARKing"—hypothesizing after the results are known—is used in psychology literature to indicate the phenomenon of constructing hypotheses after the data are analyzed, suggesting that only one hypothesis was tested while many were contemplated (30). The practice of P-hacking, a term recently coined in psychology literature and applied to a long-recognized phenomenon in modeling, refers to applying multiple statistical analyses and subanalyses until hitting upon and reporting a statistically significant result while not completely reporting how it was obtained (31).

Ultimately, inferential reproducibility might be an unattainable ideal, and in some situations not even a desirable one, because differences between scientists and their interpretations of a single or multiple studies are the means through which weaknesses or gaps in the evidence base are identified and science progresses. What is clear, however, is that none

of these types of reproducibility can be assessed without complete reporting of all relevant aspects of scientific design, conduct, measurements, data, and analysis. Such transparency will allow scientists to evaluate the weight of evidence provided by any given study more quickly and reliably and design a higher proportion of future studies to address actual knowledge gaps or to effectively strengthen cumulative evidence, rather than explore blind alleys suggested by research inadequately conducted or reported.

CONCLUSIONS

The lexicon of reproducibility to date has been multifarious and ill-defined. The causes of and remedies for what is called poor reproducibility, in any scientific field, require a clear specification of the kind of reproducibility being discussed (methods, results, or inferences), a proper understanding of how it affects knowledge claims, scientific investigation of its causes, and an improved understanding of the limitations of statistical significance as a criterion for claims. Many aspects of the new interest in research reproducibility have been salutary, but we need to move toward a better understanding of the relationship between reproducibility, cumulative evidence, and the truth of scientific claims.

REFERENCES AND NOTES

1. C. G. Begley, An unappreciated challenge to oncology drug discovery: Pitfalls in preclinical research. *Am. Soc. Clin. Oncol. Educ. Book* 466–468 (2013).
2. Open Science Collaboration, Estimating the reproducibility of psychological science. *Science* **349**, aac4716 (2015).
3. C. G. Begley, J. P. A. Ioannidis, Reproducibility in science: Improving the standard for basic and preclinical research. *Circ. Res.* **116**, 116–126 (2015).
4. J. Claerbout, M. Karrenbach, Electronic documents give reproducible research a new meaning, in *Proceedings of the 62nd Annual International Meeting of the Society of Exploration Geophysics*, New Orleans, USA, 25 to 29 October 1992.
5. R. D. Peng, F. Dominici, S. L. Zeger, Reproducible epidemiologic research. *Am. J. Epidemiol.* **163**, 783–789 (2006).
6. E. Afgan, D. Baker, M. van den Beek, D. Blankenberg, D. Bouvier, M. Čech, J. Chilton, D. Clements, N. Coraor, C. Eberhard, B. Grüning, A. Guerler, J. Hillman-Jackson, G. Von Kuster, E. Rasche, N. Soranzo, N. Turaga, J. Taylor, A. Nekrutenko, J. Goecks, The Galaxy platform for accessible, reproducible and collaborative biomedical analyses: 2016 update. *Nucleic Acids Res.* 10.1093/nar/gkw343 (2016).
7. J. Ioannidis, C. Doucouliagos, What's to know about the credibility of empirical economics? *J. Econ. Surv.* **27**, 997–1004 (2013).
8. B. Lo, Sharing clinical trial data: Maximizing benefits, minimizing risk. *JAMA* **313**, 793–794 (2015).
9. K. Bollen, J. T. Cacioppo, R. Kaplan, J. Krosnick, J. L. Olds, *Social, Behavioral, and Economic Sciences Perspectives on*

Robust and Reliable Science (National Science Foundation, Arlington, VA, 2015).
10. F. S. Collins, L. A. Tabak, Policy: NIH plans to enhance reproducibility. *Nature* **505**, 612–613 (2014).
11. D. Fanelli, W. Glänzel, Bibliometric evidence for a hierarchy of the sciences. *PLOS One* **8**, e66938 (2013).
12. M. A. Clemens, The meaning of failed replications: A review and proposal. *J. Econ. Surv.* 10.1111/joes.12139 (2015).
13. B. V. Lewenstein, W. Baur, A cold fusion chronology. *J. Radioanal. Nucl. Ch.* **152**, 273–297 (1991).
14. A. De Los Angeles, F. Ferrari, Y. Fujiwara, R. Mathieu, S. Lee, S. Lee, H.-C. Tu, S. Ross, S. Chou, M. Nguyen, Z. Wu, T. W. Theunissen, B. E. Powell, S. Imsoonthornruksa, J. Chen, M. Borkent, V. Krupalnik, E. Lujan, M. Wernig, J. H. Hanna, K. Hochedlinger, D. Pei, R. Jaenisch, H. Deng, S. H. Orkin, P. J. Park, G. Q. Daley, Failure to replicate the STAP cell phenomenon. *Nature* **525**, E6–E9 (2015).
15. Early Breast Cancer Trialists' Collaborative Group, Effects of adjuvant tamoxifen and of cytotoxic therapy on mortality in early breast cancer. An overview of 61 randomized trials among 28,896 women. *N. Engl. J. Med.* **319**, 1681–1692 (1988).
16. J. D. Schoenfeld, J. P. A. Ioannidis, Is everything we eat associated with cancer? A systematic cookbook review. *Am. J. Clin. Nutr.* **97**, 127–134 (2013).
17. R. J. Hardy, S. G. Thompson, Detecting and describing heterogeneity in meta-analysis. *Stat. Med.* **17**, 841–856 (1998).
18. E. Iorns, W. Gunn, J. Erath, A. Rodriguez, J. Zhou, M. Benzinou, The Reproducibility Initiative, Replication attempt: "Effect of BMAP-28 antimicrobial peptides on Leishmania major promastigote and amastigote growth: Role of leishmanolysin in parasite survival." *PLOS One* **9**, e114614 (2014).
19. D. T. Gilbert, G. King, S. Pettigrew, T. D. Wilson, Comment on "Estimating the reproducibility of psychological science". *Science* **351**, 1037 (2016).
20. S. N. Goodman, Toward evidence-based medical statistics. 2: The Bayes factor. *Ann. Intern. Med.* **130**, 1005–1013 (1999).
21. S. N. Goodman, Toward evidence-based medical statistics. 1: The *P* value fallacy. *Ann. Intern. Med.* **130**, 995–1004 (1999).
22. J. N. Rouder, R. D. Morey, A Bayes factor meta-analysis of Bem's ESP claim. *Psychon. Bull. Rev.* **18**, 682–689 (2011).
23. S. N. Goodman, J. Gerson, *Mechanistic Evidence in Evidence-Based Medicine: A Conceptual Framework* (Agency for Healthcare Research and Quality, Rockville, MD, 2013); http://www.ncbi.nlm.nih.gov/books/NBK154584/.
24. P. Keating, A. Cambrosio, *Cancer on Trial: Oncology as a New Style of Practice* (University of Chicago Press, Chicago, 2011).
25. S. N. Goodman, A comment on replication, *P*-values and evidence. *Stat. Med.* **11**, 875–879 (1992).
26. D. D. Boos, L. A. Stefanski, *P*-value precision and reproducibility. *Am. Stat.* **65**, 213–221 (2011).
27. A. Gelman, H. Stern, The difference between "significant" and "not significant" is not itself statistically significant. *Am. Stat.* **60**, 328–331 (2006).
28. L. C. Lazzeroni, Y. Lu, I. Belitskaya-Lévy, Solutions for quantifying *P*-value uncertainty and replication power. *Nat. Methods* **13**, 107–108 (2016).
29. R. Rosenthal, The file drawer problem and tolerance for null results. *Psychol. Bull.* **86**, 638–641 (1979).
30. N. L. Kerr, HARKing: Hypothesizing after the results are known. *Pers. Soc. Psychol. Rev.* **2**, 196–217 (1998).
31. U. Simonsohn, L. D. Nelson, J. P. Simmons, P-curve: A key to the file-drawer. *J. Exp. Psychol. Gen.* **143**, 534–547 (2014).

32. S. H. Hurlbert, Pseudoreplication and the design of ecological field experiments. *Ecol. Monogr.* **54**, 187–211 (1984).
33. K. J. Rothman, Significance questing. *Ann. Intern. Med.* **105**, 445–447 (1986).
34. J.L. Mills, Data torturing. *N. Engl. J. Med.* **329**, 1196–1199 (1993).
35. H. White, A reality check for data snooping. *Econometrica* **68**, 1097–1126 (2000).
36. A.-W. Chan, A. Hróbjartsson, M. T. Haahr, P. C. Gøtzsche, D. G. Altman, Empirical evidence for selective reporting of outcomes in randomized trials: Comparison of protocols to published articles. *JAMA* **291**, 2457–2465 (2004).
37. D. Berry, Multiplicities in cancer research: Ubiquitous and necessary evils. *J. Natl. Cancer Inst.* **104**, 1125–1133 (2012).
38. E. E. Leamer, *Specification Searches: Ad Hoc Inference with Nonexperimental Data* (Wiley, Hoboken, NJ, 1978).

Funding: This work was funded by a grant by from the John and Laura Arnold Foundation. **Competing interests:** The authors declare that they have no competing interests.

10.1126/scitranslmed.aaf5027

Citation: S. N. Goodman, D. Fanelli, J. P. A. Ioannidis, What does research reproducibility mean? *Sci. Transl. Med.* **8**, 341ps12 (2016).

3.2 Limited Reproducibility of Research Findings: Implications for the Welfare of Research Participants and Considerations for Institutional Review Boards

Barbara K. Redman and Arthur L. Caplan

This article was originally published in in IRB: Ethics & Human Research. Reprinted with permission from IRB: Ethics & Human Research and the Hastings Center.

Redman BK, Caplan AL. Limited reproducibility of research findings: Implications for the welfare of research participants and considerations for institutional review boards. IRB: Ethics & Human Research. 2016;38(4):8–10.

BY BARBARA K. REDMAN AND ARTHUR L. CAPLAN

Limited Reproducibility of Research Findings: Implications for the Welfare of Research Participants and Considerations for Institutional Review Boards

In a number of biomedical science fields, a lack of reproducibility of research results has caused alarm about wasted resources, both human and financial.[1] The inability to replicate findings has significant implications not only for the reliability of science but also for research subjects. A problem that has not drawn sufficient attention is that flawed irreproducible science can also have a negative impact on the welfare of prospective research participants by interfering with risk minimization and risk-benefit comparison, especially when participants are from vulnerable populations.

"Reproducibility" is an umbrella term covering repeatability (the question of whether repeating an original study yields the same findings), replicability (whether different data sets and their accumulation in meta-analyses by independent investigators yield the same findings),[2] and what is called "validation" (a general term for consistency with laboratory and clinical tests, guidelines, or predictive measurement instruments). Some estimates show that only 22% to 23% of published results in the biomedical sciences can be validated.[3] Others suggest that fewer than half can be.[4] There are numerous possible reasons for the inability to reproduce research methods and findings: unrecognized study variables, poor study design, poor documentation of findings, outcome reporting bias that falsely inflates the benefits of a new study, inadequate statistical analyses of study data, investigators' errors or research misconduct, and omission of Food and Drug Administration findings of data falsification or fabrication in the peer-reviewed literature.[5]

Lack of reproducibility by independent investigators may signal that research misconduct took place and that, as a result of fraudulent data, current research

participants and subsequent patients could be harmed if research and medical practices are based on such data. For example, charges of data fabrication and research misconduct have been raised against a researcher who published a family of studies about perioperative use of beta blockers for noncardiac surgery in patients with ischemic heart disease. The findings of these studies had been incorporated into practice guidelines even though systematic reviews six years earlier had identified effect sizes too large to be true.[6] Later analysis revealed that use of these medications appeared to significantly increase perioperative mortality.[7] Attempts to replicate this family of studies should have occurred much earlier, when systematic reviews revealed danger signals.

Core protections for research participants—a reasonable risk-benefit ratio, the existence of equipoise, and voluntary participation based on informed consent—assume that the research results of prior research upon which a new study is justified are valid and reproducible. With no system in place to detect that evidentiary claims justifying new studies with research participants cannot be reproduced, there is the danger of a cumulative inaccurate risk-benefit profile that could result in research-related harms to study participants.

Efforts to undertake reproducibility studies are proceeding on many fronts. For example, distressed by a lack of therapies reporting successful interventions for spinal cord injury (SCI), the National Institute of Neurological Disorders and Stroke recently funded studies to replicate several published studies.[8] Concurrently, a group of researchers established rigorously defined standard data for experiments using animal models to guide SCI research with humans.[9] Poor reproducibility caused by misidentification or contamination of cell lines is being addressed with newly required validation procedures.[10] Stunned by a series of high-profile cases

Redman BK and Caplan AL. Limited reproducibility of research findings: Implications for the welfare of research participants and considerations for institutional review boards. IRB: Ethics & Human Research 2016;38(4):8-10.

of research misconduct, leading researchers in social psychology organized initiatives to replicate published studies in their field. Of the 100 prominent papers analyzed, only 39% could be replicated unambiguously.[11] And to provide a basis upon which researchers can undertake replication studies, several journals are beginning to demand that for the peer-review process, authors submit their full data sets along with their manuscripts.

Limited reproducibility is a risk those charged with the protection of research participants need to be aware of and seek to address. Institutional review boards (IRBs) ought to require that research protocols contain explicit probability statements about likely risks and benefits, based on a comprehensive review of prior studies and meta-analyses addressing reproducibility. Such estimates are essential for IRB judgment about minimizing risk, for determining an appropriate risk-benefit ratio for presentation as a part of the informed consent process, and in seeking to facilitate the informed choices of potential research subjects.

Cumulative meta-analyses can help document the degree of reproducibility in prior trials. When researchers submit their protocol for research with humans for IRB review, they should be required to include the results of a search for such studies, as is the case for researchers conducting studies with animals.[12] Such summaries should include the risks and benefits that prior studies identified, including what is known about the likelihood, magnitude, and duration of research risks. This information will be useful in addressing whether the proposed trial will correct methodological or other issues from past trials and will contribute to improving reproducibility. Information from cumulative meta-analysis may also be useful if, during the course of the trial, information from other studies alters the initial risk-benefit ratio. For instance, a summary of more than 1500 cumulative meta-analyses of clinical intervention studies showed that systematic assessment by researchers of what was already known and replicated could have resulted in less exposure of trial participants to less effective treatments and in some instances could have undermined the rationale for new trials.[13]

In addition, concerns about serious flaws in the reliability of reagents such as antibodies could lead an IRB to require that the proposal outline steps to be taken to ensure their specificity. Rigorous experimental design and transparency in reporting specifics of data collection and analysis not only undergird reproduc-

ible science but also protect current and future research participants from unnecessary risk.

Research participants reasonably expect that their contribution to scientific research will yield progress in knowledge to solve a problem. Since prior irreproducibility can undermine this goal, it is incumbent on researchers and IRBs to flag, as best they can, concerns about reproducibility. Through their ability to obtain input from various experts, IRBs must do their best to seek evidence of reproducibility or lack of it in the line of research for individual protocols they are being asked to approve. Indeed, IRBs are more frequently being asked to judge the validity of findings from preclinical animal studies so as to make more reliable judgments about the potential risks and benefits of

With no system in place to detect that evidentiary claims justifying new studies with research participants cannot be reproduced, there is the danger of a cumulative inaccurate risk-benefit profile that could result in research-related harms to study participants.

translational trials with humans.[14] These efforts and those to assess and improve reproducibility follow from acknowledgment that scientific validity is a basic ethical requirement of research.[15] Of special concern are the high percentage of positive research findings reported in the literature and the under-reporting of harms, which make the IRB's responsibility to minimize risks and ensure reasonable risks in relation to anticipated benefits all the more difficult.

Researchers tend to overestimate potential benefits and underestimate risks, and individuals frequently don't fully understand the consequences of participating in research, making IRB protection essential. Yet one study found that research ethics committees (RECs) in Europe did not have a clear and systematic approach toward assessment of proportionality of research risks.[16] Incorporating reproducibility into REC or IRB performance can help to systematize a more rigorous estimate of proportionality.

Other research has documented that IRBs are confused about whether and how to assess the quality of the science of proposed studies and that IRB members vary in the extent to which they feel that they can ask researchers to alter a study protocol to improve the scientific quality of the research.[17] While clarification from regulators would be helpful,[18] given the evidence of the need for data from replicated studies, institutions should encourage their IRBs to conduct rigorous scientific analyses of protocols on their own or in conjunction with separate scientific review bodies.

The reproducibility issue regarding the family of beta blocker studies and other research whose results have not been replicated demonstrate an urgent need for a rapid-response safety system to apprise IRBs of concerns about reproducibility that may be associated with unexpected serious harm to research participants.[19] Research funders like the National Institutes of Health are calling for stakeholders to take the steps necessary to reset the self-corrective process of scientific inquiry.[20] In the meantime, as the entities that are required to protect the welfare of research participants, IRBs need to recognize the problem of reproducibility and take what steps they can to ensure that the studies individuals are recruited to participate in are designed and carried out on the basis of valid prior scientific findings.

■ **Barbara K. Redman, PhD, MBE,** is an associate of the Division of Medical Ethics at New York University Langone Medical Center, and **Arthur L. Caplan, PhD,** is the director of the Division of Medical Ethics at New York University Langone Medical Center.

References

1. Ioannidis J. How to make more published research true. *PLoS Medicine* 2014;11(10):1001747.
2. Dolgin E. Drug discoverers chart path to tackling data irreproducibility. *Nature Reviews Drug Discovery* 2014;13:875-876.
3. Ioannidis J. How not to be wrong. *New Scientist* 2014;22:32-33.
4. Ioannidis J. Improving validation practices in "omics" research. *Science* 2011;334:1230-1232.
5. Seife C. Research misconduct identified by the US Food and Drug Administration: Out of sight, out of the peer-reviewed literature. *JAMA Internal Medicine* 2015;175:567-577.
6. Chopra V, Eagle KA. Perioperative mischief: The price of academic misconduct. *American Journal of Medicine* 2012;125:953-955.
7. Bouri S, Shun-Shin M, Cole GD, et al. Meta-analyses of secure randomized controlled trials of beta-blockers to prevent perioperative death in non-cardiac surgery. *Heart* 2014;100:456-464.
8. Steward O, Popovich P, Diedtrich W, et al. Replication and reproducibility in spinal cord injury research. *Experimental Neurology* 2012;233:597-605.
9. Lemmon V, Ferguson AR, Popovich PG, et al. Minimum information about spinal cord injury experiment. *Journal of Neurotrauma* 2014;31:1-8.
10. Lorsch JR, Collins FS, Lippincott-Schwartz J. Fixing problems with cell biology. *Science* 2014;346:1452-1453.
11. Bohannon J. Many psychology papers fail replication test. *Science* 2015;349:910-911.
12. Animal Welfare Act 9 CFR Pt 1. Section 2.31diii.
13. Clark M, Brice A, Chalmers I. Accumulating research: A systematic account of how cumulative meta-analyses would have provided knowledge, improved health, reduced harm and saved resources. *PLoS One* 2014;9(7):e102670.
14. Kimmelman J, London AJ. Predicting harms and benefits in translational trials: Ethics and uncertainty. *PLoS Medicine* 2011;8(3):e1001011.
15. Borgerson K. Redundant, secretive, and isolated: When are clinical trials scientifically valid? *Kennedy Institute of Ethics Journal* 2014;24(4):385-411.
16. Simonsen, S. *Acceptable Risk in Biomedical Research: European Perspectives*. New York: Springer, 2012.
17. Klitzman, R. How good does the science have to be in proposals submitted to IRBs? *Clinical Trials* 2013;10(5):761-766.
18. See ref.17, Klitzman 2013.
19. Neuman M, Bosk C, Fleisher L. Learning from mistakes in clinical practice guidelines: The case of perioperative beta-blockade. *BMJ Quality and Safety* 2014;23:957-964.
20. Collins FS, Tabak LA. NIH plans to enhance reproducibility. *Nature* 2014;505:612-613.

3.3   Quality Time

Monya Baker

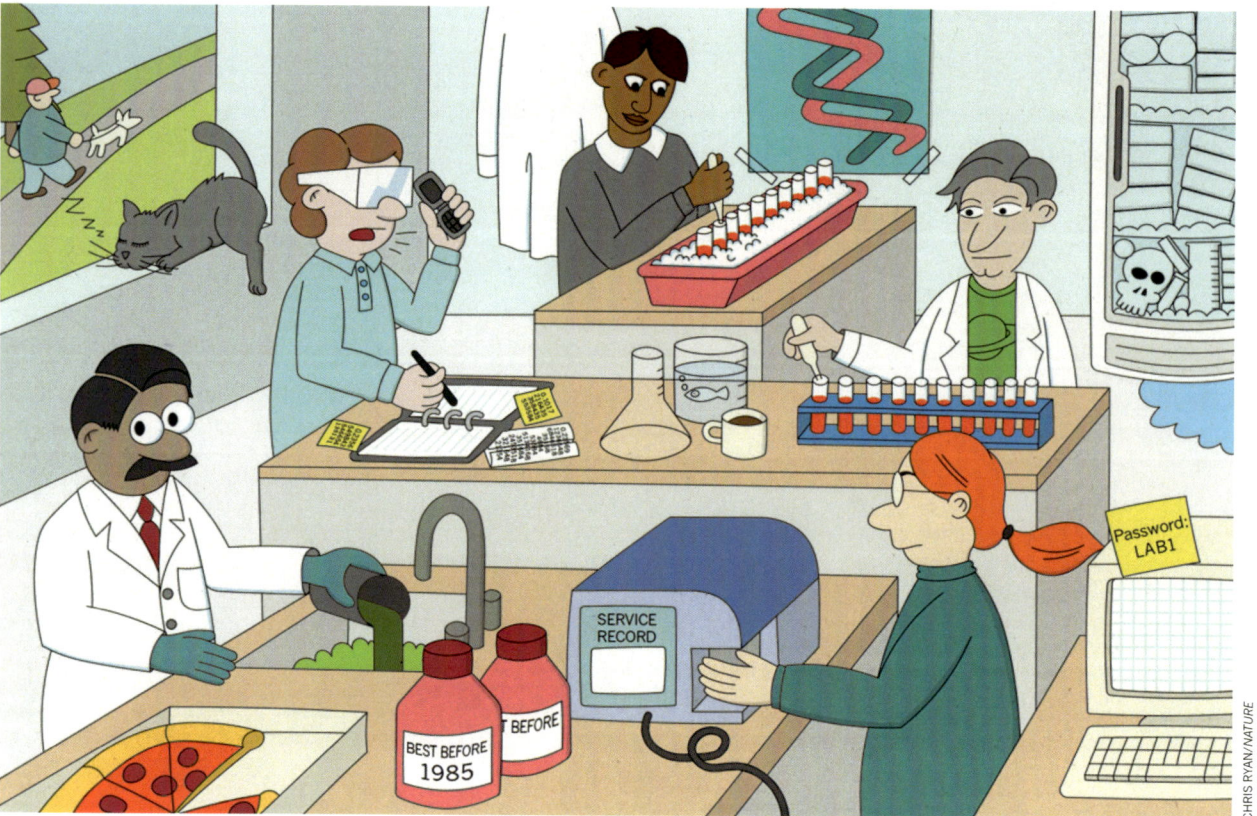

There are at least six things in this picture that a quality-assurance manager would try to improve. Can you spot them?

QUALITY TIME

IT MAY NOT BE SEXY, BUT QUALITY ASSURANCE IS BECOMING A CRUCIAL PART OF LAB LIFE.

BY MONYA BAKER

R ebecca Davies remembers a time when quality assurance terrified her. In 2007, she had been asked to lead accreditation efforts at the University of Minnesota's Veterinary Diagnostic Laboratory in Saint Paul. The lab needed to ensure that the tens of thousands of tests it conducts to monitor disease in pets, poultry, livestock and wildlife were watertight. "It was a huge task. I felt sick to my stomach," recalls Davies, an endocrinologist at the university's College of Veterinary Medicine.

She nevertheless accepted the challenge, and soon found herself hooked on finding — and fixing — problems in the research process. She and her team tracked recurring tissue-contamination issues to how containers were being filled and stored; they traced an assay's erratic performance to whether technicians let an enzyme warm to room temperature; and they established systems to eliminate spotty data collection, malfunctioning equipment and neglected controls. Her efforts were crucial to keeping the diagnostic lab in business, but they also forced her to realize how much researchers' work could improve. "That is the beauty of quality assurance," Davies says. "That is what we were missing out on as scientists."

Davies wanted to spread the word. In 2009, she got permission and financial support to launch an internal consulting group for the college, to help labs with the dry but essential work of quality assurance (QA). The group, called Quality Central, now supports more than half a dozen research labs — helping them to design systems to ensure that their equipment, materials and data are up to scratch, and helping them to improve.

She is also part of a small but growing group of professionals around the world who hope to transform basic biomedical research. Many were hired by their universities to help labs to meet certain regulatory standards, but these QA consultants have a broader vision. They are not pushing for universal adoption of formal regulatory certifications. Instead, they advocate 'voluntary QA'. With the right strategies, they argue, scientists can strengthen their research and improve reproducibility.

When Davies first started proselytizing to her fellow faculty members, the responses were not encouraging. "None of them found the idea compelling at all," Davies recalls. How important could QA be, they asked, if the US National Institutes of Health did not require it? How could anyone afford to spend money or time on non-essentials? Shouldn't they focus on the discoveries lurking in their data, and not the systems for collecting them?

But some saw the potential, based on their own experiences. Before she had heard of Quality Central, University of Minnesota virologist Montserrat Torremorell was grateful when a colleague let her use his instruments to track transmissible disease in swine. But the results made no sense. Samples from pigs experimentally infected with influenza showed extremely low levels of the virus. It turned out that her benefactor had, like many scientists, skimped on equipment maintenance to save money. "It was a real eye-opener," Torremorell recalls. "It just made me think that I could not rely on other people's equipment."

QUALITY FOR ALL

Quality systems are an integral part of most commercial goods and services, used in manufacturing everything from planes to paint. Some labs that focus on clinical applications implement certified QA systems such as Good Clinical Practice, Good Manufacturing Practice and Good Laboratory Practice for data submitted to regulatory bodies. There have also been efforts to guide research practices outside these schemes. In 2001, the World Health Organization published guidelines for QA in basic research. And in 2006, the British Association of Research Quality Assurance (now simply the RQA) in Ipswich issued guidelines for basic biomedical research. But few academic researchers know that these standards exist (Davies certainly didn't back in 2007).

Instead, QA tends to be ad hoc in academic settings. Many scientists are taught how to keep lab notebooks by their mentors, supplemented perhaps by a perfunctory training course. Investigators often improvise ways to safeguard data, maintain equipment or catalogue and care for experimental materials. Too often, data quality is as likely to be assumed as assured.

Scientific rigour has taken a drubbing in the past few years, with reports that fewer than one-third of biomedical papers can be reproduced (see *Nature* http://doi.org/477; 2015). Scientific culture, training and incentives have all been blamed for promoting sloppy work; a common refrain is that the status quo values publication counts over careful experimentation and documentation. "There is chaos in academia," says Masha Fridkis-Hareli, head of ATR, a biotechnology consultancy in Worcester, Massachusetts, that also conducts laboratory work to help move basic research into industry. For every careful researcher she has encountered, there have been others who have thought nothing of scribbling data on paper towels, repeating experiments without running controls and guessing at details months after an experiment. Davies insists that plenty of scientists are doing robust work, but there is always room for improvement (see 'Solutions'). "There are easy fixes to situations that shouldn't be happening, but are," she says.

⊃ NATURE.COM
How does your lab's
QA measure up?
go.nature.com/e6xupg

Michael Murtaugh, a swine biologist at the University of Minnesota, had tried to establish practices to beef up the reliability of his team's lab notebooks, but the attempts that he made on his own never gained traction. Then Davies got on his case. After a year or so of her "planting seeds" — as she puts it — Murtaugh agreed to work with Quality Central and implement a low-tech but effective solution.

On designated Mondays, each member of Murtaugh's lab draws a name from a paper bag to determine whose notebook to audit. The scientists check that their assigned books include relevant controls for experiments, and indicate where data are stored and which particular machine generated them. The group also makes sure that any problems noted in the previous check have been addressed. It takes about ten minutes per researcher every few weeks, but that's enough to change people's habits. Graduate student Michael Rahe says that the checks ensure that he keeps his notebook legible and up to date. "I never used to put in raw data," he says.

Albert Cirera, a technologist developing gas nanosensors at the University of Barcelona in Spain, has also embraced QA. As his lab group grew to 12 people, he found it difficult to monitor everyone's experiments, and his own efforts to implement a tracking system were inadequate. He turned to a university-based QA consulting service for help. Now, samples, equipment and their data are all linked with tracking numbers printed on stickers and recorded in individuals' notebooks, on samples and in a central tracking file. The system does not slow down experiments, and staying abreast of projects is a breeze, says Cirera. But getting to this point took about four months and frequent consultations. "It was not something that you can create from zero," he says.

> "THERE ARE EASY FIXES TO SITUATIONS THAT SHOULDN'T BE HAPPENING, BUT ARE."

MAKING A MARKET

Any scientist adopting a QA system has to wager that the up-front hassle will pay off in the future. "It is very difficult to get people to check and annotate everything, because they think it is nonsense," says Carmen Navarro-Aragay, head of the University of Barcelona quality team that worked with Cirera. "They realize the value only when they get results that they do not understand and find that the answer is lurking somewhere in their notebooks."

Even when experiments go as expected, quality systems can save time, says Murtaugh. Methods and data sections in papers practically write themselves, with no time wasted in frenzied hunting for missing information. There are fewer questions about how experiments were done and where data are stored, says Murtaugh. "It allows us to concentrate on biological explanations for results."

The more difficult data are to collect, the more important a good QA system becomes. Catherine Bens, a QA manager at Colorado State University in Fort Collins, says that she remembers getting cold, wet and dirty when she had to monitor a study involving ultrasound scans and blood samples from a population of feral horses in North Dakota. Typical animal-identification practices such as ear tagging were not allowed. So, before the collection started, Bens supported researchers as they rehearsed procedures, pre-labelled tubes, made back-up labels and recruited animal photographers and park volunteers to ensure that samples would be linked to the correct animals. Even in a snow storm with winds so loud that everyone had to shout, the team made sure that each data point could be traced.

Rare samples or not, few basic researchers are clamouring to get QA systems in place. Most are unfamiliar with the discipline, says Davies. Others are hostile. "They see it as trying to constrain them, and that you're making them do more work."

Before awarding certain grants, the Found Animals Foundation in

Los Angeles, California, which funds research on animal sterilization, requires proof that instruments have been calibrated and that written plans exist for tracing data and dealing with outliers. It can be a struggle, says Shirley Johnston, scientific director of the foundation. One grant recipient argued that QA systems were unnecessary because just looking over the data would reveal their quality.

Part of the resistance may be down to how some QA professionals present themselves. "A lot of them are there to tell you what you are doing is wrong, and a lot of them are not very nice about it," says Terry Nett, a reproductive biologist at Colorado State University who experienced this first-hand when he worked with outside consultants to incorporate Good Laboratory Practice principles in his lab. The effort was frustrating. "Instead of helping us understand, they would act like a dictator," Nett recalls. "I just didn't want them in my lab." A few years ago, however, the university hired its own quality managers, and things changed. The current manager, Bens, acts more like a partner, Nett says. She points out where labs are already using robust practices, and explains the reasoning behind QA practices that she introduces.

To win scientists over, Bens stresses that QA systems produce data that can withstand criticism. "You build a support system around any data point you collect," she says. When there is a strange result, researchers have documentation to trace its provenance. That can show whether a data point is real, an outlier or a problem — for example if a blood sample was not kept cold or was stored in the wrong tube.

Scientists need to take the lead on which QA elements they incorporate, says Melissa Eitzen, director of regulatory operations at the University of Texas Medical Branch in Galveston. "You want to give them tips that they can take or not take," she says. "If they choose it, they'll do it. If you tell them they have to do it, that's a struggle."

Rapport is paramount, says Michael Jamieson at the University of Southern California in Los Angeles, who helps other faculty members to move research towards clinical applications. Instead of talking about quality systems, he prefers to discuss concrete behaviours, such as labelling bottles with expiry dates and storage conditions. QA jargon puts scientists off, he says. "Using the term good research practice makes most researchers want to run the other way."

It's a lesson that many QA specialists have taken to heart. Some say 'assessment' or 'quality improvement' instead of 'audit'. Even 'research integrity' can be an inflammatory phrase, says Davies. "You have to find a way to communicate that QA is not punitive or guilt-inspiring."

NOT INTO TEMPTATION

Having data that are traceable — down to who did what experiment on which machine, and where the source data are stored — has knock-on benefits for research integrity, says Nett. "You can't pick out the data that you want." Researchers who must provide strong explanations about why they chose to leave any information out of their analysis will be less tempted to cherry-pick data. QA can also weed out digital meddling: popular spreadsheet programs such as Microsoft Excel can be vulnerable to errors or manipulation if not properly locked, but QA teams can set up instruments to store read-only files and prevent researchers from tampering with data accidentally or intentionally. "I can't help but think that QA is going to make fraud harder," says Davies.

And good quality systems can be contagious. Melanie Graham, who studies diabetes at the University of Minnesota, often collaborates with others to test potential treatments. More than once, she says, collaborators have sent her samples in a polystyrene tube with nothing but a single letter written on it. Graham sends it back and requests a label that specifies the sample's identity and provenance, and a range of storage temperatures. 'Keep frozen' is too vague — she will not risk

> "I CAN'T HELP BUT THINK THAT QA IS GOING TO MAKE FRAUD HARDER."

There are many things wrong with the fictitious lab shown on page 456. But, here are six that a quality-assurance manager would identify, and how they would solve them.

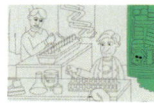
DISORGANIZED SAMPLE STORAGE
Clear labelling and proper organization are important for incubators and freezers. Everyone in the lab should be able to identify a sample, where it came from, who did what to it, how old it is and how it should be stored.

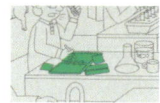
INADEQUATE DATA LOGGING
Data should be logged in a lab notebook, not scribbled onto memo paper or other detritus and carelessly transcribed. Notebooks should be bound or digital; loose paper can too easily be lost or removed.

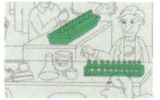
VARIABLE EXPERIMENTS
Protocols should be followed to the letter or deviations documented. If reagents need to be kept on ice while in use, each lab member must comply.

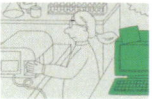
UNSECURED DATA ANALYSIS
Each lab member should have their own password for accessing and working with data, to make it clear who works on what, when. Some popular spreadsheet programs can be locked down so that manipulating data, even accidentally, is difficult.

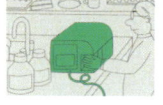
MISSED MAINTENANCE
Instruments should be calibrated and maintained according to a regular, documented schedule.

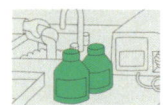
OLD AND UNDATED REAGENTS
These can affect experimental results. Scientists should specify criteria for age and storage of all important reagents.

performing uninformative experiments because reagents stored in a standard freezer were supposed to be kept at −80 °C.

When she first sent documentation requirements to collaborators, she expected them to push back. Instead, reactions were overwhelmingly positive. "It's a relief for them," says Graham. "They want us to handle their test article in a trusted way."

The benefits go beyond providing solid data. In 2013, Davies worked with Torremorell and other Minnesota faculty members on a proposal to monitor and calibrate equipment used by several labs. The plan that they put in place helped them to secure US$1.8 million to build shared lab space to deal with animal pathogens, says Torremorell. "If we want to be competitive to get funding, and if we want people to believe our data, we need to be serious about the data that we generate."

Davies is still trying to spread the word. Her invitations to give talks and review grant applications have mushroomed. She and collaborators at other institutions have been developing online training materials and offering classes to technicians, postdocs, graduate students and principal investigators. After a presentation last year, a member of the audience told her that he had reviewed a grant from one of her clients; the QA plan had made the application stand out in a positive way. Davies was delighted. "I could finally come back to my folks and say, 'It was noticed.'"

Davies knows it is still an uphill battle, but her ultimate goal is to make QA as much a part of research as peer review. It may not have the flash and dazzle of other efforts to ensure that research is robust and reproducible, but that is not the point. "A QA programme isn't sexy," says Michael Conzemius, a veterinary researcher at the University of Minnesota and another client of Quality Central. "It's just kind of become the nuts and bolts of the scientific process for us." ∎

Monya Baker *writes for* Nature *from San Francisco, California.*

References

Etz A, Vanderkerckhove J. A Bayesian perspective on the reproducibility project: psychology. PLoS One. 2016;11(2):e0149794.

Goodman SN, Fanelli D, Ioannidis JPA. What does research reproducibility mean? Sci Transl Med. 2016;8(341):1–6.

Koffel JB, Rethlefsen JL. Reproducibiity of search strategies is poor in systematic reviews published in high-impact pediatrics, cardiology and surgery journals: a cross-sectional study. PLoS One. 2016;11(9):e0163309.

Pulverer B. Reproducibility blues. EMBO J. 2015;34(22):2721–4.

Van Bavel JJ, Mende-Siedlecki P, Brady WJ, Reinero DA. Contextual sensitivity in scientific reproducibility. PNAS USA. 2016;113(23):6454–9.

Additional Suggested Reading

Begley CG, Ioannidis JPA. Reproducibility in science; improving the standard for basic and preclinical research. Circ Res. 2015;116:116–26. (*Standards for basic and preclinical research must be improved.*)

Freedman LP, Inglese J. The increasing urgency for standards in basic biologic research. Cancer Res. 2014;74(15):4024–9.

Human Subjects' Protection

4

Arthur L. Caplan and Barbara K. Redman

Federal regulations for protection of human subjects in biomedical and behavioral research have been in place since 1974. Preceded by the Belmont Report, which described ethical principles for human research, regulations known as the Common Rule (common across federal agencies) followed. They may be found at 45 CFR 46 and are administered by the Office of Human Research Protections (OHRP). Updated regulations have been approved and are expected to be in effect by early 2018.

Under these regulations, research is defined as a systematic investigation designed to produce generalizable knowledge; a human subject means a living individual involved in research (46.102). Each institution operates one or more institutional review board(s) (IRB) under policies approved by OHRP. They have the authority to approve, require modification, or disapprove research proposals; decisions are based on minimization of risk to subjects and weighed against anticipated benefits and fair subject selection. The Food and Drug Administration has similar guidelines. Detail of these requirements and description of alternative models for IRB review may be found in tables in Grady (2015). Other sources of guidance include International Ethical Guidelines for Health-related Research Involving Humans prepared by the Council for International Organizations of Medical Sciences (CIOMS), the Declaration of Helsinki by the World Medical Association, and Good Clinical Practice Guidelines by the International Conference of Harmonization.

The goal of IRB review is to assure that subjects will be protected during research. A scoping review of empirical research related to quality and effectiveness of research ethics review found no controlled trials or an underlying framework of institutional review board (IRB) effectiveness, or a systematic research agenda by which to answer these questions (Nichols et al. 2015). Literature on informed consent for research found a similar story – lack of clear evidence of potential research subjects making an informed decision. Many were thought to be enrolling in trials without an adequate understanding of fundamental concepts such as voluntariness or risks of participation, although extended one-on-one discussions appeared helpful. There are few studies of potential subjects who chose not to enroll (Hallinan et al. 2016). Despite these limitations, programs of accreditation provide evidence of quality, widely sought by IRBs.

Many institutions/trials have additional review mechanisms to assure quality. Separate scientific review committees address quality of the science and work collaboratively with the IRB. Data safety monitoring boards (DSMBs) were developed to provide close oversight of the integrity of intervention trials by ensuring objective assessment of accumulating data, monitoring trial results and data quality and safety (DeMets and Ellenberg 2016), and potentially recommending early trial termination. Neither of these mechanisms appears in federal regulations, although DSMBs may be required by funders.

Subjects protection is surely one of the most basic elements of research integrity. It requires not only a virtuous investigator who can solve ethical problems as they arise during research, but as history has taught, an effective oversight system as described above, largely structured as a form of self-regulation by peers. Now 40 years later, it is clear that the system must accommodate new issues also essential to integrity of research. These include recognition of demand on the part of potential subjects for access to clinical trials, over-protection especially of vulnerable groups such as children or prisoners which has stifled research to the groups meant to be protected, and attention to basic constructs such as risk/benefit ratio which depend as much as possible on a stable and reproducible base of prior studies.

Advice: Be informed about the research review boards (IRBs), animal care and use committees, conflict of interest, and biosafety committees in your institution. While your

4

A. L. Caplan · B. K. Redman (✉)
New York University Langone Medical Center,
New York, NY, USA
e-mail: Arthur.Caplan@nyumc.org

© Springer International Publishing AG, part of Springer Nature 2018
A. L. Caplan, B. K. Redman (eds.), *Getting to Good*, https://doi.org/10.1007/978-3-319-51358-4_4

mentor will have had much experience with them, do not hesitate to approach IRB staff during proposal preparation with your unanswered questions. It is better to get their advice now rather than after your proposal could not be approved.

4.1   A Scoping Review of Empirical Research Relating to Quality and Effectiveness of Research Ethics Review

Stuart G. Nicholls, Tavis P. Hayes, Jamie C. Brehaut, Michael McDonald, Charles Weijer, Raphael Saginur, and Dean Fergusson

Nicholls SG, Hayes TP, Brehaut JC, McDonald M, Weijer C, Saginur R, et al. (2015) AScoping Review of Empirical Research Relating to Quality and Effectiveness of Research Ethics Review. PLoS ONE 10(7): e0133639. https://doi.org/10.1371/journal.pone.0133639. Copyright: © 2015 Nicholls et al.

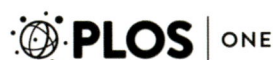

RESEARCH ARTICLE

A Scoping Review of Empirical Research Relating to Quality and Effectiveness of Research Ethics Review

Stuart G. Nicholls[1]*, Tavis P. Hayes[2], Jamie C. Brehaut[1,2], Michael McDonald[3], Charles Weijer[4], Raphael Saginur[2], Dean Fergusson[1,2]

1 School of Epidemiology, Public health and Preventive Medicine, University of Ottawa, Ottawa, Ontario, Canada, 2 Ottawa Hospital Research Institute, Clinical Epidemiology Program, Ottawa, Ontario, Canada, 3 The W. Maurice Young Centre for Applied Ethics, The University of British Columbia, Vancouver, British Columbia, Canada, 4 Rotman Institute of Philosophy, Western University, London, Ontario, Canada

* snicholl@uottawa.ca

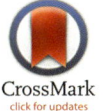

CrossMark
click for updates

Citation: Nicholls SG, Hayes TP, Brehaut JC, McDonald M, Weijer C, Saginur R, et al. (2015) A Scoping Review of Empirical Research Relating to Quality and Effectiveness of Research Ethics Review. PLoS ONE 10(7): e0133639. doi:10.1371/journal.pone.0133639

Editor: Antony Bayer, Cardiff University, UNITED KINGDOM

Received: March 24, 2015

Accepted: June 30, 2015

Published: July 30, 2015

Data Availability Statement: All relevant data are within the paper and its Supporting Information files.

Funding: This study was funded by a Canadian Institutes of Health Research Planning Grant #MPE-126678. No funders were involved in the design or conduct of the review.

Competing Interests: The authors have declared that no competing interests exist.

Abstract

Background

To date there is no established consensus of assessment criteria for evaluating research ethics review.

Methods

We conducted a scoping review of empirical research assessing ethics review processes in order to identify common elements assessed, research foci, and research gaps to aid in the development of assessment criteria. Electronic searches of Ovid Medline, PsychInfo, and the Cochrane DSR, ACP Journal Club, DARE, CCTR, CMR, HTA, and NHSEED, were conducted. After de-duplication, 4234 titles and abstracts were reviewed. Altogether 4036 articles were excluded following screening of titles, abstracts and full text. A total of 198 articles included for final data extraction.

Results

Few studies originated from outside North America and Europe. No study reported using an underlying theory or framework of quality/effectiveness to guide study design or analyses. We did not identify any studies that had involved a controlled trial - randomised or otherwise – of ethics review procedures or processes. Studies varied substantially with respect to outcomes assessed, although tended to focus on structure and timeliness of ethics review.

Discussion

Our findings indicate a lack of consensus on appropriate assessment criteria, exemplified by the varied study outcomes identified, but also a fragmented body of research. To date research has been largely quantitative, with little attention given to stakeholder experiences,

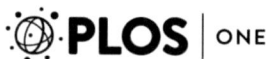

and is largely cross sectional. A lack of longitudinal research to date precludes analyses of change or assessment of quality improvement in ethics review.

Background

Research ethics review was developed by a post-WWII society to ensure that human subjects were protected from unethical research. Today ethical review is legally mandated prior to the conduct of most human subjects research [1].

While few would disagree with the general need for ethics review, existing review processes are often criticized [2]; common complaints include the amount of paperwork required [3], inconsistency of decisions between review boards, and suggestions that ethics review systems may not be equipped to properly review specific types of research [4–8]. In response to these criticisms, efforts have been made to develop standards of ethics review, and several jurisdictions have implemented accreditation processes to ensure that committees meet requirements, such as those imposed by the US Federal Policy for the Protection of Human Subjects (the 'Common Rule')[9]. However, these largely procedural standards may not necessarily reflect the goals of human subject protection that review processes were established to safeguard. To date, there is no established consensus regarding assessment criteria for evaluating research ethics review [10].

Abstract goals and evaluative frameworks have been described [11], but there remain a lack of operational definitions and consensus regarding criteria against which to perform assessments. Indeed, while there has been much discussion of the need to develop metrics or quality indicators, there has been little progress in terms of identifying and testing meaningful indicators. Despite a recent systematic review to determine what is known about how well IRBs function [12], several existing areas of study were excluded. Indeed, despite the conclusion that there is a need to clarify expectations regarding ethics review processes, and that data on the risks that research participants experience would be helpful in this regard, the authors explicitly excluded stakeholder opinions of IRB performance. Moreover, the review did not explore in detail the different methodological approaches, stakeholders involved, or theories motivating the research.

In order to progress the literature towards evidence-based assessment of ethics review processes, there is a need to examine not just procedural aspects of ethics review, but also a broader range of perspectives and descriptive accounts as well as a range of methodological approaches. In the present review we address this need through an inclusive search of the international literature, and specifically include studies targeting investigator, participant, and research board/committee perspectives with attention given to methodological approach.

Aim

To conduct a scoping review of the relevant literature regarding the evaluation of research ethics review, and to summarize the available evidence in terms of:

1. Applied theoretical frameworks relevant to evaluating research ethics review;

2. Research approaches that have been used to evaluate research ethics review;

3. Subjects of analysis within existing research to evaluate research ethics review; and

4. Research outcomes that have been used to evaluate research ethics review;

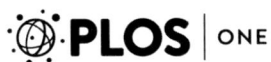

Methods

Our choice to conduct a scoping review was necessitated by the disparate body of literature regarding ethics review practices. Scoping reviews are useful to summarize and describe data from a wide range of fields which cross disciplinary and methodological lines [13]. This can include quantitative, qualitative, and review work. In keeping with the aim of scoping reviews, our approach was also informed by a desire to examine the extent, range and nature of research activity so as to provide an initial assessment of the state of the literature and identify research gaps. As per recommended practice [13, 14] we used a five step framework. The five stage process employed was:

1. Identifying the research question;

2. Identifying relevant studies;

3. Study selection;

4. Charting the data;

5. Collating, summarizing and reporting the results.

Identifying the research question

Our main question for the scoping review was: What empirical research exists that addresses the evaluation of research ethics review?

Identifying Relevant Studies

Studies were identified through an electronic search of published literature, together with citation tracking and hand searching. Electronic searches of Ovid Medline, PsychInfo, and the Cochrane DSR, ACP Journal Club, DARE, CCTR, CMR, HTA, and NHSEED, were conducted. Terms relating to research ethics boards, quality, effectiveness and evaluation were combined with terms relating to research approaches (See S1 File). The search strategy was developed through discussion with experts in the field of research ethics review, a research librarian, a previously published systematic review [12], and a narrative review of the literature. The search strategy included both Meta Subject Heading (MeSH) terms and text words as several articles identified by the narrative review did not have MeSH terms associated with them.

Study Selection

Eligibility criteria were based on the goals of our research question. While there has been much debate with respect to potential indicators of quality in research ethics review, our goal was to advance the empirical assessment of ethics review. As the motivation for the study was to move forward the research agenda on quality assessment in a meaningful way we limited our search to include only manuscripts that had attempted to develop metrics, or evaluate empirically, research ethics review processes or procedures. Studies were therefore excluded if they did not involve empirical research; did not have research ethics review (as opposed to clinical ethics review) as a core element of study; or didn't relate to humans (e.g. studies of animal research ethics). Articles were not limited by date, allowing the assessment of publication trends. Only English language studies were included.

The electronic search was conducted in June 2013 and updated in March 2014. All titles and abstracts were screened by two reviewers (TH, SN). Following the initial screen, the bibliographies of all retained articles were hand searched to identify additional studies. All articles were

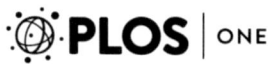

imported into Reference Manager 12 for curation. Articles were rejected on an initial screen of titles and abstracts only if the reviewers could determine that the articles did not meet the inclusion criteria. Where abstracts were not available, or where a definitive assessment could not be made, the full text of the article was retrieved. The same two authors reviewed the full texts to make a final determination of inclusion or exclusion. Any disagreements were resolved by discussion. Data extraction was conducted by one reviewer (TH), with a second reviewer (SN) screening a sample (n = 45) for comparison. Each reviewer independently extracted information from the full text manuscript and then results were compared. Differences that were qualitatively different (i.e. there had been different elements extracted) were resolved through discussion as were differences in coding applied to the data.

Charting the data

A data extraction form and process was developed based on the study aim of creating a descriptive account of the research landscape, as opposed to integrated analyses. The content of the form was developed by discussion within the team. Data extracted included: article characteristics (title, author(s), source, date of publication); description of research (type of participants, study design, data collection methods, research question, study size, dates to which data relate, region); and study outcomes.

Collating, summarizing and reporting results

Data were summarized descriptively. Qualitative data, such as individual outcomes from studies or descriptions of approaches, were collated thematically using a process of qualitative description. This is a low-inference approach to coding qualitative data in which the goal is a descriptive account of the content, as opposed to overarching concepts or abstract frameworks [15]. Themes were applied using the constant comparison method in which existing instances are revisited in light of new data. [16] Descriptive statistics were used to explore the quantitative data within the manuscripts. The data extracted are listed in Table 1.

Results

The electronic search resulted in 2939 citations for review. Review of bibliographies for initially retained papers yielded a further 1304 articles. After de-duplication a total of n = 4234 titles and abstracts were reviewed. Screening by both reviewers achieved 94% concordance. Altogether 4036 articles were excluded following screening of titles, abstracts and full text. The main reasons for exclusion were: not research ethics review (n = 3594), not empirical research

Table 1. Extracted information from retrieved articles.

Article Characteristics	Description of Research	Study Findings and Conclusions
Title	Type of Participants	Names of outcomes
Author(s)	Study Design	Results/Findings
Source	Research Questions	Theoretical framework/theory cited? If yes: definition
Date of Publication	Study Size	Authors' Conclusions
	Dates to which data relate	
	Region	
	Definition of quality	
	Definition of effectiveness	

doi:10.1371/journal.pone.0133639.t001

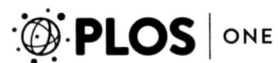

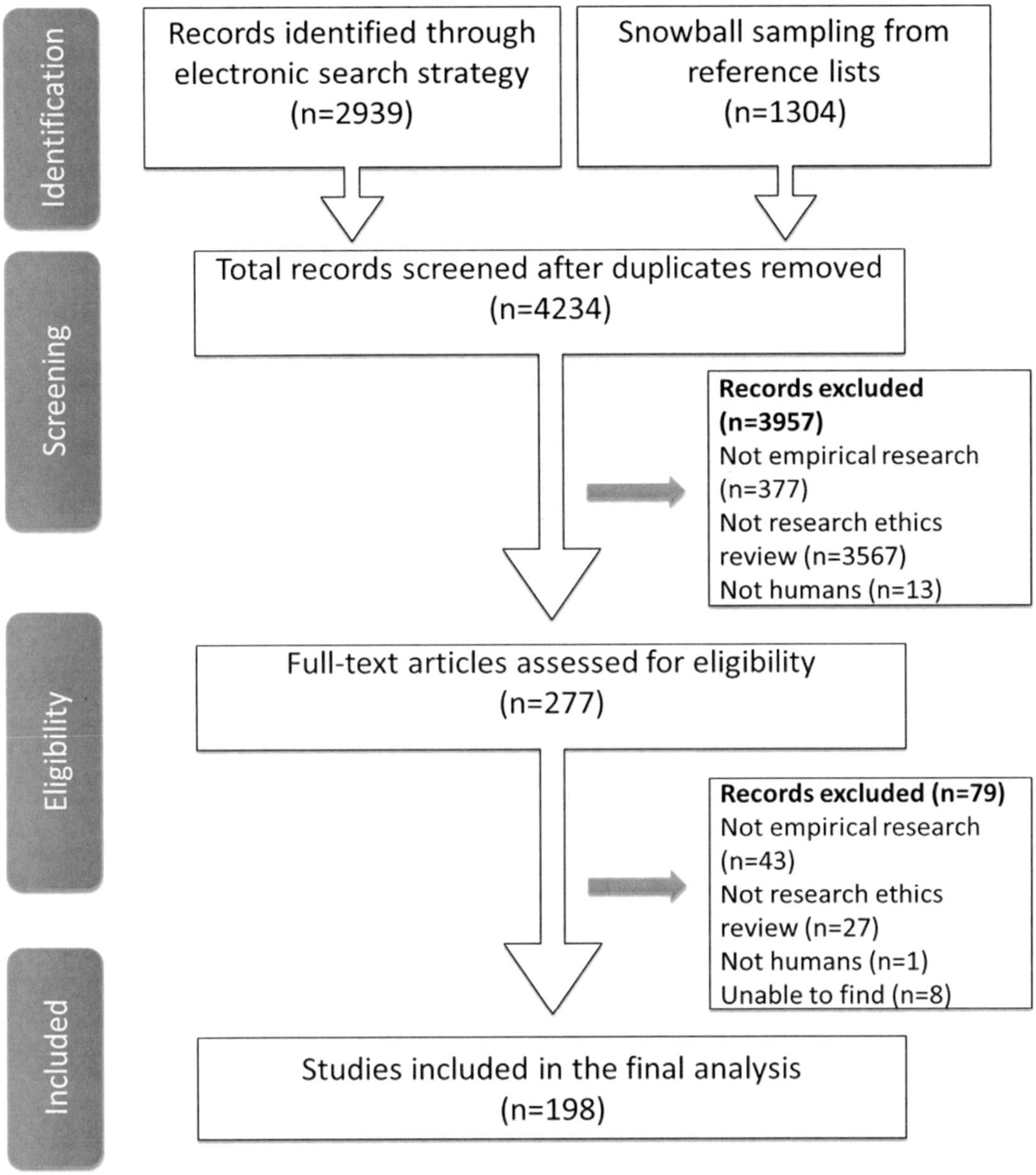

Identification

Records identified through electronic search strategy (n=2939)

Snowball sampling from reference lists (n=1304)

Screening

Total records screened after duplicates removed (n=4234)

Records excluded (n=3957)
Not empirical research (n=377)
Not research ethics review (n=3567)
Not humans (n=13)

Eligibility

Full-text articles assessed for eligibility (n=277)

Records excluded (n=79)
Not empirical research (n=43)
Not research ethics review (n=27)
Not humans (n=1)
Unable to find (n=8)

Included

Studies included in the final analysis (n=198)

Fig 1. Flowchart of screening process

doi:10.1371/journal.pone.0133639.g001

(n = 420), not human (n = 14). In addition we were unable to locate the full text of 18 articles. Consequently, a total of 198 articles were included for final data extraction (see Fig 1).

Study descriptors

Publication dates of identified studies ranged from 1979 to 2014. From 1979 through to the 1990s the number of studies identified number one to two per year. There was an increase in the number of articles per year starting in the early 2000s (from n = 6 in 2000 to n = 14 in

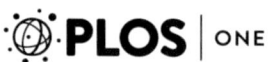

2005) with a peak in the latter part of that decade (n = 19 in 2008). Several studies did not include dates to which their data relate, precluding assessment of this. Most studies originated from North America (n = 102) or Europe (n = 62). There were relatively few authors publishing multiple articles.

Theoretical frameworks

No study reported using an underlying theory or framework of IRB quality/effectiveness to guide study design or analyses. Several studies did, however, use theories, such as grounded theory, to analyze data [17–20].

While a number of studies (n = 16) discussed quality or effectiveness of IRB decisions [7, 12, 21–34], none provided explicit operational definitions. In developing their self-assessment tool, Sleem et al., note that "there are no gold standards for determining effectiveness nor are there standards that can actually measure how well human participants are being protected by the use of standards", instead opting to use 'surrogate' metrics that they considered foundations for effectiveness and protection [30]. These surrogate metrics included: availability of policies (e.g. to deal with conflicts of interest), structural elements (such as membership composition), processes (for example, clear processes for the submission of protocols), performance measures (such as whether certain criteria were considered within the protocol review), as well as cost-related information. While the structural organization of review (for example, policies, structural elements, performance measures) is not itself a theory it does provide a framework of aspects of IRB review quality. The development of such metrics, in the absence of explicit operational definitions, was representative of many studies identified by the review.

Two studies did describe a general foundation in Procedural- and Interactional-Justice through the use of the Institutional Review Board-Researcher Assessment Tool (IRB-RAT) [35, 36]. *Procedural justice* relates to fairness of process. A fair IRB, it is argued by the authors, might display characteristics that are associated with procedural justice, such as: consistency, lack of bias, accuracy, procedures for correcting errors, representativeness, and adherence to basic ethical standards. *Interactional justice*, on the other hand, relates the behavioral aspects of the decision process. In this respect, the authors of the IRB-RAT argue for the inclusion of this aspect to evaluate the way in which people who receive decisions are treated. In essence, it is an evaluation of communication through assessment of *interpersonal sensitivity*–the degree of politeness or respect–and the substantive *justification*, that is the degree of explanation provided.

Research approaches

We did not identify any studies that had involved a controlled trial—randomised or otherwise–of ethics review procedures or processes. The two most common methods of data collection were surveys, with 92/198 (46%) manuscripts reporting results from survey research, and review of administrative data, with 79 (40%) papers (Fig 2 and S1 Table, for further details). Survey respondents varied, with manuscripts reporting on surveys with several populations. Of the 92 manuscripts reporting survey research, 63 included surveys of ethics committee/board members (69%), 28 included surveys of researchers (31%), and 4 included surveys of research participants (4%). Surveys also often focused on structural aspects of ethics review, with 52 (57%) manuscripts exploring structural or procedural aspects, 43 (47%) elements of membership, and 27 (29%) variation, while 39 (42%) explored ethics committee/board member views. Eighteen manuscripts included researcher views (20%) and 3/92 (3%) papers using surveys included participant views.

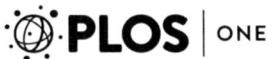

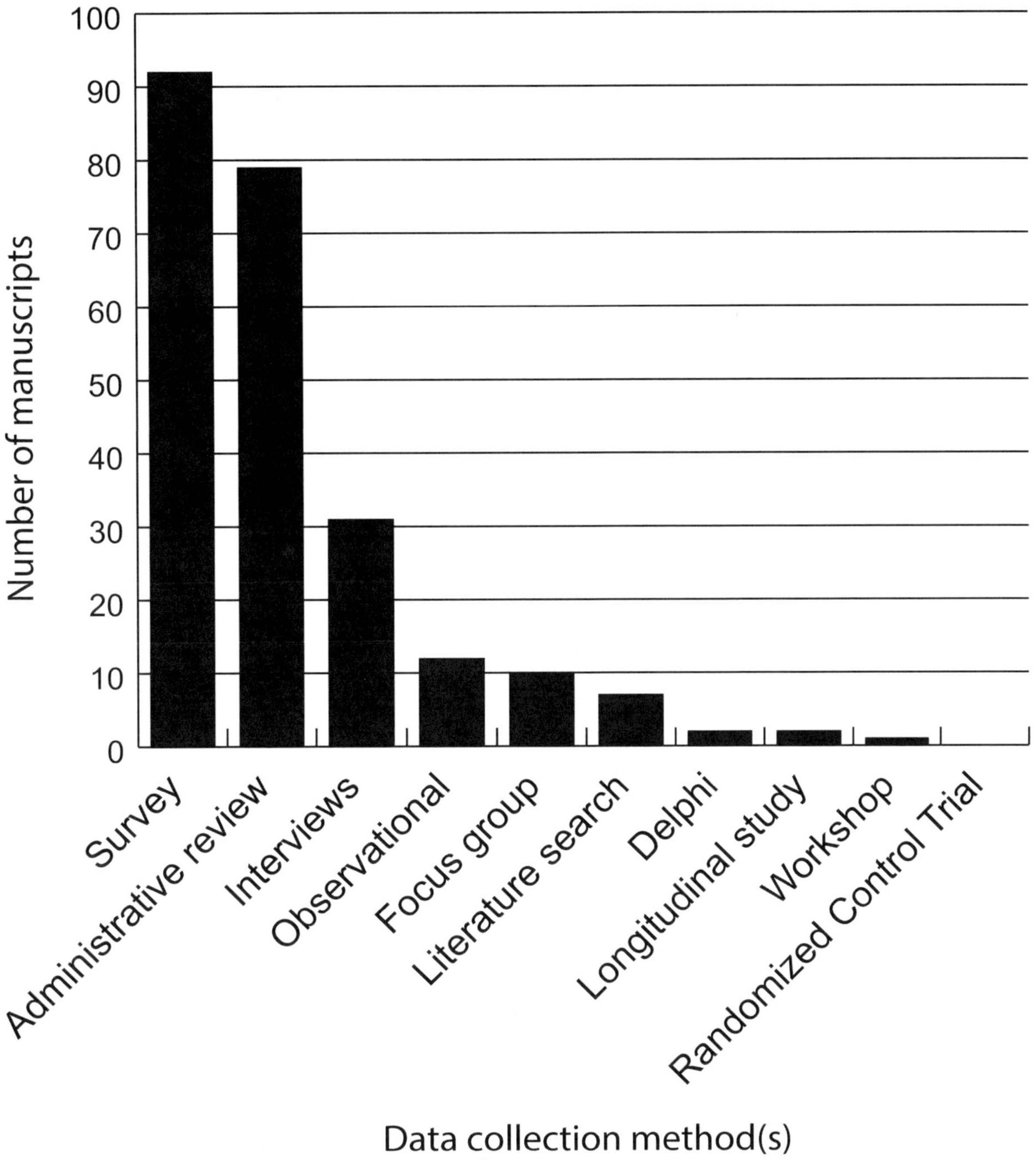

Fig 2. Data collection methods of analysed manuscripts.

doi:10.1371/journal.pone.0133639.g002

Thirty one papers (16%) reported data collected through interviews. Of these, 4 manuscripts reported interviews with research participants (13%), 8 included researchers (26%) and 24 (77%) were with ethics committee/board members. A handful of studies reported results from

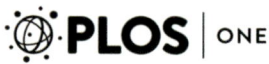
other qualitative approaches such as participant observation (n = 12; 6%) or focus groups (n = 10, 5%).

Seven papers indicated that a literature review had been undertaken: however, in only two instances were detailed search strategies and summaries of the identified literature provided [12, 29].We identified two examples of Delphi processes [26, 37] and only two studies of longitudinal data [38, 39]. Of the two longitudinal studies, Denham et al., reviewed the outcomes of studies reviewed and approved by a single research ethics committee in the UK over the period 1970 to 1978. Based on follow up they found that 43% of projects approved had been completed, 20% had been abandoned, 3% had been suspended and 26% were ongoing [38]. Allen and Waters reviewed the data on number of projects submitted, the types of study, and the numbers approved and requiring modification–including details on the types of modifications or conditions imposed by the ethics committee [39].One manuscript presented a summary of a workshop [40].

Research subject

The research subject referred to what, or who, was the subject of analysis (S1 Table). A total of 147/198 papers reported data where the assessment of administrative processes was the subject of assessment (74%), while 103 (52%) reported the views of IRB members. A total of 45 manuscripts (23%) related to analyses of review board composition, and 37 (19%) explored the views of researchers. A handful of papers included alternative subjects of study. Eight manuscripts explored the views of non-research healthcare workers who may be affected by research [37, 41–47], and only seven papers (4%) identified by the search involved research participants as the subject of study [48–54]. We identified only one study that explored the views of research sponsors[55].

Outcomes of assessment/thematic analyses

Table 2 describes the themes we identified: Membership; Time; Cost; Variation; Satisfaction; Policy Adherence; Working Hours; Outcome; Training; Knowledge; Structures and Procedures; Number of Protocols; Committee/board Member Views; Researcher Views; Participant Views; Committee/board Decision Making; Post Approval Monitoring; Number of Committee/boards in Region; and Views of Healthcare Professionals (HCPs) (see Table 2 for examples of individual outcomes included within the thematic groupings). Studies often assessed multiple outcomes.

As Fig 3 shows most outcomes were situated within the cluster relating to ethics committee/board processes and outcomes (see also S1 Table). The largest number of manuscripts assessed structures and protocols of review committees or boards (n = 104, 53%). For example, Foster et al. reviewed annual reports of UK Local Research Ethics Committees (LRECs) and sought to determine their size, gender composition, and fees charged for review [56]. Other outcomes in this more common grouping were: Committee decision making (n = 71, 36%), committee/board member views (n = 65, 33%), variation between review committees/boards (n = 61, 31%), ethics committee/board membership (n = 59, 30%); time taken for review (n = 54, 28%), outcome of review (n = 50, 25%).

Within the second cluster of outcomes–which tended to represent assessments of functional aspects of committee/board approval and monitoring—the most popular outcome was the comparison of ethics review performance against existing standards or legislation, such as the Common Rule (n = 26, 13%). Of those assessing performance against existing standards, several studies reported that different IRBs varied in their interpretation and application of the same guidelines [12, 56–59]. Some authors noted that certain criteria–such as informed

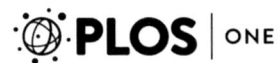

Table 2. Examples of individual study outcomes according to thematic groupings.

Thematic grouping	Examples
Membership	**Borovecki et al (2005):**1) IRB membership information: age, sex, occupation 2) Number of members in the committee
	Catania et al (2008): 1) The composition of each IRB committee administered by their office: total members per committee, number of non-institutional members, number of non-institutional members without a science background
Time	**Ahmed et al (1996):** 1) Time taken (days) to obtain ethical approval
	Al-Shahi et al (1999): Delay from application to- 1) Calling an LREC meeting 2) Initial LREC decision 3) Final LREC approval
Cost	**Byrne et al (2006):** Number of units of various resources that were used at a given IRB. 1)Travel 2)Supply and equipment purchases 3) Space used
Cost	**Chakladar et al (2011):** 1) Number of sheets of A4 paper distributed to committee members and used during requested amendments or resubmissions. 2) Paper use during IRB process. 3) Paper use during study conduct
Variation	**Angell et al (2006):** 1) Patterns of agreement in decisions, descriptively and using the kappa statistic.
	Fitzgerald et al (2006) (62): 1) Comparison between centralized and decentralized systems: administrative and the review process
Satisfaction	**Mosconi et al (2006):**1) Average level of satisfaction on the interactions with the REC for each of the following aspects: bureaucratic and secretarial, ethical, scientific and methodological, education aspects and training activities
Policy Adherence	**Abbott et al (2011)** 1) Process studies examining the extent to which federal regulations are implemented by the IRB
	Ateudjieu et al (2010) 1) Difficulties in applying regulations
Working Hours	**Ah-See et al (1998):** 1) Frequency of meetings
	Kirigia et al (2005): 1) Frequency of scheduled meetings 2) Number of times the committee actually met last year
Outcome	**Czarkowski et al (2009):** 1) Number of negative assessments given
	Russ et al (2009): 1) Frequency of formal and content-related objections in the decisions of coordinating ethics committees after first application
Training	**Ateudjieu et al (2010):** 1) Training on research ethics evaluation. 2) Types of Training. 3) Training Content. 4) Perceived importance of targeted groups for training. 5) Training objectives
Knowledge	**Banos et al (2010):** 1) Degree of improvement in the knowledge of those attending seminars
	Borovecki et al (2006): 1) Self assessment of the knowledge of each respondent in the field of biomedical ethics. 2) Participants' knowledge on the field of biomedical ethics, bioethics issues
Structures and procedures	**Foster et al (1998):** 1) Policies regarding multi-centre research
	Jones et al (1996): 1) Policies concerning scientific misconduct
Number of Protocols	**Boyce (2002)** 1) Number of new and continuing applications discussed at each meeting
	Catania et al (2008) 1) Types and volume of protocols received in the past year. 2) Total number of protocols [new and prior] 3) Number of new [all types] and of new full-committee review protocols
IRB Member Views	**Abou-Zeid et al (2009)** 1) Self-rated capacity to perform committee activities
	Allen et al (1983): 1) Present and retired IRB member general attitudes towards ethical committees and their functions
Researcher Views	**Douglass et al (1998):** 1) Researcher experiences of the ethics review process
	Kallgren et al (1996): 1) Student researcher reactions to going through the IRB process
Participant views	**Berry (1997):** 1) Did the patients know that they were research subjects? 2) Had they been given enough information and enough time to give valid consent? 3) Had they been told what to do if there was a problem?

(*Continued*)

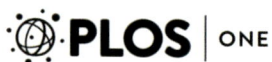
Table 2. (*Continued*)

Thematic grouping	Examples
	Karunaratne et al (2006):1) Were there any parts which you found difficult to understand? 1) Which activities do you think ethics committees are involved in?
IRB Decision Making	**Boyce (2002):** 1) Reasons for condition approval/deferral
	Czarkowski et al (2009): 1) Basis on which decisions concerning research projects were made. 2) Basis for reviewing applications
Post Approval Monitoring	**Arda (2000):** 1) Methods used to monitor the progress of projects
	Gibson et al (2008) 1) Assessment of need for ongoing monitoring of registry by REB 2) Types of information that would need to be reported
Number of RECs in Region	**Vulcano (2012)** 1) Assessment of the number IRBs using a database
Views of HCPs	**Allen et al (1983):** 1) Doctors who have never been members of an ethical committee views towards ethical committees and their functions

doi:10.1371/journal.pone.0133639.t002

consent–received much greater consideration than others, such as risk minimization or data monitoring requirements [58]. Others report variation in the requirements of ethics applications, even within the same jurisdiction [59]. Other outcomes within this cluster were costs (n = 24, 12%), researcher views (n = 23, 12%), post approval monitoring (n = 23, 12%), training undertaken by review board members (n = 22, 11%), working hours (n = 20, 10%), and number of protocols reviewed (n = 18, 9%).

Least studied were outcomes relating to human subjects protections, and the conduct of others involved in the research ethics enterprise. Notably, the views of healthcare professionals not directly involved in research and research participants were rarely studied.

Nine studies identified assessed ethics committee/board member knowledge. As above, multiple approaches were often employed, with seven studies using surveys to explore knowledge, three focus groups, one study using an observational design, and another conducting interviews. These studies ranged with respect to the areas of knowledge being evaluated and how this was assessed. Allen, for example, explored IRB member knowledge of processes and procedures for reviewing genetics protocols [60] while others explored committee/board member knowledge of methodology [42] and ethical principles [42, 61–63] and procedures [55, 63, 64].

We identified four studies (2%) that specifically explored the views of research participants, and one that assessed the views of healthcare professionals not directly involved in research [41]. Studies of participant views ranged in focus, from evaluating IRB consent decisions by exploring participant experiences and understanding of the research in which they were involved [48, 50, 54] to surveying research participants regarding their views as to the roles and purposes of ethics committees [51].

Existing tools

A number of tools were identified that could potentially provide standardized assessments of ethics boards/committees (S2 Table). These include: the IRB-RAT [35, 36], the Training and Resources in Research Ethics Evaluation (TRREE)[65], the Research Ethics Committee (REC) Quality Assurance Self-Assessment Tool[30], an assessment tool developed by Tsan et al., for evaluating research protection programs in the Department of Veterans Affairs [32, 33], and a draft evaluation instrument for use in convened NIH IRB meetings [63].

However, there has been little–if any–validation of these tools. Only one tool–the IRB-RAT–has been used in a replication study, although Tsan et al., have applied their tool at

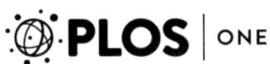

several time points to evaluate the same population [32, 33]. While the NIH instrument is reported as something that will be used to evaluate four of the NIH's 14 IRBs, no follow up reports were identified by our review.

Discussion

While research ethics review is a cornerstone of ethical research practice, there are no gold standards against which to evaluate research ethics review processes. This lack of standards

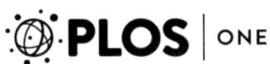

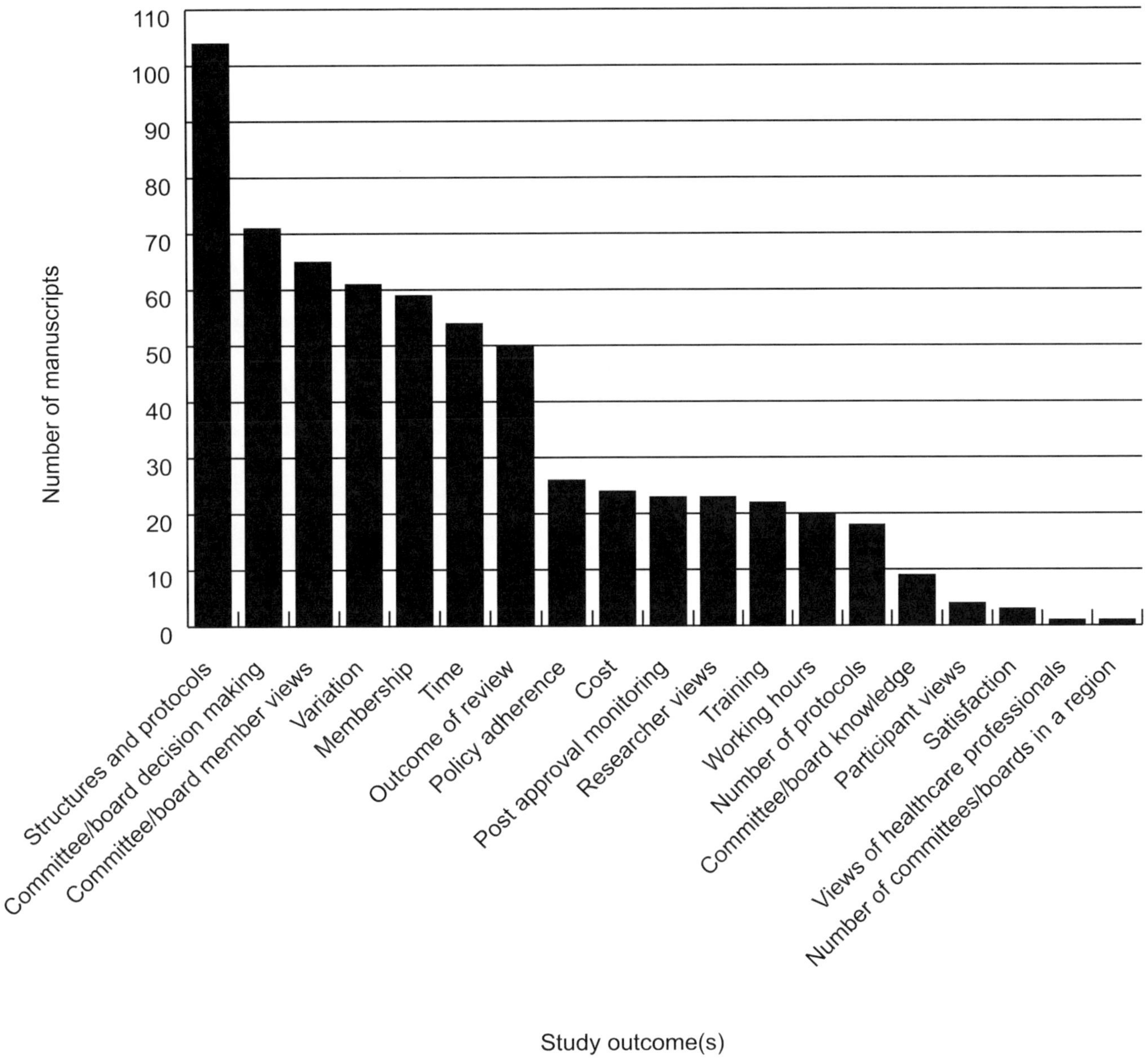

Fig 3. Instances of outcomes present in analysed manuscripts.

doi:10.1371/journal.pone.0133639.g003

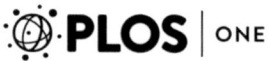

stems, at least in part, from the lack of consensus regarding assessment criteria, but may also indicate a lack of emphasis on the evaluation of ethics review processes.

The findings of our scoping review indicate that until the turn of the 21st Century there has been little in the way of published research on the subject of assessment of research ethics review. What published research there has been has varied in terms of methodological approaches, subjects of assessment, and the outcomes evaluated. Most research has been conducted into procedural aspects of research ethics review such as committee composition, variation in review outcomes or time to approval, and that the majority of research has been conducted using quantitative approaches such as surveys or administrative review of quantitative data. The majority of research that was identified in this review has been conducted in North America and Europe.

Research approaches

The majority of studies retained in our review were quantitative in nature. As a result there has tended to be a focus on descriptive research; studies have documented how committees are composed, and the number of studies reviewed, or the amount of variation between committees reviewing the same protocol. There is much less explanatory research: why do committees make the decisions they do? How do the dynamics of committees play into decisions? Qualitative studies that include ethnographic methods could help to elucidate decision making models or objects of concern that are not easily or readily accessible through structured quantitative approaches.

A second notable gap in the existing literature is the lack of long-term–or longitudinal–assessment. The lack of longitudinal research is problematic if a goal is to protect human subjects or derive a net benefit for clinical research: as the study of de Jong et al., indicates, research outcomes, adverse events, or publications may not be immediately accessible and only through longitudinal studies would these outcomes be amenable to evaluation. Indeed, their finding that studies that had more correspondence with an ethics committee were less likely to achieve publication [66] is something that should motivate a greater degree of research into post approval monitoring.

The lack of longitudinal research may be symptomatic of the lack of a coherent research agenda with respect to developing evaluation frameworks or tools against which to assess research ethics review processes. Moreover, there may be barriers to the conduct of such research. A study by McKenzie et al., that sought to conduct long term follow up of studies receiving ethical approval itself faced difficulties in obtaining ethical approval on the grounds that the researchers were not obtaining informed consent from the trialists to view their ethics application [67].There is a need for leadership in this area, but also greater collaboration. Important questions need to be asked of researchers, administrators and funders. Funding will be central, but will also generate questions of responsibility and management: given the vagaries of short term contract research and associated funding, should the collection of information on ethics review processes be centrally resourced and conducted by ethics review committees themselves? Does this need to be done by an independent oversight body such as the Association for the Accreditation of Human Research Protection Programs (AAHRP), and if so how should this be managed and reported? These questions cannot be addressed in isolation, and need all relevant stakeholders to be at the table.

Research subjects

Our results indicate that there has been limited research with key stakeholders beyond the membership of ethics committees/boards and the researchers that interact with them; the

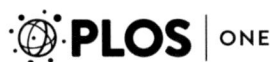

views of research participants have been largely missing from existing research. If a goal is to develop evaluation tools to assess research ethics review processes against their remit of protecting human subjects, then further research is warranted with those individuals who are subject to research. Indeed, current research is lacking several stakeholders who may be considered relevant to the debate. McDonald et al., have argued that research ethics review is but one part of the research ethics lifecycle, and that there are a broader range of perspectives that need to be considered beyond the researcher-ethics committee/board dyad [68]. We found little research with healthcare professionals outside the research context, and only one study that included the views of research sponsors. Identifying and including all relevant stakeholders in the review process; be they researchers, IRB members, policy-makers, legislators, research funders, institutional-sponsors, or research participants, will be key to identifying shared goals of research ethics review that are appropriate for, and amenable to, assessment. As such, we suggest that more research is needed that includes additional stakeholders beyond the IRB-researcher dyad.

Research outcomes

Given that research ethics review has been established to minimize harms to research participants, and that existing guidelines, regulations and research indicate that the protection of human subjects is a continued goal, we found a paucity of research exploring the experiences of research participants.Greater involvement of participants (and the public) may provide greater support for the decisions made, and could potentially lead to increased trust in the decision-makers and decision-making process as well as improved decisions [69]. Moreover, exploring participants' experiences may identify factors that contribute to potential negative effects, and facilitate modifications to the review process that may mitigate future repetition.

While calls for the development of metrics for measuring the quality of ethics review appear to have been heeded to the extent that some instruments were identified within the review, there has, to date, been little evaluation of these tools. Existing instruments reflect a fragmented research program in which individual researchers have developed custom data collection tools. This has not only limited assessments of reliability or validity, but has led to competing and contrasting data collection tools being developed.

Tools developed in other areas relating to core ethical principles could be useful for the evaluation of ethics review processes and should be considered for evaluation. In a recent review of measurement instruments in clinical and research ethics, Redman identified 10 validated instruments measuring ethical constructs [70].This included two measures of informed consent; the Multi-Dimensional Measure of Informed Choice [71], and the Quality of Informed Consent [72] instruments, but only one instrument that directly related to research. This tool, the Reactions to Research Participation Questionnaires for Children and for Parents (RRPQ-C and RRPQ-P), was developed to evaluate experiences of participating in research, as opposed to incorporating this within a framework for the evaluation of research ethics review [73]. Using tools such as this within a framework to evaluate research ethics review processes could allow for consistent metrics of assessment while specifically addressing the important goals of human subject protections. Moreover, the focus of measures such as this would clearly address the present research gap on participant experiences. However, further development and evaluation is needed to evaluate if such a tool is appropriate, together with consideration of whether this should be a researcher driven evaluation, or something undertaken by review boards themselves.

Limitations

Our results must be interpreted within the context of the limitations of the study. Firstly, our sampling frame was limited to a specific number of databases. As such, some articles, such as

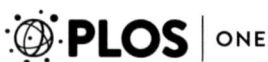

articles from social science databases or grey literature, may be missing based on the limits and boundaries of the included databases. A second caveat is the specificity of the search strategy itself: while steps were taken to ensure that key articles were included, the sensitivity of the search strategy was limited in order to generate a manageable number of articles. However, our review may have been overly-calibrated toward identified key articles. We attempted to mitigate these limitations through reviewing the reference lists of articles, which was not limited by the original databases or the terms within the search strategy. The substantial number of articles achieved through this process indicates the utility of this approach in a heterogeneous area such as the evaluation of research ethics review. Finally, our search strategy was limited to English language publications. This may have biased our results towards countries where this is the predominant language of publication and may account, in part, for the larger number of articles retrieved from certain countries or geographic regions.

Conclusion

There is a continued call for, and interest in, the development of quality indicators for research ethics review. Our review indicates a lack of consensus on appropriate assessment criteria, exemplified by the varied study outcomes identified, but also a fragmented body of research. To date research has been largely quantitative, with little attention given to stakeholder experiences, and cross sectional. On the basis of our review we make the following recommendations for future research developments:

1. Assessment of long-term outcomes following research ethics review to identify variation within and between ethics review committees and to allow time for the identification of potential trends.

2. Engagement with a broader range of stakeholders, including research participants, in order to avoid viewing research ethics solely as ethics review, as opposed to a broader research ethics lifecycle [74].

3. The development of theoretical foundations upon which to base empirical investigations of research ethics review

4. The creation of review strategies and structures that facilitate the systematic search of the diverse literature around the evaluation of research ethics review including high quality databases of peer-reviewed publications across the range of disciplines and a common interface and search language.

Supporting Information

S1 File. Search Strategy.
(DOC)

S1 Table. Articles retrieved.
(DOC)

S2 Table. Identified measures or tools for evaluating research ethics review.
(DOC)

Acknowledgments

Disclaimer: The paper presents the views of the authors and should not be taken to be representative of the funding agency nor the authors' institutions.

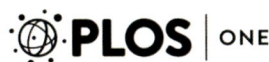

We would like to thank Heather Colquhoun for her comments on the reporting of scoping reviews and Kelly Carroll for her input in developing the data extraction procedures. We would also like to thank the Canadian Institutes of Health Research (CIHR) who funded a two day workshop on the topic of evaluation of ethics review, as well as all the participants at the workshop.

Author Contributions

Conceived and designed the experiments: SGN JCB DF MM RS CW. Performed the experiments: SGN TPH JCB. Analyzed the data: SGN TPH JCB. Wrote the paper: SGN JCB DF TPH MM RS CW.

References

1. Heimer CA, Petty J. Bureaucratic Ethics: IRBs and the Legal Regulation of Human Subjects Research. Annual Review of Law and Social Science. 2010; 6(1):601–26.

2. Joffe S. Revolution or reform in human subjects research oversight. J Law Med Ethics. 2012;Winter: :922–9.

3. Jamrozik K. Research ethics paperwork: what is the plot we seem to have lost? Br Med J. 2004; 329:236–7.

4. Schrag Z. The case against ethics review in the social sciences. Res Ethics. 2012; 7(4):120–31.

5. De Vries R, DeBruin DA, Goodgame A. Ethics review of social, behavioral, and economic research: where should we go from here? Ethics & Behaviour. 2004; 14(4):351–68. Epub 2006/04/22.

6. Wynn LL. Ethnographers' Experiences of Institutional Ethics Oversight: Results from a Quantitative and Qualitative Survey. J Policy Hist. 2011; 23(01):94–114.

7. Beagan B, McDonald M. Evidence-based practice of research ethics review? Health Law Rev. 2005:62–8. PMID: 16459416

8. McDonald M, Cox S. Moving Toward Evidence-Based Human Participant Protection. J Acad Ethics. 2009; 7(1–2):1–16.

9. Association for the Accreditation of Human Research Protection Programs Inc. AAHRPP Accreditation Standards. 2009.

10. Emanuel EJ, Wood A, Fleischman A, Bowen A, Getz KA, Grady C, et al. Oversight of human participants research: Identifying problems to evalute reform proposals. Ann Intern Med. 2004; 141:282–91. PMID: 15313744

11. Emanuel EJ, Wendler D, Grady C. What makes clinical research ethical? JAMA. 2000; 283:2701–11. PMID: 10819955

12. Abbott L, Grady C. A systematic review of the empirical literature evaluating IRBs: what we know and what we still need to learn. J Empir Res Hum Res Ethics. 2011; 6(1):3–19. Epub 2011/04/05. doi: 10. 1525/jer.2011.6.1.3 PMID: 21460582

13. Arksey H, O'Malley L. Scoping studies: towards a methodological framework. Int J Soc Res Methodol. 2005; 8:19–31.

14. Levac D, Colquhoun H, O'Brien KK. Scoping studies: advancing the methodology. Implement Sci. 2010; 5:69. Epub 2010/09/22. doi: 10.1186/1748-5908-5-69 PMID: 20854677

15. Sandelowski M. Whatever happened to qualitative description? Res Nurs Health. 2000; 23:334–40. PMID: 10940958

16. Strauss AL. Qualitative analysis for social scientists: Cambridge University Press; 1996.

17. Valdez-Martinez E, Turnbull B, Garduño-Espinosa J, Porter JDH. Descriptive ethics: a qualitative study of local research ethics committees in Mexico. Dev World Bioeth. 2006; 6(2):95–105. PMID: 16594973

18. Klitzman R. The ethics police?: IRBs' views concerning their power. PLoS One. 2011; 6(12).

19. Klitzman R. "Members of the same club": challenges and decisions faced by US IRBs in identifying and managing conflicts of interest. PLoS One. 2011; 6(7):e22796. Epub 2011/08/11. doi: 10.1371/journal. pone.0022796 PMID: 21829516

20. Klitzman R. US IRBs confronting research in the developing world. Dev World Bioeth. 2012; 12(2):63–73. doi: 10.1111/j.1471-8847.2012.00324.x PMID: 22515423

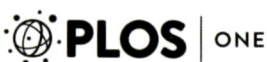
21. Angell E, Sutton AJ, Windridge K, Dixon-Woods M. Consistency in decision making by research ethics committees: a controlled comparison. J Med Ethics. 2006; 32(11):662–4. Epub 2006/11/01. PMID: 17074825

22. Byrne MM, Speckman JL, Getz KA, Sugarman J. Variability in the costs of Institutional Review Board oversight. Acad Med. 2006; 81:708–12. PMID: 16868423

23. Dal-Ré R, Espada J, Ortega R. Performance of research ethics committees in Spain. A prospective study of 100 applications for clinical trial protocols on medicines. J Med Ethics. 1999; 25:268–73. PMID: 10390685

24. Feldman JA, Rebholz CM. Anonymous self-evaluation of performance by ethics board members: a pilot study. J Empir Res Hum Res Ethics. 2009; 4(1):63–9. Epub 2009/04/23. doi: 10.1525/jer.2009.4.1.63 PMID: 19382879

25. Fitzgerald MH, Phillips PA. Centralized and non-centralized ethics review: a five nation study. Account Res. 2006; 13(1):47–74. Epub 2006/06/15. PMID: 16770859

26. Geisser ME, Alschuler KN, Hutchinson R. A Delphi study to establish important easpects of ethics review. J Empir Res Hum Res Ethics. 2011; 6(1):21–4. doi: 10.1525/jer.2011.6.1.21 PMID: 21460583

27. Maskell NA. Variations in experience in obtaining local ethical approval for participation in a multi-centre study. QJM. 2003; 96(4):305–7. PMID: 12651975

28. Norton K, Wilson DM. Continuing ethics review practices by Canadian research ethics boards. IRB. 2008; 30(3):10–4. PMID: 18814440

29. Silberman G, Kahn KL. Burdens on research imposed by Institutional Review Boards: The state of the evidence and its implications for regulatory reform. Milbank Q. 2011; 89(4):599–627. doi: 10.1111/j.1468-0009.2011.00644.x PMID: 22188349

30. Sleem H, Abdelhai RA, Al-Abdallat I, Al-Naif M, Gabr HM, Kehil ET, et al. Development of an accessible self-assessment tool for research ethics committees in developing countries. J Empir Res Hum Res Ethics. 2010; 5(3):85–96; quiz 7–8. Epub 2010/09/14. doi: 10.1525/jer.2010.5.3.85 PMID: 20831423

31. Taylor HA, Chaisson L, Sugarman J. Enhancing communication among data monitoring committees and institutional review boards. Clin Trials. 2008; 5:277–82. doi: 10.1177/1740774508091262 PMID: 18559418

32. Tsan MF, Smith K, Gao B. Assessing the quality of human research protection programs: the experience at the Department of Veterans Affairs. IRB. 2010; 32(4):16–9. Epub 2010/09/22. PMID: 20853799

33. Tsan M-F, Nguyen Y, Brooks R. Using quality indicators to assess human research protection programs at the Department of Veterans Affairs. IRB. 2013; 35(1):10–4. PMID: 23424821

34. Wagner TH, Cruz AME, Chadwick GL. Economies of Scale in Institutional Review Boards. Med care. 2004; 42(8):817–23. PMID: 15258484

35. Reeser JC, Austin DM, Jaros LM, Mukesh BN, McCarty CA. Investigating Perceived Institutional Review Board Quality and Function Using the IRB Researcher Assessment Tool. J Empir Res Hum Res Ethics. 2008; 3(1):25–34. Epub 2009/04/24. doi: 10.1525/jer.2008.3.1.25 PMID: 19385780

36. Keith-Spiegel P, Koocher GP, Tabachnick B. What scientists want from their research ethics committee. J Empir Res Hum Res Ethics. 2006; 1(1):67–82. doi: 10.1525/jer.2006.1.1.67 PMID: 19385866

37. Wu MH, Liao CH, Chiu WT, Lin CY, Yang CM. Can we accredit hospital ethics? A tentative proposal. J Med Ethics. 2011; 37(8):493–7. Epub 2011/06/04. doi: 10.1136/jme.2010.038836 PMID: 21636607

38. Denham MJ, Foster A, Tyrrell DAJ. Work of a district ethical committee. Br Med J. 1979; 2:1042–5. PMID: 519278

39. Allen PA, Waters WE. Development of an ethical committee and its effect on research design. Lancet. 1982:1233–6.

40. Davies H, Wells F, Czarkowski M. Standards for research ethics committees: purpose, problems and the possibilities of other approaches. J Med Ethics. 2009; 35(6):382–3. Epub 2009/06/02. doi: 10.1136/jme.2008.027722 PMID: 19482984

41. Allen P, Waters WE. Attitudes to research ethical committees. J Med Ethics. 1983; 9:61–5. PMID: 6876098

42. Banos JE, Lucena MI, Seres E, Bosch F. Reflections on running training workshops for research ethics committee members in Spain between 2001 and 2008. Croat Med J. 2010; 51(6):552–9. Epub 2010/12/17. PMID: 21162168

43. Carline JD, O'Sullivan PS, Gruppen LD, Richardson-Nassif K. Crafting successful relationships with the IRB. Acad Med. 2007; 82(10 Suppl):S57–S60. PMID: 17895692

44. Chaudhry SH, Brehaut JC, Grimshaw JM, Weijer C, Boruch R, Donner A, et al. Challenges in the research ethics review of cluster randomized trials: International survey of investigators. Clin Trials. 2013; 10:257–68. doi: 10.1177/1740774513475530 PMID: 23539109

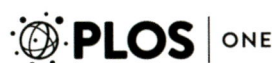 ONE

45. Lynöe N, Sandlund M, Jacobsson L. Research ethics committees: a comparative study of assessment of ethical dilemmas. Scand J Public Health. 1999; 27(2):152–9. PMID: 10421726

46. Mosconi P, Colombo C, Labianca R, Apolone G. Oncologists' opinions about research ethics committees in Italy: an update, 2004. European Journal of Cancer Prevention. 2006; 15:91–4. PMID: 16374238

47. Sarpel U, Hopkins MA, More F, Yavner S, Pusic M, Nick MW, et al. Medical students as human subjects in educational research. Med Educ Online. 2013; 18:1–6. Epub 2013/02/28.

48. Berry J. Local research ethics committees can audit ethical standards in research. J Med Ethics. 1997; 23:379–81. PMID: 9451608

49. Howe A, Delaney S, Romero J, Tinsley A, Vicary P. Public involvement in health research: a case study of one NHS project over 5 years. Prim Health Care Res Dev. 2009; 11(01):17.

50. Karunaratne AS, Myles PS, Ago MJ, Komesaroff PA. Communication deficiencies in research and monitoring by ethics committees. Intern Med J. 2006; 36(2):86–91. Epub 2006/02/14. PMID: 16472262

51. Kent G. The views of members of Local Research Ethics Committees, researchers and members of the public towards the roles and functions of LRECs. J Med Ethics. 1997; 23:186–90. PMID: 9220334

52. McGrath MM, Fullilove RE, Kaufman MR, Wallace R, Fullilove MT. The limits of collaboration: a qualitative study of community ethical review of environmental health research. Am J Public Health. 2009; 99 (8):1510–4. Epub 2009/06/23. doi: 10.2105/AJPH.2008.149310 PMID: 19542033

53. Nelson K, Garcia RE, Brown J, Mangione CM, Louis TA, Keeler E, et al. Do patient consent procedures affect participation rates in health services research? Med care. 2012; 40:283–8.

54. Skrutkowski M, Weijer C, Shapiro S, Fuks A, Langleben A, Freedman B. Monitoring informed consent in an oncology study posing serious risks to subjects. IRB. 1998; 20(6):1–6. PMID: 11657586

55. Simek J, Zamykalova L, Mesanyova M. Ethics Committee or Community? Examining the identity of Czech Ethics Committees in the period of transition. J Med Ethics. 2010; 36(9):548–52. Epub 2010/08/03. doi: 10.1136/jme.2009.034298 PMID: 20675735

56. Foster CG, Marshall T, Moodie P. The annual reports of Local Research Ethics Committees. J Med Ethics. 1995; 21:214–9. PMID: 7473640

57. Driscoll A, Currey J, Worrall-Carter L, Stewart S. Ethical dilemmas of a large national multi-centre study in Australia: time for some consistency. J Clin Nurs. 2008; 17(16):2212–20. Epub 2008/08/19. doi: 10. 1111/j.1365-2702.2007.02219.x PMID: 18705740

58. Lidz CW, Appelbaum PS, Arnold R, Candilis P, Gardner W, Myers S, et al. How closely do institutional review boards follow the common rule? Acad Med. 2012; 87(7):969–74. Epub 2012/05/25. doi: 10. 1097/ACM.0b013e3182575e2e PMID: 22622205

59. Larson E, Bratts T, Zwanziger J, Stone P. A survey of IRB process in 68 U.S. hospitals. J Nurs Scholarsh. 2004; 36(3):260–4. PMID: 15495496

60. Allen HJ. Genetic protocols review by Institutional Review Boards at National Cancer Institute-designated cancer centers. Genet Test. 1998; 2(4):329–36. PMID: 10464612

61. Borovecki A, ten Have H, Orešković S. Ethics and the structures of health care in the European countries in transition: hospital ethics committees in Croatia. Br Med J. 2005; 331:227–30.

62. Brahme R, Mehendale S. Profile and role of the members of ethics committees in hospitals and research organisations in Pune, India. Indian J Med Ethics. 2009; 6(2):78–84. PMID: 19517650

63. Wichman A, Kalyan DN, Abbott LJ, Wesley R, Sandler AL. Protecting human subjects in the NIH's Intramural Research Program: a draft instrument to evaluate convened meetings of its IRBs. IRB. 2006; 28 (3):7–10. Epub 2006/10/14. PMID: 17036438

64. Kass N, Dawson L, Loyo-Berrios NI. Ethical oversight of research in developing countries. IRB. 2003; 25(2):1–10. PMID: 12833901

65. Ateudjieu J, Williams J, Hirtle M, Baume C, Ikingura J, Niare A, et al. Training needs assessment in research ethics evaluation among research ethics committee members in three African countries: Cameroon, Mali and Tanzania. Dev World Bioeth. 2010; 10(2):88–98. Epub 2009/11/17. doi: 10.1111/j. 1471-8847.2009.00266.x PMID: 19912281

66. de Jong JP, Ter Riet G, Willems DL. Two prognostic indicators of the publication rate of clinical studies were available during ethical review. J Clin Epidemiol. 2010; 63(12):1342–50. Epub 2010/06/19. doi: 10.1016/j.jclinepi.2010.01.018 PMID: 20558034

67. McKenzie JE, Herbison GP, Roth P, Paul C. Obstacles to researching the researchers: a case study of the ethical challenges of undertaking methodological research investigating the reporting of randomised controlled trials. Trials. 2010; 11:28. Epub 2010/03/23. doi: 10.1186/1745-6215-11-28 PMID: 20302671

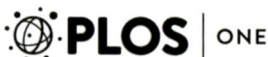

68. McDonald M, Pullman D, Anderson J, Preto N, Sampson H. Research ethics in 2020: strengths, weaknesses, opportunities, and threats. Health Law Rev. 2011; 19(3):36–55.

69. Bruni RA, Laupacis A, Martin DK. Public engagement in setting priorities in health care. CMAJ. 2008; 179(1):15–8. Epub 2008/07/02. doi: 10.1503/cmaj.071656 PMID: 18591516

70. Redman BK. Review of measurement instruments in clinical and research ethics, 1999–2003. J Med Ethics. 2006; 32(3):153–6. Epub 2006/03/02. PMID: 16507659

71. Marteau TM, Dormandy E, Michie S. A measure of informed choice. Health Expect. 2001; 4:99–108. PMID: 11359540

72. Joffe S, Cook EF, Cleary PD, Clark JW, Weeks JC. Quality of Informed Consent: a new measure of understanding among research subjects. J Natl Cancer Inst. 2001; 93:139–47. PMID: 11208884

73. Kassam-Adams N, Newman E. The reactions to research participation questionnaires for children and for parents (RRPQ-C and RRPQ-P). Gen Hosp Psychiatry. 2002; 24:336–42. PMID: 12220800

74. Anderson JA, Sawatzky-Girling B, McDonald M, Pullman D, Saginur R, Sampson HA, et al. Research ethics broadly writ: beyond REB review. Health Law Rev. 2011; 19(3):12–24.

4.2   Pharmaceuticalisation and Ethical Review in South Asia: Issues of Scope and Authority for Practitioners and Policy Makers

Bob Simpson, Rekha Khatri, Deapica Ravindran, and Tharindi Udalagama

Simpson, B, Khatri, R, Ravindran, D, Udalagama, T. Pharmaceuticalisation and ethical review in South Asia: Issues of scope and authority for practitioners and policy makers. *Social Science and Medicine* 131, 247–254 (2015).

Social Science & Medicine 131 (2015) 247–254

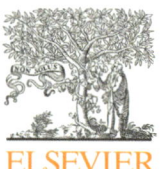

Contents lists available at ScienceDirect

Social Science & Medicine

journal homepage: www.elsevier.com/locate/socscimed

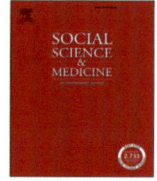

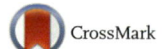

Pharmaceuticalisation and ethical review in South Asia: Issues of scope and authority for practitioners and policy makers

Bob Simpson [a,*], Rekha Khatri [b,c], Deapica Ravindran [c,d], Tharindi Udalagama [c,e]

[a] Department of Anthropology, Durham University, Dawson Building, Lower Mountjoy, Stockton Rd., Durham DH1 3LE, UK
[b] Social Science Baha, Nepal
[c] Biomedical Health Experimentation in South Asia Project
[d] Anusandhan Trust/Centre for Studies in Ethics and Rights, Mumbai, India
[e] University of Colombo, Sri Lanka

ARTICLE INFO

Article history:
Received 12 September 2013
Received in revised form
6 February 2014
Accepted 19 March 2014
Available online 24 March 2014

Keywords:
Ethical review
South Asia
ICH-GCP
Clinical trials
Capacity-building

ABSTRACT

Ethical review by expert committee continues to be the first line of defence when it comes to protecting human subjects recruited into clinical trials. Drawing on a large scale study of biomedical experimentation across South Asia, and specifically on interviews with 24 ethical review committee [ERC] members across India, Sri Lanka and Nepal, this article identifies some of the tensions that emerge for ERC members as the capacity to conduct credible ethical review of clinical trials is developed across the region. The article draws attention to fundamental issues of scope and authority in the operation of ethical review. On the one hand, ERC members experience a powerful pull towards harmonisation and a strong alignment with international standards deemed necessary for the global pharmaceutical assemblage to consolidate and extend. On the other hand, they must deal with what is in effect the double jeopardy of ethical review in developing world contexts. ERC members must undertake review but are frequently made aware of their responsibility to protect interests that go beyond the 'human subject' and into the realms of development and national interest [for example, in relation to literacy and informed consent]. These dilemmas are indicative of broader questions about where ethical review sits in institutional terms and how it might develop to best ensure improved human subject protection given growth of industry-led research.

Crown Copyright © 2014 Published by Elsevier Ltd. This is an open access article under the CC BY license (http://creativecommons.org/licenses/by/3.0/).

From time to time, terms appear in the social sciences which help in capturing a biomedical *zeitgeist*. Notions such as 'medicalization' and 'geneticisation' (Lipmann, 1991; Hedgecoe, 1998; Have, 2001) have in the past provided a simple shorthand for the ways that social, economic and technological changes begin to reshape the landscape of health care and the experience of those that pass through it. In similar fashion, pharmaceuticalisation has entered social science discourse. Williams et al. (2011) provide a critical evaluation of this concept and its utility in understanding the pervasive impact of pharmaceuticals within medical systems, economies and societies (also see (Abraham, 2011)). Consistent with their intention to give greater specificity to the pharmaceuticalisation thesis, we set out in this article to interrogate some of the 'upstream (macro) level processes' (2011: 712) that come

within the ambit of pharmaceuticalisation. The arena we consider is one which is increasingly important in understanding the growth and development of pharmaceuticals in society but one that is often lost in a bias towards Euro-American accounts of this process. Here we bring together globalisation, governance and the ethical review of clinical trials involving human subjects in the developing world. The main sites we consider are research ethics committees and the responses of their members to a growing number of protocols for industry-sponsored clinical trials. What we show through this analysis is the way that the growing engagement with pharmaceutical interests across South Asia produces significant tensions for ERC members. Beneath the documentary and procedural claims to standardised measurement, rules and disinterested evaluation in ethical review, industry-sponsored clinical trials generate concerns about scope, legitimacy and authority for those whose job it is to undertake and develop credible ethical review (*cf* Timmermans and Almeling, 2009; Timmermans and Epstein, 2010). Whilst such tensions are likely to be evident in any context where research

* Corresponding author.
   E-mail address: robert.simpson@durham.ac.uk (B. Simpson).

http://dx.doi.org/10.1016/j.socscimed.2014.03.016

248   *B. Simpson et al. / Social Science & Medicine 131 (2015) 247–254*

ethics and economic interest coalesce, we argue that in developing world settings there are other factors in play that give these questions a particular urgency and complexity.

Our stepping off point in considering the relationship between ethical review and clinical trials in South Asia is a question posed by Rachel Douglas–Jones in her doctoral thesis on capacity-building in ethical review in Asia: 'what are the problems to which the ethics committee is a solution?' [2013, p34]. The question is an important one. Ethical review committees play a crucial role in the regulation of experimentation involving human beings. In the most basic of terms, the approval of a formally constituted body of experts should ensure that research is beneficial, scientifically valid, and, above all, safe for those who participate. Yet, whereas in Europe and North America ERCs may have reached a degree of institutional integration and stability, they are still very much in a state of development in parts of the world that have only recently been drawn into the rapidly growing demand for experimentation involving human subjects. South Asia is a case in point. Capacity for ethical review is rapidly developing across the region and ERCs currently follow a broadly similar institutional and procedural format. Regional capacity-building has developed in association with organisations like the Forum for Ethical Review Committees in Asia and the Western Pacific (FERCAP), the Strategic Initiative for Developing Capacity in Ethical Review (SIDCER) and the Global Forum on Bioethics (GFB) all of which work to build capacity when it comes to the review of projects locally. Affiliation to these organisations and the establishment of local branches [for example, FERC – Sri Lanka and FERC – India] is an important route to harmonisation and the dissemination of good practice. Arguably however, the more powerful source of standardisation for review of industry conducted trials has been the ICH-GCP guidelines which aim to provide 'a more economical use of human, animal and material resources, and the elimination of unnecessary delay in the global development and availability of new medicines whilst maintaining safeguards on quality, safety and efficacy, and regulatory obligations to protect public health' (ICH, 2005). Drawing on a genealogy of crisis reaching back to the Declaration of Helsinki, the ICH-GCP lays down detailed benchmarks for the ethical and scientific conduct of trials. Yet, linking the work of ERCs with a genealogy of universal human rights in this way provides significant cover for the extension of commercial pharmaceutical research (Abraham, 2007; Abraham and Reed, 2002). In this view, ERCs are the handmaiden rather than the governor of trial activity with ethical review seen as essentially procedural, bureaucratic and rule observing. Earlier studies suggest that in countries that have embraced standard guidelines and particularly the ICH-GCP guidelines, ERCs are apt to operate in ways that appear to be more about legal defence of researchers rather than actual protection of subjects (Bosk, 2007; Kleinman, 1999; Stark, 2012). Our analysis confirms these concerns, and shows ethics committee members raising issues that are not limited to human subject protection *per se* but drawing in a range problems which afflict large numbers people in their society [for example, poor access to resources, corruption, illiteracy, inequality to name but a few]. These issues are articulated at a variety of scales [the person, the hospital, the University, the research community, the vulnerable, the nation state, the developing world and so forth]. Yet, the reality faced by many ERC members is one of growing pressure to accomplish human subject protection by narrowing the focus of ethical review such that it is clearly in line with industry specified guidelines.

1. Methods

The data on which this paper is based are drawn from a study of the growth of clinical trials and human experimentation in South

Table 1
The BHESA interview data-set.

Category	Nepal	India	Sri Lanka	US, UK	Total
PIs and Co-Is	10	31	11	3	55
Clinical research assistants	14	18	11	0	43
Other trial staff	24	22	39	0	85
Collaborators	0	3	1	1	5
Sponsors and CRO staff	0	35	1	13	49
Ethics committee members	6	14	6	0	26
Regulators	2	7	2	6	17
Other key informants	17	18	9	13	57
Total	73	148	80	36	337

Asia [India, Nepal and Sri Lanka].[1] In this study we identified key actors in the conduct, management and regulation of clinical trials in a variety of settings (See Table 1).

In total we carried out 337 semi-structured interviews, the vast majority of which were recorded, translated into English where necessary, and transcribed. The resulting dataset was entered into Atlas.ti for coding. The codes were generated by an iterative process at a workshop held in Mumbai with all coders present; trial codings were carried out and a selection of interviews was recoded to ensure consistency.

Here we draw principally on extended interviews with a small sub-set of Ethical Review Committee [ERC] members from India [14], Sri Lanka [6] and Nepal [6]. In many respects, the sample is unrepresentative of the wider body of reviewers at work in each of these countries as it was self-selecting and therefore tended to be made up of people who were knowledgeable, articulate and keen to express their views on the rights and wrongs of clinical trials, the work of ERCs and their less responsible colleagues. They were also mostly from Institutional [hospital] and University settings. Nonetheless, consideration of their accounts of topics such as ethical review, operation and composition of committees, capacity building, training for reviewers and approaches to informed consent provides a useful indicator of the major challenges faced by committed ERC members in the settings identified. We also draw to a lesser extent on interviews with regulators, policy-makers, academics and investigators involved in developing ethical review infra-structure. Before considering these responses in detail it is necessary to consider briefly the three contexts in which our study took place.

2. India

India has a well-established pharma industry dating back to the 1950s. The thrust of this industry has been the production of generics for local markets. This infrastructure, combined with large numbers of English speaking doctors and technicians, as well as large populations of treatment naive people with a range of disorders of interest in the west [e.g. cancers, cardio-vascular disease, diabetes] has stimulated much interest in clinical trials. Trials are outsourced by western pharmaceutical industries as well as conducted by local companies keen to move into global markets for their products. Acceleration in this sector of activity has overwhelmed existing machinery for ethical review and monitoring which previously catered mostly for locally conducted research. Along with Ethical Guidelines for Biomedical research Involving Human Subjects Indian Council of Medical Research (2000), the

---

[1] The research was funded by the Economic and Social Research Council of the United Kingdom in collaboration with the Department for International Development [ESRC/DfID nbrRES-167-25-0503]. Ethical approval for the study was initially given by the School of Social and Political Sciences Research Ethics Committee, University of Edinburgh [13/10/2010]. Ethical clearance was then gained from local ERCs for research to be carried out in India, Nepal and Sri Lanka.

B. Simpson et al. / Social Science & Medicine 131 (2015) 247–254 249

ICH-GCP guidelines have provided the framework for the conduct of ethical and scientific conduct of trials. In 2001, ICH-GCP India were created (CDSCO, 2001), adapting the generic guidelines to fit local circumstances. In 2005, the 'Schedule Y' amendment of the Drugs and Cosmetic Act provided further guidance on the constitution and responsibilities of ethics committees. To date, ERCs have largely operated within the institutions in which the trials have taken place. The ICMR has launched various initiatives to encourage the take up of standard operating procedures against a backdrop of poor regulation and variable quality of the review process. The Forum for Ethical Review Committees — India [FERCI] was established under the auspices of FERCAP to improve quality and standards and held its first conference in 2011. In 2007, the ICMR established its own clinical trials registry.[2] At the time of writing, there over 650 ERCs registered via the Clinical Trials Registry of India.[3] The workload of ERCs is unevenly spread with a relatively small number of ERCs dealing with the majority of trials and a disproportionate number using independent ERCs.

3. Sri Lanka

Sri Lanka has neither the population nor the pharmaceutical industry that India has. Not surprisingly therefore, the development of ERCs looks very different. All the major medical faculties and teaching hospitals currently have their own institutional ethical review committees, making for some 15 committees (Dissanayake et al., 2006). The Sri Lanka Medical Association (SLMA) formed its ethics committee in 1991 and began considering research projects carried out by its members in 1999. In 2005, the Forum for Ethical Review Committees in Sri Lanka [FERCSL] was established along with Uniform Guidelines for ethical review (Dissanayake et al., 2006). However, take-up of the guidelines appears patchy with considerable variation in standard operating procedures in evidence. The increase in the number of ERCs and the quality of their capacity to review projects was in part driven by an increase in international collaborative research being conducted in Sri Lanka as well as by the desire to create robust research governance of the kind needed to attract trials in the future. Sri Lanka has also recently created its own clinical trials registry.[4] As in India, ERCs are a key mechanism in the regulation of trial activity but they are also identified as having serious weaknesses that need to be addressed if they are to be effective (Karunananyake, 2012).

4. Nepal

Nepal is by far the smallest player in the emergence of human experimental activity in Asia and consequently has a very recent and modest history of ethical review. The central body regulating research studies in Nepal is the apex Ethical Review Board (ERB) of Nepal Health Research Council. The 20 Institutional Review Committees (IRCs) that operate mostly in the medical schools have been approved by the national ERB. The IRCs came in existence because

of increasing volume of local research studies seeking approval from ERB. IRCs are not currently authorised to review international trials which must be reviewed at ERB level. National Ethical Guidelines for Health Research in Nepal were published in 2001. A National Guideline on Clinical Trials with the use of Pharmaceutical Products was published in 2005. Phase I and Phase II trials are not currently allowed and as a consequence Nepal has not been a target for growth in these activities with the increase in research mostly being carried out by international charities, NGOs and academic bodies (Khatri et al., nd).

5. The rise of human experimentation in Asia

The earlier attitude was that we should block it [clinical trials development] because as I told you it was a nation of traders at that time and now because our own people are innovating, we want the innovation to be there, we want to be landscaped for the innovation, so the trials are to be permitted but then at the same time the ethical standards have moved up, benchmarks have increased, every trial has to be put on the web and everything has to be on the web, so it is an open system, so in that you don't feel threatened; not at all but the only thing, I feel heavy as a person. Senior Government of India Official [022]

...[the government].. want to promote clinical trials more as a money making exercise than anything else I guess, because clinical trials are big money, and we have a good receptive population here, educated and also the free health care which means that people need not bother about funding health care for the patients with side effects or anything, that automatically falls on the state to fund all that, so it's a very practical place for clinical trials. Sri Lanka ERC member [71]

Before 1990, there are people who brought medicines in bags and distributed but after the formation of Nepal Health Research Council in 1991, every health research in the country should take ethical approval from them. I am dead against clinical trials. My soul just doesn't agree to it. There are vulnerable groups like poor people, army, students, handicapped people who are being tested. We should not encourage it [clinical trials]...[]... Newer biological products should not be tested in humans. There are also DDA regulations to be cleared in Nepal. NepalERC member [03]

In the three quotations given above, something of the ambivalence that those with responsibility for ethical review feel about clinical trials sponsored by commercial trials organisations is evident. On the face of it, the economics of experimentation are undoubtedly attractive. Saving costs on drug development, opening up new markets and even developing entirely new drugs using local expertise has the potential to reconfigure the shape of the pharmaceutical industry across the globe. In anticipation of such developments, extravagant claims have been made for the contribution that clinical trials will, in due course, make to economies in the region and particularly in India. These claims have stimulated the promotion of trials, training of personnel and capacity building in the knowledge and expertise needed to conduct trials in accordance with international standards. Much of this activity is intended to create a climate in which home-grown as well as outsourced clinical trials will thrive; the promise is nothing short of a pharmaceutical El Dorado.

On the way to this El Dorado, however, serious concerns have been raised. Many of these concerns are by now familiar and well-rehearsed; they draw attention to the potential for abuse and exploitation of 'human subjects' in trials. This may range from the inadequacy of informed consent procedures through to physical

---

[2] The Clinical Trials Registry India. http://www.who.int/ictrp/network/ctri/en/index.html accessed 23rd July 2013 http://www.who.int/ictrp/network/ctri/en/index.html accessed 23rd July 2013.

[3] Details of registered ERCs can be found on the website of the Central Drugs Standard Control Organisation: http://www.cdsco.nic.in/forms/Default.aspx accessed 5th Feb 2014.

[4] The Sri Lanka Clinical Trials Registry (SLCTR) is a Registry for clinical trials involving human subjects, conducted in Sri Lanka or overseas. The SLCTR is a Primary Registry linked to the Registry Network of the International Clinical Trials Registry Platform of the WHO (WHO-ICTRP). It is a not-for-profit Registry, with free and open access to researchers, clinicians, and the general public'. http://www.slctr.lk/accessed 21st July 2013.

harm and even death as a result of adverse drug reactions for which there may then be little or no compensation, giving rise to charges that local populations are used as 'guinea pigs' with 'double standards' in operation (Macklin, 2004). There are concerns that groups rendered vulnerable by their marginality, poverty and lack of literacy are being caught up in the 'global search for human subjects' (Petryna, 2009). In the ensuing debates, ERCs figure as both a key mechanism in enabling trials as well as a site of potential activism aimed at drawing attention to abuses and the broader issues of inequality that often underpin these. ERC members frequently indicated their awareness of vulnerable research subjects and their duties and responsibilities in ensuring their protection:

> …. the people who are in the ethics committee, they really see to it that the patient's rights are properly taken care of … because they don't know anything scientifically India, ERC member [003]

The problems identified, however, were not just downward facing ones. ERC members in each country spoke of their responsibilities to feed issues and concerns up into legal and policy-making machinery. Here, the concerns were much more about 'national' interest and how it might be sidelined, undermined or over-ridden in the quest for viable experimental economies. One informant spoke of 'research coolies', an emotive term intended to invoke parallels with other arena in which domination and exploitation of developing world populations is underway. This was particularly so in India following a change of law in 2005 which allowed easier access to pharmaceutical companies to local populations (see Nundy and Gulhati, 2005). Similar, sentiments were evident in Sri Lanka:

> … the problem is we need to upgrade our societal knowledge levels, preparedness must be upgraded, if that [successful engagement with international clinical trials] is to actually work in that way, otherwise it won't, it will be a new kind of colonialism. That's the problem. Sri Lanka ERC member [074]

In response to these problems, members of ERCs spoke optimistically of a progressively stronger, more confident and better organised infrastructure out of which robust and consistent responses could be applied to international and locally sponsored research proposals

> …… we have a strong procedure right now. Earlier there was hardly any procedures and now we have an application form, even including a standard operating procedure is available for the investigators to check..[].. one of the biggest advantages came for the ethics review parties the ICMR guidelines which came in 2004, '05 which actually helped a lot to formulate how an ethics committee should function in the country. India ERC member [009]

> … ethics committees have evolved. The type of questions that we use to ask and the issues we used to raise 10 years ago are different from what we raise now. And by and large the bar has risen. And therefore even investigators have refused trials, I know. And in fact many of them involve me in that pre-nup discussion. You know, before they firm up with the company they will, they have ethical issues they want to know from me also whether these are ethical issues, whether these will cause problems. So they do want to iron it out. …[].. the investigator community needs to be convinced that the ethics committee is a policeman, but a strict policeman, but not somebody who is against us. But [someone] who wants to promote good ethical research. And has ultimately got the patient's good at heart. India ERC member [002]

Yet, despite these claims to progress, there was a sense in which the work of committee members was a small response in the face of a much bigger problem. Most of the ERC members interviewed were voluntary. Their work involved long hours and exacting work dealing with an unfeasible workload with the threat of possible hostility from researchers in the background should they give unfavourable decisions. Nonetheless, many of those interviewed expressed strong commitment and dedication to their work. Indeed, some spoke with enthusiasm bordering on evangelical zeal about the importance of ethical review and the need to extend its scope and improve its thoroughness.

However, the management of ethical review in practice was likely to be rather more pragmatic and tactical. As a comment from a member of an ethics committee in India makes clear, social and humanitarian concerns are less in evidence as other priorities take over

> …. according to me if a person is recruited as a subject of research and it is deemed by a component ethical review board and set of researchers, that there is no ethical wrong or scientific wrong in that person being recruited I don't see why Indian subjects can't be recruited for clinical trials. So, yes, ok Indian patients are being made guinea pigs for molecules. If it is being done in the right way I don't see anything wrong…[].. I suppose there are many agencies which are conducting clinical trials which are not earlier into ethical standards or scientific standards that is required. I don't know about that. But as far as we are concerned I don't see anything wrong. India ERC member [001]

In this rather straight up and down reading of ethical review, the scope and function of ERCs is simple and clearly limited to the research protocol and the assurances given therein. The attraction of this approach, particularly among younger researchers, appeared to be that it offers both procedural efficiency and authoritative outcomes in circumstances where complexity and the sheer volume of work might otherwise overwhelm. In the midst of this tension, our research identified a powerful and emerging alignment. In managing the growing volume of protocols to review, ERCs appeared to be cleaving to ICH-GCP as a route to procedural clarity. At the same time, they also found themselves in competition with a new breed of 'independent' and, indeed, internationally sponsored ERCs.

These organisations were beginning to feature in the ethical review landscape of India and to a lesser extent in Sri Lanka. Constituted and practicing in conformity with ICH-GCP from their inception, they offer a commercial route to ethical approval. Their emergence causes concern to those who have laboured to develop capacity and rigour in the work of institutional review bodies. Concerns expressed were twofold. First, the guidelines followed can be interpreted quite minimally and specifically and whilst scientific rigour is likely to be guaranteed [because otherwise the validity of the data would be compromised] issues of patient safety are likely to be treated in a more procedural fashion.

Furthermore, a route to ethical approval which circumvents a more politicised reading of ethics and what it means to protect a 'subject' is highly attractive to those wishing for a speedy review. This tension is most evident in industry sponsored clinical trials which are likely to be multi-centred. Here industry standards enshrined in the ICH GCP create expectations of high levels of conformity between trials. ERCs have less of a role to play in such trials, primarily because the protocols are less negotiable but also because large pharma companies, particularly foreign ones, have both the resources and the experience to draft scientifically sound and ethically plausible protocols. As one PI on a commercial trial in

India put it: '*Sponsors are very clear. They want safety data, efficacy in the Indian population. That's all. Nothing more*' India Clinical Trial PI [004]. In the drive towards procedural efficiency and auditable outcomes, trialists, both commercial and non-commercial, end up paying less attention to the wider socio-economic contexts in which trials take place. Complex questions of just what is informed consent and how to get it, and what the benefits are for those who participate in research are apt to be occluded in the face of pharma induced proceduralism. This is not to say that these issues are absent from protocols but rather that, in the complex chains of responsibility and accountability that lie between a professionally crafted and ethically approved application and its implementation on the ground, there is much scope for the interests of trial participants to become secondary to the conduct of the trial and the data it sets out to generate. This problem is further compounded by the fact that it is often junior staff with minimal training who are responsible for the implementation of agreed protocols at the level of day to day interaction with research participants.

The emergence of independent ethics committees within the ERC landscape adds further momentum to this process, with concerns being expressed about their independence (Karam and Karandikar, 2012); also see (Emanuel et al., 2006). For many of those interviewed, ethical review was not a legitimate area for commercial activity because of the tension it creates between robustness of review procedures on the one hand and the likelihood of future use of particular ERCs by CROs and their sponsors on the other:

.. If an independent ethics committee is very cautious, and they fear that if they don't approve, it [the trial] easily goes elsewhere and they get the approval from there. Like EC shopping. There is nothing to prevent that. India ERC member [002].

The minute they realize that there is something going wrong, when we ask uncomfortable questions, they just go to some other committee India ERC member [001]

At the time of writing [Jan 2014] the Drug Controller General of India has forbidden independent ethics committees from approving clinical trial protocols following complaints about procedural irregularities.[5] Further steps have been taken by the Supreme Court of India to establish more stringent monitoring of trials including registration and accreditation of ERCs which will, in future, also have increased responsibilities for monitoring and reporting.[6] Neither Sri Lanka nor Nepal has the kind of demand that would currently make independent ethics committees viable. Nonetheless, as we will see in the next section the issues of legitimacy and jurisdiction that their existence raises is much wider than India alone.

6. ERCs and the question of legitimacy and authority

ERCs feature in a complex landscape of interests and concerns. These are at once economic and humanitarian; legal and social; national and international. Procedural legitimacy and authority is drawn from their location within particular institutions. These include Universities, Professional Associations, Hospitals and government departments and institutes with committees assembled out of suitably representative experts. ERCs also derive their

authority from a patchwork of guidelines and regulations that emanate from different sources: government, industry, academia and international NGOs. Reference to these sources enables ERCs to gain credibility and acceptance among local and international researchers. They provide members with an ethical charter of sorts which validates and legitimates action.

We are SIDCER approved, and basically ...[]..., there is the FERCSL national guidelines on writing your standard operating procedures and doing the ethics review and we basically follow that to the letter, so our SOPs is already readily available you can find it or I can give you a copy, everything is in writing and it's very easy to understand, it's all tick boxes and check lists and we are very transparent in the whole review, so really that's what we follow and at the moment we are reviewing our SOPs also, and probably that's of course just our procedures I think you may have to also look at our criteria for review and see whether we can improve on that. It is very standard everybody does the same thing within our EC. Sri Lanka ERC member [071].

... we have developed our SOP's based on ICMR, ICH and FERCAP guidelines, so we follow those. And now because we have a SOP we are stronger in saying certain things — India ERC member [156].

Unlike in Sri Lanka and Nepal, there is an expectation in India that the responsibilities that figure in a research application will be legally recognised and approved:

Interviewer: *In India CRO PI, investigator and director all sign an agreement relating to the collaboration?*

Respondent: *Yes. That is reviewed. But it comes to the ethics committee; it also goes to our legal expert. You have a (hospital ethics committee) legal expert. He also clarifies that, gets things done the way the hospital is supposed to have it legally and it also comes to the ethics committee to have a final look at that. This goes simultaneously; when they put in support for the scientific review they will immediately send the CTA to the legal expert office.* India ERC member [156].

Whilst these forms of regulatory triangulation increase confidence, they also raise concerns about over-excessive and disabling regulation among researchers. ERCs as mechanisms that enable and facilitate better research, give way to rather more antagonistic readings of the role of ERCs among researchers with concerns expressed that ERCs address problems that are not within their sphere of responsibility:

I mean we are talking about ethics; we are talking about bad science which is impeaching on ethics. They do ask, 'who are you, what is this? This is (name of the respondent)'s EC please, we should try to avoid it'. So we have people like that. So it's not that simple. ... whoever has to work as regulators are never popular people, by definition. India ERC member [002]

However, in contexts where authority is weak and mistrust is high, invoking rhetorics of legitimacy, such as audit, monitoring, surveying and certification by higher authorities, is one of the few strategies available to persuade outsiders of the committee's authority to make legitimate pronouncements on the ethics of research. Such credentials are essential when it comes to an ERCs ability to act as what Stark has referred to as a 'declarative body', that is, one capable of making judgements and evaluations but, most critically, decisions which will be accepted as emerging from a democratic process (Stark, 2012, pp. 4–5).

---

[5] http://pharmabiz.com/ArticleDetails.aspx?aid=76984&sid=1   accessed   13th August 2013.

[6] Government set to tighten clinical trial norms. Times of India 3/01/2014. http://articles.timesofindia.indiatimes.com/2014-01-03/india/45834762_1_clinical-trials-accreditation-council-ethics. accessed 10th Jan 2014.

The power of ERCs is, therefore, largely negotiated rather than absolute, based on guidelines rather than laws and persuasion rather than instruction. Whilst great strides have been made in channelling more research through ERCs and cultivating the confidence of researchers, there remain anxieties about the limits of their power and a sense that all their good work might be undone once the project passes beyond the ERC and into its implementation phase. For example, in Nepal and Sri Lanka, once a project is approved it is very much a matter of trust and investigators' willingness to self-report on how the trial is implemented. For one of our informants, this issue was further linked with lack of capacity within the committee:

> … *there's no training, we don't have people who have trained in it [ethical review], it needs training, monitoring, for the moment we have done the consent monitoring and then we have depended on adverse events from the investigators, ..[]… We do not have the staffing or the training.* Sri Lanka ERC member [076]

For this ERC member, establishing a functioning ERC, simply served to highlight the partiality of the process; there was an awareness that many further steps would need to be taken to ensure that monitoring was both comprehensive and rigorous. The committee simply made apparent the magnitude of the problem of policing projects once approved.

Problems of ERC scope, however, are not just about jurisdiction. Other concerns arise for ERC members when they consider the limits of their roles and responsibilities towards subjects who they will never know. The moral complexity of the issues that they are expected to deal with are substantial. As one of our Indian informants candidly put it:

> …. *I find it very difficult to put myself in the feet of the completely uneducated women from Uttar Pradesh. I find it impossible to do so. Which means to know how she would think and how she would react to a situation is impossible for me? Which means then we need them [ERC members] to discuss this, to come up with a guidance document. Like I told you, to talk to this cancer survivor, completely different thought process came in to my mind, that you have to think of it from too many different sources.* India ERC member [002].

What this quotation points to, is a profoundly humanistic conception of the role of ERCs but one that is often lost to procedure and pragmatism. The starting point for any application is a research protocol. The style of the protocol is invariably technical and constructed in such a way that researchers and 'subjects' are described impersonally and with maximum detachment — socially and culturally these documents are flat, and intentionally so. It is the skill of the person drafting the research protocol, and particularly in pharmaceutically sponsored multi-centred trials, to produce such documents. However, through ethical review, there is some presumption that the social imagination of the reviewers will be brought into play. It is, in theory at least, the task of the ethics committee to animate the protocol, that is, to try to imagine the people who are likely to end up in the trial and the worlds in which they live. Arguably, this is why social scientists and lay people are brought on to ERCs and why there is currently a great deal of interest in community advisory boards as ways of amplifying the voice of those who end up in trials (Weijer and Emmanuel, 2000). The purpose of such a mechanism is precisely to help stimulate acts of imagination and empathy capable of invoking the people and relationships with which the protocol will ultimately engage.

> … *you can't define risk only as physical risk. People just forget social risks, economic risks and psychological risks.* India ERC member [002].

However, putting oneself in another's shoes in the context of a busy ERC is both challenging, time consuming and deemed by some to be wholly misplaced. Consequently, there is a danger that the human subject that features at the heart of an ERC's deliberations will not be any actual person in a real place and time but the trans-cultural, trans-historical, universal subject which features in all protocols. At this juncture, ICH-GCP offers an attractive route to consistency in the conduct of clinical trials and particularly its focus on the informed consent transaction as the primary index of ethical conduct. However, the economic and cultural questions that exercise some ERC members are apt to be obscured or overlooked.

In India in particular, limitations in terms of resources, training and the absence of clearly defined statutory duties render the limits of ERC responsibilities fuzzy at the margins. Indeed, the scale and complexity of activity means that the possibilities for breaches of regulation are rife. A current concern of a number of informants was the potential for moving activity to the edges of regulatory reach whether this be in terms of the regions in which trials are conducted or the committees through which trials are put. As a result there have been calls for ERCs to have 'teeth' and a clearer articulation with law and state regulation. Proposals to amend the Drugs and Cosmetics Act [1940], as mentioned above, have specified that ethical approval for clinical trials can only be given by ERCs that have been registered with the licensing authority. This development further ties in the practice of clinical trials with the ICH-GCP India Guidelines via the formal registration of ERCs. The amendment also gives the Central Drugs Standard Control Organisation the power to inspect the documentation of an ERC at any time.

7. Conclusion

We began our considerations of ERC members' views with a question: if ethics committees are the solution what is the problem? In reflecting on the impacts of industry sanctioned models and strategies for ethical review in the developing world it would seem that there are a range of problems, some of which extend the business of human subject protection beyond the immediate engagement between a trial participant and a treatment being tested in an RCT. In this article we have provided insights from those who are, in many respects, at the eye of the storm when it comes to the governance of clinical trial activity. On the one hand, ERC members articulate a need for contextualisation and localisation in the attempt to render trials ethical in developing world settings (cf Emanuel et al., 2004; Lavery et al., 2007). Here, ERC members we interviewed, allude to issues that confound their efforts to protect subjects, such as poverty, literacy and structural inequality. Achieving a satisfactory ethical review might, in other words, inspire advocacy and social critique. On the other hand, however, they face considerable pressure. Their workload is substantial, they are under-resourced and there is a strong push to standardise and regularise the work of ethical review in ways that remove the independence of reviewers to set the scope of their concerns.

These tensions are not just national or indeed regional phenomena but are fuelled by changes that are taking place in Europe and US which are aimed at increasing research capacity and velocity by means of an alignment between ethical review and industry standards and procedures. For example, at the time of writing, the EU is proposing to replace the existing clinical trials directive with a new regulation aimed at accelerating application procedures and harmonising administrative requirements for multi-centre trials across the European Union and in countries participating in trials beyond the EU (Den Boer and Schipper, 2013). In the US, Food and Drugs Administration (FDA) proposed that the

International Conference on Harmonisation - Good Clinical Practice (ICH-GCP) be designated as the new regulatory standard which in effect sidelined the Declaration of Helsinki for trials carried out outside the US (Goodyear et al., 2009). Both of these developments have significant implications for the role that ethical review might play in attempts to safeguard trial participants from harm and exploitation. Given that ethics committees may not be able to provide the kinds of protection that vulnerable people need we ought to ask a further question: if ethic committees are the problem, what is the solution?

That ethics committee are currently a problem in the countries considered might be inferred from the ways in which clinical trials activity has generated debate, stimulated activism and stirred those responsible for the governance of research to put forward improved regulatory responses. For example, since our data was collected, responses to public concerns over clinical trial regulation in India have resulted in a wide range of new regulations coming from the Supreme Court, the Office of Drugs Controller General of India and a series of expert panels. Registration of ethics committees, audio-video recoding of the informed consent procedures and clearer rules regarding compensation for deaths and injuries that occur during clinical trials are all now mandatory.[7] In Sri Lanka, the drafting of a new Clinical Trials Act has provoked controversy as it is believed by some to lower the regulatory threshold thereby making it easier to conduct clinical trials (Siribaddana and Bandara, 2013). In Nepal, whilst debates about commercial trials have only just begun, there is much interest in regulating research activities and promoting ethical standards in the conduct of both clinical and public health research. Significantly, in each of these places, ERCs are identified as the problem but they are also identified as the solution when it comes to better research governance.

Yet, when it comes to what constitutes effective and legitimate ethical review, the language of ICH-GCP is a strong card to play. One of the reasons for this is the ease with which techniques of verification such as monitoring, audit, record keeping, documenting and other evidence making procedures familiar to scientists, can be imported into the practice of ethical review. However, the failure of ethical review to protect human subjects beyond the informed consent transaction does not result in a change of method but typically better monitored replications of the same process (cf McGoey, 2010). One consequence of this move in the US has been a tendency to replicate the evidential turn in science through an evidence-based ethics in that it would similarly, '.... emphasize the importance of data in informing decision and decision-making about the ethical issues inherent in clinical medicine and research' (Sugarman, 2004, p. 495). The tendency to instrumentalise ethics in this way was evident in the accounts of a number of researchers interviewed. Rather than seeing the directives of an ERC as the beginning of an ongoing awareness of the wide-ranging vulnerability of their subjects, many researchers spoke of ethics as a kind of object; something obtained from, or 'given' by, the ERC which then enabled them to continue with a clear conscience.

Acknowledgements

We would like to acknowledge Vajira Dissanayake, Ian Harper, Roger Jeffery, Amar Jesani, Neha Madhiwala, Salla Sariola, Jeevan Raj Sharma and other members of the Biomedical Health Experimentation in South Asia project for their help in developing this paper. To Rachel Douglas—Jones and Gerard Porter for their various suggestions. Its development was also facilitated by participation at the end of project dissemination event held at University of Edinburgh [September 2012]. We would also like to express our sincere thanks to the many people who generously gave of their time in interviews and discussions. The research was funded by the Economic and Social Research Council/Department for International Development [RES-167-25-0503].

References

Abraham, J., 2007. Drug trials and evidence bases in international regulatory context. BioSocieties 2 (1), 41–56.

Abraham, J., 2011. Evolving sociological analyses of 'pharmaceuticalisation': a response to Williams, Martin and Gabe. Sociology of Health & Illness 33, 726–728.

Abraham, J., Reed, T., 2002. Progress, innovation and regulatory science in drug development: the politics of international standard setting. Social Studies of Science 32, 337–369.

Bosk, C.L., 2007. The new bureaucracies of virtue or when form fails to follow function. PoLar: Political and Legal Anthropology Review 30 (2), 192–209.

Central Drugs Standard Control Organisation, 2001. Good Clinical Practices for Clinical Research in India. India. http://cdsco.nic.in/html/GCP1.html (accessed 11.08.13.).

Den Boer, A., Schipper, I., 2013. New EU regulation on clinical trials: the impact on ethics and safeguards for Participants. Indian Journal of Medical Ethics 10 (2), 106–109.

Dissanayake, V.J., Lanerolle, R., Mendis, N., 2006. Research ethics and ethical review committees in Sri Lanka: a twenty-five year journey. Ceylon Medical Journal 51 (3), 110–113.

Douglas-Jones, R., 2013. Locating Ethics: capacity building, ethics review and research governance across Asia (PhD thesis). University of Durham. February 2013.

Emanuel, E.J., Lemmens, T., Elliot, C., 2006. Should society allow research ethics boards to be run as for-profit enterprises? PLoS Med 3 (7), e309 http://dx.doi.org/10.1371/journal.pmed.0030309 (accessed 23.07.13.).

Emmanuel, E.J., Wendler, D., Killen, J., Grady, C., 2004. What makes clinical research in developing countries ethical? The benchmarks of ethical research. Journal of Infectious Diseases 189, 930–937.

Goodyear, M., Lemmens, T., Sprumont, D., Tangwa, G., 2009. Does the FDA have the authority to trump the declaration of Helsinki? British Medical Journal 338. http://dx.doi.org/10.1136/bmj.b1559.

ten Have, H.A.M.J., 2001. Genetics and culture: the geneticization thesis. Medicine, Health Care and Philosophy 4 (3), 295–304.

Hedgecoe, A., 1998. Geneticization, medicalisation and polemics. Medicine, Health Care and Philosophy 1, 235–243.

Indian Council of Medical Research. 2000. Ethical Guidelines for Biomedical Research Involving Human Subjects. Indian Council of Medical Research. http://www.stvincent.org/uploadedFiles/Medical_Services/Research_and_Clinical_Trials/EthicalGuidelinesforBiomedicalResearchonHumanSubjects-India.pdf (accessed 23.07.13.).

International Conference on Harmonisation, 2010. ICH 20th Anniversary Value Benefits of ICH to Drug Regulatory Authorities — Advancing Harmonization for Better Health. ICH Secretariat, Geneva. http://www.ich.org/fileadmin/Public_Web_Site/News_room/C_Publications/ICH_20_anniversary_Value_Benefits_of_ICH_for_Regulators.pdf (accessed Friday, 05.08.11.).

Jesani, A., 2012. Ethics of expert opinion and the observations of the department-related parliamentary standing committee on the CDSCO. Journal of Pharmacology and Pharmacotherapeutics 3 (4), 297–299.

Jesani, A., 2013. New regulations on compensation for injury and death in drug trials. Indian Journal of Medical Ethics X (2), 77–79.

Kadam, R., Karandikar, S., 2012. Ethics committees in India: facing the challenges! Ethics 3 (2), 50–56.

Karunanayake, P., 2012. Effective Participant Protection Must be Ensured. The Sunday Island (Sri Lanka). Sept 6th.

Khatri, R., Sharma, R.J., Harper, I. nd Evolution and growth of health research and experimentation in Nepal: emerging trends, actors and modalities. European Bulletin of Himalayan Research.

Kleinman, A., 1999. Moral experience and ethical reflection: Can ethnography reconcile them? 'A quandary for the new bioethics'. In: Kleinman, A., Fox, R., Brandt, A. (Eds.), Bioethics and Beyond. Daedalus 128, vol. 4, pp. 69–97.

Lavery, J.V., Grady, C., Wahl, E.R., Emanuel, E.J., 2007. Ethical Issues in International Biomedical research: a Casebook. Oxford University Press, Oxford.

Lippman, A., 1991. Prenatal genetic testing and screening: constructing needs and reinforcing inequities. American Journal of Law and Medicine 17, 15–50.

Macklin, R., 2004. Double Standards in Medical Research in Developing Countries. Cambridge University Press, Cambridge.

McGoey, L., 2010. Profitable failure: antidepressant drugs and the triumph of flawed experiments. History of Human Sciences 23 (1), 58–78.

Nundy, S., Gulhati, C.M., 2005. A new colonialism? Conducting clinical trials in India. New England Journal of Medicine 352 (16), 1633–1636.

---

[7] Panel recommends sweeping changes in clinical trials, The Hindu Sept 18, 2013. http://www.thehindu.com/sci-tech/health/panel-recommends-sweeping-changes-in-clinical-trials/article5141590.ece accessed 20th Jan 2014, http://www.thehindu.com/sci-tech/health/panel-recommends-sweeping-changes-in-clinical-trials/article5141590.ece accessed 20th Jan 2014. Also see (Jesani, 2102, 2013).

Petryna, A., 2009. When Experiments Travel: Clinical Trials and the Global Search for Human Subjects. Princeton University Press, New Jersey.

Siribaddana, S., Bandara, W., 2013. Clinical trials in Sri Lanka: new act at the behest of the pharmaceutical industry? Indian Journal of Medical Ethics X (4), 268–270.

Stark, L., 2012. Behind Closed Doors: IRB's and the Making of Ethical Research. University of Chicago Press, Chicago and London.

Sugarman, J., 2004. Determining the appropriateness of including children in clinical research: how thick is the ice? Journal of the American Medical Association 291 (4), 494–496.

Timmermans, S., Almeling, R., 2009. Objectification, standardization, and commodification in health care: a conceptual readjustment. Social Science & Medicine 69, 21–27.

Timmermans, S., Epstein, S., 2010. A world of standards but nota standard world: toward a sociology of standards and standardization. Annual Review of Sociology 36, 69–89.

Weijer, C., Emanuel, E., 2000. Protecting communities in biomedical research. Science 289, 1142–1144.

Williams, S.J., Martin, P., Gabe, J., 2011. The pharmaceuticalisation of society? A framework for analysis. Sociology of Health and Illness 33 (5), 710–725.

4.3   Understanding the Functions and Operations of Data Monitoring Committees: Survey and Focus Group Findings

Karim A. Calis, Patrick Archdeacon, Raymond Bain, David DeMets, Miriam Donohue, M. Khair Elzarrad, Annemarie Forrest, John McEachern, Michael J. Pencina, Jane Perlmutter, and Roger J. Lewis

Calis, K, et al. Understanding the functions and operations of data monitoring committees: Survey and focus group findings. *Clinical Trials* 14(1), 59–66 (2017).

Article

CLINICAL
TRIALS

Clinical Trials
1–7
© The Author(s) 2017

Reprints and permissions:
sagepub.co.uk/journalsPermissions.nav
DOI: 10.1177/1740774517707743
journals.sagepub.com/home/ctj

§SAGE

Recommendations for data monitoring committees from the Clinical Trials Transformation Initiative

Karim A Calis[1,2], Patrick Archdeacon[1], Raymond Bain[3], David DeMets[4], Miriam Donohue[5], M Khair Elzarrad[6], Annemarie Forrest[7], John McEachern[8], Michael J Pencina[9], Jane Perlmutter[10] and Roger J Lewis[11]

Abstract

Background/aims: Use of data monitoring committees to oversee clinical trials was first proposed nearly 50 years ago. Since then, data monitoring committee use in clinical trials has increased and evolved. Nonetheless, there are no well-defined criteria for determining the need for a data monitoring committee, and considerable variability exists in data monitoring committee composition and conduct. To understand and describe the role and function of data monitoring committees, and establish best practices for data monitoring committee trial oversight, the Clinical Trials Transformation Initiative—a public–private partnership to improve clinical trials—launched a multi-stakeholder project.

Methods: The data monitoring committee project team included 16 individuals charged with (1) clarifying the purpose of data monitoring committees, (2) identifying best practices for independent data monitoring committee conduct, (3) describing effective communication practices, and (4) developing strategies for training data monitoring committee members. Evidence gathering included a survey, a series of focus group discussions, and a 2-day expert meeting aimed at achieving consensus opinions that form the foundation of our data monitoring committee recommendations.

Results: We define the role of the data monitoring committee as an advisor to the research sponsor on whether to continue, modify, or terminate a trial based on periodic assessment of trial data. Data monitoring committees should remain independent from the sponsor and be composed of members with no relevant conflicts of interest. Representation on a data monitoring committee generally should include at least one clinician with expertise in the therapeutic area being studied, a biostatistician, and a designated chairperson who has experience with clinical trials and data monitoring. Data monitoring committee meetings are held periodically to evaluate the unmasked data from ongoing trials, but the content and conduct of meetings may vary depending on specific goals or topics for deliberation. To guide data monitoring committee conduct and communication plans, a charter consistent with the protocol's research design and statistical analysis plan should be developed and agreed upon by the sponsor and the data monitoring committee prior to patient enrollment. We recommend concise and flexible charters that explain roles, responsibilities, operational issues, and how data monitoring committee recommendations are generated and communicated. The demand for data monitoring committee members appears to exceed the current pool of qualified individuals. To prepare a new generation of trained data monitoring committee members, we encourage a combination of didactic educational programs,

[1]Office of Medical Policy, Center for Drug Evaluation and Research, US Food and Drug Administration, Silver Spring, MD, USA
[2]Office of the Clinical Director, National Institute of Child Health and Human Development, National Institutes of Health, Bethesda, MD, USA
[3]Merck & Co., Inc., Kenilworth, NJ, USA
[4]Department of Biostatistics and Medical Informatics, University of Wisconsin–Madison, Madison, WI, USA
[5]Quintiles IMS Holdings, Inc., Durham, NC, USA
[6]Office of Science Policy, National Institutes of Health, Bethesda, MD, USA
[7]Clinical Trials Transformation Initiative, Durham, NC, USA
[8]PAREXEL International, Waltham, MA, USA
[9]Duke Clinical Research Institute, Durham, NC, USA
[10]Ann Arbor, MI, USA
[11]Harbor-UCLA Medical Center, Torrance, CA, USA

Corresponding author:
Annemarie Forrest, Clinical Trials Transformation Initiative, 300 W. Morgan Street, Suite 800, Durham, NC 27701-2183, USA.
Email: ctti@mc.duke.edu

practical experience, and skill development through apprenticeships and mentoring by experienced data monitoring committee members.

Conclusion: Our recommendations address data monitoring committee use, conduct, communication practices, and member preparation and training. Furthermore recommendations form the foundation for ongoing efforts to improve clinical trial oversight and enhance the safety and integrity of clinical research. These recommendations serve as a call to action for implementation of best practices that benefit study participants, study sponsors, and society.

Keywords
Data monitoring committees, clinical trials, data and safety monitoring boards

Introduction

The use of data monitoring committees (DMCs) to oversee clinical trials has increased and evolved since the concept was introduced in 1967 by the Greenberg Report.[1] Initial recommendations in that report were applied in National Institutes of Health (NIH)-sponsored cardiovascular trials to monitor trial conduct and safety and to recommend trial modifications or closure. Today, DMCs are occasionally used across therapeutic areas to oversee single trials, groups of trials, or entire portfolios of research related to an investigational intervention. Safeguarding clinical trial participants and monitoring interim safety and efficacy outcomes data in ongoing trials remain paramount responsibilities for DMCs, but variation in the structure and organization of DMCs exist. Membership and responsibilities of DMCs also may vary depending on the nature and goals of the trial.

The Clinical Trials Transformation Initiative, a public–private partnership whose mission is to develop and drive adoption of practices that will increase the quality and efficiency of clinical trials, initiated the DMC Project to address the identified issues in understanding the role, importance, and conduct of DMCs, and to recommend best practices for DMCs and for sponsors working with DMCs. The DMC Project Team included 16 representatives from a broad cross section of the clinical trials enterprise, including regulators, government and industry sponsors of clinical research, academics, contract research organizations, patient representatives, and clinical investigators. The project team developed recommendations for DMC use and conduct (Supplementary Appendix 1) based on their expertise and analysis of the findings from the project's evidence-gathering activities. Our recommendations may apply to any DMC that is charged with monitoring an interventional trial regardless of sponsorship or funding source. While these recommendations focus on external DMCs (defined as an independent group of individuals, external to the sponsor, that conduct its activities outside of the sponsor organization), many of the principles and recommendations may also apply to internal DMCs that conduct similar activities within the sponsor organization.[2]

The objectives of the DMC Project were to (a) clarify the purpose of DMCs and the rationale for their use; (b) develop best-practice recommendations for the operation and optimal conduct of independent DMCs; (c) describe effective communication practices between independent DMCs and trial stakeholders (e.g. sponsors, investigators, and institutional review boards); and (d) identify strategies for preparing the next generation of DMC members.[3]

Methods

Approach

To address the objectives, the DMC Project Team employed three research strategies: a survey of 143 DMC members and organizers, a series of focus group discussions with 43 participants, and a 2-day expert meeting. Detailed methods and results of the survey and focus group discussions are described elsewhere.[3]

The expert meeting[4] was conducted in July 2015 among 54 stakeholders representing academia, government agencies, industry, contract research organizations, patient representatives, and professional societies. Findings and key themes from the survey and focus group discussions were presented. The DMC Project Team used discussion from the meeting to refine recommendations through an iterative process based on consensus-building guidelines[5] that focus on core values of inclusiveness, shared control, and flexibility.

Described herein are the primary outcomes of the DMC Project with emphasis on consensus-based, multi-stakeholder recommendations (Supplementary Appendix 1) for optimizing the operation and conduct of contemporary DMCs.

Results

Clarifying the role of the DMC

As use of DMCs has increased and evolved, confusion has emerged regarding the role of the DMC, which may contribute to unclear expectations between DMCs and other trial stakeholders. We sought to clarify the unique role of DMCs relative to roles of other groups involved in oversight of clinical trials.

The key difference between a DMC and other research oversight groups is that DMCs perform periodic benefit–risk assessments using available efficacy and safety outcomes data gathered during the course of a trial in order to provide the most optimal recommendations and advice to the sponsor and trial leadership. This necessitates close monitoring of the trial for "early definitive evidence of benefit, convincing evidence of harm, or sufficient evidence of no potential benefit to render continuation of the trial to be futile."[6] To adequately perform this important function, DMC members require full access to the unmasked safety and efficacy outcomes data during the course of the trial. The DMC must be able to review the accumulating data by treatment group to assess the benefit–risk balance for trial participants. We emphasize that interim analyses of unmasked trial data require thoughtful consideration and the utmost of care. Various statistical monitoring methods exist but were not discussed in this project and are beyond the scope of this article.

When reviewing trial data, bias must be minimized particularly in the assessment of study outcomes and attribution of adverse events. Therefore, independence from the trial sponsor is critical for the DMC to fulfill its central role of protecting vulnerable study participants from unpredictable harm that may arise during the course of a trial. Occasionally, this may require unscheduled meetings of the DMC and/or additional analyses without alerting the sponsor or study investigators.

Best practices for DMC conduct

Composition. The composition of a DMC must be carefully balanced to ensure effective monitoring of clinical trials. Representation on a DMC, at minimum, should include a clinician with expertise in the therapeutic area being studied and a biostatistician with expertise in statistical monitoring plans and analysis of clinical trial data. The designated chairperson—whether a clinician or statistician—must have experience with clinical trials and data monitoring. Other types of expertise (e.g. pharmacology, toxicology, and behavioral science) also may be required, and some trials by nature have challenging social, cultural, and ethical implications and may benefit from added expertise and diverse perspectives for effective evaluation and monitoring. In light of the increased complexity of clinical trials and interventions being evaluated, the inclusion of bioethicists and patient advocates should also be considered, particularly for trials evaluating high-risk interventions or involving vulnerable populations. Knowledge of research methodology and data analysis, and experience in clinical research are skills generally considered essential for any DMC member.

Selection of an effective DMC chairperson is critically important. The pivotal role of the DMC chair is not limited to trial monitoring, but extends to organizing the operational aspects of the committee and ensuring that DMC members have adequate resources and flexibility to do their work without hindrance or undue interference, particularly from sponsors and others with a vested interest in the trial outcome. Prior experience as a DMC member is essential for the chair. Importantly, the chair should be an accomplished leader and effective communicator who can skillfully manage meetings and create an environment that encourages cooperation and active participation of all DMC members. The chair should be capable of bringing consensus without being overbearing or forceful with personal conclusions or opinions. In addition, the DMC chair should have the necessary interpersonal skills to draw from the collective talents of all members in order to thoughtfully and effectively guide the process of monitoring and oversight.

Conflicts of interest. Prospective DMC members may have potential financial or intellectual conflicts of interest that could compromise their ability to objectively monitor a trial. Thus, conflict of interest must be regularly disclosed, assessed, and managed for all DMC members. At each meeting, members should be asked to declare any new conflicts, and report activities or connections with any parties that may introduce bias and influence their conduct. Activities or relationships deemed to have the potential to undermine independence of DMC members may result in disqualification from DMC service; therefore, both actual and perceived conflicts should be disclosed. Even the perception of a conflict of interest can damage the credibility of the DMC and raise questions about its conduct and recommendations.

Conversely, it is important to note that not all previous interactions with a sponsor are necessarily disqualifying. In some cases, identifying experts with highly specific skills and knowledge but without any connections to the study sponsor or investigators can be difficult. If concerns about conflicts of interest are taken to extremes, few qualified members would be available to serve on DMCs. Many minor conflicts that are unlikely to introduce bias (e.g. prior DMC service for the same sponsor for a different treatment intervention) can be addressed and managed by proper disclosures to the sponsor and other DMC members. However, some conflicts are so significant that they cannot be mitigated by the usual means and may require exclusion from DMC service for certain trials.

It should be emphasized that not all conflicts of interest are financial in nature. Scientists can have vested intellectual or research interests in the results of a given trial, which might impede their impartiality.

Such conflicts must also be addressed on a case-by-case basis and may preclude service on a DMC.

Statistical Data Analysis Center. To support the DMC in fulfilling its role, a Statistical Data Analysis Center capable of preparing reports for or performing additional analyses that may be requested by the DMC is typically utilized. For the DMC to make optimal recommendations regarding the trial to the sponsor and trial leadership, planned interim analyses (based on the DMC Charter, trial protocol, and the statistical analysis plan) may necessitate unplanned analyses to provide insight regarding the interim safety and/or efficacy findings. Therefore, the Statistical Data Analysis Center should have access to all accumulating trial data beginning at trial initiation, possibly necessitating coordination between the Statistical Data Analysis Center and the trial's data management group. It is not acceptable for the sponsor—either by requirement or by financial contract—to limit the scope of statistical work that is to be conducted by the Statistical Data Analysis Center. Instead, the Statistical Data Analysis Center contracts should allow for reasonable adjustments after trial initiation to ensure the sponsor does not unduly influence or restrict the type of work the Statistical Data Analysis Center conducts in support of the DMC. This approach would also minimize the chance that a sponsor is inadvertently informed about additional analyses requested by the DMC in the course of trial monitoring.

The Statistical Data Analysis Center should receive scheduled data transfers both prior to scheduled data reviews and during the period between reviews. Flexibility in the timing of these transfers is essential to aid the DMC in fulfilling its responsibilities. The tables, listings, and figures to be provided to the DMC during its meeting should be specified in advance and the templates approved by the DMC prior to its first data review. Changes to these templates may be requested during the trial, and there should be enough flexibility by the Statistical Data Analysis Center to implement these modifications.

DMC meetings. A best practice for DMC meetings is to hold an initial organizational meeting in order to orient and familiarize DMC members with their roles and responsibilities. All DMC meetings should be held at a neutral venue, avoiding sponsor offices or lavish accommodations. The inaugural meeting should ideally be held in person prior to the start of patient recruitment to allow DMC members to meet each other and review the DMC charter, protocol, and planned Statistical Data Analysis Center report templates. The protocol and statistical analysis plan should be readily available. The DMC members should have minimal

sponsor interactions outside of the formal DMC meetings.

In addition to the DMC members, another key participant in the DMC meetings is the Statistical Data Analysis Center biostatistician. As the Statistical Data Analysis Center reports to and serves the DMC directly, the Statistical Data Analysis Center biostatistician should have an in-depth understanding of the data and how it is acquired, as well as comprehensive knowledge of the statistical analysis plan and protocol.

We recommend a face-to-face DMC meeting at least annually, but other meetings can be held via teleconference or web-based conferencing. Meetings can consist of open sessions (meetings in which individuals not directly involved in the DMC operations may attend) or closed sessions (meetings in which only DMC members and the Statistical Data Analysis Center statistician are permitted). Only blinded data are reviewed in open sessions. Regardless of trial sponsorship (i.e. commercial, government, or private foundation), review of unblinded data can only occur in the closed sessions without any representation or undue influence from the sponsor. Even during open sessions in which blinded data are reviewed and study progress is discussed, sponsor and trial leadership attendees generally should be limited to a few designated officials who are directly responsible for overseeing the trial for the sponsoring organization.

Effective communication practices

Charter. To inform DMC communication practices and address the overall oversight process, a charter that is carefully aligned with the research protocol and the statistical analysis plan should be developed by the sponsor in collaboration with the trial executive committee and with substantive input from the DMC. This important document should be agreed upon by the sponsor, executive committee, Statistical Data Analysis Center, and the DMC members prior to patient enrollment. After careful review of the charter, the protocol, and the statistical analysis plan, feedback from the DMC should be incorporated into the charter. The charter should clearly state the rationale for use of a DMC, broad goals, and the roles, responsibilities, and operational structure of the DMC relative to other clinical trial oversight groups. In addition, the charter should clearly describe the decision-making process of the DMC, describe how DMC recommendations are made, and include the following items: (1) composition, including the number and expertise areas of its members; (2) scheduled data transfers from the trial's data management group to the Statistical Data Analysis Center; (3) the format (face-to-face, tele- or video-conference, open and closed session, etc.) and frequency (e.g. every 6 months) of meetings; and (4) the relationship and communication between DMC and Statistical

Data Analysis Center, and other trial committees and stakeholders, including the trial sponsor.

The content of a DMC charter and the principles underlying it are not identical to those of the protocol and statistical analysis plan. By design, the latter documents are meant to be strictly followed, and any deviations need to be documented with substantive changes requiring amendments. In contrast, the DMC charter should be a succinct and user-friendly document that outlines a set of guiding principles for conduct of the DMC. While clearly aligned with the protocol and statistical analysis plan, the charter should avoid rigidity and legalism since it is not possible to anticipate and address all potential scenarios that could emerge during the course of an ongoing trial. Lengthy elements, such as table and figure templates to be included in DMC reports, should be relegated to the appendix section of the charter. Given the broad and flexible nature of the charter, amendments to this document should be infrequent. A critical aspect of the DMC charter is the monitoring guidelines for efficacy and safety outcomes.

DMC recommendations. The recommendation to continue, modify, or terminate a trial is the most important communication provided to the sponsor and trial leadership by the DMC. The DMC makes its recommendations based on benefit–risk assessments, and it is the sponsor who is ultimately responsible for acting upon these recommendations. Consensus should be sought among DMC members, and voting is generally discouraged. If differences of opinion persist, these are documented in the DMC minutes, and it is acceptable to describe these differences without attribution when issuing a statement or other formal communication.

As previously described, sponsors—and particularly the project team(s) directly involved in trial operations—often have a vested interest that may lead to a biased perspective on the research. Therefore, DMC trial recommendations and proposed modifications should be provided to a steering committee or sponsor leadership group authorized to act on these recommendations, and not to those directly involved with implementation of the trial.

The primary and preferred method of communicating the DMC's recommendations to the sponsor is in written form. The DMC may also verbally brief the sponsor and/or trial leadership after the closed session, and the recommendations should be conveyed clearly and concisely.

When in agreement with the DMC's recommendations, the sponsor should report these within an appropriate time period to institutional review boards and, in the case of trials performed under regulatory guidance, to the relevant regulatory authorities. Minor operational recommendations do not necessarily require regulatory reporting. Procedures for managing disagreements between the sponsor and the DMC should be described in the charter. Although consensus between the sponsor and DMC with respect to the recommendations is highly desirable, in case of an impasse, it is the sponsor's decision whether to accept or reject the recommendations. The sponsor may choose to respond to the DMC through written comments, especially in the case of disagreement with the DMC's recommendations. If the sponsor rejects the recommendations, this decision and its rationale should be reported promptly along with the written DMC recommendations to institutional review boards and to the appropriate regulatory agencies if the trial is under regulatory purview. Based on the information provided, the regulatory agencies and institutional review boards may reach their own independent conclusions and act accordingly within their respective authorities. At the end of the trial, all minutes and reports from the DMC meetings should be made available to the sponsor and trial leadership, as needed.

Preparing the next generation of DMC members

The pool of qualified individuals available to serve as DMC members may soon be inadequate to meet the current needs of the research enterprise, as demand for trained and qualified DMC members has risen and may continue to grow. In 2013, the Office of Inspector General at the US Department of Health and Human Services reported that the NIH faces challenges in the recruitment and training of DMC members. As a result, the Office of Inspector General[7] recommended that NIH develop ways to recruit and train new DMC members. Although training is highly desirable prior to serving on a DMC, the vast majority of our survey respondents indicated that they had not received training and were unaware of DMC-specific training programs.[3]

The DMC Project also identified a growing need to prepare a new generation of qualified DMC members so that the pool of properly trained and experienced individuals does not dwindle. Preparing individuals to serve as DMC members is challenging because of the complexity of data monitored in clinical trials and the interpretation relative to the monitoring guidelines. Knowledge of research, familiarity with the study design, and unstructured on-the-job training are not sufficient to ensure that prospective DMC members are adequately qualified to serve on a DMC. While the skills needed for prospective DMC members are described in the literature, to date, nationally recognized training programs have not been established.

Effective training for DMC members should consist of a combination of didactic educational programs and practical experience. Didactic elements could include a review of the fundamentals of clinical trials, study design, data analysis, and the functions and responsibilities of DMCs. They should also focus on the aspects of DMC work that are different from the work conducted by those who operate the trial. One of the realities of DMC operations involves the real-time analysis of emerging study data that has yet to undergo the full quality-control checks to ensure completeness and accuracy of the data.

However, didactic training and review of case studies, alone, may be insufficient. Effective training of prospective DMC members should also incorporate formal, supervised longitudinal apprenticeships in the setting of actual DMC proceedings, including closed sessions during which the most critical and sensitive issues are addressed. The adoption and endorsement of this type of comprehensive training by sponsors and other key stakeholders will help ensure that a new generation of DMC members is adequately prepared.

To advance this effort, stakeholders with an interest in the role and function of DMCs (e.g. professional, scientific, and medical societies and organizations) should consider developing and maintaining databases of qualified DMC members that include a listing of their experience and relevant expertise.[8] In compliance with confidentiality provisions for a given trial, DMC members should also be encouraged to submit interesting and instructive DMC case studies to peer-reviewed journals in order to raise awareness of important issues and challenges that can arise during a clinical trial. Legal and contractual issues concerning service on a DMC (e.g. indemnification) require thoughtful discourse but were not formally addressed in our DMC project.

Discussion

The rationale for using a DMC in clinical trial monitoring is predicated on the need for periodic assessment of the risks and benefits in an ongoing trial guided by a well-defined DMC charter that is aligned with the research protocol and statistical analysis plan. Similarly, our recommended best practices for DMC oversight and communication are intended to ensure the validity and sensitivity of this monitoring process to detect early evidence of avoidable harm, futility, or benefit, and to communicate DMC recommendations in a manner that is actionable when necessary and maintains trial integrity to the greatest extent possible.

An independent, knowledgeable, and well-trained DMC serves the trial sponsor, trial leadership, investigators, and study participants through this periodic assessment of risks and benefits. DMCs have an important and unique role in trial oversight that is substantially distinct from institutional review boards, ethics committees, or trial steering committees, which do not see unblinded interim results. Thus, the role of the

DMC cannot be delegated or shared with other entities without the potential for substantially increased risk to trial integrity, and thus also to study participants and sponsors.

The choice of DMC members should be thoughtfully considered, and the role of the chair should never be bestowed on an individual solely by virtue of their position or status in academia or as a key opinion leader. Previous experience acting as a member of a DMC should be a primary consideration, as this experience is invaluable for effectively leading the DMC and providing guidance to newly trained members. Our recommendation for apprenticeship and mentoring necessitates close interaction among DMC team members.

The composition of the DMC is especially important in light of its responsibility to make the best possible recommendations unbiased by the sponsor or commercial interests with relatively sparse information, given that their recommendations often result in irreversible actions being taken. For example, if a trial is stopped and the sponsor and trial leadership is unmasked to treatment assignment, that action cannot be undone. Even if trial enrollment is only suspended for a potential safety concern, it is often difficult or impossible for the prior rate of patient enrollment or investigator enthusiasm to be regained should trial enrollment be resumed.

While our recommendations for DMC use, conduct, communication, and member training form the foundation for improved oversight of clinical trials and enhanced participant safety, it is the effectiveness of the implementation of these recommendations that will determine whether the potential benefits are realized. Several recommendations proposed by us are well aligned with those of the NIH, specifically regarding the importance of DMC access to the unmasked trial data, the need to identify and adequately train new DMC members, and the restriction of attendance at the closed sessions to DMC members only.[7] Our recommendations should, ideally, serve as a call to action, encouraging all those involved in clinical trial design and conduct to ensure the DMC structure, charter, membership, and implementation are all consistent with these recommendations. Doing so will ultimately benefit study participants, study sponsors, investigators, and society.

Acknowledgements

The authors wish to acknowledge the contributions of the DMC Project Team and Zachary Hallinan (Clinical Trials Transformation Initiative). Medical writing assistance was provided by Kelly Kilibarda, PhD, in affiliation with Whitsell Innovations, Inc. All authors are considered equal contributors.

Declaration of conflicting interests

The views expressed in this publication are those of the authors and do not necessarily reflect the official policies of the Department of Health and Human Services, nor does any mention of trade names, commercial practices, or organization imply endorsement by the US Government.

Funding

Funding for this manuscript was made possible, in part, by the Food and Drug Administration through grant R18FD005292 and cooperative agreement U19FD003800. Partial funding was also provided by pooled membership fees from the Clinical Trials Transformation Initiative's member organizations.

References

1. Organization, review, and administration of cooperative studies (Greenberg Report): a report from the Heart Special Project Committee to the National Advisory Heart Council, May 1967. *Control Clin Trials* 1988; 9: 137–148.

2. SCT Working Group on Data Monitoring, Dixon DO, Freedman RS, et al. Guidelines for data and safety monitoring for clinical trials not requiring traditional data monitoring committees. *Clin Trials* 2006; 3: 314–319.

3. Calis KA, Archdeacon P, Bain RP, et al. Understanding the functions and operations of data monitoring committees: survey and focus group findings. *Clin Trials* 2017; 14: 59–66.

4. Clinical Trials Transformation Initiative. CTTI data monitoring committees project expert meeting, https://www.ctti-clinicaltrials.org/briefing-room/meetings/ctti-data-monitoring-committees-project-expert-meeting (2015, accessed 25 July 2016).

5. American Heart Association. Consensus-based decision-making processes, https://www.heart.org/idc/groups/heart-public/@wcm/@mwa/documents/downloadable/ucm_454080.pdf (accessed 5 August 2016).

6. DeMets DL and Ellenberg SS. Data monitoring committees – expect the unexpected. *New Engl J Med* 2016; 375: 1365–1371.

7. Office of Inspector General. *Data and safety monitoring boards in NIH clinical trials meeting guidance, but facing some issues.* Washington, DC: Department of Health and Human Services, Office of Inspector General, 2013.

8. Duke Clinical Research Institute (DCRI). DCRI leadership in data monitoring committees, http://dmc.dcri.org/ (accessed 8 September 2016).

4.4 Women and Fetuses First? An Ethical Case for Giving Priority in Clinical Research Testing of Zika Vaccines to Pregnant Women

Kelly McBride Folkers and Arthur L. Caplan
   Unpublished.

Women and fetuses first:

An ethical case for giving priority in clinical research testing of Zika vaccines to

pregnant women

Introduction

The rapid emergence of the Zika virus has been described as "unprecedented" because the virus can spread through both a mosquito vector and sexually, causing severe neurological birth defects and miscarriages in humans.[1] Though 80 percent of people infected with Zika are asymptomatic, Zika virus infection can cause microcephaly and other severe birth defects in developing fetuses and neurological developmental defects in infants.[2] The long-term effects of Zika virus infection on both mother and child are not yet known, but it is likely that some deleterious effects in children born to mothers with Zika virus infection will not be apparent until later in their childhood.[3] Additionally, Zika virus infection has been associated with an increase in the number of cases of Guillain-Barré syndrome in Rio de Janeiro, Brazil, and Puerto Rico.[4,5]

Because Zika virus infection can lead to these severe health problems, it is prudent for the public health community to develop a vaccine prior to the next major outbreak. As of September 2017, there were approximately 32 vaccine candidates in various stages of the drug development pipeline.[6] However, Zika vaccine development has slowed in recent months for several reasons. The summer of 2017 saw a decrease in the number of documented Zika virus infections in the Americas,[7] which means that researchers face difficulties in reliably determining the efficacy of vaccine candidates as herd immunity has likely contributed to a decline in Zika infections. In November 2016, the World Health Organization (WHO) stated that microcephaly and other neurological disorders caused by Zika were no longer a public health emergency of international concern.[8] Vaccine developers may have interpreted the November statement as a "downgrade" in the seriousness of the problem. Indeed, Sanofi Pasteur, one of the only major pharmaceutical company working on a vaccine, withdrew from developing its candidate in September of 2017.[9]

And phase II vaccine testing that was scheduled to take place in Puerto Rico will likely be temporarily halted as the region recovers from extensive damage from Hurricane Maria in 2017.

Nevertheless, Zika remains a public health concern and could re-emerge in the foreseeable future. How to effectively prepare for a Zika outbreak and identifying which target populations should receive a vaccine before its received regulatory approval remain open questions. An editorial in *The Lancet Infectious Diseases* argues that Zika vaccine development must receive higher strategic planning priority from the World Health Organization so that vaccines can be rolled out quickly in the event of an outbreak.[9] Delays in vaccine development now may lead to hastening the enrollment of participants for trials later, so it is still very important to consider who should be enrolled. Recent population-level modeling data suggest that Zika virus vaccination with a moderate to highly effective vaccine could virtually eliminate prenatal infections if a vaccine were to be approved.[10]

As of April 2018, no Zika vaccine trials were enrolling pregnant women. Because the population most affected by Zika are infants and unborn children, the public health and clinical research communities are presented with difficult ethical challenges in developing safe and effective prophylactic vaccines. This challenge is especially acute given the "vulnerable" subject status of pregnant women and fetuses as research participants. The Common Rule, a set of federal ethical regulations that U.S. government-funded research sponsors must follow, states that vulnerable populations, including pregnant women and neonates, should receive additional protections in order to enroll them in research to ensure their welfare.[11] In April of 2018, the U.S. Food and Drug Administration (FDA) released new draft guidance on the safe and ethical inclusion of pregnant women in clinical research, which states that failing to study the safety and

3

efficacy of new drugs on pregnant women creates uncertainty that may damage their health and that of their fetuses.[12]

Zika vaccine development raises several important questions about the ethical conduct of research. First, do women and fetuses belong in Zika vaccine trials? Others in the bioethics community have responded to this important question with a resounding "yes." The Ethics Working Group on ZIKV Research & Pregnancy has established a set of recommendations that put first the needs of pregnant women, who have historically not been represented adequately as research participants.[13,14] We agree with their recommendations, particularly that researchers should "pursue and prioritize development of ZIKV vaccines that will be acceptable for use by pregnant women in the context of an outbreak."[13] To augment this group's influential work, we believe it's important to answer a set of related questions: Why should pregnant women be prioritized as a population to study in these trials? How does this priority affect public health responses in future outbreaks of the virus? How should researchers handle priority enrollment?

Justifying the inclusion of pregnant women and fetuses in Zika vaccine trials

Testing a vaccine candidate in pregnant women may be ethically justifiable. Indeed, others have made this claim.[13,14] The goal of priority enrollment of a pregnant population is to ensure that only vaccines that are expected to be safe for testing during pregnancy and that have been thoroughly examined on a pregnant population should receive regulatory approval for general usage. We believe that pregnant women should be included in trials and receive priority access to enrollment in clinical trials that test the safety and efficacy of Zika vaccine candidates, at phase II or later, which is reflected in these guidelines.

4

Several guidance documents provide ethical justification for the safe inclusion of pregnant women in research that can guide future study design. FDA draft guidance issued in April of 2018 states that pregnant women should be included in clinical research when nonclinical research on pregnant animals has been previously conducted, and there is a prospect of direct benefit for the pregnant mother and/or the fetus.[12] Guideline 19 of the International Ethical Guidelines for Health-related Research Involving Human Subjects, updated in 2016, asserts the need to study certain interventions that can specifically benefit pregnant women: "Pregnant and breastfeeding women have distinctive physiologies and health needs. Research designed to obtain knowledge relevant to the health needs of the pregnant and breastfeeding woman must be promoted."[15] The CIOMS guideline states that research ethics committees "may permit a minor increase above minimal risk" when the social value that the research will provide is strong enough to improve to lives of pregnant women or their fetuses; short-term and long-term follow-up may be required, depending on the study intervention's potential risks. This guideline responds to the obligation of researchers to enroll members of populations in research studies that are expected to benefit from the results of the study. However, none of these guidelines provide justification for how to *prioritize* the involvement of pregnant women in research for a situation like Zika vaccine trials.

A moral imperative to prevent vertical transmission of infectious disease justifies the priority inclusion of pregnant women and fetuses in Zika vaccine trials. Verweij *et al.* describe pregnancy as an "immunologically altered state that can render women more susceptible to infections than they are when they are not pregnant."[16] Maternal immunization is justified if the vaccination provides direct protection for pregnant women, prevents disease transmission, can provide passive immunity to the newborn child, and/or can reduce infant mortality that results from infectious disease transmission.[16] The authors justify these claims by suggesting a more reasonable version of the precautionary principle, which dictates that for activities that may cause irreversible harm, precautionary measures are warranted.[16] In the case of maternal immunization, the authors suggest that adverse event reporting and disease surveillance measures be strengthened so that vaccination be offered when there are "concrete, severe risks of disease for mother and child."[16] The risk of severe birth defects, as occurs with Zika, fits this description.

Why do pregnant women and fetuses deserve priority enrollment in Zika vaccine trials?

The statement that pregnant women and fetuses deserve priority enrollment in Zika vaccine trials does not answer the most pressing questions for sponsors of these trials: Why is priority enrollment necessary, and how exactly should it work? Adding to the work of the Ethics Working Group on ZIKV Research & Pregnancy, we argue that pregnant women should be enrolled first and that spots for enrollment in these trials be reserved specifically for pregnant women.

To strengthen the argument for the inclusion of pregnant women in Zika vaccine trials, it is prudent to consider that unapproved vaccine candidates may need to be authorized for emergency use in the event of an outbreak in the future. In such an instance, available doses of Zika vaccine candidates that have been made for usage in clinical trials could fall short for covering the entire at risk population. Available doses will need to be rationed. In the case of a Zika outbreak, those that are at the greatest risk for serious health issues related to the virus have the strongest need for access to a vaccine that may help. A just and fair public health regulatory authority will provide those in dire need with the resources to meet that need.

Because of the aforementioned risks of viral infection, pregnant women and fetuses should be first in line to receive experimental Zika vaccine candidates in an emergency situation. The plausibility of such an outbreak is not unreasonable to envision in the near future. Hurricane recovery efforts in Puerto Rico and the U.S. Virgin Islands, in the wake of 2017's Hurricane Maria, have been slow. A lack of electricity and standing water, combined with increasing global temperatures, could create optimal breeding conditions for disease-carrying mosquitos.

Furthermore, women of childbearing age in areas of the world where Zika has been endemic often do not have safe or legal access to abortion if they were to become pregnant while infected with the virus. Thus, if a pregnant woman believes she may be infected with Zika, she may have no choice but to carry her child to term, which may lead to lifelong financial, medical, and social challenges that particularly affect socioeconomically disadvantaged communities. According to the Pew Research Center, 26% of countries included in a recent analysis of abortion regulation worldwide only allow abortions to save the life of the mother.[17] 42% of countries, including Brazil, only allow abortions when the mother's life is at risk or for at least one other specific reason, such as the desire to terminate a pregnancy that resulted from rape or incest.[17] If abortion is not a feasible option for pregnant women who have contracted a Zika virus infection, it is ethically required to offer them an experimental vaccine that is believed to have some chance of protecting a fetus from neurological devastation or birth defects.

Finally, if there is going to be emergency use authorization of an experimental Zika vaccine, more data gathered from pregnant women and fetuses would be helpful, or perhaps necessary, to guide the administration of the vaccine in an outbreak. In some cases of compassionate use, where a pharmaceutical sponsor makes its product available to patients without other treatment options outside of a clinical trial setting, sponsors are unwilling to provide an experimental product if there is no data on a specific population that may desire early access to an intervention in development (personal communication). Thus, in preparing for public health responses in the future, it is important to gather data before the anticipation of emergency use authorizations.

Discussion

We believe that giving pregnant women and fetuses priority enrollment, first and foremost, in Zika vaccine trials is a sensible path forward for countermeasure development in the event that the virus re-emerges to cause an outbreak. In general, it is ethically sound to conduct research on populations that would need access first in an emergency situation. Public health emergencies, though unanticipated, are not unforeseeable. Setbacks in timely Zika vaccine development, combined with the exclusion of pregnant women from phase II and III testing of the candidates that are moving forward in the development pipeline, will only further contribute to healthcare injustices for the populations most affected by Zika.

One might ask why it is necessary to further justify that pregnant women need to be enrolled in Zika vaccine trials first. Developing a transparent rationing strategy of available vaccine doses ahead of an outbreak will balance the competing approaches of utilitarianism and egalitarianism and will garner more public support than leaving these decisions to the last minute. Pregnant women carrying developing fetuses will be first in line to receive an experimental vaccine, so the public health community needs to know with some degree of confidence if a vaccine candidate demonstrates some efficacy in those populations.

The argument for priority enrollment of populations likely to be most affected by a particular infectious disease is applicable to other areas of public health concern. For example,

H7N9 avian influenza is zoonotic and spreads from human contact with infected birds. If this virus is able to spread between humans, it will become pandemic.[18] Immunocompromised individuals, the elderly, and the very young are particularly susceptible to mortality from influenza.[18] Research studies that test new interventions against the standard of care should be sure to enroll members of these groups first, after phase I studies in healthy volunteers demonstrate a feasible immune response. In the event that pandemic flu results, it has been suggested vaccines be rationed according to medical neediness first, followed by random selection for the rest of the population.[19] This method of rationing follows an egalitarian principle that is rooted in social justice, which could similarly be applied for a Zika vaccine rationing strategy.[19]

Ultimately, priority enrollment of the most at-risk populations in research studies for interventions that may benefit them is not just an argument that relates to Zika vaccine development. When sponsors consider populations from which to sample in the development of therapeutic agents for infection disease, they should put first the people who are most likely to benefit from the experimental intervention. This is important because institutional review board (IRB) professionals need to understand priority enrollment as well. Though IRBs mostly are concerned with the protection of human participants from risks inherent in biomedical research participation like undue inducement, exploitation, and coercion, there is a role for them to facilitate safe access to research that will benefit populations with unmet medical needs that are at high risk for an infectious illness.

The prioritization argument challenges the precautionary principle, which dictates that in the absence of scientific understanding of the safety and efficacy of an intervention, the potential risks of that using that intervention should be diminished by any means possible. A strict

9

interpretation of this principle may leave pregnant women in Zika-endemic areas – or to give

other examples, those with a high risk of influenza mortality or those who are at risk of acquiring

resistance to HIV medication – with little to no options to meet their medical needs.[16] A softened

version of the precautionary principle would balance the needs of these populations with

facilitated access to experimental interventions in emergent situations, in which quick regulatory

decisions must be made based on available evidence. Priority access to research participation

must become an essential component of public health policy strategy so that these decisions can

be made with as much information possible. Inclusion is important, but frequently in vaccine

research eligibility is not enough to ensure enrollment in a study. Public health officials,

sponsors, and regulators need to also determine who goes first.

References

1.   Frieden TR, Schuchat A, Petersen LR. Zika Virus 6 Months Later. *JAMA.* 2016;316(14):1443-1444.
2.   Rasmussen SA, Jamieson DJ, Honein MA, Petersen LR. Zika Virus and Birth Defects--Reviewing the Evidence for Causality. *N Eng J Med.* 2016;374(20):1981-1987.
3.   Marrs C, Olson G, Saade G, et al. Zika Virus and Pregnancy: A Review of the Literature and Clinical Considerations. *Am J Perinatol.* 2016;33(7):625-639.
4.   Ferreira da Silva IR, Frontera JA, Moreira do Nascimento OJ. News from the battlefront: Zika virus-associated Guillain-Barre syndrome in Brazil. *Neurology.* 2016;87(15):e180-e181.
5.   Dirlikov E, Medina NA, Major CG, et al. Acute Zika Virus Infection as a Risk Factor for Guillain-Barre Syndrome in Puerto Rico. *JAMA.* 2017;318(15):1498-1500.
6.   Scutti S. Sanofi stops work on Zika vaccine while others forge forward. *CNN* 2017; http://www.cnn.com/2017/09/07/health/sanofi-discontinues-zika-vaccine-development/index.html. Accessed 23 October 2017.
7.   Pan American Health Organization. Regional Zika Epidemiological Update (Americas) August 25, 2017. 2017; http://www.paho.org/hq/index.php?option=com_content&view=article&id=11599:regional-zika-epidemiological-update-americas&Itemid=41691. Accessed 23 October 2017.
8.   World Health Organization. Fifth meeting of the Emergency Committee under the International Health Regulations (2005) regarding microephaly, other neurological disorders and Zika virus. 2016;

http://www.who.int/mediacentre/news/statements/2016/zika-fifth-ec/en/. Accessed 23 October 2017.

9. The Lancet Infectious Diseases. Vaccine against Zika must remain a priority. *The Lancet Infectious Diseases.* 2017;17(10):1003.

10. Durham DP, Fitzpatrick MC, Ndeffo-Mbah ML, Parpia AS, Michael NL. Evaluating Vaccination Strategies for Zika Virus in the Americas. *Ann Inter Med.* 2018;156(11):ITC6-1.

11. Ribeiro LS, Marques RE, Jesus AM, Almeida RP, Teixeira MM. Zika crisis in Brazil: challenges in research and development. *Curr Opin Virol.* 2016;18:76-81.

12. U.S. Food and Drug Administration. Pregnant Women: Scientific and Ethical Considerations for Inclusion in Clinical Trials, Guidance for Industry. Silver Spring, MD, 2018.

13. The Ethics Working Group on ZIKV Research & Pregnancy. Pregnant Women & the Zika Virus Vaccine Research Agenda: Ethics Guidance on Priorities, Inclusion, and Evidence Generation. June 2017 ed. Baltimore, MD, 2017.

14. Faden RR, Krubiner CB, Lyerly AD, et al. Ethics, pregnancy, ZIKV vaccine research & development. *Vaccine.* 2017;35(49 Pt B):6819-6822.

15. Berciano J, Sedano MJ, Pelayo-Negro AL, et al. Proximal nerve lesions in early Guillain-Barre syndrome: implications for pathogenesis and disease classification. *J Neurol.* 2016;264(2):221-236.

16. Verweij M, Lambach P, Ortiz JR, Reis A. Maternal immunisation: ethical issues. *The Lancet Infectious Diseases.* 2016;16(12):e310-e314.

17. Theodorou AE, Sandstrom A. How abortion is regulated around the world. 2015; http://www.pewresearch.org/fact-tank/2015/10/06/how-abortion-is-regulated-around-the-world/. Accessed 23 October 2017.

18. Tanner WD, Toth DJ, Gundlapalli AV. The pandemic potential of avian influenza A(H7N9) virus: a review. *Epidemiology and Infection.* 2015;143(16):3359-3374.

19. Zimmerman RK. Rationing of influenza vaccine during a pandemic: ethical analyses. *Vaccine.* 2007;25(11):2019-2026.

11

4.5   Rethinking the Belmont Report?

Phoebe Friesen, Lisa Kearns, Barbara Redman, and Arthur L. Caplan

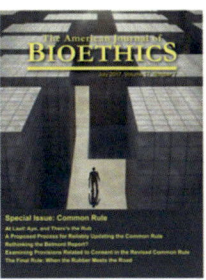

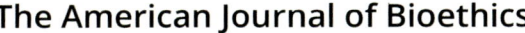
The American Journal of Bioethics

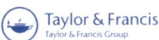

ISSN: 1526-5161 (Print) 1536-0075 (Online) Journal homepage: http://www.tandfonline.com/loi/uajb20

Rethinking the Belmont Report?

Phoebe Friesen, Lisa Kearns, Barbara Redman & Arthur L. Caplan

To cite this article: Phoebe Friesen, Lisa Kearns, Barbara Redman & Arthur L. Caplan (2017) Rethinking the Belmont Report?, The American Journal of Bioethics, 17:7, 15-21, DOI: 10.1080/15265161.2017.1329482

To link to this article: http://dx.doi.org/10.1080/15265161.2017.1329482

The American Journal of Bioethics, 17(7): 15–21, 2017
Copyright © Taylor & Francis Group, LLC
ISSN: 1526-5161 print / 1536-0075 online
DOI: 10.1080/15265161.2017.1329482

Target Article

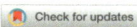

Rethinking the Belmont Report?

Phoebe Friesen, NYU School of Medicine
Lisa Kearns, NYU School of Medicine
Barbara Redman, NYU School of Medicine
Arthur L. Caplan, NYU School of Medicine

This article reflects on the relevance and applicability of the Belmont Report nearly four decades after its original publication. In an exploration of criticisms that have been raised in response to the report and of significant changes that have occurred within the context of biomedical research, five primary themes arise. These themes include the increasingly vague boundary between research and practice, unique harms to communities that are not addressed by the principle of respect for persons, and how growing complexity and commodification in research have shed light on the importance of transparency. The repercussions of Belmont's emphasis on the protection of vulnerable populations is also explored, as is the relationship between the report's ethical principles and their applications. It is concluded that while the Belmont Report was an impressive response to the ethical issues of its day, the field of research ethics involving human subjects may have outgrown it.

Keywords: research ethics, Belmont Report, autonomy, beneficence, justice, human subjects research

As the new revisions to the Common Rule take their place, it seems timely to reflect on the significant document that gave shape to the regulations both at its inception and now. Since its release in 1978 and publication in 1979, the Belmont Report (National Commission for the Protection of Human Subjects of Biomedical and Behavioral Research 1979) has had an enormous impact on the way research with human subjects has been conducted in the United States and in many other nations. This article explores some of the more significant criticisms that have been raised in response to the report, as well as changes that have reshaped many questions central to research ethics since its publication, and asks whether the report still holds up nearly four decades later. Part I briefly summarizes the central components of the Belmont Report, describes the ethical climate at the time, and provides clarification about what the report was and was not meant to achieve. Part II explores several criticisms that have been leveled against the report and situates many of them within the dynamic landscape of biomedical research. Finally, Part III offers a discussion of whether the Belmont Report is in need of a 21st-century overhaul.

PART I: THE BELMONT REPORT

The 11 members of the National Commission for the Protection of Human Subjects of Biomedical and Behavioral Research who authored the Belmont Report

worked on it from 1974 to 1978, including four intensive working days at the Smithsonian Institution's Belmont Conference Center in 1976. The Secretary of Health, Education, and Welfare (now Health and Human Services [HHS]) gave them four primary tasks: identify the boundary between research and practice, determine the role of risk–benefit analyses in human subjects research, outline appropriate guidelines for subject selection, and provide criteria for what constitutes truly informed consent (National Commission for the Protection of Human Subjects of Biomedical and Behavioral Research 1979). Both the organization and the content of the Belmont Report reflect these directives. The first section of the report addresses the first task; it defines "practice" as an intervention solely meant to enhance a patient's well-being, and "research" as "an activity designed to test an hypothesis, permit conclusions to be drawn, and thereby to develop or contribute to generalizable knowledge" (National Commission for the Protection of Human Subjects of Biomedical and Behavioral Research 1979). The second section describes three ethical principles that are "particularly relevant" to research involving human subjects: respect for persons, beneficence, and justice (National Commission for the Protection of Human Subjects of Biomedical and Behavioral Research 1979). The third links each of these principles to the remaining three tasks, suggesting that respect for persons should be the guiding principle behind informed consent, that beneficence should underlie

Address correspondence to Arthur L. Caplan, New York University Langone Medical Center, Division of Bioethics, 227 E. 30th St., Seventh Floor, New York, NY 10016, USA. E-mail: Arthur.Caplan@nyumc.org

The American Journal of Bioethics

risk–benefit analyses, and that justice ought to be the central principle behind subject selection.

To understand the Belmont Report, one must understand the ethical climate in which it was written. Three decades earlier, the Nuremberg Code, a set of research ethics principles to guide human experimentation, had been promulgated, at the conclusion of the "Doctors Trial" of Karl Brandt and 22 other Nazi defendants (The Nuremberg Code 1949). The verdict, with some modifications, was later endorsed by the World Medical Association as a code of ethics meant to guide research involving human subjects: the Declaration of Helsinki (WMA General Assembly 1996). While there is certainly ethical overlap between these documents and the Belmont Report, the ethical emphases of the latter are drawn from particular concerns that were paramount in the United States at the time. Especially important were the revelations contained in the now famous exposé on subject abuses penned by Henry Beecher in the *New England Journal of Medicine* and the publicity surrounding the Tuskegee Syphilis Experiment, which continued to track the progression of untreated syphilis in hundreds of poor black men long after a cure had become widely available (Beecher 1966). The public outcry in 1972, triggered by an African American whistleblower at the Centers for Disease Control (McCallum et al. 2006), led Congress to establish the National Commission for the Protection of Human Subjects of Biomedical and Behavioral Research.

The content of the Belmont Report reflects the committee's fears that research subjects would continue to be deceived, harmed, or otherwise exploited by investigators, a point that has often been overlooked by critics. As one Belmont author explains, the Belmont Report was meant to be "a proclamation that had to ring true in the ears of scientists, policymakers, politicians, ethicists, journalists, and judges" (Jonsen 2005). As well as being a proclamation, the Belmont Report was primarily intended to be a statement of a general, principled moral framework that would help prevent abuses such as Tuskegee from occurring in research involving human subjects in the future (Beauchamp 2008). Although some have expressed concern that the report is "not easily understood or fathomed" (Vanderpool 2001), and that its principles are often misinterpreted as direct action guidelines (Levine 2005), the authors maintain that there "was never any ambition or attempt to make this document specific and practical" (Beauchamp 2005) and that the report "was not to be a philosophical treatise nor was it to be a set of guidelines" (Jonsen 2005). The Belmont Report was not written as an extension of any particular moral theory (Levine 2005), and was both principlist and casuist at the same time (Beauchamp 2005).[1] This may seem somewhat unambitious given the stakes involved, but the goal of the report was only to offer a preliminary, protective ethical

framework. A national Ethics Advisory Board was meant to act as a standing agency to continue to grapple with practical ethical issues related to human subjects research (Jonsen 2005; National Commission for the Protection of Human Subjects of Biomedical and Behavioral Research 1978, January 13), and indeed many remaining issues were explored in 16 volumes the National Commission later produced (Beauchamp 2008). Despite its modest goal, the Belmont Report was an impressive response to the ethical issues facing human subject researchers when considered in the very troubling context in which it was written.

PART II: CRITICISMS AND CHANGES

Several significant changes have occurred within the field of human subjects research since the publication of the Belmont Report, and many concerns about the adequacy of the report have been raised in the literature in the intervening years. Five key themes that arise are the distinction between research and practice, harms to communities, the importance of transparency, implications of protectionism, and the relationship between Belmont's ethical principles and their applications.

Research and Practice

Although the commission knew it could not adequately delineate the complicated boundary between research and practice, it did manage to capture paradigmatic features of each. The report states that research is meant to contribute to generalizable knowledge, while practice is meant to contribute to patient well-being. The authors recognized that there often could be overlap between the two; for example, practice could contain significant risks and require oversight, or could involve goals beyond the well-being of individual patients (Beauchamp and Saghai 2012). However, in the decades since the publication of the report, the line between research and practice has become even more vague.

Institutional review boards (IRBs), charged with the protection of human research subjects, have long relied on the report's distinction to determine what is and is not within their purview, but today face an increasing number of examples of novel "practice" involving significant risks and therefore in need of significant oversight (e.g., pre-approval, or "compassionate" access to drugs; innovative treatment design; innovative surgeries), as well as a growing number of cases of "research" involving only minimal risk (e.g., retrospective analysis of deidentified data, some forms of survey research, the use of biospecimens) (Faden et al. 2013). These examples illuminate the difficulties in drawing a boundary between research and practice on the basis of the aim of either creating generalizable knowledge or seeking patient well-being. This boundary also limits what information is gained, since practitioners often abstain from collecting data during routine care or innovative practice as a result of the perceived burdens of research oversight (Rhodes 2010). As a result, risky interventions take place with no oversight and no data

---

1. One of the authors of the report, A. R. Jonsen, has noted that the Belmont Report was written as if guided primarily by principles, but constructed on the basis of casuistry (Jonsen 1988.)

collection, while minimal-risk research is delayed or forgone due to the difficulty of securing regulatory approval. In response, some have argued that unique guidelines for innovative practice are needed (Taylor 2010), especially since disadvantaged groups are particularly at risk of being enrolled in such therapies (Sherwin 2005). Others suggest that research and practice should be integrated into a single, comprehensive learning health care system (Faden et al. 2013).

Harms to Communities

Another criticism of the Belmont Report is that it fails to account for the unique harms to communities that can occur due to research (Weijer 1999; Weijer and Anderson 2002; Emanuel and Weijer 2005). These are not simply the aggregate of harms to individuals within a community, but harms suffered by a community as a whole. Many communities have endured a long history of abuses at the hands of researchers, leading them to doubt the likelihood that they will be beneficiaries of research conducted on them, while others do not share the goals of the researchers. These groups include poor communities, racial and ethnic minorities, those living with mental or physical illness or disabilities, and other stigmatized groups. Harm to these groups cannot be mitigated simply by securing informed consent from individuals according to Belmont's principle of respect for persons. This principle fails to take into account the unique harms that can be done to communities *qua* communities, such as violating widespread trust or taking ownership of a community's stories. For example, in the case of the controversial Human Genome Diversity Project, several indigenous communities expressed reluctance to help researchers in their development of a theory that may offer them no benefit and may serve as evidence to debunk their beliefs about their creation beliefs and histories (Weijer and Anderson 2002). This has led some to argue that there are "special issues related to the religious beliefs, cultural traditions, and history of aboriginal communities" that are not addressed by the report (Weijer and Anderson 2002). Others suggest adding a principle of respect for cultures (Levine 1982) or expanding respect for persons to "respect for persons and communities" (Lebacqz 2005).

Transparency in Research

Concerns about transparency in research have become paramount in the years since the publication of the Belmont Report. Protocols submitted to IRBs have become increasingly elaborate, while biomedicine has become much more commodified, raising issues of conflicts of interest.

When the report was written, most submissions to IRBs were for government-funded, National Institutes of Health (NIH) projects taking place at a single site. Now committees often review complex protocols that are privately sponsored and global in scope (Emanuel 2015). Further issues complicating transparency are worries about the composition of IRBs and their scope of responsibilities

as additional committees devoted to research oversight have been created, such as data safety and monitoring boards (DSMBs) and institutional biosafety committees (IBCs). Biomedicine has also seen tremendous growth in the value of patents, devices, and stock.

The majority of biomedical research in the United States is funded by industry, tying the profit motive to every stage of the research process (Taylor 2010), and making transparency much more difficult to attain. This has made the task of identifying and managing conflicts of interest increasingly important (Dumit 2012). Some have argued that the principles offered by the Belmont Report are unable to uphold research integrity, since they do not provide "a clear basis for investigators to keep promises, tell the truth, and avoid killing" (Veatch 2005).

Another significant development that compromises transparency has been the rise of new technologies that pose novel and sometimes unpredictable risks to research participants' privacy and confidentiality of data. These risks can arise throughout all stages of research: participant recruitment through social media, the development of digital monitoring devices that collect data on unwitting bystanders, the use of vast amounts of data being collected and analyzed by companies without individual consent, and the potential to reidentify data using the wealth of personal information available online or through the use of genetic data (Kelly et al. 2013; Gelinas et al. 2017; Benitez and Malin 2010; Metcalf and Crawford 2016).

Critics have noted the Belmont Report's limitations with regards to transparency, suggesting that the report pays little attention to the importance of trust and openness within research (Faden, Mastroianni, and Kahn 2005). Many of these issues, unheard of in the 1970s, threaten the ethical principles espoused in the report, especially that of beneficence. Obstacles to transparency may limit the ability of members of IRBs, DSMBs, and IBCs to adequately analyze the risks and benefits involved in a given study, if they lack access to a significant portion of past research, as a result of publication biases or trade secrets, or if they are unaware of all known risks to participants, as a result of a lack of full disclosure by private sponsors.

Implications of Protectionism

Given the Tuskegee Syphilis Experiment's role in the creation of the Belmont Report, it is understandable that the protection of vulnerable populations took center stage in the report, including those who are vulnerable due to a lack of autonomy, such as children and individuals who are mentally disabled, and those vulnerable for other reasons, such as "racial minorities, the economically disadvantaged, the very sick, and the institutionalized" (National Commission for the Protection of Human Subjects of Biomedical and Behavioral Research 1979). Certainly, protecting vulnerable research participants from exploitation or abuse is an essential task of any research ethics framework. In retrospect, however, the weight the report places on protectionism has both helped

The American Journal of Bioethics

and hindered epistemic and ethical progress in research. One negative result of the emphasis on protectionism is that some groups considered vulnerable have been left out of the research process and health data relevant to them are now lacking (e.g., pregnant women, children, embryos, the institutionalized, the elderly) (Beauchamp 2008; Rhodes 2010; Sherwin 2005; King 2005). Additionally, as the AIDS epidemic showed, being protected from research is not always desired by members of vulnerable groups (Beauchamp 2008; King 2005; Rogers and Lange 2013).

Today, the desire in many communities to move away from protectionism can be seen in the increasing demands for pre-approval access to investigational drugs, in participants' insistence that they receive active agents and not placebos in clinical trials, and in concerns about the under-representation of minorities in late-stage clinical research (Rogers and Lange 2013). This raises questions about how much autonomy those interested in participating in research should be allowed and whose interpretation of risk/benefit analysis—the IRB member's, the researcher's, or the potential participant's—should take precedence.

Concerns about how groups are characterized as "vulnerable" in the report have also been voiced. Some worry that the term is not explicitly defined (Rogers and Lange 2013; Levine et al. 2004) and that the reasons for particular groups' vulnerabilities are not explored (King 2005; Luna 2009), leading to a widespread assumption that all individuals in a vulnerable group lack autonomy (Rhodes 2010). Others have suggested that identifying groups or individuals as vulnerable can trigger paternalism and stereotyping (Rogers and Lange 2013; Luna 2009), while others note the failure of the report to spell out different guidelines for groups facing consent-based and fairness-based vulnerability (Nickel 2006).

Ethical Principles and Applications

A final criticism concerns the relationship between ethical principles and their applications. Belmont advocates for a deductive relationship, in that each principle is matched with one aspect of the research process: Respect for persons applies to informed consent, beneficence to risk/benefit analysis, and justice to subject selection.[2]

---

2. It should be noted that there is some disagreement among members of the commission about whether the principles were meant to have a deductive relationship with the applications (Beauchamp 2008; Levine 2005). The report itself, however, is quite explicit about the relationship: "Just as the principle of respect for persons finds expression in the requirements for consent, and the principle of beneficence in risk/benefit assessment, the principle of justice gives rise to moral requirements that there be fair procedures and outcomes in the selection of research subjects." The report also suggests that "other principles may also be relevant", but maintains that these three are comprehensive in themselves (National Commission for the Protection of Human Subjects of Biomedical and Behavioral Research 1979).

Many criticisms of the report stem from this deductive relationship, as they unpack the implications of putting forward principles with such a narrow scope. For example, several authors suggest that the principle of respect for persons is often taken to represent autonomy, consent, and individual choice, when in fact it ought to have (and some say it used to have) a much broader meaning—concern for a patient and respect for the dignity of each individual, regardless of his or her capacity for autonomous choice (Lebacqz 2005; Faden, Mastroianni, and Kahn 2005; Cassell 2005). A narrow focus on autonomy ignores the way in which people are embedded in relationships, and so does not capture the lived experience of many potential participants (Lebacqz 2005). Similarly, the report's concept of beneficence has been criticized for failing to encompass the related principle of nonmaleficence (Beauchamp 2005; Lebacqz 2005), or for being ambiguous in terms of whether it includes non-maleficence (Veatch 2005). It has also been observed that beneficence has shifted away from meaning the good of the whole patient over time toward a much narrower meaning, measured by the good done in the short run to some dimension of the patient (Cassell 2005). Likewise, the report's discussion of the principle of justice has received heated criticism for its lack of breadth and its narrow focus on subject selection (King 2005). The principle, it has been argued, fails to take into account social justice, including historical patterns of oppression and domination (Shore 2006; Sherwin 1992), and compensatory justice for those injured in research and for groups excluded from the research process (Vanderpool 2001; Lebacqz 2005; King 2005). Justice Belmont-style also does not address procedural justice such as involving vulnerable groups in the process of establishing research agendas (Sherwin 2005; King 2005), or key aspects of distributive justice, especially how the benefits of research will be made available to participants and to underserved populations (Vanderpool 2001).

Questions about how to apply the report's ethical principles are especially pertinent to discussions of IRBs. In an empirical exploration of how IRBs function, investigators found a significant portion of committee discussion revolved around the process of informed consent, while issues related to confidentiality, subject selection, risk/benefit analysis, adverse event reporting, and the minimization of risks were overlooked (Lidz et al. 2012).[3] Transcripts from meetings of the National Commission show its concern for mechanisms for the evaluation and monitoring of IRB performance, yet its suggestions include only process measures (site visits, audits of IRB records, and the like), and they were never addressed or published (National Commission for the Protection of Human Subjects of Biomedical and Behavioral Research 1978, March 10–11).

---

3. See also Klitzman (2015).

PART III: MOVING BELMONT INTO THE 21ST CENTURY—IS A TOTAL OVERHAUL NEEDED?

The Line Between Research and Practice Is Insufficient

Defining research and practice as interventions aimed at knowledge and interventions aimed at well-being is incompatible with Belmont's own principles of respecting persons, maximizing beneficence, and ensuring justice. The boundaries around what requires oversight should be defined pragmatically, so that knowledge production and benefits to all communities are maximized and harms to participants are minimized. Oversight should be required for any research or intervention involving novel, significant risks that are not part of the standard of care. This would encourage low-risk data collection during routine practice and ensure that innovative therapies are regulated and their findings disseminated. Investigators ought to be permitted to engage in low-risk or minimally risky research with minimal oversight, while regulatory mechanisms for experiments with significant risks should be kept in place. Regulation ought to be proportionate to novelty and level of risk, rather than derived from intent.

Unique Harms to Communities Remain Unacknowledged

The Belmont Report's failure to consider the potential for harms to communities should be taken into account in the design of any research protocol. This oversight could be overcome if harms to communities were explicitly acknowledged, whether as a new principle or as an extension of the principle of respect for persons. Such a principle "would obligate researchers to respect the values and interests of the community in research and, wherever possible, to protect the community from harms" (Weijer and Anderson 2002). These goals can be achieved by conducting research that is more participatory, by taking into account the needs and interests of the community involved throughout the development of a research agenda, in stages of research collection and analysis, and during the dissemination of results (Weijer and Anderson 2002). A move toward this goal was taken in the recent Common Rule updates, which state that the official governing body of American Indian/Alaska Native tribes can establish additional protections and use of a single IRB (Federal Policy for the Protection of Human Subjects 2017). There is no simple way to define a community, but relevant factors would include self-definition, shared health data and outcomes, group-based vulnerabilities, and historical relationships with prior research.

The Report Fails to Address Current Concerns Involving Transparency

In order for regulatory agencies to operate with the principle of beneficence in mind, they must understand, to the fullest extent possible, the risks and benefits involved in a given research protocol. To achieve this goal, each stage of the research process must strive for greater transparency. By adopting an additional principle of transparency, or making explicit the principle of nonmaleficence, a revised framework could better address issues that arise in the wake of the commodification of biomedicine. Some advances toward this goal are already taking place, such as the Food and Drug Administration (FDA) requirement that details of all clinical trials be reported on ClinicalTrials.gov (Piller 2015). As industry funding continues to outpace government investments in research, transparency will remain an important tool for minimizing conflicts of interest.

A Focus on Protectionism Is Incompatible With Today's Emphasis on Participation

The Belmont Report's emphasis on researchers' duty to protect participants is admirable and necessary. Yet this duty should be augmented by a duty to include individuals from excluded and vulnerable groups in the research process. Inclusion should be understood to mean including those who have been left out not only as participants but as research partners who can help shape the research goals and protocols. This broader understanding of inclusion is likely to be more effective at reducing the inequalities in both knowledge and opportunity to obtain benefits that exist between those who have been overly protected and those who have not. This move away from protectionism and toward participation, from subjects to partners, is supported by both the principle of beneficence, since it may lead to greater positive health outcomes, and the principle of respect for persons, since many individuals desire to be more involved in research. This also aligns with the recently released Common Rule updates, which now exclude pregnant women and those with physical disabilities from those "potentially vulnerable due to undue influence" (Federal Policy for the Protection of Human Subjects 2017), and the revised Council for the International Organizations of Medical Sciences (CIOMS) International Ethical Guidelines for Health-related Research Involving Humans, which recognize that a judgment of vulnerability "requires empirical evidence to document the need for special protections" (CIOMS 1993). Of course, care must still be taken to ensure that each stage of the research process is not exploitative. Especially important is that participants receive reasonable compensation for harms and injuries they might sustain within an experiment, a problem that remains unsolved to this day.

The Deductive Relationship Between Single Ethical Principles and Applications Espoused by the Report Is Too Limited

Although the Belmont Report suggested that the relationship between individual principles and applications be understood as a deductive one, this unnecessarily

The American Journal of Bioethics

limits the principles to narrow aspects of the research process; the principles instead ought to be understood as applying broadly to all aspects of research involving human subjects. Each principle should be kept in mind by investigators, oversight committees, and regulators throughout each stage of research design, development, implementation, and distribution. Respect for persons should no longer be thought of as a principle that is captured merely by the process of informed consent, but as one that guides the entire research process. In practice, this would involve determining eligibility criteria with this principle in mind, so that individuals are not excluded for trivial reasons (e.g., extra time required for a translator) and those deemed eligible would be likely to benefit from the results (e.g., individuals living below the poverty level are less likely to benefit from an investigation of a novel device not covered by Medicaid). This would also imply that specific informed consent can sometimes be forgone in favor of "broad consent" (Federal Policy for the Protection of Human Subjects 2017; Council for International Organizations of Medical Sciences 2002).[4] Similarly, follow-up should be conducted with the principle of respect for persons in mind; test results should be given directly to a participant's primary care physician when requested, and someone from the study team should be available to answer questions for a reasonable period of time once data collection is complete.

CONCLUSION

The Belmont Report was an impressive and inspiring response to the ethical issues of its day. Since its release, the field of research involving human subjects has developed in complex and unexpected ways, challenging the report's ethical framework to respond not only to the fears related to research abuses that it stemmed from, but also to the increasing commodification of biomedicine, the exclusion of many groups from research, the globalization of research, the desires of many to have access to experimental drugs, the lack of generalizability and reproducibility of many research findings, and the unique harms and histories that communities have experienced as a result of research. While these challenges are likely to continue to shift and expand in the coming years, there are several areas where the report comes up short today. Considering the important role the Belmont Report has played and continues to play in research ethics today (Federal Policy for the Protection of Human Subjects 2017), it is time for a tune-up, if not a complete overhaul. ∎

---

4. In fact, the recently released Common Rule acknowledges that feedback on the previously proposed policy of requiring informed consent for the use of biospecimens was insufficient in that it emphasized "respect for persons with little regard for the principles of beneficence and justice" (Federal policy for the protection of human subjects 2017).

REFERENCES

Beauchamp, T. L. 2005. The origins and evolution of the Belmont report. In *Belmont revisited: Ethical principles for research with human subjects*, ed. J. F. Childress, E. M. Meslin, and H. T. Shapiro, 12–25. Washington, DC: Georgetown University Press.

Beauchamp, T. L. 2008. The Belmont report. In *The Oxford textbook of clinical research ethics*, ed. E. J. Emanuel, 149–55. New York, NY: Oxford University Press.

Beauchamp, T. L., and Y. Saghai. 2012. The historical foundations of the research-practice distinction in bioethics. *Theoretical Medicine and Bioethics* 33 (1):45–56.

BEECHER, H. 1966. ETHICS AND CLINICAL RESEARCH. *NEW ENGLAND JOURNAL OF MEDICINE* 274 (24):1354.

Benitez, K., and B. Malin. 2010. Evaluating re-identification risks with respect to the HIPAA privacy rule. *Journal of the American Medical Informatics Association* 17 (2):169–77.

Cassell, E. J. 2005. The principles of the Belmont report: How have respect for persons, beneficence, and justice been applied in clinical medicine? In *Belmont revisited: Ethical principles for research with human subjects*, ed. J. F. Childress, E. M. Meslin, and H. T. Shapiro, 77–95. Washington, DC: Georgetown University Press.

Council for International Organizations of Medical Sciences. 1993. International ethical guidelines for biomedical research involving human subjects. http://www.cioms.ch/publications/guidelines/guidelines_nov_2002_blurb.htm.

Council for International Organizations of Medical Sciences. 2002. International ethical guidelines for biomedical research involving human subjects. *Bulletin of Medical Ethics* Oct. (182):17.

Dumit, J. 2012. *Drugs for life: How pharmaceutical companies define our health.* Durham, NC: Duke University Press.

Emanuel, E. J. 2015. Reform of clinical research regulations, finally. *New England Journal of Medicine* 373 (24):2296–99.

Emanuel, E. J., and C. Weijer. 2005. Protecting communities in research: From a new principle to rational protections. In *Belmont revisited: Ethical principles for research with human subjects*, ed. J. F. Childress, E. M. Meslin, and H. T. Shapiro, 165–83. Washington, DC: Georgetown University Press.

Faden, R. R., N. E. Kass, S. N. Goodman, P. Pronovost, S. Tunis, and T. L. Beauchamp. 2013. An ethics framework for a learning health care system: A departure from traditional research ethics and clinical ethics. *Hastings Center Reports* 43 (s1):S16–27.

Faden, R. R., A. C. Mastroianni, and J. P. Kahn. 2005. Beyond belmont: Trust, openness, and the work of the advisory committee on human radiation experiments. In *Belmont revisited: Ethical principles for research with human subjects*, ed. J. F. Childress, E. M. Meslin, and H. T. Shapiro, 41–54. Washington, DC: Georgetown University Press.

Federal policy for the protection of human subjects. 2017. *Federal Register* 82 (12):7150, 7158, 7204.

Gelinas, L., R. Pierce, S. Winkler, and B. Bierer. 2017. Using social media as a research recruitment tool: Ethical issues and recommendations. *American Journal of Bioethics* 17 (3):3–14.

Jonsen, A. R. 1988. *The abuse of casuistry.* Berkeley, CA: University of California Press.

Jonsen, A. R. 2005. On the origins and future of the Belmont Report. In *Belmont revisited: Ethical principles for research with human subjects*, ed. J. F. Childress, E. M. Meslin, and H. T. Shapiro, 3–11. Washington, DC: Georgetown University Press.

Kelly, P., S. J. Marshall, H. Badland, et al. 2013. An ethical framework for automated, wearable cameras in health behavior research. *American Journal of Preventive Medicine* 44 (3):314–19.

King, P. A. 2005. Justice beyond Belmont. In *Belmont revisited: Ethical principles for research with human subjects*, ed. J. F. Childress, E. M. Meslin, and H. T. Shapiro, 136–47. Washington, DC: Georgetown University Press.

Klitzman, R. 2015. *The ethics police?: The struggle to make human research safe*. New York, NY: Oxford University Press.

Lebacqz, K. 2005. We sure are older but are we wiser? In *Belmont revisited: Ethical principles for research with human subjects*, ed. J. F. Childress, E. M. Meslin, and H. T. Shapiro, 99–110. Washington, DC: Georgetown University Press.

Levine, C., R. Faden, C. Grady, D. Hammerschmidt, L. Eckenwiler, and J. Sugarman. 2004. The limitations of "vulnerability" as a protection for human research participants. *American Journal of Bioethics* 4 (3):44–9.

Levine, R. J. 1982. Validity of consent procedures in technologically developing countries. In *Human experimentation and medical ethics: Proceedings of the 15th CIOMS Round Table Conference*, ed. Z. Bankowski and R. J. Levine, 16–30. Geneva, Switzerland: Council for International Organizations of Medical Sciences.

Levine, R. J. 2005. The National Commission's ethical principles with special attention to beneficence. In *Belmont revisited: Ethical principles for research with human subjects*, ed. J. F. Childress, E. M. Meslin, and H. T. Shapiro, 126–35. Washington, DC: Georgetown University Press.

Lidz, C., P. Appelbaum, R. Arnold, et al. 2012. IRBs: How closely do they follow the Common Rule. *Academic Medicine* 87:1–6.

Luna, F. 2009. Elucidating the concept of vulnerability: Layers not labels. *International Journal of Feminist Approaches to Bioethics* 2 (1):121–39.

McCallum, J. M., D. M. Arekere, B. L. Green, R. V. Katz, and B. M. Rivers. 2006. Awareness and knowledge of the U.S. public health service syphilis study at Tuskegee: Implications for biomedical research. *Journal of Health Care for the Poor and Underserved* 17 (4):716–33.

Metcalf, J., and K. Crawford. 2016. Where are human subjects in big data research? *The emerging ethics divide*. Big Data and Society, May 14.

National Commission for the Protection of Human Subjects of Biomedical and Behavioral Research. 1978, March 10–11. Meeting Transcript, Tab 2, Box 30. Georgetown University Archives, Washington, DC.

National Commission for the Protection of Human Subjects of Biomedical and Behavioral Research. 1978, January 13. Meeting Transcript, Tab 2, Box 33. Georgetown University Archives, Washington, DC.

National Commission for the Protection of Human Subjects of Biomedical and Behavioral Research. 1979. The Belmont report: Ethical principles and guidelines for the protection of human subjects of research. Available at: http://www.hhs.gov/ohrp/regulations-and-policy/belmont-report

Nickel, P. J. 2006. Vulnerable populations in research: The case of the seriously ill. *Theoretical Medicine and Bioethics* 27 (3):245–64.

The Nuremberg Code. 1949. In *Trials of war criminals before the Nuremberg Military Tribunals under Control Council Law No. 10*, vol. 2, 181–82. Washington, DC: U.S. Government Printing Office.

Piller, C. 2015. Failure to investigate: A STAT investigation of clinical trial reporting. *STAT News*, December 13. Available at: https://www.statnews.com/2015/12/13/clinical-trials-investigation/

Rhodes, R. 2010. Rethinking Research Ethics. *American Journal of Bioethics* 5(1): 7–28.

Rogers, W., and M. M. Lange. 2013. Rethinking the vulnerability of minority populations in research. *American Journal of Public Health* 103 (12):2141–46.

Sherwin, S. 1992. *No longer patient: Feminist ethics and health care*, 72–79. Philadelphia, PA: Temple University Press.

Sherwin, S. 2005. Belmont revisited through a feminist lens. In *Belmont revisited: Ethical principles for research with human subjects*, ed. J. F. Childress, E. M. Meslin, and H. T. Shapiro, 148–64. Washington, DC: Georgetown University Press.

Shore, N. 2006. Re-conceptualizing the Belmont report: A community-based participatory research perspective. *Journal of Community Practice* 14 (4):5–26.

Taylor, P. L. 2010. Overseeing innovative therapy without mistaking it for research: A function-based model based on old truths, new capacities, and lessons from stem cells. *Journal of Law, Medicine & Ethics* 38 (2):286–302.

Vanderpool, H. Y. 2001. Unfulfilled promise: How the Belmont report can amend the Code of Federal Regulations Title 45 Part 46—Protection of human subjects. *National Bioethics Advisory Commission [NBAC] Ethical and Policy Issues in Research Involving Human Participants Volume II: Commissioned Papers*. Rockville, MD: National Bioethics Advisory Commission.

Veatch, R. M. 2005. Ranking, balancing, or simultaneity: Resolving conflicts among the belmont principles. In *Belmont revisited: Ethical principles for research with human subjects*, ed. J. F. Childress, E. M. Meslin, and H. T. Shapiro, 184–204. Washington, DC: Georgetown University Press.

Weijer, C. 1999. Protecting communities in research: philosophical and pragmatic challenges. *Cambridge Quarterly of Healthcare Ethics* 8 (4):501–13.

Weijer, C., and J. A. Anderson. 2002. A critical appraisal of protections for aboriginal communities in biomedical research. *Jurimetrics* 42 (2):187–98.

WMA General Assembly. 1996. *WMA Declaration of Helsinki—Ethical principles for medical research involving human subjects*. Somerset West, South Africa: World Medical Association.

References

DeMets DL, Ellenberg SS. Data monitoring committees – expect the unexpected. N Engl J Med. 2016;375(14):1365–71.

Grady C. Institutional review boards; purpose and challenges. Chest. 2015;148(5):1148–55.

Hallinan A, Forrest A, Uhlenbrauck G, Young S, McMinney R. Barriers to change in the informed consent process: a systematic literature review. IRB. 2016;38(3):1–10.

Nicholls SG, Hayes TP, Brehaut JC, McDonald M, Weijer C, Saginur R, Fergusson D. A scoping review of empirical research relating to quality and effectiveness of research ethics review. PLoS One. 2015;10(7):E013639.

Additional Suggested Reading

The Belmont Report: Ethical principles and guidelines for the protection of human subjects of research. 1979. (*This is a foundational document which describes the ethical basis for human subjects protection in research.*)

Grady C. Institutional review boards; purpose and challenges. Chest 2015;148(5):1148–1155. (*Provides a clear description of institutional review boards and the policies under which they operate.*)

Hallinan Z, Forrest A, Uhlenbrauck G, Young S, McKinney R. Barriers to change in the informed consent process: A systematic literature review. IRB. 2016 ;38(3):1–10. (*Reviews research on informed consent in research and suggests steps to make it more robust.*)

Responsible Authorship

Arthur L. Caplan and Barbara K. Redman

While authorship is perhaps the major source of credit for scientific work, it also carries major ethical responsibilities of vouching for the accuracy and integrity of the conduct of research and the resulting publications. Authorship credit can be highly contested with few guidelines or sources for the adjudication of disputes. Still, even without a single algorithm to determine authorship, addressing authorship and authorship priority at the beginning of an inquiry can reduce the potential for disagreements and disappointment later.

Author order and inclusion/exclusion are major issues. In a few fields, author order is alphabetical; in others practices vary, making it difficult to determine relative credit and responsibility. International Council of Medical Journal Editors (ICMJE) criteria suggest that authorship requires being responsible for ideas and/or data acquisition and analysis, and/or drafting text (Matheson 2016). All authors must give final approval of the work and guarantee their belief in its overall integrity. Honorary authorship, in which individuals are named as authors but do not meet the criteria for contributing, is common and rarely contested, especially by junior authors who are dependent on mentors. The practice is customary in some labs, frowned upon in others. Ghost authorship fails to name as author someone who fulfilled the criteria, who often is a professional writer hired by the funder. A study of nursing journals found a 42% prevalence of honorary authorship and a 28% prevalence of ghost authorship (Kennedy et al. 2014). A survey of authors in chemistry found half of those queried believed they were not given appropriate credit in papers for their work (Seeman and House 2015).

Addressing the integrity of authorship requires understanding the integrity of editors and publishers, since many incentives are set by these organizations/individuals. With the explosion in open access publishing, a not insignificant number of journals exhibit characteristics that lead them to be labeled as "predatory." They are pay to publish outlets. This means that they have little or poor peer review, charge large fees to publish, refuse to allow manuscript withdrawal, refuse to retract or correct articles, and may not be digitally preserved. All of these practices undermine responsible authorship. Again in one sample field, nursing, 57% of journals could be classified as predatory (Oermann et al. 2016).

Finally, several mechanisms are used to correct the scientific record. Article retraction should be made in cases of "pervasive error" or unsubstantiated or irreproducible data. Authors (usually requiring agreement of all authors) can request correction or retraction of a published article. The US Office of Research Integrity (ORI) sometimes requires article correction or retraction in a finding of research misconduct. In many instances editors can retract for sufficient cause with or without author agreement.

Since publications are prime sources of scientific credit, research integrity requires strong norms about authorship responsibility, likely best addressed through effective self-regulation by scientific communities. Authors must exercise caution and diligence in seeking to avoid publication in predatory, pay to publish publications.

Advice: Pre-study, written agreement about authorship including order and responsibility is the best practice – ask for one and be sure the parties involved sign off on it. As an author, you should have access to raw data, its analyses, and interpretation, in order to vouch for the study. You should always sign off on the final version of a manuscript before it is submitted to a journal and after revisions, for resubmission. Third party sign-off for you is not acceptable.

Be sure to check with mentors which journals in your field are predatory and stay away from them. Solicitation of manuscripts through social media from strangers is a sign of likely predatory publication outlets.

A. L. Caplan · B. K. Redman (✉)
New York University Langone Medical Center,
New York, NY, USA
e-mail: Arthur.Caplan@nyumc.org

© Springer International Publishing AG, part of Springer Nature 2018
A. L. Caplan, B. K. Redman (eds.), *Getting to Good*, https://doi.org/10.1007/978-3-319-51358-4_5

5.1   The Problem of Publication-Pollution Denialism

Arthur L. Caplan

Caplan A. The problem of publication-pollution denialism. Mayo Clinic Proceedings 2015; 90(5):565–566.

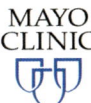

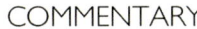

The Problem of Publication-Pollution Denialism

Arthur L. Caplan, PhD

The world is facing a huge threat from pollution. The scientific community seems unable or unwilling to do anything about the problem and appears to be in a state of denial. The pollution crisis I'm describing is not the warming of the Earth's atmosphere due to an accumulation of greenhouse gasses. It is not the tragedy of plastic materials accumulating in the oceans. It is not the air pollution that is overwhelming many major urban areas and contributing to respiratory and other diseases in the local populations. It is, instead, the pollution of science and medicine by plagiarism, fraud, and predatory publishing. If the medical and scientific communities continue to remain in publication pollution denial, the trustworthiness, utility, and value of science and medicine will be irreparably damaged.

Harvard researcher Mark Shrime recently wrote an article entitled "Cuckoo for Cocoa Puffs?: The Surgical and Neoplastic Role of Cacao Extract in Breakfast Cereals." The fake authors he chose for the piece were Pinkerton A. LeBrain and Orson Welles. Shrime submitted this fake article to 37 journals. At last count, 17 had accepted the obviously phony, nonsensical paper.[1] John Bohannon[2] did the same thing with a completely phony paper, with even more depressing results in terms of peer-reviewed acceptance to journals. The journals that took these gibberish-laden, concocted articles were scam, author-must-pay, profit-driven entities that nevertheless have every appearance of being legitimate journals.

Jeffrey Beall, a librarian at the University of Colorado at Denver, maintains a list of what he terms *predatory publishers*. These publishers produce fake journals that recruit authors whom they will publish for pay, primarily for the purpose of providing profit for the publishers. These publishers are different from legitimate, indexed, peer-reviewed journals that use author-pay financial models to underwrite journal peer review, processing, and publication costs (eg, the PLOS family of journals). Predatory publishers are the direct descendants of vanity presses—book publishers whose authors pay for the privilege of publishing to give the false impression that they have written a book that has been vetted by a mainstream, reputable publisher. Beall estimates that 25% of all open-access journals are predatory.[3]

Why the recent proliferation of polluting journals? As Sarwar and Nicolaou observe, "Arguably, many researchers and departments may have equated the concept of 'quantity' rather than 'quality' with research success. The association between the number of publications and suitability for funding or career progression has been with us for a while. When applying for senior posts, surgical trainees are continuously questioned on the number of publications achieved, disregarding the quality of the publication or journal. ... this attitude has predisposed to a massive rise in journal titles, many of which are of low quality and are poorly maintained."[4]

The problems generated by phony, predatory journals that use substandard or no peer review are enormous. Not only do they provide opportunities for the unscrupulous in academia and industry to pad their curriculum vitaes and bibliographies with bogus articles and editorial appointments, they also make it difficult for those involved in the assessment and promotion of scholars to discern value from junk.[5] The impact of publication pollution does not end there. Predatory, pay-to-publish, non—peer-reviewed journals flood disciplines with bad or fake science, making it hard, much as light pollution does, to see the real stars. Worse, publication pollution lessens the impact of legitimate science in the formation of public policy, undermining public health, weakening the overall value of legitimate publications in influencing policy, and creating opportunities for the continued power of crackpot views that corrode many areas of public life, such as vaccination, fluoridation, and the prevention and treatment of diseases, such as autism, AIDS, and cancer.

The pay-for-publication practices and inadequate peer review of phony journals are major sources of publication pollution but not the only sources. Misconduct is

From the Division of Medical Ethics, Langone Medical Center, New York University, New York, NY.

polluting the fabric of science and medicine as well.

Studies are making it into print that have been condemned by the Food and Drug Administration, other regulators, and legitimate authors and review groups. My colleague Charles Seife found in a review of Food and Drug Administration inspection reports between 1998 and 2013 that of nearly 60 clinical trials in which regulators had uncovered violations serious enough to earn the agency's most severe classification ("official action indicated"), 78 articles using data from these trials were published. Seife[6] believes that there could well be more.

A recent analysis of the prevalence of research misconduct by Daniele Fanelli looked at "scientific behaviors that distort scientific knowledge" and found that 2% of the scientists surveyed admitted to serious misconduct (falsification or fabrication of data) at least once and nearly 34% admitted other questionable research practices. When participants were asked about their colleagues' practices, the results were much worse: 14% for falsification of data and 72% for other questionable practices.[7]

Fraud, however, pales in comparison to plagiarism as a means of polluting science and medicine. An article in *Nature* about the use of plagiarism-searching software found, during a few months in 2010,[8] "staggering levels of plagiarism, from self-plagiarism, to copying of a few paragraphs, or the wholesale copying of other articles." Editor friends of mine from many fields of medicine and science tell me that they must spend inordinate amounts of time checking for plagiarism in submissions they receive. Unfortunately, the plagiarism problem appears to be increasing even as various computer software programs emerge to detect it.

All these polluting factors detract from the ability of scientists and physicians to trust what they read, devalue legitimate science, undermine the ability to reproduce legitimate findings, impose huge costs on the publication process, and take a toll in terms of disability and death when tests, treatments, and interventions are founded on faulty claims. Once pollution enters the waters of legitimate publication, it is difficult to expunge it from reader's minds, even if the articles have been retracted as flawed or bogus.[9] As is so often true of pollution, publication pollution has a very long half-life.

Publication pollution is corroding the reliability of science and medicine and yet neither the leadership nor those who rely on the truth of science and medicine are sounding the alarm loudly or moving to fix the problem with appropriate energy.

The currency of science is fragile, and allowing counterfeiters, fraudsters, bunko artists, scammers, and cheats to continue to operate with abandon in the publishing realm is unacceptable. Talk of free speech and the power of the marketplace of ideas to sort out the wheat from the chaff is naive. When the marketplace is full of dangerous and defective goods, there is no free market because the trust requisite to support a market has evaporated.[10] The time for a serious, sustained international effort to halt publication pollution is now. Otherwise scientists and physicians will not have to argue about any issue—no one will believe them anyway.

Correspondence: Address to Arthur L. Caplan, PhD, Division of Medical Ethics, Langone Medical Center, New York University, New York, NY 10016 (arthur.caplan@nyumc.org).

REFERENCES

1. Segran E. Why a fake article titled "Cuckoo for Cocoa Puffs?" was accepted by 17 medical journals. Body Week website. http://www.fastcompany.com/3041493/body-week/why-a-fake-article-cuckoo-for-cocoa-puffs-was-accepted-by-17-medical-journals. Accessed February 10, 2015.
2. Bohannon J. Who's afraid of peer review? *Science*. 2013; 342(6154):60-65.
3. Beall J. Predatory publishers are corrupting open access. *Nature*. 2012;489(9):179.
4. Sarwar U, Nicolaou M. Fraud and deceit in medical research. *J Res Med Sci*. 2012;17(11):1077-1081.
5. Balon R. Perilous terra incognita: open-access journals. *Acad Psychiatry*. 2014;38(2):221-223.
6. Seife C. Research misconduct identified by the US Food and Drug Administration: out of sight, out of mind, out of the peer-reviewed literature [published online February 9, 2015]. *JAMA Intern Med*. http://dx.doi.org/10.1001/jamainternmed.2014.7774.
7. Fanelli D. How many scientists fabricate and falsify research? a systematic review and meta-analysis of survey data. *PLoS One*. 2009;4(5):e5738.
8. Butler D. Journals step up plagiarism policing: cut-and-paste culture tackled by CrossCheck software. *Nature*. 2010; 466(7303):167.
9. Whitley WP, Rennie D, Hafner AW. The scientific community's response to evidence of fraudulent publication: the Robert Slutsky case. *JAMA*. 1994;272(2):170-173.
10. Fleischacker S. *On Adam Smith's Wealth of Nations: A Philosophical Companion*. Princeton, NJ: Princeton University Press; 2004.

5.2 Addressing Research Misconduct and Detrimental Research Practices: Current Knowledge and Issues

National Academy of Sciences

National Academy of Sciences. Addressing research misconduct and detrimental research practices: current knowledge and issues. Washington, DC: National Academies Press; 2017, Chapter 7, Fostering Integrity in Research; p.114–119. Copyright © National Academy of Sciences. All rights reserved.

Reprinted with permission from the National Academy of Sciences, courtesy of the National Academies Press.

AUTHORSHIP-RELATED CHALLENGES TO RESEARCH INTEGRITY

Nature and Scope of the Problem

As discussed in other parts of this report, published papers are the currency of science. Through such papers, science is communicated, critiqued, and assessed. The number and quality of published articles credited to a scientist, especially peer-reviewed articles, are major criteria for promotion and tenure, and so have a powerful impact on scientific careers. Authorship designates who is willing to take responsibility for an article and who bears responsibility for the

PREPUBLICATION COPY—UNEDITED PROOFS

ADDRESSING RESEARCH MISCONDUCT AND DETRIMENTAL RESEARCH PRACTICES   115

work in case of error or allegations of misconduct. Authorship credit is therefore an integral part of the scientific enterprise as a professional system.

Chapter 3 discusses how changes in the research environment such as technological advances that have transformed many aspects of performing and reporting research, the growing importance of collaborative and interdisciplinary research, and the globalization of research are affecting authorship practices and conventions. Several of the most difficult challenges to research integrity involve authorship abuses, particularly authorship credit misallocations/misappropriations (Martinson and Master, 2015). As discussed in Chapter 4, plagiarism is one category of authorship credit misallocation that is included in the definition of research misconduct by the U.S. federal government and by most other countries. For the most part, other categories of authorship credit misallocation are considered detrimental research practices for the purposes of this report. This section will describe some of the most pressing challenges related to authorship and research integrity and consider the advantages and disadvantages of alternative approaches to addressing them.

Authorship can be misused in several ways. Gift, guest, or honorary authorship involves listing an author who made no substantive contribution to the research reported. For example, researchers may add the name of a prominent researcher to a paper in the belief that it will increase its odds of being accepted by a prestigious journal. Gift authorship can happen with or without the knowledge or permission of the researcher being "honored." When the gift author had no role in the conducting or writing of the article, listing his or her name is a misallocation of credit. In cases where work is fabricated or falsified, questions are raised about the responsibilities of coauthors whose contributions may or may not have merited authorship. The stem cell case at Seoul National University and the University of Pittsburgh, described in Appendix D, discusses these issues.

A senior scientist may demand or be granted an authorship designation for a "specialized" service such as providing biological materials or specimens, helping to secure funding for the research, or serving as head of the laboratory or department where the research is undertaken. Insistence by a scientist in a position of authority that he or she be listed as an author on all papers submitted to journals by subordinates, including articles in which the senior scientist has played no direct role, is known as "coercive authorship."

As data and code sharing become part of the usual practice of science, reuse of these scholarly outputs is increasingly common. The expectation is that the use or reuse of data and/or code produced by another researcher will be appropriately cited. Such recognition rewards the producer of the data and code while improving, extending, and building on these objects in their own right. It is inappropriate to condition data or code reuse on coauthorship when there is no other contribution to the paper. This is a coercive practice that slows the advancement of science when other mechanisms are in place to reward data and code contributors, such as citation. The practice of conditioning data use on coauthorship is more widespread in some disciplines than in others but should not exist in any discipline. This is separate from, and not to be confused with, a data or code contributor who is or becomes part of the research team and collects novel data or builds code for the purposes of a research project or series of projects. Coercive authorship practices occur when coauthorship is conditioned on using data and code associated with a previous or different project rather than the only expectation being citation for downstream use.

Another detrimental authorship practice is unacknowledged or "ghost" authorship, in which researchers who have made a substantial contribution to a research article are not listed as

PREPUBLICATION COPY—UNEDITED PROOFS

authors. Not all unacknowledged authorship fits into this category. For example, reporting someone else's research results as one's own without designating that person as an author and without their knowledge is a form of plagiarism. A professional writer whose only involvement in the research is participation in writing the paper is not considered to be an author in most contexts, but many journals require that professional writers be acknowledged.

A problematic form of ghost authorship arises when researchers who are directly involved in all phases of the research are not acknowledged (Fugh-Berman, 2010). For example, a pharmaceutical company may finance and undertake research that supports a non-FDA-approved use of one of its products, prepare the paper, and recruit prominent medical researchers to sign on as authors. The corporate support and industry authors may not be disclosed. In some cases, the listed academic authors will have had some involvement with the research, but sometimes they do not. In these latter cases, ghost authorship also becomes a type of honorary authorship.

While the immediate motivation for this form of ghostwriting is to hide the financial interest of the sponsor and ghost authors in the work, it has also been associated with other detrimental research practices such as selective reporting and suppression of some findings. In the Paxil case described in Appendix D, data falsification was admitted by the sponsor and ghost authors but denied by the listed authors. If data are falsified or the reported results are misleading in such clinical studies and the listed authors are not able to vouch for the integrity of the data or results, using the study as a basis for treating patients may present serious health and safety risks.

In addition to the Paxil case, several other examples of alleged ghostwriting that involved other alleged detrimental research practices led to legal consequences for both medical industry sponsors and ghostwriters (Feely, 2012; Fugh-Berman, 2010). In one case, documents were released showing that Pfizer's Wyeth Pharmaceutical Company had not disclosed its role in preparing journal articles supporting the used of Prempro, a hormone drug, and recruiting academic authors (Fugh-Berman, 2010). In 2012, Pfizer had paid $896 million to settle only about half of the cases alleging Prempro had caused cancer (Feeley, 2012). In addition to Paxil and Prempro, ghostwriting has "been documented in the promotion of 'Fen-phen', Neurontin, Vioxx and Zoloft" (Fugh-Berman, 2010). The companies that produce these drugs have paid millions to billions of dollars in lawsuit settlements.

This form of ghostwriting has been condemned as an "example of fraud" and "a disturbing violation of academic integrity standards, which form the basis of scientific reliability" (Bosch and Ross, 2012; Stern and Lemmens, 2011). The practice is not currently equated with plagiarism and so is not within ORI's power to regulate. Bosch and Ross (2012) suggest that ORI include ghostwriting in its definition of research misconduct so that it can be investigated and addressed under the federal research misconduct policy. The International Committee of Medical Journal Editors (ICMJE) (2010) established criteria against which to determine appropriate assignment of biomedical authorship and recommends that those who do not meet all of the criteria only be listed in the acknowledgments sections. The Committee on Publication Ethics (COPE) (2011) also recommends that specific rules be implemented to prevent ghostwriting, which is explicitly defined as misconduct in its guidelines. The pharmaceutical industry itself has promulgated guidelines for clinical trials that specify adherence to the ICMJE authorship criteria (PhRMA, 2014).

All of the authorship abuses described above undermine research integrity. Even when the research that is reported is correct and of high quality, inaccurate and misleading authorship

PREPUBLICATION COPY—UNEDITED PROOFS

ADDRESSING RESEARCH MISCONDUCT AND DETRIMENTAL RESEARCH PRACTICES   *117*

designations can lead to misallocation of credit, rewards, and future resources. They can damage the conduct of science if, for example, authorship credit without deep knowledge or skill in the science involved helps promote an honorary author to a position of authority. They can also obscure responsibility for reported work and make it more difficult to address other forms of misconduct, such as data fabrication. Indeed, there is evidence that engaging in authorship credit misrepresentation increases the risk that researchers will engage in research misconduct later (Martinson and Master, 2015). Several cases discussed in Appendix D, including the Paxil case and the stem cell case at Seoul National University and the University of Pittsburgh involve authorship.

Over the past several decades, surveys and meta-analyses have shed light on how prevalent inaccurate and misleading authorship designations are. A 2011 meta-analysis of research on authorship found that an average of 29 percent of respondents had experienced some problems with misuse of authorship (Marusic–*PLOS ONE*, 2011). An international survey of authors of articles published in six general medical journals in 2008 found that 21 percent of papers had honorary and/or ghost authors, down from 29 percent in 1996 (Wislar et al., 2011). Both the 2011 and 1996 surveys used the ISMJE definition of authorship (to be discussed in more detail below). Almost two-thirds of the 2011 respondents resided in the United States or Canada, with most of the rest residing in Europe. Even if other fields have a much lower incidence of authorship misrepresentation than biomedical research, the overall incidence would be disturbingly high, since biomedical research constitutes a large fraction of overall research funding and publishing.

More recent work presented at a scientific meeting and reported in the media found significantly higher rates of guest and ghost authorship than the results cited above (Jaschik, 2015).

Addressing Authorship Credit Misrepresentation

Stakeholders in the research enterprise widely recognize that more vigorous efforts are needed to reduce and ultimately eliminate authorship credit misrepresentation. In recent years, a number of journals and professional groups such as the Council of Science Editors, COPE, and ICMJE have updated and clarified their authorship criteria to prohibit honorary and ghost authorship. Journals also are adopting practices such as author contribution statements and are requiring independent approval of all coauthors on articles as mechanisms to discourage inaccurate authorship designation. In a 2009 report, the Institute of Medicine called on academic medical centers and teaching hospitals to prohibit medical ghostwriting (IOM, 2009).

A 2012 editorial in *Science* called for renewed attention to the problem of honorary authorship and advocated that more journals adopt the use of author contribution statements (Greenland and Fontanarosa, 2012). The editorial also called on research institutions to combat honorary authorship more directly and proactively, pointing out that institutions such as Washington University in St. Louis define honorary authorship as misconduct in their policies (Washington University, 2009). For example, junior researchers need to know who to notify and the appropriate procedures to follow when they are coerced into listing a noncontributing co-author.

Several alternative approaches might be considered to address this challenge. One would be to treat some forms of authorship credit misrepresentation in addition to plagiarism as

PREPUBLICATION COPY—UNEDITED PROOFS

research misconduct. A footnote in the 1992 *Responsible Science* report states that "it is possible that some extreme cases of noncontributing authorship may be regarded as misconduct because they constitute a form of falsification" (NAS-NAE-IOM, 1992). *Responsible Science* also noted that, in 1989, a Public Health Service annual report of its activities to address research misconduct included several abuses of authorship as examples of misconduct, such as "preparation and publication of a book chapter listing co-authors who were unaware of being named as co-authors" and "engaging in inappropriate authorship practices on a publication and failure to acknowledge that data used in a grant application were developed by another scientist." It should be noted that this formulation predated the 2000 federal policy on research misconduct. In 1989, the PHS definition of research misconduct was "fabrication, falsification, plagiarism, or other serious deviations from commonly accepted research practices." None of the specific terms was further defined.

Authorship misrepresentation other than plagiarism is clearly not included in the definition of falsification specified in the current U.S. federal research misconduct policy (OSTP, 2000). A change in the definition of falsification would be needed for inaccurate or misleading authorship designations to be treated as research misconduct by the federal government.

Implementation of such a change would face a number of practical obstacles. To begin with, although the authorship standards of COPE, the Council of Science Editors, and ICMJE are widely respected, disciplines vary widely in authorship standards and practices. For example, ICMJE defines authors as those who have fulfilled the following criteria: (1) substantial contributions to the conception or design of the work; or the acquisition, analysis, or interpretation of data for the work; (2) drafting the work or revising it critically for important intellectual content; (3) final approval of the version to be published; and (4) agreement to be accountable for all aspects of the work in ensuring that questions related to the accuracy or integrity of any part of the work are appropriately investigated and resolved (ICMJE, 2013b). However, in research fields involving work on complex instruments and the generation of large amounts of data, it is possible to imagine circumstances where articles are published in which no one qualifies as an author according to the ICMJE criteria. The same circumstances might imply author credit misrepresentation in one field and acceptable practice in another. This would make it difficult to develop a workable definition of falsification that could be applied in a consistent way.

Professional disputes and legal allegations over the denial of rightful authorship or a lack of rightful authorship credit have become a growing issue within the research enterprise. While academic theft is a serious transgression, it may be difficult to determine how, or from whom, an idea originated. There are numerous examples of researchers, often postdocs and junior scientists, proving that their research had been published without their name credited as an author or without their knowledge at all, both inside and outside of academia. However, there are also instances in which graduate students or junior scientists perform research with a mentor who developed the same research idea years earlier. In 1995 a graduate student, Pamela Berge, won over $1 million in a lawsuit claiming academic theft against her mentors; however, it was later revealed that the research had been ongoing for several years before Berge entered the research laboratory and the verdict was overturned (Woolston, 2002). Clear communication and discussion of how authorship roles are to be determined at the onset of research may avoid later questions of authorship credit.

PREPUBLICATION COPY—UNEDITED PROOFS

Another practical difficulty in addressing authorship credit misrepresentation other than plagiarism through the research misconduct policy framework involves the sheer scale of the phenomenon. Suppose that the study cited above is correct and more than 20 percent of biomedical research articles have honorary and/or ghost authors (Wislar et al., 2011). There are roughly 50,000 biomedical articles published by U.S. authors per year (NSB, 2012). If current practices were to continue, therefore, roughly 10,000 additional incidents of research misconduct would occur each year in just one discipline. While these incidents would certainly not all be reported or investigated, even 2,000 to 3,000 additional cases per year is more than an order of magnitude greater than the current combined number of cases now handled by NSF-OIG and ORI per year, which itself reflects substantial recent increases. By expanding the scope of the federal research misconduct definition in this way, implementing the recommendation might require significant additional resources for ORI, NSF-OIG, and perhaps other agencies.

Also, since the federal misconduct policy only applies to federally funded research, as discussed above, a change in interpretation of the research misconduct definition would not address honorary, coercive, or ghost authorship in purely privately funded research except as an exemplar and spur to raise standards across the board. The problem of ghostwriting discussed above, for example, largely concerns research that is funded by companies.

An alternative approach to reducing and ultimately eliminating authorship credit misrepresentation would rely on identifying best practices for researchers, institutions, sponsors, and journals, and encouraging that these stakeholders accelerate adoption of these practices. For example, at the disciplinary level, societies and journals could work to update and specify their authorship standards. Sponsors and journals could more actively discourage ghost and guest authorship. A pathway toward strengthening authorship standards is discussed in Chapter 8. Chapter 9 discusses best practices, and Chapter 10 covers findings and recommendations addressing these issues.

5.3   Exploring New Approaches

National Academy of Sciences

National Academy of Sciences. Exploring new approaches. Washington, DC: National Academies Press; 2017, Chapter 8, Fostering Integrity in Research; p.129–133. Copyright © National Academy of Sciences. All rights reserved.

Reprinted with permission from the National Academy of Sciences, courtesy of the National Academies Press.

STRENGTHENING AUTHORSHIP STANDARDS AND PRACTICES

What additional steps should stakeholders in the research enterprise take to address the challenges discussed in Chapter 7? For example, how should detrimental research practices related to authorship, such as coercive authorship, gift authorship, and unacknowledged ghost authorship, be discouraged and reduced? These practices impair the usefulness and reliability of authorship as the central institution for assigning credit for reported work, fixing responsibility for that work's quality and integrity, and communicating critical information that allows other researchers to replicate, extend, and where necessary correct that work.

The status quo is increasingly problematic. Although some disciplines have developed clear guidelines, authorship practices and conventions are largely left to individual institutions and journals. Greater clarity at the disciplinary level about the roles that merit authorship, the contributions that do not merit authorship, the significance of author order, and the responsibilities of a primary or corresponding author would be very helpful in facilitating appropriate decisions and practices in labs and collaborations. Universal condemnation (i.e., by all disciplines) of gift or honorary authorship, coercive authorship, and ghost authorship would also contribute to changing the culture of research environments where these practices are still accepted. Universal adoption of the requirement that all authorship roles be disclosed, as is the case for a growing number of journals, and commitment to the principle that all contributors who merit authorship should be listed would also be positive steps.

A Framework for Disciplinary and Interdisciplinary Authorship Standards

As discussed above, a number of scientific societies, journals, associations, and research institutions have developed or updated their authorship criteria and guidelines in recent years. Some of these criteria and guidelines explicitly call for an end to such practices as ghost and gift authorship.

We have good examples of authorship guidelines and standards set at the field or disciplinary level or by individual journals. Standards may also describe the responsibilities of authors in areas such as data sharing, as well as the roles and responsibilities of reviewers. For, example, the journal *Neurology* has a very detailed set of authorship guidelines on its "Information for Authors" page (*Neurology*, 2016). The World Association of Medical Editors and the International Committee of Medical Journal Editors also have developed authorship standards. As explained above, these standards have some important differences. The committee favors an approach that authorship should be established through a significant intellectual contribution to the work in at least one area, such as planning, performing, analyzing, or writing. All authors should have the opportunity to approve the final manuscript.

The committee recognizes that flexibility in the development and implementation of authorship guidelines is needed due to the significant differences between disciplines. For example, in many disciplines, research is performed in complex collaborations of large, distributed groups that perform highly specialized tasks. The recent article reporting on the first observation of gravitational waves, which had been hypothesized by Einstein, is a good example of such work (Abbott, et al., 2016). The article has around 1,000 authors. In such efforts, researchers who perform critical tasks in conceptualizing the work or parts of the work may not participate in collecting or analyzing data. Likewise, it is impractical for hundreds or thousands of co-authors to play meaningful roles in writing or editing a journal article. Disciplines need to be able to define for themselves what a significant intellectual contribution is. Also, manuscript approval and specification of author roles may need to be implemented by groups or subgroups of authors through a defined procedure rather than by individuals.

The process of developing and promulgating authorship guidelines may differ by discipline. For example, the Guidelines for Responsible Conduct Regarding Scientific Communication adopted by the Society for Neuroscience (SfN) in 2010 are very detailed and cover a range of issues (SfN, 2010). An SfN working group developed the guidelines, which were approved by the SfN Council. Other fields and disciplines might also develop standards through a leading society, through a coalition of societies and journals, or through another process aimed at ensuring broad buy-in by the community. Standards could also be developed in interdisciplinary areas where there is enough research activity and enough disparity in practices between the collaborating disciplines to warrant such a step. In developing interdisciplinary standards, scientific societies, interdisciplinary journals (e.g., *Science, Nature, PNAS, PLOS*), and sponsors of interdisciplinary research can play important roles.

Research institutions can make an important contribution to stronger authorship standards. A number of institutions already have adopted guidelines that prohibit practices such as guest or honorary authorship, with Harvard Medical School being a good example (Harvard Medical School, 1999).

PREPUBLICATION COPY—UNEDITED PROOFS

The committee believes that the widespread development and dissemination of such standards will make a significant contribution to research integrity, and urges the research enterprise to continue and accelerate progress.

The following framework for developing authorship standards outlines several baseline requirements and might be useful to disciplines that are developing or updating their standards. At the same time, the framework is flexible enough to accommodate the significant differences that exist between disciplines in their authorship practices. The committee recommends that disciplines adopt standards compatible with this framework.

Standards should specify the appropriate roles that merit designation as an author:
- Substantial intellectual contribution to conceiving, designing, or planning the research to be reported;
- Substantial intellectual contribution to acquiring, analyzing, or interpreting the primary data;
- Substantial intellectual contribution to drafting or revising the article reporting the research in question.

Standards should specify the contributions that do not merit authorship but may merit acknowledgment and/or citation:
- Securing funding for the research;
- Providing general supervisory or administrative support for the research;
- Technical writing, editing, and proofreading of the article reporting the research;
- Making available data collected for previously reported work, or providing materials or specimens.

Standards should explicitly identify detrimental authorship practices that are unacceptable:
- Gift or honorary authorship, coercive authorship, and ghost authorship.

Standards should also specify:
- That all authors should approve the final manuscript;
- That one or more authors who are accountable for the entire work should be identified;
- That the roles of each of the listed authors should be specified, including which authors or groups of authors are responsible for which aspects of the reported work;
- The types of work being covered by the standards (e.g., only primary research articles or other types of work as well);
- The process for gaining approval of articles for publication and the principle underlying the approval process (e.g., all listed authors must individually approve a manuscript prior to submission, or an alternative approval mechanism for large collaborations);
- The meaning of "substantial intellectual contributions" to relevant research in that discipline;
- The significance (if any) of author order.

PREPUBLICATION COPY—UNEDITED PROOFS

Alternative Approaches

The committee considered several alternatives to its recommended approach. One possible alternative would be for this committee or another body to develop and implement a more detailed uniform authorship standard across all disciplines. As covered above in the discussion considering whether forms of authorship misrepresentation other than plagiarism should be included in a revised federal research misconduct definition, developing a uniform authorship standard that would be meaningful and at the same time applicable to current conditions in all fields and disciplines would be impractical and probably counterproductive.

Another alternative would be to move away from the concept of authorship entirely toward a new principle for assigning credit and responsibility for reported research. The institution of authorship within research emerged with the first scientific journals in 17th-century Europe. From that time until fairly recently, the predominant mode of research production was for an individual investigator to report on experiments or observations, perhaps assisted by students, in a laboratory or field setting. As discussed in Chapter 3, some research still fits this traditional paradigm, but a growing proportion of scientific activity does not. The past several decades have seen a notable shift toward larger teams, collaborations between groups dispersed throughout the world, and increased specialization. The challenges that the research enterprise faces in the area of authorship are exacerbated by a tension between the conventions of authorship, which assume a unitary authority who can vouch for the entirety of the work, will receive most of the credit for it, and decide who else will be recognized and how, and the way a significant fraction of research activity is actually undertaken today.

Some experts have advocated that the institution of authorship be replaced by a new concept known as *contributorship*. In a contributorship framework, all the contributions to reported work are identified within an agreed taxonomy. An example of work in this area is the Contributor Roles Taxonomy project (Project CRediT), which was launched following a 2010 workshop at Harvard University and aims to "provide transparency to the contributions of researchers to scholarly published work, to enable discoverability and to improve attribution, credit, and accountability" (CASRAI, 2016). Table 8-1 shows an early version of the contributorship taxonomy (Brand, et al., 2015). It specifies a number of roles that are included in traditional definitions of authorship, such as conceptualization and validation, and also lists contributions such as securing funding and general supervision that are not considered appropriate author roles but might be included in acknowledgments today. The taxonomy is now being tested; Cell Press is encouraging authors to describe their contributions in this way.

An additional advantage of contributorship is that it would take advantage of the emerging digital infrastructure that automates recognition and verification systems through mechanisms like unique author (or contributor) identifiers. These systems have the potential to connect researchers with their research products so that datasets and other nonarticle contributions can be more easily utilized, and researchers who make these contributions can receive credit (CASRAI, 2016). Since the contributorship approach is inherently more transparent and less hierarchical than traditional authorship, moving in this direction might ameliorate some of the problems that have been identified in recent years related to misuse of bibliometric indicators such as the Journal Impact Factor (Alberts, 2013).

PREPUBLICATION COPY—UNEDITED PROOFS

EXPLORING NEW APPROACHES   *133*

TABLE 8-1 Project CRediT Terms

Contributor Role	Role Definition
Conceptualization	Ideas; formulation or evolution of overarching research goals and aims.
Methodology	Development or design of methodology; creation of models.
Software	Programming, software development; designing computer programs; implementation of the computer code and supporting algorithms; testing of existing code components.
Validation	Verification, whether as a part of the activity or separate, of the overall replication/reproducibility of results/experiments and other research outputs.
Formal Analysis	Application of statistical, mathematical, computational, or other formal techniques to analyze or synthesize study data.
Investigation	Conducting a research and investigation process, specifically performing the experiments, or data/evidence collection.
Resources	Provision of study materials, reagents, materials, patients, laboratory samples, animals, instrumentation, computing resources, or other analysis tools.
Data Curation	Management activities to annotate (produce metadata), scrub data, and maintain research data (including software code, where it is necessary for interpreting the data itself) for initial use and later reuse.
Writing – Original Draft Preparation	Creation and/or presentation of the published work, specifically writing the initial draft (including substantive translation).
Writing – Review and Editing	Preparation, creation, and/or presentation of the published work by those from the original research group, specifically critical review, commentary, or revision—including pre- or postpublication stages.
Visualization	Preparation, creation, and/or presentation of the published work, specifically visualization/data presentation.
Supervision	Oversight and leadership responsibility for the research activity planning and execution, including mentorship external to the core team.
Project Administration	Management and coordination responsibility for the research activity planning and execution.
Funding Acquisition	Acquisition of the financial support for the project leading to this publication.

Source: Brand et al., 2015.

The committee believes that Project CRediT and other efforts to develop new models to modify or replace authorship are worthwhile and have the potential to make a significant contribution. They can help improve the transparency and accuracy of how credit and accountability for scientific work are assigned and recognized. The committee decided not to recommend that the research enterprise adopt the contributorship concept at this time, due to concern about including traditional author roles and other contributions within a single framework. Some committee members also strongly believe that a credit/responsibility framework for science needs to identify one or more individuals who are accountable for the entire work.

PREPUBLICATION COPY—UNEDITED PROOFS

5.4 A Systematic Review of Research on the Meaning, Ethics and Practices of Authorship across Scholarly Disciplines

Ana Marusic, Lana Bosnjak, and Ana Jeroncic

Marusic, A, Bosnjak, L, Jeroncic, A. A systematic review of research on the meaning, ethics and practices of authorship across scholarly disciplines. *PLoS One* 6(9), e2347 (2011). Copyright: 2011 Marusic et al.

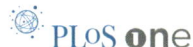

A Systematic Review of Research on the Meaning, Ethics and Practices of Authorship across Scholarly Disciplines

Ana Marušić[1]*, Lana Bošnjak[2], Ana Jerončić[1]

1 Department of Research in Biomedicine and Health, University of Split School of Medicine, Split, Croatia, 2 Office for Science and Department of Research in Biomedicine and Health, University of Split School of Medicine, Split, Croatia

Abstract

Background: The purpose of this systematic review was to evaluate evidence about authorship issues and provide synthesis of research on authorship across all research fields.

Methods: We searched bibliographical databases to identify articles describing empirical quantitive or qualitative research from all scholarly fields on different aspects of authorship. Search was limited to original articles and reviews.

Results: The final sample consisted of 123 articles reporting results from 118 studies. Most studies came for biomedical and health research fields and social sciences. Study design was usually a survey (53%) or descriptive study (27%); only 2 studies used randomized design. We identified four 4 general themes common to all research disciplines: authorship perceptions, definitions and practices, defining order of authors on the byline, ethical and unethical authorship practices, and authorship issues related to student/non-research personnel-supervisor collaboration. For 14 survey studies, a meta-analysis showed a pooled weighted average of 29% (95% CI 24% to 35%) researchers reporting their own or others' experience with misuse of authorship. Authorship misuse was reported more often by researcher outside of the USA and UK: 55% (95% CI 45% to 64%) for 4 studies in France, South Africa, India and Bangladesh vs. 23% (95% CI 18% to 28%) in USA/UK or international journal settings.

Interpretation: High prevalence of authorship problems may have severe impact on the integrity of the research process, just as more serious forms of research misconduct. There is a need for more methodologically rigorous studies to understand the allocation of publication credit across research disciplines.

Citation: Marušić A, Bošnjak L, Jerončić A (2011) A Systematic Review of Research on the Meaning, Ethics and Practices of Authorship across Scholarly Disciplines. PLoS ONE 6(9): e23477. doi:10.1371/journal.pone.0023477

Editor: Tom Jefferson, Cochrane Acute Respiratory Infections Group, Italy

Received June 29, 2011; **Accepted** July 19, 2011; **Published** September 8, 2011

Funding: This study was funded by a research grant from the Committee on Publication Ethics (COPE). The sponsor had no role in the study, including data collection and analysis, manuscript preparation or authorization for publication.

Competing Interests: The authors have declared that no competing interests exist.

* E-mail: ana.marusic@mefst.hr

Introduction

Recently, PubMed – the largest bibliographical database in biomedicine made a new record in the number of authors on the byline of an indexed article: 2080 authors needed 165 lines on the PubMed site to spell out their surnames and initials. The paper was from high energy physics [1] and the number of authors probably did not surprise any physicist. It also probably did not surprise those involved in clinical trials, where the number of authors can also reach thousands [2]. But researchers in many areas of social sciences and humanities may expect to be sole authors, or perhaps discuss the senior authorship between a supervisor and a doctoral student [3].

Regardless of the practices in the number of authors, authorship and publication credit is the currency system of research and academic community, with both positive and negative implications [4]. To improve the practices of responsible authorship, it is important to understand the definition(s) of authorship, its impact on research productivity and roles of different stakeholders in the allocation of publication credit. The purpose of this systematic review was to evaluate evidence about authorship issues and provide a synthesis of research on authorship across research fields.

Methods

Selection Criteria

All articles describing empirical quantitive or qualitative research from all scholarly fields on the definition of or criteria for authorship, authors' contribution to the research and manuscript, order of authors on the byline, opinions of researchers and/or editors on different aspects of authorship were selected for the review. We excluded articles describing research that used journal articles and their authors for analyzing collaborative or citation networks; authorship in the context of citation analysis; analysis of research collaboration outputs of institutions, groups, research fields; trends in authorship in journals, groups of journals, fields, institutions, countries, geographical regions; gender of authors in journals, groups of journals, fields, institutions, countries, geographical regions. Articles describing research on authorship attribution in literature, taxonomy, and psychology/cognitive research were also excluded. Articles that did not provide methodological and/or numerical information (such as found in letters and conference proceedings) were also excluded.

Database Search and Retrieval of Articles

Electronic databases were searched on 17 January 2011 using a general text search term 'authorship' to increase the sensitivity of the search. Where possible, the search was limited to original research articles and reviews. The search included all databases available from the on-line source of the Croatian Academic Network (CARNet): Databases included Agricola (1970 to 2011 Week 3); Business Source Complete (since 1886); CINAHL (since 1981); Current Contents (1993 Week 27 to 2011 Week 3); EBM reviews (2005 to 2011 Week 3), including Cochrane Database of Systematic Reviews, ACP Journal Club, DARE, CCTR, CMR, HTA, and NHSEED; ERIC (1965 to 2011 Week3); GeoRef (since 1966); Food Science and Technology Abstracts (1969 to 2011 Week 3); INSPEC (1969 to 2011 Week 3); Library, Information Science & Technology (since mid-1960ties); MEDLINE (1950 to 2011 Week 3); PsycINFO (1967 to 2011 Week 3); SCOPUS (1960 to 17 Jan 2011); and Web of Knowledge (1991 to 17 Jan 2011), including Science Citation Index Expanded (SCI-EXPANDED), Social Sciences Citation Index (SSCI) and Arts & Humanities Citation Index (A&HCI). There were no language restrictions. There was no attempt to search grey literature because our study was focused on authorship research in the mainstream science. Hand search of relevant journals was not performed because authorship topics are published in a variety of journals and because we used a sensitive rather than specific search; only the theme issues of JAMA, related to peer review conferences were searched by hand.

The titles and available abstracts of retrieved records were examined for possible inclusion in the review. Selected full text articles were used as a starting point for the berrypicking search, a technique which included footnote, citation and author searching [5], as well as searching of 'Related citations' feature in MEDLINE, where appropriate. Our own work and knowledge of the literature, as well as other experts in the field, were also used to find possible articles for inclusion.

Titles and abstracts of all retrieved articles were screened by one author to determine if they met inclusion criteria, and the selection was verified by the other author. Disagreements were discussed and full text articles were retrieved in cases of doubt for review and decision on inclusion. Full texts of the articles were reviewed by both authors; disagreements were resolved by discussion. A description of the population and extractable data were the minimum for the inclusion in the systematic review.

Analysis and presentation of findings

We used a data collection form (Table S1) to extract study type, intervention, setting, participant demographics, and outcome measures. Study quality was assessed on the basis of study design, sample size and sampling frame, response rate, and outcome measures. Disagreements in the assessment and data extraction were resolved by discussion and consensus. As most of the included studies were observational studies with heterogeneous measurements, we could not perform a statistical pooling of the results. Instead, we performed a qualitative synthesis of the results, providing a narrative description of the results. We also identified themes arising from the study results and assigned the studies to these defined categories.

For the percentage (proportion) of respondents who recalled their own problems or problems of colleagues with authorship issues (n = 14 studies), we were able to perform quantitative data synthesis. The data were transformed with Freeman-Tukey variant

of the arcsine square root [6]. Pooled effect size was calculated as the back-transform of weighted mean of the transformed proportions, using DerSimonian-Laird weights for random effects model [6]. Homogeneity was tested with Cochran's Q test based upon inverse variance weights [7]. Differences between groups of studies were tested with Mann-Whitney U test using inverse variance weighted averages. Publication bias was assessed with funnel plot Harbord bias indicator [6]. The statistical analyses were run on an SPSS software package 17 for Windows (SPSS Inc., Chicago, IL, USA), using the 'MeanES', 'MetaF' and 'MetaReg' macros by David B. Wilson [7].

Results

8988 references were retrieved from the bibliographic database search (FIGURE 1). After excluding 7703 overlapping records, 1285 abstracts were screened for eligibility. After excluding 1109 records, 176 full text articles were assessed for the inclusion in systematic review. Out of these, 61 articles were excluded on the basis of full-text assessment because they did not present research results (n = 32), did not address authorship as defined in the inclusion criteria (n = 22) or had no extractable data (n = 7). The berrypicking search of full articles yielded 8 articles, and no additional relevant articles were identified by experts in the field. Thus the total number of included articles with original data was 123 [8–130], presenting 118 studies (list of articles in Table S2). All articles were published in English except 1 in Spanish, 1 in Portuguese and 1 in Dutch.

Most of the articles were published in health sciences (n = 66), including 52 studies from general medicine and/or biomedicine (1 study was presented in 2 articles [38,52]), 6 from nursing, and 7 from more than one research field. There were 33 articles from social sciences, including 12 studies from psychology, 12 from economics/business/marketing, 3 from social work, 2 from education research, 1 from information research and 3 from more than one research field. Out of 9 articles from natural sciences, 3 were from physics (results from 1 study presented in 2 articles [79,101]), 3 from chemistry (1 study presented in 3 articles [119,126,127]) and 1 each in agriculture and ecology. There were 15 articles covering more than one scientific area, where 2 articles presented results from 1 study [8,9]. No studies on authorship in humanities could be identified.

Most of the studies were performed in international science journals (n = 47) or in the USA (46 studies reported in 49 articles). Five studies were performed in Canada, 4 in Australia, 2 in South Africa, 2 in the Netherlands and 1 (2 articles) in the international physics laboratory in Europe (CERN). A study was performed in each of the following countries: Bangladesh, Brazil, Croatia, France, India, Iran, Pakistan, Spain, Sweden and UK. Finally, 1 study had respondents from both the US and Canada, and for 1 study it was not clear whether it was performed in the UK, US or both countries.

The design of most studies was cross-sectional survey (63 studies published in 65 articles), with response rates ranging from 16% to 100%. There were 32 descriptive studies (published in 34 articles), mainly literature analysis. One involved mathematical modeling [43], 1 was a test-retest study [94] and 1 combined a survey and intervention design [93]. Five studies were qualitative (1 published in 2 articles) [34,79,101,104,116,128] and 2 randomized [86,102]; there were 3 before-and-after studies [90,106,121] and 1 cohort study [92].

Many studies (n = 85) had methodological limitations. Out of 65 studies involving survey designs, 27 did not report details on survey development or testing. All before-and-after studies had no

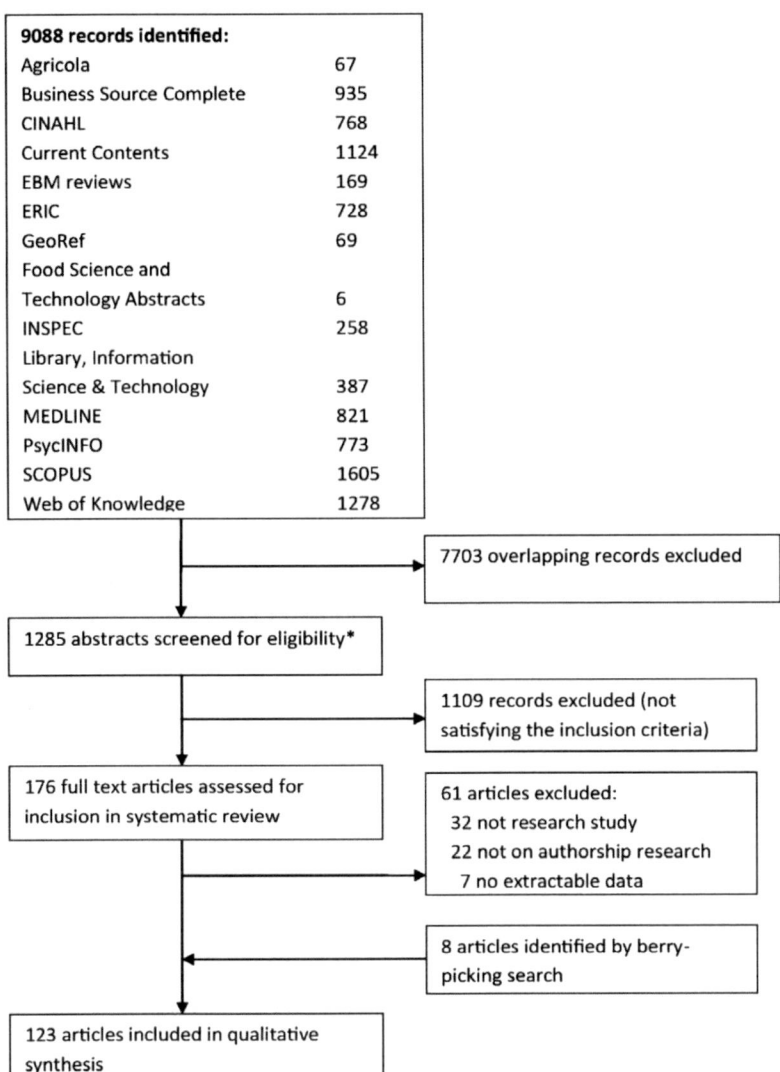

Figure 1. Selection of the articles for the systematic review. Search keyword was 'authorship', limited to article as a publication type, search performed 15 January 2010. Asterisk : inclusion criteria – quantitive or qualitative research on the definition of or criteria for authorship, authors' contribution to the research and manuscript, order of authors on the byline, opinions of researchers and/or editors on authorship criteria, opinions of researchers and/or editors on authorship order; exclusion criteria: 1. research topics which use journal articles and their authors as a starting point for studying: collaborative or citation networks; authorship in the context of citation analysis; analysis of research collaboration outputs of institutions, groups, research fields; trends in authorship in journals, groups of journals, fields, institutions, countries, geographical regions; gender of authors in journals, groups of journals, fields, institutions, countries, geographical regions; 2. analysis of authorship attribution in literature, taxonomy, and psychology/cognitive research.
doi:10.1371/journal.pone.0023477.g001

controls. Out of 6 articles on qualitative studies, 5 did not report on the protocol and details of the sample or data analysis procedure or independent confirmation of identified themes and their analysis. Randomized studies involved questionnaires and were single blinded; 1 described piloting of the questionnaire. Quality assessment of the articles (Table S2) revealed that most studies had clearly stated objectives, but the description of the sample and sampling procedures sometimes lacked detail. Study findings were stated with varying levels of detail and in some reports it was difficult to discern the findings of qualitative and quantitive analyses.

The first identified study addressed the differences in name ordering of Nobel laureates from different disciplines in comparison to their colleagues in 1967 [8,9], followed in 1970 by a study on name ordering in physiology journal [10] and a seminal survey of publication credit assignment practices in psychology [11]. In the 80ties, there were only 7 studies across all disciplines, whereas the 90ties witnessed the increasing trend in authorship research, particularly in health sciences (FIGURE 2).

We identified 4 general themes studied across research disciplines: authorship perceptions, definitions and practices (n = 58 articles), defining order of authors on the byline (n = 45), ethical and unethical

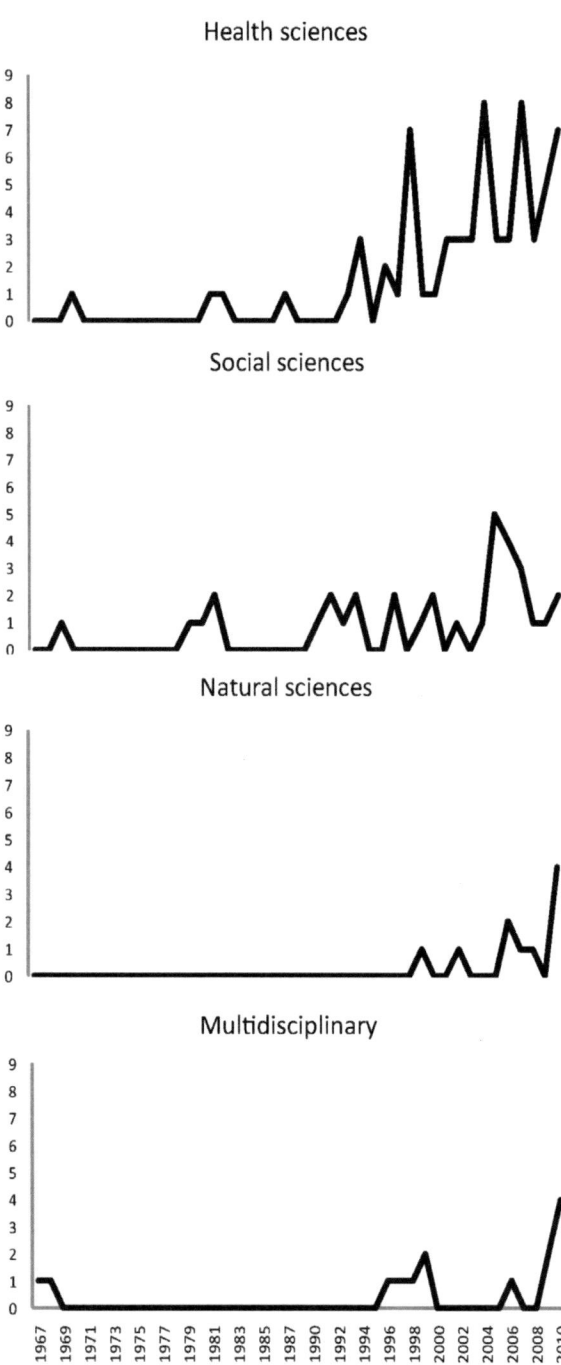

Figure 2. Trends in publications on authorship research in different research areas since 1967, when the first research report was identified [8]. No studies were identified in humanities.
doi:10.1371/journal.pone.0023477.g002

authorship practices (n = 46), and authorship issues related to student/non-research personnel-supervisor collaboration (n = 19). Most of the articles explored one of these themes (n = 90), 21 explored 2, 11 explored 3 and 1 article addressed all 4 themes.

Authorship definitions, perceptions and practices

Fifty-four studies examined the perceptions of authorship buy different stakeholders, authorship definitions in use and actual practices, and contributions for deserving authorship (TABLE 1 and TABLE S3): 31 studies from the health research field [13,16,23,25,26,31,35,36,39,41,47,50,52,54,57,60,65,66,77,80,82-,94,100,102–104,106,110–112,121];12 studies from social sciences [11,12,14,18,24,27,33,34,48,49,55,91], 6 studies from more than one research field [29,45,90,116,122,128] and 5 studies from natural sciences, published in 6 articles [46,58,79,101,119,126].

Conception of research/research design and writing the manuscript were identified as most qualifying contributions for authorship across different sciences, geographical regions and the time span from 1970ties to present [12,16,18,23,24,26,27,35,47–50,66,82,110]. Deserving authorship was not restricted or granted to researchers but to other member of the research team who made important contribution [13,14,16,36,41,55,126]. Recently, collective or community authorship has emerged in different disciplines involved in research with Indigenous communities [116]. In health research, the position of medical writers and statisticians/methodologists has been explored in more detail. Most professional medical writers would expect authorship when they contributed to the collection and/or analysis of data and contribute to the manuscript writing [103] but authorship as acknowledgment for medical writing assistance was reported by 16% or authors [52]. Methodologists were recognized as authors in 65% to 88% articles in general medical journals [54], and editorial teams of Cochrane review groups for systematic review/meta-analyses made important contributions to published articles [57].

Five surveys asked for a single contribution that would qualify for authorship: the most frequent choice for psychologists was choice of statistical method and data analysis (55%) [11], manuscript drafting for nursing professionals (53%) [13], design of the study for postdoctoral fellows from different disciplines (92%) [29], providing statistical advice on an ongoing basis for researchers at a medical school (92%) [31] and data interpretation or doing 20–50% of the work for business/non-business faculty (90%) [33]. In the latter study, more business than non-business faculty would grant authorship for only final preparation and submission of a manuscript (44% vs. 21%).

Several studies explored if stakeholders in research provided authorship guidance. A 1999 study of the professional organizations in the USA showed that up to 56%of them had non-specific statements but that only 17% had clear criteria for authorship [45]. A recent study from Australia demonstrated that, even when there are national authorship policies, the universities do not fully comply with them [122]. Biomedical journals, which generally declare to follow the authorship criteria of the International Committee of Medical Journal Editors (ICMJE) [131], often do not explicitly state these criteria in their guidelines for authors or have outdated versions [60,100,111,112]. It is thus not surprising that just over 60% of authors in health research journals satisfy authorship criteria [24,39,41] and that many authors and editors are not familiar with such criteria or think they are not realistic or fair [31,39,41,65,66,77]. Similar lack of knowledge or use of guidelines was demonstrated for postdoctoral fellows or active researchers in physics in the USA [46,58] and faculty and students in psychology [48]. A study of postdoctoral fellows at the National Institutes of Health in the USA in 2007 showed that training in responsible conduct of research did not significantly change the awareness and use of authorship guidelines [90]. For faculty in departments of chemistry in the USA, the factors that explained the variance in influences on authorship decisions was graduate

Table 1. Definitions of authorship, contributions for deserved authorship and authorship practices*.

Article	Study population	Study topic
Spiegel, 1970 [11]	Psychologists in USA	Single contribution that qualifies for authorship; Preferred solution to multiple authorship
Bridgewater,[a] 1981 [12]	Academic psychologists in USA	Agreement of respondents on qualifying contributions for authorship
Werley,[a] 1981 [13]	Nursing professionals in USA	Single contribution that qualifies for authorship; Preferred solution to multiple authorship
von Glinow, 1982 [14]	Professionals associated with management journals in USA	Opinion of editors vs. editorial review board on collection of data as deserving authorship contribution
Waltz,[a] 1985 [16]	Health professionals in nursing in USA	Contributions that do not deserve authorship
van der Kloot, 1991 [18]	Social psychologists and psychometricians in The Netherlands	Scores on a continuum scale of deserving authorship for different contributions
Diguisto, 1994 [23]	University research staff in Australia	Value of contributions for deserving authorship
Floyd, 1994 [24]	Authors of articles published in management journals	Importance of contributions for authorship
Goodman, 1994 [25]	First authors or research articles in general medical journal	Prevalence of authors who satisfied ICMJE authorship criteria
Shapiro, 1994 [26]	First authors from USA of research articles in general medical journal	Most frequent contributions by all authors as reported by first author
Wagner, 1994 [27]	Single, first or second author in a psychology journal	Contribution importance for authorship
Eastwood, 1996 [29]	Postdoctoral fellows at a university	Sufficient contribution for authorship
Bhopal, 1997 [31]	Staff from university medical school in UK	Reported agreement with ICMJE authorship criteria; Contributions that alone merit authorship
Hamilton, 1997 [33]	Business and non-business university faculty in USA	Deserving joint authorship for a single contribution
Netting, 1997 [34]	University faculty and student in focus groups in USA	Emerging themes in authorship
Almeida, 1998 [35]	Mental health professionals (physicians and non-physicians) in Brazil	Opinions of physicians vs. non-physicians on contributions valid for granting authorship
Butler, 1998 [36]	Nurses expected to publish research in Canada	Agreement among nurses of different professional status on different authorship scenarios
Hoen, 1998 [39]	Authors of articles published in national general medical journal in The Netherlands	Awareness and fulfilment of ICMJE criteria
White, 1998 [41]	First authors of papers on nursing research from USA	Knowledge of authorship guidelines; Reported contributions to different aspects of manuscript; Prevalence of articles with all authors qualifying for authorship
Rose, 1999 [45]	Ethics statements from scientific professional organizations in USA	Prevalence of statements on authorship in ethics codes
Tarnow, 1999 [46]	Postdoctoral fellows in physics in USA	Knowledge of association authorship guidelines; Discussion of authorship criteria with supervisor; Criteria for designating postdocs or others as authors
Yank, 1999 [47]	Articles in general medical journal	Contributions declared for authors and persons in acknowledgment lists
Bartle, 2000 [48]	Faculty and students from psychology departments in USA	Most important contributions for authorship; Opinion of students vs. faculty on APA ethical guidelines
Hart, 2000 [49]	Co-authors of papers in library science	Importance of research tasks for authorship
Price, 2000 [50]	Faculty from institutions granting graduate degrees in nursing in USA	Criteria most important for authorship; Opinion on number of criteria needed for authorship; Role of journals in authorship issues
Phillips,[b] 2001 [52]	Authors of articles in large and small medical journals	Acknowledgement of medical writing assistance as authorship
Altman, 2002 [54]	Authors of articles in general medical journals	Recognition of a methodologist as an author
Laband, 2002 [55]	Authors in economic and agricultural economics journals	Fraction of production team given authorship rights in economics vs. agricultural economics
Mowatt, 2002 [57]	Corresponding authors of Cochrane systematic reviews	Contributions of authors vs. Cochrane editorial team
Tarnow, 2002 [58]	Members of American Physical Society (APS)	Use of APS authorship guidelines; Preference of authorship guidelines
Foote, 2003 [60]	Biomedical journals	No. journals without definition of authorship in guidelines
Cohen, 2004 [65]	Members of US and Canadian Academy of Pathology (USCAP)	Use of authorship guidelines; Expressed preference of authorship guideline
Etemadi, 2004 [66]	Editors of medical journals in Iran	Opinions on criteria for authorship
Pignatelli, 2005 [77]	Senior clinical researchers in France	Practices in authorship; Agreement with ICMJE criteria
Birnholtz, 2006 [79]	Researchers in high energy physics	Themes in authorship in high energy physics
Burbonniere, 2006 [80]	Researchers at a clinical centre in Canada	Satisfaction with use of in-house authorship guideline
Dhaliwal, 2006 [82]	Faculty in teaching hospital in India	Acceptable criteria for authorship

Table 1. Cont.

Article	Study population	Study topic
Funk, 2007 [90]	NIH postdoctoral fellows in USA	Awareness and use of authorship guidelines after RCR training
Geelhoed, 2007 [91]	Authors of research articles in clinical psychology journals	Most common opinions on authorship decision process
Ilakovac, 2007 [94]	Authors of research articles in general medical journal	Reliability of contribution declaration form for corresponding author
Wager, 2007 [100]	Guidelines for authors in medical journals	Presence of authorship guidance; Reference to ICMJE authorship criteria
Birnholtz,[c] 2008 [101]	Researchers in high energy physics	Emerging themes in authorship
Ivaniš, 2008 [102]	Authors of research articles in general medical journal	Prevalence of authors satisfying ICMJE criteria when declaring contributions in a binary vs. ordinal rating scale
Lang, 2008 [103]	Experienced medical writers from USA	Opinion on deserved authorship for medical writers
Louis, 2008 [104]	High profile researchers in biomedicine in USA	Identified guiding factors for authorship decisions
Baerloccher, 2009 [106]	Original research articles in general medical journals	Number of authors after introduction of contribution disclosure requirement
Pulido, 2009 [110]	Spanish authors in health who publish in international journals	Most important contributions for any author vs. first author; Knowledge of ICMJE criteria
Rowan-Legg, 2009 [111]	Guidelines published in biomedical journals	Prevalence of journals with authorship addressed in guidelines
Samad, 2009 [112]	Pakistani medical and dental journals	Prevalence of journals with no guidance on authorship
Castleden, 2010 [116]	Researchers involved in research with Indigenous communities in Canada	Collective/community authorship as emerging practice
House,[d] 2010 [119]	Faculty from departments of chemistry in USA	Factors explaining deserved authorship; Factors explain and influences on authorship
McDonald, 2010 [121]	Articles from medical journals	Influence of authorship restriction policies on number of authors, 1986 to 2006
Morris, 2010 [122]	All (n = 39) Australian universities	No. universities with authorship policy and policy rating
Seeman,[d] 2010 [126]	Faculty from departments of chemistry in USA	Situational differences in authorship decisions
Street, 2010 [128]	Staff and doctoral candidates in health research at Australian universities	Emerging themes in authorship

*Abbreviations: ICMJE, International Committee of Medical Journal Editors; APA, American Psychological Association; NIH, National Institutes of Health, USA; RCR, responsible conduct of research.
[a]Partial or full replication or modification of questionnaire by Spiegel and Keith Spiegel, 1970 [11].
[b]Sub-analysis of data from Flanagin et al [38].
[c]The same study as Birnholtz, 2006 [79].
[d]House and Seeman [119] and Seeman and House [126] present results from the same study.
doi:10.1371/journal.pone.0023477.t001

school education (31%), institutional or other sources (19%) and personal values (14%) [119]. Experience from a medical setting in Canada indicated that researchers may be satisfied with guidelines developed in-house [80], whereas a study of authors from clinical psychology journals demonstrated that the satisfaction with both the process and outcomes of authorship decisions significantly increases with the use of guidelines [91]. Authors from clinical psychology journals identified the first authors as the most common deciders on co-authorship, and indicated factors other than effort and contributions which affected authorship decisions: taking project leadership, loyalty or obligation, power issues, and publish or perish pressures, with tenured faculty giving significantly less value to these factors, being more satisfied with the process and perceiving themselves to have more power relative to others [91]. One study described the influence of a specific subfield, number of publications, county of PhD degree, and previous experiences with authorship in providing credit research contributions on the academic chemistry environment in the USA [126].

Although psychologists used to declare their contributions in published articles already in the 1970ties [11], contribution declaration was implemented by many medical journals only 20 years later [132]. This policy did not show any effect on the number of authors [106,121] and a test-retest study demonstrated that the reliability of contribution declaration forms used in

journals is too low to warrant their use in making conclusions on authorship [94]. A randomized study in a medical journals demonstrated that using ordinal rating scale instead of binary 'yes-no' declaration of contributions significantly increased the number of authors satisfying the ICMJE authorship criteria [102].

Four studies, published in 5 articles, qualitatively explored authorship issues [34,79,101,104,128]. Although most of them had methodological limitations, they identified emerging themes on authorship in social sciences, high energy physics, biomedicine, and multidisciplinary teams in health research. All studies identified common social factors in authorship decisions, best summarized in the study of Louis et al from 2008 [104], which identified fairness, reciprocity and sponsorship as main guiding factors in making authorship decision by high-profile researchers in biomedicine. For high energy physics, where collaborations increase to thousand co-authors [1], the individual still remains the unit of the research effort but larger collaborations increases the range of contributions and includes both infrastructure and discovery efforts [79,101]. In such situation, it is particularly difficult for a young researcher to balance the practice of attributing credit to a large group with their individual need for recognition and promotion, so they have to develop pragmatic strategies for professional survival.

Table 2. Order of authors on the byline*.

Article	Study population	Study topic
Zuckerman, 1967 [8]	Nobel laureates in USA and matched scientists	1st authorship of laureates vs. others
Zuckerman,[a] 1968 [9]	Nobel laureates in USA and matched scientists	Ratio observed/expected frequency of papers with 6 or more authors and name order pattern for laureates vs. others
Over, 1970 [10]	Articles published in *J Physiol* 1961–1964	Percent authors with A–E vs. P–Z surnames in a journal with alphabetical author listing
Spiegel, 1970 [11]	Psychologists in USA	Preferred method for authorship order when contributions are equal
Werley,[b] 1981 [13]	Nursing professionals in USA	Preferred method for authorship order when contributions are equal
von Glinow, 1982 [14]	Professionals associated with management journals in USA	Preferred method for ordering authors
Over, 1982 [15]	Articles in psychology journals	Change in number of articles with alphabetical ordering of authors from 1949 to 1979
Waltz,[b] 1985 [16]	Health professionals in nursing in USA	Preferred method for authorship order when contributions are equal
Gay,[b] 1987 [17]	Educators in nursing USA	Methods for determining authorship
McCarl, 1993 [21]	Citations in 5 journals on agricultural economics	Chance of having a citation when first-author has a Z or A surname
Shulkin, 1993 [22]	Articles by chairs of department of medicine in USA	Last-authorship papers of short-term vs. long-term chairs
Shapiro, 1994 [26]	First authors from USA of research articles in general medical journal	No. and type of contributions of first vs. last author
Wagner, 1994 [27]	Single, first or second author in a psychology journal	Mean percent contributions for different authorship positions
Davies, 1996 [28]	Chairs of pediatric departments and deans of medical faculties in Canada	Opinions on value of first author contribution in individual or group authorship
Slone, 1996 [30]	First authors from USA on papers from a radiology journal	Reported contributions of first authors vs. 5th–10th author
Butler, 1998 [36]	Nurses in Canada, expected to publish research	Agreement among nurses that order of authorship should be based on contributions, not status
Drenth, 1998 [37]	Authors of articles in general medical journal 1975–1995	Prevalence of senior level authors as last authors in 1975 vs. 1995
White, 1998 [41]	First authors from USA on papers on nursing research	Knowledge of agency or institution guidelines for authorship sequencing
Engers, 1999 [43]	Articles from journals on law, economics, social sciences, natural sciences or medicine	Prevalence of alphabetical ordering of authors
Yank, 1999 [47]	Articles in general medical journal	Contributions for different authorship byline position
Hart, 2000 [49]	Co-authors of papers in library science	Most prevalent method of ordering authors
Chambers, 2001 [51]	Articles in general medical journal	Most common letters for surnames of first authorship
Laband, 2002 [55]	Authors of articles in economic and agricultural economics journals	Prevalence of alphabetized co-authorship
Mowatt, 2002 [57]	Corresponding authors of Cochrane systematic reviews	Reported practices in deciding on authors' order
Tarnow, 2002 [58]	Members of American Physical Society (APS)	Probability of change after initial authorship list is determined
Bhandari, 2003 [59]	Editorial board members of medical journal in USA	Agreement on method for authorship order
Bhandari, 2004 [63]	Chairs of surgery or medicine departments in Canada	Change in assignment of authorship credit to first or last author when they are corresponding authors
Cohen, 2004 [65]	Members of US and Canadian Academy of Pathology (USCAP)	Probability of change after initial authorship list is determined
Meyer, 2004 [68]	Editorial members of accounting journals and young accounting faculty members in USA	Perceived behaviour appropriateness and occurrence and actual knowledge of occurrence of co-authorship issues
Apgar, 2005 [72]	Members of Society for Social Work and Research in USA	Opinions on authorship order
Hilmer, 2005 [74]	Faculty members of agricultural economics departments in USA and their publications	Prevalence of alphabetical authorship in co-authored vs. multi-authored articles; Estimated annual salary return to an additional article depending on alphabetical authorship
Pignatelli, 2005 [77]	Senior clinical researchers in France	Practice of ordering authorship
Brown, 2006 [81]	Multiauthored articles from academic institutions published n marketing journals	Percent alphabetical ordering of authors
Einaw, 2006 [83]	Faculty of economic or psychology departments, Econometric Society (ES) fellows, Nobel laureates and Clark Winners, authors of articles in economics journals in USA	Increase in probability for tenure status with each letter closer to the front of the alphabet; Percent multiauthored articles with alphabetical authorship in economics journals
Laband, 2006 [84]	Articles in journals from medicine, natural sciences, economics, social sciences and general journals	Mean change in prevalence of alphabetical authorship in co-authored articles from 1974 to 1999
Manton, 2006 [85]	Business faculty in USA	Opinion on method of listing authors
Moore, 2006 [87]	Authors of articles in educational research journals	Preferred method of authorship order

Table 2. Cont.

Article	Study population	Study topic
Baerlocher, 2007 [89]	Articles in general medical journals	Satisfaction of ICMJE criteria 1 and 2, depending on byline position
Kurichi, 2007 [95]	Chairs of surgery departments in USA medical schools	Likelihood for authorship position in regard to serving as chair
Manton, 2007 [96]	Faculty of colleges of business in USA	Preferred method of listing co-authors
van Praag, 2008 [105]	Articles published in mainstream economics journals	Prevalence of articles with alphabetical authorship
Hu, 2009 [107]	Articles in biomedical or multidisciplinary journals	Increase in prevalence of equal first authorships
Maciejeovsky, 2009 [108]	Faculty members and advanced graduate students from economics, marketing and psychology in USA/UK	Prevalence of alphabetical authorship; Preferences for credit to a position in multiauthored papers; Inferences based on authorship order
Akhabue, 2010 [115]	Original research articles from general medical journal	Trends in equal authorships from 2000 to 2009
Chan, 2010 [117]	Multi-authored original research articles from academic real estate journals	Prevalence of alphabetical authorship from 1990 to 2006; Likelihood for alphabetical authorship
Frandsen, 2010 [118]	Articles from economics, library information science (LIS) and high-energy physics (HEP) journals	Yearly change in share of articles with alphabetic authorship from 1978 to 2007
Walker, 2010 [129]	Corresponding authors of original research articles in medical journals	Opinion on authorship position with greatest merit for promotion; Practice of ordering authorship position

*Abbreviations: ICMJE, International Committee of Medical Journal Editors.
aThe same study as Zuckerman, 1967 [8].
bPartial or full replication or modification of questionnaire by Spiegel and Keith Spiegel, 1970 [11].
doi:10.1371/journal.pone.0023477.t002

Authorship order

The order of authors on the byline was specifically addressed by 46 studies (TABLE 2 and TABLE S4): 22 studies from the health research field [10,13,16,17,22,26,28,30,36,37,41,47,51,57,59,63,65,77,89,95,115,129], 18 studies from social sciences [11,14,15,21,27,49,55,60,72,74,81,83,85,87,96,105,108,117], 5 studies from more than one research field [8,9,43,84,118] and 1 study from natural sciences [58].

For researchers in most sciences, the amount of work and not prestige or position were the preferred method for determining authorship order [10,11,13,15–17,36,49,51,57,59,72,77,85,87,96,108]. Notable exceptions were the fields of management research [14] and most areas of economy [21,43,55,74,81,83,84,105,108,117,118], where alphabetical ordering of authors has been the norm for a long time. Economists calculated that with each letter closer to the front of the alphabet there was an increase in the probability to be tenured at top economy departments and receive professional recognition [83], as well as a significant increase of 0.41% in estimated salary return for an additional article with alphabetical authorship [74] and a 3.3% chance that 1% lower ranked alphabet letter would increase total and annual publication output in mainstream economics journals [105]. In real estate journals, likelihood for alphabetical authorship was greater in higher quality articles or higher academic ranking of authors or with authors from Europe [117]. Greater academic ranking or prestige, such as Nobel prize, was associated with more generosity in giving prominent place to collaborators or accepting alphabetical authorship [8,9,83]. Nobel laureates had more first authorship at 20 years of age but less when they were 40, compared to scientists matched in discipline, age, type of affiliation, and initial letter of the surname [8]. Alphabetical authorship seems to be a constant feature of economics journals and perhaps and emerging one for social sciences journals, with a mean increase in prevalence of 9.9% and 18.6%, respectively, from 1974 to 1999, compared to a sharp decrease of 47.8% in general journals such as *Science* and *Nature*, 82% in medical journals, and 39.1% in natural science journals in the same period [84]. A recent study analyzing changes from 1978 to 2007 confirmed that alphabetical authorship was stable in economics and common for authors in high energy physics, but decreasing for articles in library information research [118].

Several studies explored the importance of the author's position on the byline, particularly in the field of biomedical research. Most prestige and greatest contribution was expected from the first author [26,28,30,47,59,63,89,129], whereas seniority brought prestige with the last author position [22,26,37,47,59,63,95]. In medicine and multidisciplinary journals, there is a recent trend of equal authorship of the first 2 or more authors [107,115].

Most of the researchers psychology, nursing and social work favored pre-study agreement as the best policy for ordering names on the byline [11,13,16,72]. In medicine, this was reported as a common practice [129]. Only 5% of first authors from the USA on nursing research papers reported that they were aware of any agency or institution guidelines for authorship sequencing [41]. In physics, the probability of change after initial authorship list was determined was 4% for decrease and 12% for increase [58], similar to pathology researchers in medicine (3% and 18%, respectively) [65].

Ethics of authorship

Ethical and unethical practices in authorship and perceptions about them were analyzed in 51 studies (TABLE 3 TABLE S5): 34 studies from the health research field [13,16,17,30,31,36,38,41,42,50,53,56,57,61,62,64,65,67,69,70,73,75,77,82,86,92,93,97,99,109,114,120,123,125], 10 studies from social sciences [11,14,18,33,68,71,76,85,91,96], 3 studies from natural sciences [46,58,127] and 4 studies from more than one research field [29,90,107,113].

In 4 studies that used variations of the same survey questionnaire [11], researchers in psychology and nursing showed agreement in their opinion on ethical authorship decisions: not giving authorship to a colleague who failed to keep agreement on study work and multiple publications from the same study, provided that there is indication that they are part of the same study [11,13,16,17]. Across disciplines, adding undeserving authors or excluding deserving authors was considered unethical

Table 3. Ethical and unethical authorship practices*.

Article	Study population	Study topic
Spiegel, 1970 [11]	Psychologists in USA	Ethical practices in granting authorship
Werley,[a] 1981 [13]	Nursing professionals in USA	Ethical practices in granting authorship
von Glinow, 1982 [14]	Professionals associated with management journals in USA	Ethical practices in granting authorship
Waltz,a 1985 [16]	Health professionals in nursing in USA	Ethical practices in granting authorship
Gay,[a] 1987 [17]	Health professionals in nursing in USA	Ethical practices in granting authorship and publishing multiple publications from the same study
van der Kloot, 1991 [18]	Social psychologists and psychometricians in The Netherlands	Agreement about authorship between professors and junior researchers
Eastwood, 1996 [29]	Postdoctoral fellows at a university in USA	Willingness to engage in giving undeserved authorship
Slone, 1996 [30]	First authors from USA on papers from a radiology journal	Reported undeserved authorship for co-authors; Reasons for undeserved authorship; Time of decision on authorship
Bhopal, 1997 [31]	Staff from university medical school in UK	Reported problems with authorship; Gift authorship
Hamilton, 1997 [33]	Business and non-business university faculty in USA	Views on unethical authorship practices
Bulter, 1998 [36]	Nurses expected to publish research in Canada	Agreement among nurses about ethical issues in authorship
Flanagin, 1998 [38]	Corresponding authors from USA on articles in large and small medical journals	Reported prevalence of research articles with undeserved or undisclosed or ghost authorship
White, 1998 [41]	First authors from USA on papers on nursing research	Reported issues, problems and concerns about author inclusion or ordering
Wilcox, 1998 [42]	Cases brought to university ombuds office in USA	Authorship issues in cases 1991/92 vs. 1996/97
Tarnow, 1999 [46]	Postdoctoral fellows in physics in USA	Reported papers where supervisor did not satisfy APS guidelines; Reasons for inappropriate authorship
Price, 2000 [50]	Faculty from institutions granting graduate degrees in nursing in USA	Experiences and opinions on unethical authorship practices
Reidpath, 2001 [53]	Authors of articles published in general medical journal	Reported authorship was among stipulations for sharing data-set from their article
Mainous, 2002 [56]	Corresponding authors of research articles in medical journals	Personal or professional concerns in authorship; Opinion on effective ways for authorship decisions
Mowatt, 2002 [57]	Corresponding authors of Cochrane systematic reviews	Prevalence of honorary authors or ghost and honorary authors
Tarnow, 2002 [58]	Members of American Physical Society (APS)	Probability that an additional author is inappropriate; Comfort for younger vs. older respondent to deny undeserving authorship
Hwang, 2003 [61]	Research articles in medical journal	Prevalence of undeserved ICMJE authorship
Bates, 2004 [62]	Research articles in medical journals with different contribution declaration forms	Prevalence of undeserved ICMJE authorship
Buchkowsky, 2004 [64]	Clinical trials published in medical journals	Increase in author affiliation with industry from 1981/1984 to 1997/2000
Cohen, 2004 [65]	Members of US and Canadian Academy of Pathology (USCAP)	Probability that an additional author is inappropriate; Reported denying undeserved authorship
Marušić, 2004 [67]	Research articles in general medical journal	Prevalence of undeserved ICMJE authorship
Meyer, 2004 [68]	Editorial members of accounting journals and young accounting faculty members in USA	Perceived behaviour appropriateness/behaviour occurrence/actual knowledge of occurrence of co-authorship issues
Procyshyn, 2004 [69]	Research articles on antipsychotic drugs in medical journals	Prevalence of authors affiliated with 3 pharmaceutical firms
Szirony, 2004 [70]	Nursing faculty members in USA	Formal teaching to graduate students about authorship credit in publications; Ethical decisions in authorship
Apgar, 2005 [71]	Members of Society for Social Work and Research in USA	Unethical granting of authorship
Freda, 2005 [73]	Editors of nursing journals	Reported prevalence of ethical issues about authorship encountered in editorial work
Joubert, 2005 [75]	Authors of research papers from university in South Africa	Reported prevalence of ethical issues in authorship
Mixon Jr, 2005 [76]	Articles published in more and less prestigious economics journals	Ratio between number of authors and contributors in acknowledgment
Pignatelli, 2005 [77]	Senior clinical researchers in France	Opinions and reported experience on gift and ghost authorship

Table 3. Cont.

Article	Study population	Study topic
Dhaliwal, 2006 [82]	Faculty in teaching hospital in India	Reported conflict over authorship
Manton, 2006 [85]	Business faculty in USA	Reported experience of unethical granting of authorship
Marušić, 2006 [86]	Authors of articles in general medical journal	Prevalence of authors not satisfying ICMJE criteria in different forms of contribution declaration
Funk, 2007 [90]	NIH postdoctoral fellows in USA	Ethically appropriate responses to case vignettes at 3 time points after training on RCR
Geelhoed, 2007 [91]	Authors of articles in clinical psychology journals	Experiences about fairness and ease of authorship decision process
Gotsche, 2007 [92]	Clinical trial protocols and publications from Sweden	Prevalence of ghost authorship
Hren, 2007 [93]	Medical students with or without instruction on ICMJE criteria, physicians and medical faculty in Croatia	Opinions on eligible contributions for authorship
Manton, 2007 [96]	Faculty of colleges of business in USA	Reported that co-authors did very little/no work
Peppercorn, 2007 [97]	Articles on breast cancer clinical trials in medical journals	Prevalence of pharmaceutical company authorship on published studies
Tungaraza, 2007 [99]	Published clinical trials on psychiatric drug treatment	Prevalence of industry-authored studies
O'Brien, 2009 [109]	Corresponding authors of original research articles in general medical journals	Reported experience or opinion unethical authorship
Wager, 2009 [113]	Editors of journals published by Blackwell	Reported experience of ethical issues in authorship
Ahmed, 2010 [114]	Participants in bioethics course in Bangladesh	Experiences of authorship conflicts
Lacasse, 2010 [120]	Public policies of academic medical centres in USA	Prevalence of policies banning ghostwriting
Nastasee, 2010 [123]	Articles in medical journals	Increase in acknowledgment of medical writing from 2000 to 2007
Rose, 2010 [125]	Clinical trials published in oncology journal	Odds for authors reporting financial ties to industry:
Seeman,[b] 2010 [127]	Faculty from departments of chemistry in USA	Experience of unethical behaviour in authorship

*bbreviations: NIH, National Institutes of Health, USA; RCR, responsible conduct of research.
[a]Partial or full replication or modification of questionnaire by Spiegel and Keith Spiegel, 1970 [11].
[b]The same study as House and Seeman [119] and Seeman and House [126].
doi:10.1371/journal.pone.0023477.t003

[14,33,36,50,68,70,71,77,90,109], but was reported to be a practice by 10% to 89% of the respondents [18,31,41, 46,50,58,65,68,75,82,85,91,96,109,114,127]. Prestige was an important factor in deciding on authorship, as articles from more prestigious economics journals had more authors and fewer contributors in the acknowledgement then those from less prestigious journals [76]. The reasons for agreeing on inappropriate authorship were similar across disciplines and included the feeling of obligation, crediting past and future relationships, team responsibility, power relations [45,56,68]. In two studies that assessed the opinions of physicists and pathologists about ICMJE authorship criteria and authorship guidelines of the American Physical Society (APS), the probability that an additional author would not satisfy APS or ICMJE criteria was 23% vs. 67% for physicists [58], and 45% vs. 65% for pathologists [65].

Journal editors also reported experiences with authorship disputes, from 5% in nursing journals [73] to 30% in journals from a major publisher [113]. Despite the reported prevalence of authorship problems, editors did not consider them to be severe and were confident in their management of the problems [68,113]. Authorship disputes were reported as an increasing problem for institutions [42], but ethics training at institutions may not have effect on the willingness to engage in giving undeserved authorship [29]. In biomedicine, authors often asked for authorship as a stipulation for sharing data-sets [53].

In medicine, the number of authors who did not satisfy widely accepted ICMJE authorship criteria ranged from less than 1% to 63% [38,57,61,62,67,86]. The variation may be due to the difference in counting the third ICMJE criterion ('Approval of the article before publication') as satisfied by default [38,57,61,62] or checking if authors really declared on this criterion [67,86]. The prevalence of undeserving authors also depended on the form of contribution declaration in medical journals: it was 21.5% in the journal with a list of contributions to choose from, 9.5% in the journal that provided for open-ended answers, and only 0.5% in the journal that instructed which and how many contributions are needed for each of the 3 ICMJE authorship criteria [62]. The results of this observations study were confirmed in a randomized study with three different declaration forms in a single general medical journal [86]. Undeserved authorship was considered to have potential adverse effects both for the undeserving author and the co-authors, as well as for patient care [109].

Industry relationship and ghost authorship were other important issues for medical journal. Increasing author affiliations with industry were reported in several studies [64,97,99], as well as increased odds for authors reporting financial ties to industry [125]. The prevalence of ghost authorship was reported in the range from 2% to 75% [38,50,57,92,113]. The highest prevalence was found in clinical trial protocols that were later published [92]. Editors considered that there was an increasing trend of ghost authorship, but did not perceive it as a severe problem in their work [113]. Although a recent study demonstrated increasing acknowledgments of medical writing [123], only 20% of academic medical centers in the USA had policies that explicitly banned ghostwriting [120].

Only a few studies looked at the possible interventions to prevent undeserved authorship. The measures proposed by

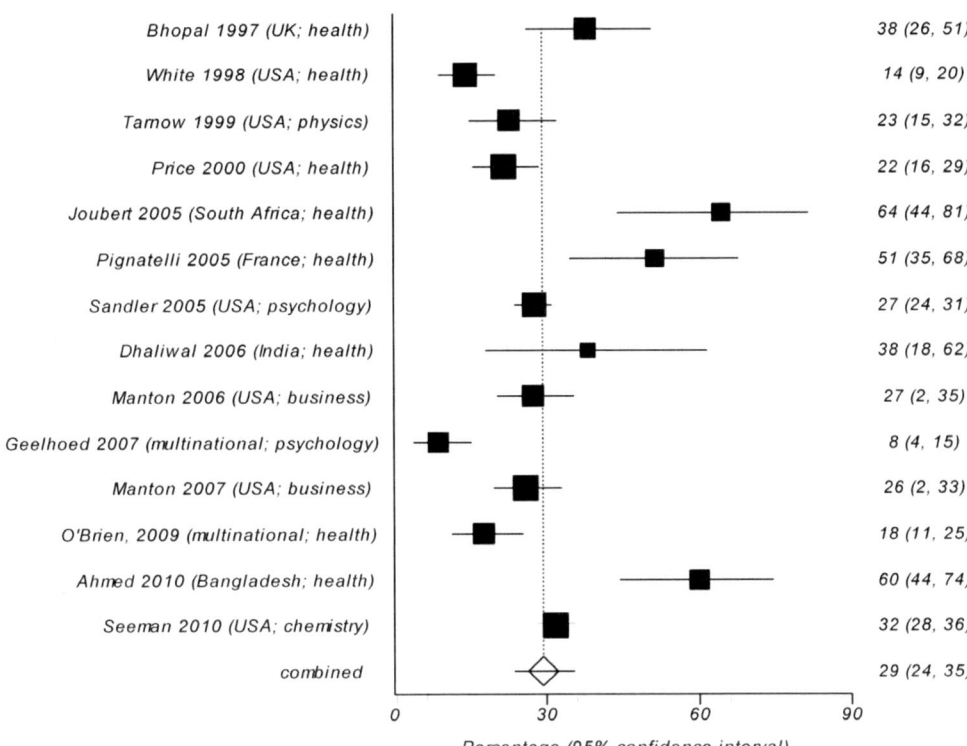

Figure 3. Forest plot of reported rates of problems with or misuse of authorship in self- or non-self reports in 14 survey studies [31,41,46,50,75,77,78,82,85,91,96,109,114,126]. The area of a square represent sample size, horizontal lines are 95% confidence interval, diamond and vertical dotted line show the pooled weighted estimate.
doi:10.1371/journal.pone.0023477.g003

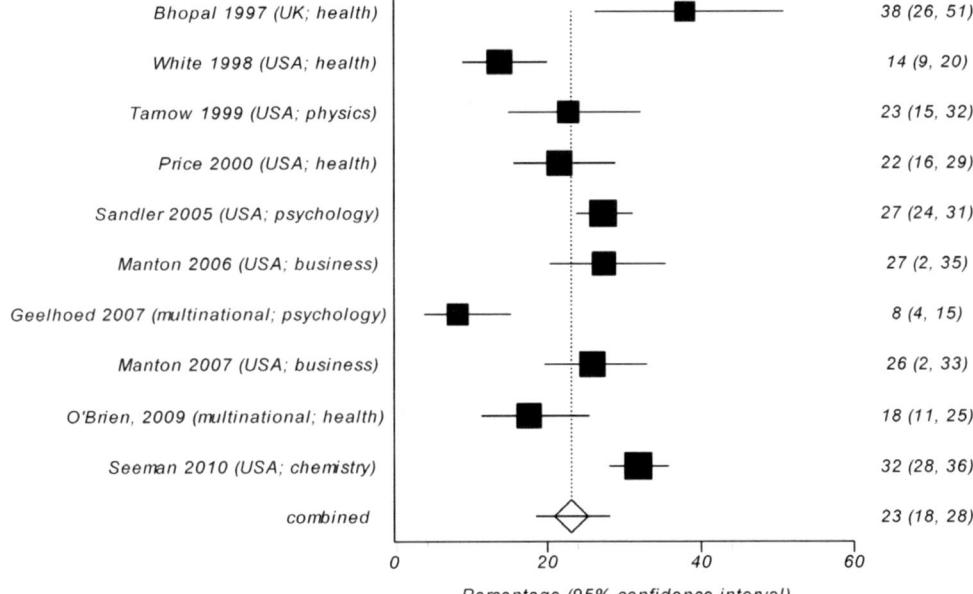

Figure 4. Forest plot of reported rates of problems with or misuse of authorship in self- or non-self reports in 12 survey studies from USA, UK or international journals [31,41,46,50,78,85,109,126]. The area of a square represent sample size, horizontal lines are 95% confidence interval, diamond and vertical dotted line show the pooled weighted estimate.
doi:10.1371/journal.pone.0023477.g004

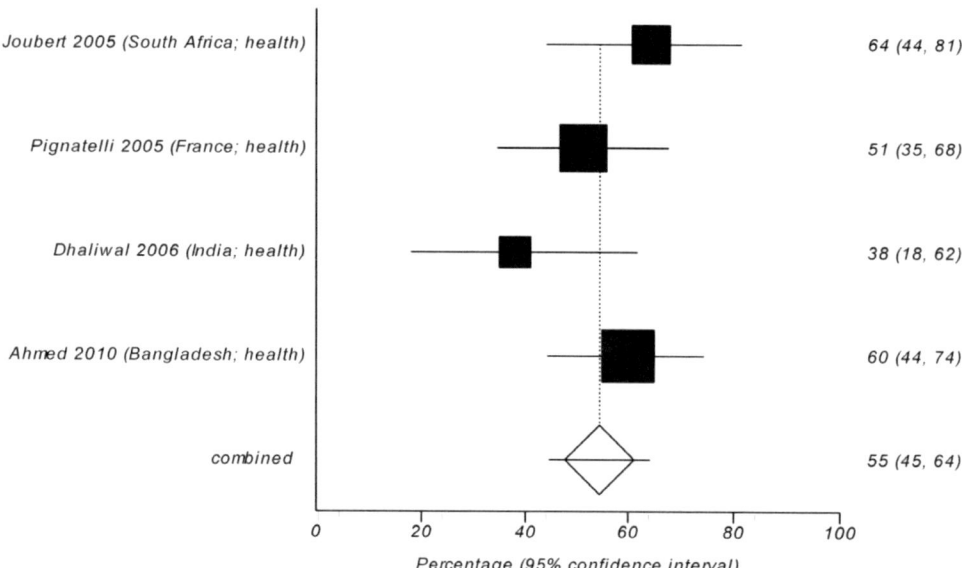

Figure 5. Forest plot of reported rates of problems with or misuse of authorship in self- or non-self reports in 4 survey studies from South Africa, France, India, or Bangladesh [75,77,82,114]. The area of a square represent sample size, horizontal lines are 95% confidence interval, diamond and vertical dotted line show the pooled weighted estimate.
doi:10.1371/journal.pone.0023477.g005

researchers in medicine were publishing the statements on authors' contributions or limiting the number of authors on a byline [31,56]. When authors made decision about authorship during planning rather than later stages, the prevalence of undeserving authors was smaller, 23% vs. 47% [30]. Although only 44% nursing faculty members in the USA reported formal teaching to graduate students about authorship credit [70], instruction on authorship criteria may increase awareness of ethical decisions about authorship. In a study that looked at how medical students rated different contributions which were both eligible or not eligible for ICMJE authorship criteria, students without any instruction rated critical revision of the manuscript and final approval significantly lower than students with such instruction [93]. In the cluster analysis of ratings by medical students with or without instruction on ICMJE criteria, physicians, and medical faculty, conception/design, analysis/interpretation, and manuscript drafting clustered together, with final approval clustering only for students with instruction [93].

Fourteen survey studies asked the participants if they personally experienced problems and/or misuse of authorship or observed it for other colleagues [31,41,46,50,75,77,78,82,85,91,96,109, 114,126]. Between 1.5% and 71% of respondents replied affirmatively (crude unweighted mean = 31%, 95% CI = 21% to 41%). Meta-analysis yielded a pooled weighted estimate of 29% (95% CI 24% to 35%), with significant heterogeneity (Cochran's $Q = 11.26$, df = 13, $P < 0.0001$) (FIGURE 3). The indicators of publication bias were not significant (Harbord bias = 1.54 (92.5% CI −1.83 to 4.91), $P = 0.391$). There was no difference in reported prevalence between studies from health and non-health research fields (W = 36; Z = −1.16; $P = 0.245$; inverse variance weighted Mann-Whitney U-test). However, the comparison between the groups of studies with different locations (USA/UK/international journals vs. non-USA/UK) demonstrated that non-USA/UK studies had significantly higher proportion of reported problems with authorship (W = 55; Z = −2.83; P = 0.002; inverse variance

weighted Mann-Whitney U-test). Pooled weighted estimate for USA/UK/international studies was 23% (95% CI 18% to 28%) (FIGURE 4), compared with 55% (95% CI 45% to 64%) for non-USA/UK studies (FIGURE 5), with significant heterogeneity in the USA/UK/international sample (Cochran's $Q = 61.23$, df = 9, $P < 0.0001$), which persisted even after stratifying studies by location. Non-USA/UK studies were homogeneous (Cochran's $Q = 3.98$, df = 3, P = 0.264). The indicators of publication bias were not significant for both study groups (Harbord bias = −3.26 (92.5% CI −7.22 to 0.69), $P = 0.130$, for USA/UK/international group and −3.78 (92.5% CI −18.25 to 10.69), $P = 0.463$, for non-USA/UK group).

Power issues in authorship

The practices and perceptions about authorship decisions in supervisor/professor – student/non-research persons was assessed in 19 studies (TABLE 4 and TABLE S6): 11 studies from social sciences [11,19,20,44,48,68,71,78,91,98,130], 4 studies from the health research field [13,16,17,70], 2 studies from more than one research field [32,40] and 2 studies from natural sciences [88,124].

Fairness of the research collaboration between professor-supervisor and a student was an important issue in psychology. Surveys since 1970 showed that psychologists generally regard students as sufficiently expert to warrant the 1st authorship on their master or doctoral theses, even when faculty makes significant contribution to the work and manuscript writing [11,19,44,48,98]. They also generally regarded that any collaborator, regardless of their position or payment for the work, deserved authorship if they made substantial contribution to most aspects of research and writing [11]. Similar perceptions were reported in nursing [13,16,17,70],multidisciplinary areas [32,40], accounting research [68], social work [71], ecology [88], agriculture, and education research [130].

Using critical incident technique, psychologists identified "taking other's ideas or manuscripts", "failure to give credit"

Table 4. Authorship in researcher – student/non-researcher collaborations*.

Article	Study population	Study topic
Spiegel, 1970 [11]	Psychologists in USA	Opinion on deserved authorship for students/non-researchers; Preferred outcome for student-professor collaboration
Werley,[a] 1981 [13]	Nursing professionals in USA	Opinion on deserved authorship for students/non-researchers; Preferred outcome for student-professor collaboration
Waltz,[a] 1985 [16]	Health professionals in nursing in USA	Opinion on deserved authorship for students/non-researchers
Gay,a 1987 [17]	Educators in nursing in USA	Opinion on deserved authorship for students/non-researchers
Costa, 1992 [19]	Psychology students and faculty in USA	Faculty vs. students views of authorship order for published dissertation with different level of faculty input
Goodyear, 1992 [20]	Editorial board members and authors of psychology journals in USA	Reported critical incidents related to student research
Brown-Wright, 1997 [32]	Graduate assistants and faculty members in USA	Assistance in analysis of research data warrants authorship for graduate assistant – faculty vs. Assistants
Rose, 1988 [40]	Graduate students in physics, biological, engineering and social sciences in USA	Opinion on deserved authorship for students; Perceived reporting of authorship problems
Louw, 1999 [44]	Academic and non-academic psychologists and masters' degree students in South Africa	Deserving first authorship by academics, non-academics and students
Bartle, 2000 [48]	Faculty and students from psychology departments in USA	Agreement of faculty vs. students on authorship from student-faculty collaboration
Meyer, 2004 [68]	Editorial members of accounting journals and young accounting faculty members in USA	Perceived behaviour appropriateness/behaviour occurrence/actual knowledge of occurrence of co-authorship issues between faculty and students
Szirony, 2004 [70]	Nursing faculty members in USA	Opinions on unethical authorship in student-professor collaboration
Apgar, 2005 [71]	Members of Society for Social Work and Research in USA	Opinions on unethical authorship in student-professor collaboration
Sandler, 2005 [78]	APA members and students with a publication from student-faculty collaboration in USA	Involvement in and reporting of perceived unethical or unfair authorship assignment
Weltzin, 2006 [88]	Participants of ecology meeting in USA	Opinion on first authorship in student-professor collaboration
Geelhoed, 2007 [91]	Authors of articles in clinical psychology journals	Opinion of students vs. faculty on influences on authorship decision making
Tryon, 2007 [98]	Doctoral students in school psychology in USA	Different opinions on first authorship in publications from dissertations
Picard, 2010 [124]	Students and supervisors from agriculture school in Australia	Agreement on authorship issues between students and professors
Welfare, 2010 [130]	Students and faculty from US universities with graduate studies in education	Opinion of students vs. faculty for common and recommended practices in authorship

*Abbreviations: APA, American Psychological Association.
[a]Partial or full replication or modification of questionnaire by Spiegel and Keith Spiegel, 1970 [11].
doi:10.1371/journal.pone.0023477.t004

and "giving unwarranted credit" as most important problems in faculty-student collaboration [20]. Doctoral students in psychology considered it more desirable and ethical for a student to develop the dissertation idea and also though that it was desirable and ethical for the student rather than advisor to be first authors [98]. Although authorship problems occurred [40,68,78], students were not likely to, or considered it effective to talk to the dean, file a complaint or contact a journal [40]. The reported reasons for no action were fear of negative consequences, events instigated by respondent, or incident not reaching the level of importance [78]. More psychology students than faculty thought that power differences influenced authorship and saw themselves as having less power than other authors [91]. For students in education research, all recommended authorship practices in offered scenarios was greater than perceived practice [130]. Also, students put a significantly higher authorship value to the research tasks usually given to students, such as collection of qualitative data, entering data into statistical program or analyzing them, writing literature review for the introduction section or writing methods section, and the total time spent on a project.

Discussion

To the best of our knowledge, this is the first systematic review of research on authorship across all scholarly disciplines. Our search did not identify any systematic review in individual disciplines, although there were a number of overviews and theoretical discussions, including the recent series of the authorship history, current practices, and educational activities in social sciences, engineering and biomedical and life sciences [133–137]. The review of 118 studies reported in 123 articles revealed the absence of experimental research on authorship but also outlined our current knowledge about authorship across research disciplines. The available evidence demonstrated the diversity of authorship perceptions but also universal themes: there was a common perception that the conception of research/research design and writing the manuscript were the most important qualifying contributions for authorship – across disciplines, geographical regions and time. Also, respondents from most disciplines would grant authorship not only to the researchers but also to all members of the research team who had made an important contribution. Authorship order emerged as an important but formally undefined issue across disciplines, with clear difference between the minority enforcing alphabetical authorship, such as economy research, and the majority allocating the position on the byline according to the type and quantity of contribution. Power issues in authorship, especially in regard to the relationship between the supervisor/professor and students or non-research members of the team were particularly important in social sciences. Taking other's ideas or manuscripts, failure to give credit and giving unwarranted credit were identified as most important problems in faculty-student collaboration but were rarely reported.

Ethical issues in authorship were common to all disciplines. For the subset of 14 studies that reported results of surveys asking researchers about their own or others' experience of problems with or misuse of authorship, we were able to perform a meta-analysis, the first such analysis for authorship. On average, 29% of the respondents acknowledged such experience. This prevalence of ethical problems in authorship is more than 10-fold greater than the 2% prevalence of research misconduct of fabrication, falsification or data modification, reported in the recent meta-analysis [7]. While authorship misuse is not considered misconduct but a 'questionable research practice' by many official research integrity bodies, including the Office of Research Integrity (ORI) in the USA [138], the prevalence estimated in our meta-analysis indicates that authorship problems may have a greater impact on research than 'classical' misconduct activities of fabrication, falsification and plagiarism. Furthermore, it can be argued that omitting or adding authors on an article represents falsification or fabrication which directly damages the integrity of the research process, particularly because authorship credit is the foundation of career advancement, esteem in scientific community and funding for research [133]. Although authorship as a research topic is dominant in biomedicine and health [132], we did not find differences in reported problems with authorship between studies from health and other areas. However there was a clear difference between 23% authorship misuse prevalence reported in surveys conducted in the USA or UK settings or international journals with dominant US/UK authorship [91,109] and 55% in settings outside of USA and UK, from France to South Africa and Bangladesh and India. The reasons why authorship problems are more prevalent in some countries and not in others is not clear. While the USA has two formal bodies to oversee and direct research integrity activities [139,140], UK does not have a formal body [141], so official structures for preventing misconduct could not be an explanation for the observed difference. France, as most of the countries in Europe except for Scandinavian countries [142], does not have such national bodies, and we could find no evidence for similar national bodies in South Africa, Bangladesh and India. A possible explanation for the high prevalence of authorship misuse in these countries may rather be their position in the mainstream science, either because of the smallness of their scientific communities or language barriers [143].

The results of our systematic survey and meta-analysis are limited primarily by the poor methodological quality of retrieved studies and their heterogeneity. Of the 118 studies, 95 (81%) were either surveys or descriptive studies. Many studies did not report on the construction and pre-testing of surveys of their sampling frames and often with unclear or incomplete reporting of study findings; examples include the lack of interval range for Likert scales and reporting of only means without measures of variability. There were only 8 studies that evaluated some kind of intervention in authorship [86,90,93,94,102,106,121] but all had methodological limitations, so the conclusions on the effects sizes of any

intervention to promote responsible authorship practices were not possible. The two single-blinded randomized studies [86,102] and a test-retest study [94] of authorship declarations demonstrated that currently used forms for declaring authorship contributions as defined by the ICMJE criteria [131], most widely accepted in biomedical and health fields [4,132,136], were not reliable instruments to make conclusions on authorship. They also indicated that were several cognitive problems involved in reporting authorship contributions either for oneself or for others. This may in part explain the findings from several studies that researchers often were not familiar with ICMJE criteria or thought that they were not realistic or fair [34,39,41,65,66,77]. These findings were also confirmed by qualitative studies, which identified issues in authorship that could not be addressed by normative instructions provided by formal authorship definitions and policies [34,79,101,104,116,128].

We deliberately performed a systematic review with a wide scope, sensitive but not specific search, inclusive of all study designs and focused on mainstream publications in international bibliographical indexes because we wanted to provide the synthesis of existing evidence in all research fields and to identify gaps in knowledge. Despite the limitations of the review and retrieved evidence, the results provide an outline of common themes for future research across disciplines. To study authorship definitions, perceptions and practice, there appears to be little scope for conducting more small descriptive surveys or descriptive studies with heterogeneous methodology. To understand how authorship credit is awarded, we may benefit from methodologically rigorous qualitative studies, as well as studies to identify sociological factors associated with authorship and its use and misuse. All these studies would be more powerful if they were conducted across multiple sites and disciplines. This would be particularly relevant to address the observed differences in prevalence of authorship misuse among different geographical settings in the meta-analysis. Testing different sample characteristics in larger, multi-site studies with standardized methodology may reveal important correlates of misconduct in authorship.

As the evidence shows that decisions on authorship are often not made according to the official criteria, there is a need for research into the role of moral vs. normative judgments on authorship [144]. Our recent analysis of authorship statements and definitions in scholarly journals and ethics codes of professional organizations showed that the tone of authorship statements in journals was mostly aspirational, formulating suggestions for best or desired practices, while the statements in ethics codes predominantly used a normative language, conveying minimal standards for practice in authorship [145]. Further research into these differences may provide better tools to promote the moral autonomy of individual researchers and an environment where ethical behaviour in authorship is the norm.

The nature of authorship decisions is also relevant for educational interventions to promote integrity in authorship, which is a rather neglected area both in education and in research [133]. For example, if authorship issues are exclusively a matter of convention, then educational interventions should aim at informing students about authorship criteria and providing opportunities for applying them in practice. If, on the other hand, authorship is, at least partially, a moral issue, then educational interventions targeting moral judgment would be more appropriate [146,147].

Research avenues outlined here are not possible without collaboration among different stakeholders and across geographical regions and research disciplines. Given the social responsibility of science and its collective impact on human lives, regardless of the discipline, professional development for responsible authorship and other aspects of research should be subjected to the same valid and rigorous forms of evaluation and testing expected for health interventions, such as medicines and medical devices.

Supporting Information

Table S1   Data extraction form.
(DOC)

Table S2   Overview of included studies.
(DOC)

Table S3   Results of studies addressing the definition of authorship, contributions for deserved authorship and authorship practices.
(DOC)

Table S4   Results of studies addressing the order of authors on the byline.
(DOC)

Table S5   Results of studies addressing ethical authorship practices.
(DOC)

Table S6   Results of studies addressing authorship in researcher – student/non-researcher collaborations.
(DOC)

Acknowledgments

The authors thank Dario Sambunjak, MD, PhD, for his critical comments during the review of articles. This study was presented in part at the Committee on Publication Ethics (COPE) Seminar in London, 18 March 2011.

Author Contributions

Conceived and designed the experiments: AM. Performed the experiments: AM LB AJ. Analyzed the data: AM LB AJ. Contributed reagents/materials/analysis tools: AM LB AJ. Wrote the paper: AM. Critical revision of the manuscript: LB AJ.

References

1. Khachatryan V, Sirunyan AM, Tumasyan A, Adam W, Bergauer T, et al. (2010) First Measurement of Bose-Einstein Correlations in Proton-Proton Collisions at root s = 0.9 and 2.36 TeV at the LHC. Physical Review Letters 105: 032001.
2. King C (2007) Multiauthor paper redux: a new peak at new peaks. Science Watch Nov–Dec. Available at http://scientific.thomsonreuters.com/m/pdfs/klnl/848096/swmultiauthor.pdf. Accessed: 1 August 2011.
3. Fine M (2003) Reflections on the intersection of power and competition in reflecting teams as applied to academic settings. J Marital Fam Ther 29: 339–351.
4. Claxton LD (2005) Scientific authorship. Part 2. History, recurring issues, practices, and guidelines. Mutat Res 589: 31–45.
5. Bates MJ (1989) The design of browsing and berry-picking techniques for the online search interface. Online Review 13: 407–412.
6. Field AP, Gillett R (2010) How to do a meta-analysis. Br J Math Stat Psychol 63: 665–694.
7. Fanelli D (2009) How many scientists fabricate and falsify research? A systematic review and meta-analysis of survey data. PLoS ONE 4: e5738.
8. Zuckerman H (1967) Nobel laureates in science: patterns of productivity, collaboration, and authorship. American Sociological Review 32: 391–403.
9. Zuckerman HA (1968) Patterns of name ordering among authors of scientific papers - study of social symbolism and its ambiguity. American Journal of Sociology 74: 276–291.
10. Cleverdon CW, Davies D, Over R, Smallman S (1970) Citation idiosyncrasies. Nature 228: 1356–1357.
11. Spiegel D, Keith-Spiegel P (1970) Assignment of publication credits - ethics and practices of psychologists. American Psychologist 25: 738–747.
12. Bridgwater CA, Bornstein PH, Walkenbach J (1981) Ethical issues and the assignment of publication credit. American Psychologist 36: 524–525.
13. Werley HH, Murphy PA, Gosch SM, Gottesmann H, Newcomb BJ (1981) Research publication credit assignment - nurses' views. Research in Nursing & Health 4: 261–279.
14. Von Glinow MA, Novelli L (1982) Ethical standards within organizational behavior. Academy of Management Journal 25: 417–436.
15. Over R (1982) Collaborative research and publication in psychology. American Psychologist 37: 996–1001.
16. Waltz CF, Nelson B, Chambers SB (1985) Assigning publication credits. Nursing Outlook 33: 233–238.
17. Gay JT, Lavender MG, McCard N (1987) Nurse educator views of assignment of authorship credits. Image - the Journal of Nursing Scholarship 19: 134–137.
18. Van der Kloot W, Willemsen T (1991) Authorship and the order of authorship: Academic psychologists' assessments of the usefulness of contributions to a research project. [in Dutch]. Nederlands Tijdschrift voor de Psychologie en haar Grensgebieden 46: 368–378.
19. Costa MM, Gatz M (1992) Determination of authorship credit in published dissertations. Psychological Science 3: 354–357.
20. Goodyear R, Crego C, Johnston M (1992) Ethical issues in the supervision of student research: A study of critical incidents. Professional Psychology: Research and Practice 23: 203–210.
21. McCarl B (1993) Citations and individuals: first authorship across the alphabet. Review of Agricultural Economics 15: 307–312.
22. Shulkin DJ, Goin JE, Rennie D (1993) Patterns of authorship among chairmen of departments of medicine. Academic Medicine 68: 688–692.
23. Digiusto E (1994) Equity in authorship - a strategy for assigning credit when publishing. Social Science & Medicine 38: 55–58.
24. Floyd SW, Schroeder DM, Finn DM (1994) Only if I'm 1st author - conflict over credit in management scholarship. Academy of Management Journal 37: 734–747.
25. Goodman NW (1994) Survey of fulfilment of criteria for authorship in published medical research. BMJ 309: 1482.
26. Shapiro DW, Wenger NS, Shapiro MF (1994) The contributions of authors to multiauthored biomedical research papers. JAMA 271: 438–442.
27. Wagner MK, Dodds A, Bundy MB (1994) Psychology of the Scientist. 67. Assignment of authorship credit in psychological research. Psychological Reports 74: 179–187.
28. Davies HD, Langley JM, Speert DP (1996) Rating authors' contributions to collaborative research: the PICNIC survey of university departments of pediatrics. Pediatric Investigators' Collaborative Network on Infections in Canada. CMAJ 155: 877–882.
29. Eastwood S, Derish P, Leash E, Ordway S (1996) Ethical issues in biomedical research: Perceptions and practices of postdoctoral research fellows responding to a survey. Science and Engineering Ethics 2: 89–114.
30. Slone RM (1996) Coauthors' contributions to major papers published in the AJR: Frequency of undeserved coauthorship. American Journal of Roentgenology 167: 571–579.
31. Bhopal R, Rankin J, McColl E, Thomas L, Kaner E, et al. (1997) The vexed question of authorship: Views of researchers in a British medical faculty. BMJ 314: 1009–1012.
32. Brown-Wright DA, Dubick RA, Newman I (1997) Graduate assistant expectation and faculty perception: Implications for mentoring and training. Journal of College Student Development 38: 410–416.
33. Hamilton JI, Greco A (1997) Ethical questions regarding joint authorship: business and nonbusiness faculty perceptions on noncontributing authorship. Journal of Education for Business 72: 325–330.
34. Netting FE, Nichols-Casebolt A (1997) Authorship and collaboration: Preparing the next generation of social work scholars. Journal of Social Work Education 33: 555–564.
35. Almeida O (1998) Authorship of scientific articles: What do such authors actually do? [in Portuguese]. Revista ABP-APAL 20: 113–116.
36. Butler L, Ginn D (1998) Canadian nurses' views on assignment of publication credit for scholarly and scientific work. Canadian Journal of Nursing Research 30: 171–183.
37. Drenth JPH (1998) Multiple authorship - The contribution of senior authors. JAMA 280: 219–221.
38. Flanagin A, Carey LA, Fontanarosa PB, Phillips SG, Pace BP, et al. (1998) Prevalence of articles with honorary authors and ghost authors in peer-reviewed medical journals. JAMA 280: 222–224.
39. Hoen WP, Walvoort HC, Overbeke AJPM (1998) What are the factors determining authorship and the order of the authors' names? - A study among authors of the Nederlands Tijdschrift voor Geneeskunde (Dutch Journal of Medicine). JAMA 280: 217–218.
40. Rose M, Fischer K (1998) Do authorship policies impact students' judgments of perceived wrongdoing. Ethics & Behavior 8: 59–79.
41. White AH, Coudret NA, Goodwin CS (1998) From authorship to contributorship. Promoting integrity in research publication. Nurse Educator 23: 26–32.
42. Wilcox LJ (1998) Authorship - The coin of the realm, the source of complaints. JAMA 280: 216–217.
43. Engers M, Gans JS, Grant S, King SP (1999) First-author conditions. Journal of Political Economy 107: 859–883.

44. Louw DA, Fouche JB (1999) Authorship credit in supervisor-student collaboration: assessing the dilemma in psychology. South African Journal of Psychology 29: 145–148.
45. Rose M (1999) What professionals expect: scientific professional organizations' statements regarding authorship. Science Editing & Information Management. pp 15–22.
46. Tarnow E (1999) The authorship list in science: Junior physicists' perceptions of who appears and why. Science and Engineering Ethics 5: 73–88.
47. Yank V, Rennie D (1999) Disclosure of researcher contributions: A study of original research articles in The Lancet. Annals of Internal Medicine 130: 661–670.
48. Bartle SA, Fink AA, Hayes BC (2000) Psychology of the scientist: LXXX. Attitudes regarding authorship issues in psychological publications. Psychological Reports 86: 771–788.
49. Hart RL (2000) Co-authorship in the academic library literature: A survey of attitudes and behaviors. Journal of Academic Librarianship 26: 339–345.
50. Price JH, Dake JA, Oden L (2000) Authorship of health education articles: Guests, ghosts, and trends. American Journal of Health Behavior 24: 290–299.
51. Chambers R, Boath E, Chambers S (2001) The A to Z of authorship: analysis of influence of initial letter of surname on order of authorship. BMJ 323: 1460–1461.
52. Phillips S, Carey L, Biedermann G (2001) Attitudes toward writing and writing assistance in peer reviewed articles. AMWA Journal: American Medical Writers Association Journal 16: 10–16.
53. Reidpath DD, Allotey PA (2001) Data sharing in medical research: An empirical investigation. Bioethics 15: 125–134.
54. Altman DG, Goodman SN, Schroter S (2002) How statistical expertise is used in medical research. JAMA 287: 2817–2820.
55. Laband DN (2002) Contribution, attribution and the allocation of intellectual property rights: economics versus agricultural economics. Labour Economics 9: 125–131.
56. Mainous AG, 3rd, Bowman MA, Zoller JS (2002) The importance of interpersonal relationship factors in decisions regarding authorship. Family Medicine 34: 462–467.
57. Mowatt G, Shirran L, Grimshaw JJM, Rennie D, Flanagin A, et al. (2002) Prevalence of honorary and ghost authorship in Cochrane reviews. JAMA 287: 2769–2771.
58. Tarnow E (2002) Coauthorship in physics. Science and Engineering Ethics 8: 175–190.
59. Bhandari M, Einhorn TA, Swiontkowski MF, Heckman JD (2003) Who did what? (Mis)perceptions about authors' contributions to scientific articles based on order of authorship. Journal of Bone and Joint Surgery -American Volume 85A: 1605–1609.
60. Foote M (2003) Review of current authorship guidelines and the controversy regarding publication of clinical trial data. Biotechnology Annual Review 9: 303–313.
61. Hwang SS, Song HH, Baik JH, Jung SL, Park SH, et al. (2003) Researcher contributions and fulfilment of ICMJE authorship criteria: Analysis of author contribution lists in research articles with multiple authors published in Radiology. Radiology 226: 16–23.
62. Bates T, Anić A, Marušić M, Marušić A (2004) Authorship criteria and disclosure of contributions - Comparison of 3 general medical journals with different author contribution forms. JAMA 292: 86–88.
63. Bhandari M, Busse JW, Kulkarni AV, Deveraux PJ, Leece P, et al. (2004) Interpreting authorship order and corresponding authorship. Epidemiology 15: 125–126.
64. Buchkowsky SS, Jewesson PJ (2004) Industry sponsorship and authorship of clinical trials over 20 years. Annals of Pharmacotherapy 38: 579–585.
65. Tarnow E, De Young BR, Cohen MB (2004) Coauthorship in pathology, a comparison with physics and a survery-generated and member-preferred authorship guideline. Med Gen Med 6: 1–2.
66. Etemadi A, Raiszadeh F, Alaeddini F, Azizi F (2004) Views of Iranian medical journal editors on medical research publication. Saudi Medical Journal 25: S29–S33.
67. Marušić M, Božikov J, Katavić V, Hren D, Kljaković-Gašpić M, et al. (2004) Authorship in a small medical journal: A study of contributorship statements by corresponding authors. Science and Engineering Ethics 10: 493–502.
68. Meyer M, McMahon D (2004) An examination of ethical research conduct by experienced and novice accounting academics. Issues in Accounting Education 19: 413–442.
69. Procyshyn RM, Chau A, Fortin P, Jenkins W (2004) Prevalence and outcomes of pharmaceutical industry-sponsored clinical trials involving clozapine, risperidone, or olanzapine. Canadian Journal of Psychiatry 49: 601–606.
70. Szirony TA, Price JH, Wolfe E, Telljohann SK, Dake JA (2004) Perceptions of nursing faculty regarding ethical issues in nursing research. Journal of Nursing Education 43: 270–279.
71. Apgar DH, Congress E (2005) Authorship credit: A national study of social work educators' beliefs. Journal of Social Work Education 41: 101–112.
72. Apgar DH, Congress E (2005) Ethical beliefs of social work researchers: Results of a national study. Journal of Social Service Research 32: 61–80.
73. Freda MC, Keamey MH (2005) Ethical issues faced by nursing editors. Western Journal of Nursing Research 27: 487–499.
74. Hilmer CE, Hilmer MJ (2005) How do journal quality, co-authorship, and author order affect agricultural economists' salaries? American Journal of Agricultural Economics 87: 509–523.
75. Joubert G (2005) Practices and experiences in the Faculty of Health Sciences of the University of the Free State. South African Family Practice 47: 57–60.
76. Mixon JF, Swyer W (2005) Contribution, attribution and the assignment of intellectual property rights in economics. Journal of Economic Studies 32: 382–386.
77. Pignatelli B, Maisonneuve H, Chapuis F (2005) Authorship ignorance: views of researchers in French clinical settings. Journal of Medical Ethics 31: 578–581.
78. Sandler JC, Russell BL (2005) Faculty-student collaborations: Ethics and satisfaction in authorship credit. Ethics & Behavior 15: 65–80.
79. Birnholtz JP (2006) What does it mean to be an author? The intersection of credit, contribution, and collaboration in science. Journal of the American Society for Information Science and Technology 57: 1758–1770.
80. Bourbonniere MC, Russell DJ, Goldsmith CH (2006) Authorship issues: One research center's experience with developing author guidelines. American Journal of Occupational Therapy 60: 111–117.
81. Brown C, Chan K, Lai P (2006) Marketing journal coauthorships: an empirical analysis of coauthor behaviour. Journal of Marketing Education 28: 17–25.
82. Dhaliwal U, Singh N, Bhatia A (2006) Awareness of authorship criteria and conflict: survey in a medical institution in India. Med Gen Med 8: 52.
83. Einav L, Yariv L (2006) What's in a surname? The effects of surname initials on academic success. Journal of Economic Perspectives 20: 175–187.
84. Laband D, Tollison R (2006) Alphabetized coauthorship. Applied Economics 38: 1649–1653.
85. Manton E, English D (2006) Reasons for co-authorship in business journals and the extent of guest or gift authorships. Delta Pi Epsilon Journal 48: 86–95.
86. Marušić A, Bates T, Anić A, Marušić M (2006) How the structure of contribution disclosure statements affects validity of authorship: a randomized study in a general medical journal. Current Medical Research and Opinion 22: 1035–1044.
87. Moore M, Griffin B (2006) Identification of factors that influence authorship name placement and decisions to collaborate in peer-reviewed, education-related publications. Studies in Educational Evaluation 32: 125–135.
88. Weltzin JF, Belote RT, Williams LT, Keller JK, Engel EC (2006) Authorship in ecology: attribution, accountability, and responsibility. Frontiers in Ecology and the Environment 4: 435–441.
89. Baerlocher MO, Newton M, Gautam T, Tomlinson G, Detsky AS (2007) The meaning of author order in medical research. Journal of Investigative Medicine 55: 174–180.
90. Funk C, Barrett K, Macrina F (2007) Authorship and publication practices: evaluation of the effect of responsible conduct of research instruction to postdoctoral trainees. Accountability in Research - Policies and Quality Assurance 14: 269–305.
91. Geelhoed RJ, Phillips JC, Fischer AR, Shpungin E, Gong YJ (2007) Authorship decision making: An empirical investigation. Ethics & Behavior 17: 95–115.
92. Gotzsche PC, Hrobjartsson A, Johansen HK, Haahr MT, Altman DG, et al. (2007) Ghost authorship in industry-initiated randomised trials. PLoS Medicine 4: 47–52.
93. Hren D, Sambunjak D, Ivaniš A, Marušić M, Marušić A (2007) Perceptions of authorship criteria: effects of student instruction and scientific experience. Journal of Medical Ethics 33: 428–432.
94. Ilakovac V, Fišter K, Marušić M, Marušić A (2007) Reliability of disclosure forms of authors' contributions. CMAJ 176: 41–46.
95. Kurichi JE, Sonnad SS (2007) Authorship patterns of surgical chairs. Surgery 141: 267–271.
96. Manton E, English D (2007) The extent of gift authorships in business journals. Journal of Organizational Culture, Communications & Conflict 11: 29–36.
97. Peppercorn J, Blood E, Winer E, Partridge A (2007) Association between pharmaceutical involvement and outcomes in breast cancer clinical trials. Cancer 109: 1239–1246.
98. Tryon G, Bishop J, Hatfield T (2007) Doctoral students' beliefs about authorship credit for dissertations. Training and Education in Professional Psychology 1: 184–192.
99. Tungaraza T, Poole R (2007) Influence of drug company authorship and sponsorship on drug trial outcomes. British Journal of Psychiatry 191: 82–83.
100. Wager E (2007) Do medical journals provide clear and consistent guidelines on authorship? MedGenMed 9: 16.
101. Birnholtz J (2008) When authorship isn't enough: lessons from CERN on the implications of formal and informal credit attribution mechanisms in collaborative research. Journal of Electronic Publishing 11: 1.
102. Ivaniš A, Hren D, Sambunjak D, Marušić M, Marušić A (2008) Quantification of authors' contributions and eligibility for authorship: Randomized study in a general medical journal. Journal of General Internal Medicine 23: 1303–1310.
103. Lang T (2008) What do you think constitutes authorship? AMWA Journal: American Medical Writers Association Journal 23: 65–67.
104. Louis KS, Holdsworth JM, Anderson MS, Campbell EG (2008) Everyday ethics in research: Translating authorship guidelines into practice in the bench sciences. Journal of Higher Education 79: 88–112.
105. Van Praag M, Van Praag B (2008) The benefits of being economics professor A (rather than Z). Economics 75: 782–796.

106. Baerlocher MO, Gautam T, Newton M, Tomlinson G (2009) Changing author counts in five major general medicine journals: effect of author contribution forms. Journal of Clinical Epidemiology 62: 875–877.

107. Hu X (2009) Loads of special authorship functions: Linear growth in the percentage of "equal first authors" and corresponding authors. Journal of the American Society for Information Science and Technology 60: 2378–2381.

108. Maciejovsky B, Budescu DV, Ariely D (2009) The researcher as a consumer of scientific publications: how do name-ordering conventions affect inferences about contribution credits? Marketing Science 28: 589–598.

109. O'Brien J, Baerlocher MO, Newton M, Gautam T, Noble J (2009) Honorary coauthorship: does it matter? Can Assoc Radiol J 60: 231–236.

110. Pulido M, Gonzalez JC, Sanz F (1994) Original articles published in Medicina Clinica (1962–1992) - number of authors, interval between acceptance and publication, and references [in Portugese]. Medicina Clinica 103: 770–775.

111. Rowan-Legg A, Weijer C, Gao J, Fernandez C (2009) A comparison of journal instructions regarding institutional review board approval and conflict-of-interest disclosure between 1995 and 2005. Journal of Medical Ethics 35: 74–78.

112. Samad A, Khanzada TW, Siddiqui AA (2009) Do the instructions to authors of Pakistani medical journals convey adequate guidance for authorship criteria? Pakistan Journal of Medical Sciences 25: 879–882.

113. Wager E, Fiack S, Graf C, Robinson A, Rowlands I (2009) Science journal editors' views on publication ethics: results of an international survey. Journal of Medical Ethics 35: 348–353.

114. Ahmed HS, Hadi A, Choudhury N (2010) Authorship conflict in Bangladesh: an exploratory study. Learned Publishing 23: 319–325.

115. Akhabue E, Lautenbach E (2010) "Equal" contributions and credit: an emerging trend in the characterization of authorship. Annals of Epidemiology 20: 868–871.

116. Castleden H, Morgan VS, Neimanis A (2010) Researchers' perspectives on collective/community co-authorship in community-based participatory indigenous research. Journal of Empirical Research on Human Research Ethics 5: 23–32.

117. Chan K, Hardin IW, Liano K (2010) Author order conditions and co-authorship in real estate journals. Journal of Real Estate Literature. pp 1841–1851.

118. Frandsen TF, Nicolaisen J (2010) What is in a name? Credit assignment practices in different disciplines. Journal of Informetrics 4: 608–617.

119. House MC, Seeman JI (2010) Credit and authorship practices: educational and environmental influences. Accountability in Research-Policies and Quality Assurance 17: 223–256.

120. Lacasse JR, Leo J (2010) Ghostwriting at elite academic medical centers in the united states. PLoS Medicine 7: e1000230.

121. McDonald RJ, Neff KL, Rethlefsen ML, Kallmes DF (2010) Effects of author contribution disclosures and numeric limitations on authorship trends. Mayo Clinic Proceedings 85: 920–927.

122. Morris S (2010) Cracking the code: Assessing institutional compliance with the Australian code for the responsible conduct of research. Australian Universities Review 52: 18–26.

123. Nastasee SA (2010) Acknowledgment of medical writers in medical journal articles: a comparison from the years 2000 and 2007. Current Medical Research and Opinion 26: S6–S6.

124. Picard M, Wilkinson K, Wirthensohn M (2010) Perceptions and expectations of authorship: Towards development of an e-learning tool facilitating discussion and reflection between post-graduate supervisors and candidates. Ergo - The Journal of the Education Research Group of Adelaide 1: 21–33.

125. Rose SL, Krzyzanowska MK, Joffe S (2010) Relationships between authorship contributions and authors' industry financial ties among oncology clinical trials. Journal of Clinical Oncology 28: 1316–1321.

126. Seeman JI, House MC (2010) Influences on authorship issues: An evaluation of receiving, not receiving, and rejecting credit. Accountability in Research-Policies and Quality Assurance 17: 176–197.

127. Seeman JI, House MC (2010) Influences on authorship issues: An evaluation of giving credit. Accountability in Research-Policies and Quality Assurance 17: 146–169.

128. Street JM, Rogers WA, Israel M, Braunack-Mayer AJ (2010) Credit where credit is due? Regulation, research integrity and the attribution of authorship in the health sciences. Social Science & Medicine 70: 1458–1465.

129. Walker RL, Sykes L, Hemmelgarn BR, Quan HD (2010) Authors' opinions on publication in relation to annual performance assessment. BMC Medical Education 10: 21.

130. Welfare L, Sackett C (2010) Authorship in student-faculty collaborative research: Perceptions of current and best practices. Journal of Academic Ethics 8: 199–215.

131. International Committee of Medical Journal (2010) Uniform requirements for manuscripts submitted to biomedical journals: Ethical considerations in the conduct and reporting of research: authorship and contributorship. Updated April 2010. Available at at http://www.icmje.org/ethical_1author.html. Accessed 15 May 2011.

132. Rennie D, Yank V, Emanuel L (1997) When authorship fails - A proposal to make contributors accountable. JAMA 278: 579–585.

133. Kalichman MW (2011) Overview: Underserved areas of education in the responsible conduct of research: Authorship. Science and Engineering Ethics Science and Engineering Ethics 17: 335–339.

134. Borenstein J (2011) Responsible authorship in engineering fields: An overview of current ethical challenges. Science and Engineering Ethics 17: 355–364.

135. Plemmons D (2011) A broader discussion of authorship. Science and Engineering Ethics 17: 389–398.

136. Macrina FL (2011) Teaching authorship and publication practices in the biomedical and life sciences. Science and Engineering Ethics 17: 341–354.

137. Bebeau MJ, Monson V (2011) Authorship and publication practices in the social sciences: Historical reflections on current practices. Science and Engineering Ethics 17: 365–388.

138. Steneck N (2006) Fostering integrity in research: definitions, current knowledge, and future direction. Science and Engineering Ethics 12: 53–74.

139. Department of Health and Human Services (2005) Public Health Service policies on research misconduct. Federal Register 70: 28369–28400.

140. National Science Foundation (2002) Research misconduct. Federal Register 67: 11936–11939.

141. Marcovitch H (2011) Is research safe in their hands? BMJ 342: d284.

142. Bosch X (2008) Integrity: Croatia's standards unusual in much of Europe. Nature 454: 574.

143. Marusic A, Katavic V, Marusic M (2007) Role of editors and journals in detecting and preventing scientific misconduct: strengths, weaknesses, opportunities, and threats.. Medicine and Law 26: 545–566.

144. Turiel E (1983) The development of social knowledge: Morality and convention. Cambridge: University Press.

145. Bosnjak L, Marusic A (2011) Prescribed practices of authorship in scholarly publications: survey of codes of ethics from professional bodies and journal guidelines across disciplines. Submitted manuscript.

146. Self DJ, Olivarez M, Baldwin DC (1998) The amount of small-group case-study discussion needed to improve moral reasoning skills of medical students. Academic Medicine 73: 521–523.

147. Haidt J (2001) The emotional dog and its rational tail: a social intuitionist approach to moral judgment. Psychology Review 108: 814–834.

5.5 The Disposable Author: How Pharmaceutical Marketing is Embraced within Medicine's Scholarly Literature

Alastair Matheson

Matheson, A. The disposable author: How pharmaceutical marketing is embraced within medicine's scholarly literature. *Hastings Center Report* 6(4), 31–37 (2015).

THE DISPOSABLE
AUTHOR

How Pharmaceutical Marketing Is Embraced
within Medicine's Scholarly Literature

BY ALASTAIR MATHESON

In an ethics framed by the narrative of medicine's victimhood by the pharmaceutical industry, medicine's journals have escaped adequate scrutiny, and the advocacy-based marketing they host has been insulated from reform.

The creatures outside looked from pig to man, and from man to pig, and from pig to man again; but already it was impossible to say which was which.

—*George Orwell,* Animal Farm*, 1945*

Is medicine the manipulated victim of the pharmaceutical corporations, or their colleague in corruption? The answer, of course, is both. Sometimes medicine is pharma's unwitting dupe, sometimes its eager bedfellow. The best studies have recognized the ambiguous nature of the relationship.[1] Yet most scholarship has pursued a simpler, more saleable narrative in which pharma is a scheming villain and medicine its maidenly victim. This framing is exemplified in titles such as *The Truth about the Drug Companies: How They Deceive Us* and *Bad Pharma: How Drug Companies Mislead Doctors.*[2] Much of this scholarship, not least, in these two works, is excellent, but I argue that such crude moral framing blunts understanding of the murky realities of medicine's relationship with pharma and, in consequence, holds back reform. My goal in this article is to put matters right in respect to one critical area of scholarly interest, the medical journal publication.

Pharma relies on peer advocacy to sell its wares to prescribing doctors. This is an arrangement in which clinicians' qualified colleagues, including "key opinion leaders," are recruited by pharmaceutical corporations and marketing agencies to deliver commercially expedient content to their professional fellows. A more technical definition of peer advocacy is provided at the end of this essay, but precisely how this practice works in the setting of publications is not well understood because ethicists studying the problem have made too much of the narrative of corporate villainy and medical victimhood. Accordingly, criticism of industry publications has been preoccupied with the crudely dishonest practices of ghostwriting, ghost authorship, and "ghost management," vices condemned as "dirty little secrets"

Alastair Matheson, "The Disposable Author: How Pharmaceutical Marketing Is Embraced within Medicine's Scholarly Literature," *Hastings Center Report* 46, no 4 (2016): 31-37. DOI: 10.1002/hast.576

perpetrated from "behind the scenes" with the connivance of academic "shills" or "guest authors," in contempt of standards set by the International Committee of Medical Journal Editors (ICMJE).[3] This account is appealing, and yet it is wrong or, at the very least, seriously incomplete, with only limited relevance to the actualities of contemporary industry practices. In truth, many commercial publications are not developed in secret but fashioned within a culture of open collaboration, where academic authors make substantial, independent contributions; pharmaceutical companies are showcased rather than hidden; and medicine's editorial standards assist rather than impede the workings of commerce. Ghostly practices are real and important, but publications-based marketing works with a broader canvas, involving a culture of influence and accommodation that naturalizes the presence of commerce within medicine and normalizes the vice of peer endorsement. For want of a rubric, I refer to this here as "mainstream marketing."

Bad Pharma, Good Pharma: My Experience

Many scholars have looked at these cultural dimensions of industry's relations with medicine, and Arnold Relman, Richard Horton, Richard Smith, Trudo Lemmens, David Healy, and Carl Elliott have all influenced the ideas I discuss here.[4] My own professional experiences have been equally important, though. Following a brief career as a biologist, I worked in pharmaceutical marketing between 1994 and 2010, first in a "medical communications" company and then as a freelance consultant working directly or indirectly for most of the major pharmaceutical corporations and over thirty marketing agencies in North America and Europe. I worked on over one hundred drugs, most of which were, in my estimation, mediocre products that could be better pitched if a more persuasive scientific angle could be

found for them. I visited corporate headquarters and congresses; analyzed markets, products, and competitors; groomed key opinion leaders; ghostwrote manuscripts; developed publications plans; and devised marketing strategies.

This experience has afforded me detailed inside understanding of how industry and medicine work together on clinical research and publications. It has also left me with a bivalent attitude toward industry. On the one hand, it remains my belief that pharmaceutical research and development efforts are capable of great good. I think highly of the work on molecular medicines in virology and oncology, for example. Many clinical trials are interesting and informative, and numerous negative trial results representing commercial failures are published every month.[5] Critics should be prepared to acknowledge the good, if only to better understand the bad; and indeed, every last "pharmascold" will swallow, inject, or infuse pharma's wares at some point in his or her life.

On the other hand, pharmaceutical *marketing* is anathema to science, corrupting to medicine, wasteful to economies, and harmful to patients, and I must acknowledge the moral difficulty that for many years I sold my intellect in its service. Pharma itself, of course, has never truly acknowledged its underbelly of secrets, half-truths, corruption, power, and death, and it flaunts the language of ethics like a silk cummerbund over a paunch. If it is a lie to dissemble, distort, or omit, then pharma must be considered a liar whose subtle falsehoods stock the annals of medicine. It is to these annals—the peer-reviewed journals of the academic medical profession—that I now turn.

Advocacy Marketing and the Committed, Disposable Academic

In order to clarify how advocacy-based marketing works within mainstream medical literature, the

first step is to adopt a systematic rather than metaphorical approach and to ask with each article,

- Who are the stakeholders, and what are their stakes?
- How was this article financed, planned, and placed?
- How was the content determined?
- How is it attributed?

The lead stakeholders are of course pharma companies, but academic authors and institutions have agendas, too, as do journals and publishers. Industry articles emerge from a process of negotiation that must gratify all parties. I return to this theme below. As for finance and planning, industry often plays a secret and indeed ghostly role in determining the themes, topline content, authorship, and placement of articles, without the articles' academic authors, let alone readers, knowing about it.[6] Overall, however, the balance between secret planning and public negotiation varies. In large clinical trials, for instance, academic institutions are frequently contracted to help organize the research, and doctors and senior academics often head the study and publications committees, helping plan and place articles in this capacity.[7]

It is when we come to the third question, concerning content, that the significance of multiple stakeholders becomes critical. Throughout my experience of commercial publications planning, crude ghostwriting was extremely rare. Many industry articles do not rely on ghostwriters, and when they do, one or more academic authors generally amend the text produced by the writing team. The notion that academics are passive "guests" or "shills" is a misunderstanding of their function: their contributions should be both substantive and independent, stamping publications with intellectual distinctiveness and credibility. The art of publications development lies not in coating commercial content with an academic veneer, but in meshing commercial positioning and academic expertise as deeply as possible, creating content that is scientifically compelling but instilled with subtle commercial valence. Nonetheless, a diagnostic feature of this literature is that academic recruits and their institutions are readily replaceable by others without any decisive impact on the published product. Alternative academics and institutions might add varying intellectual content to the work, but its commercial functions will be served just as well. The leading problem with the use of academic authors in today's industry publications is not passivity but *disposability*. Only the corporate project itself is fundamental, and particular academic contributions are exchangeable details.

How, then, are the commercial dimensions of industry literature delivered? They are not prefabricated, as "ghost" metaphors suggest, but woven into text using a variety of interventions. These include in-house planning, as related above; selection of reliable authors and institutions whose contributions can be broadly anticipated; well-documented techniques for manipulating the design and analysis of clinical trials;[8] commercial ownership and analysis of data; documentary guidance for manuscript development in the form of article outlines, clinical study reports, or results summaries; review and discussion of emerging content; and the use of company employees as coauthors on most clinical trials.[9] On some articles trade writers are used as well. Sometimes these commercial writers draft text, but in other cases they develop outlines, compile bibliographies, add details such as tables, or collate or amend text. Not all such contributions qualify as "ghostwriting," but all of them influence content. These numerous options for subtle steerage and framing are alloyed with the bona fide contributions of academic recruits to yield a product that works commercially but enables academics to feel a sense of intellectual ownership. Some key opinion leaders knowingly accommodate commercial positioning, but

most do not feel especially compromised. They stand foursquare behind their work, and the companies smile.

Collective Misattribution

It is with the final question—concerning the attribution of industry-financed literature—that the language of "ghosting" is most misleading. To appreciate why, one must first keep in mind that, correctly understood, attribution involves more than mere authorship. Every feature of an article that communicates information to readers about its stakeholders, planning, and development should be considered part of its attribution. Furthermore, readers' perceptions are crucial, and articles in which important disclosures are made but the disclosures are in vague language, endnotes, or small print should be considered poorly attributed.

The attribution of commercial journal articles is nuanced. Marketing based on peer advocacy demands that academics are portrayed as the masters; but far from hiding companies, mercantile literature also uses corporate display so that the article promotes not only the drug but also the company—as academic medicine's trustworthy partner. As with content development, these attributional goals are achieved through a bricolage of subtle interventions. Academics are commonly placed at the front of bylines, company employees in the middle, and commercial writers in the small print. An effect functionally analogous to ghostwriting can be achieved when content is heavily influenced by industry coauthors while the conspicuous lead authorship position is assigned to

an academic. Content control and academic endorsement can thereby be delivered without any recourse to ghostwriting or guest authorship.

Beyond the author byline, the spin continues. Frequently, readers are simply not told what drug is being promoted, whether the work was instigated by the "sponsor," and whether the data are the company's private property. The company is regularly described as a provider of "support" or "funding," and when accounts of its role are given, these are often sketchy or in small print, while commercial writers are credited with "assistance," leaving their precise contribution obscure. "Contributor" listings, which describe in small print what tasks were carried out by whom, help record accountability,[10] but considered as a means of attribution, these lists merely enable the academic-dominated author byline to command readers' attention. Through a patchwork of diminutions, aggrandizements, omissions, euphemisms, fudges, and misnomers, academics are positioned as masters, and proprietors as their worthy aides. The company is placed in the shop window—but nobody is told it owns the shop.

Such devices are widespread in medicine's peer-reviewed journal literature.[11] But who is behind them, and whose interests are served? Here we come to the crux. *Everyone* is behind them, and each party benefits in its own way. Companies get the elixir of endorsement on which advocacy marketing depends; academics reap the rewards of authorial status and generally feel that they deserve top billing; journals sell reprints; and culturally, I believe, academic medicine and its journals crave the sense

> **The medical journal article should be a point of resistance and distinction between commerce and academia, but it operates instead as one of merger and ratification. The commercial-academic landscape is continuous.**

that the research scene remains in their hands. It is customary for academic "investigators" to be placed at the front of the byline, and indeed, it is understandable that readers who will prescribe the drug want to read the opinions of qualified peers who have used it in their patients. But when the project is not in truth an academic one but wholly or partly commercial, these sentiments open the door to advocacy marketing. The language of corporate "sponsorship" and academic "investigators" and superficial arrangements of trial committees suggest that companies merely provide finance and that independent academic institutions are in true command, while the actual role of commerce in instigation, analysis, framing, writing, and data ownership is politely shepherded into the margins by diverse attributional tricks—and that is how medicine likes it. A former head of publications at Merck has noted that industry articles may be more likely to secure publication in prestigious journals if their authorship is led by academic authors, whereas articles fronted by industry authors have been scorned by readers, who expect academic-led fare.[12] Advocacy-based marketing is a disgrace to medicine and its journals, but it has, to use an Orwellian phrase, long been "too normal to be noticed"[13]—perhaps above all for the simple reason that doctors like to feel in charge.

Finally, although it is beyond the scope of this essay to consider the matter in detail, medicine's editorial guidelines lend support to this culture of misattribution. In previous work I and others showed how the ICMJE authorship formula supports commercial byline avoidance.[14] All the forms of spin I have discussed in this section are overlooked, tolerated, or mandated by ICMJE requirements. By complying with ICMJE diktats, industry literature may lay claim to the highest ethical standards. Far from a dirty little secret, drug marketing is ostentatiously robed in the standards of medicine itself.

The VIGOR Study: Still a Paradigm for Mainstream Marketing

These practices are illustrated by the publication in the *New England Journal of Medicine* of the Vioxx Gastrointestinal Outcomes Research study (VIGOR), which compared the analgesic rofecoxib (Vioxx) with an older generic drug, naproxen, in patients with rheumatoid arthritis.[15] VIGOR was organized and financed and its data owned and analyzed by Merck. In a major clinical and commercial setback, the trial detected an excess of cardiovascular events in the Vioxx group. The company's response was to pursue the hypothesis that the difference between the treatment groups was not caused by a harmful effect of Vioxx but, rather, a hypothetical "protective" effect of naproxen.[16] When VIGOR was published, this interpretation was central to the manuscript, which reported that the incidence of cardiovascular events was "lower in the naproxen group," rather than higher with Vioxx, and explicable as a cardioprotective effect. Yet the manuscript was not ghostwritten: the academics contributed substantively alongside industry colleagues and forthrightly defended the publication when criticized.[17] There is no reason to doubt their sincerity—but the article delivered just the interpretation the company wanted.

How, then, was VIGOR attributed? Notwithstanding the role of the company in financing and organizing the trial, influencing the themes of the paper, owning and analyzing the data, and developing the manuscript, only two of the fourteen authors were company employees, the lead and corresponding author were academic, and the journal declared that the report came "from" a list of institutions, the first and most visible being academic. A footnote stated, "Supported by a grant from Merck." It is not known whether the impression of academic leadership persuaded any readers who might otherwise have thought twice to trust the "cardioprotective" interpretation.

What is known is that Merck ordered a vast number of reprints—allegedly over 900,000—the journal's publisher profited handsomely, the reprints were used to market Vioxx to prescribing doctors, and many thousands of patients were killed before Vioxx was withdrawn from sale.[18]

VIGOR was published sixteen years ago, but pharmaceutical marketing is still based on this form of subtle peer advocacy, in which commercially functional content is presented under the leadership of honest academics. The ICMJE has introduced piecemeal reforms over the years, several of which have been beneficial, but the basic calculus of advocacy has remained intact. Companies still instigate the work, own the data, provide low-profile coauthors and editorial teams, and obtain the framing they want. Academics still dominate author bylines and front the research. Journals still state frequently that articles come "from" academic institutions and omit to tell readers who instigated the work, who owns the data, and what is being marketed. There is little to stop a publication like VIGOR from happening again.

"Ghost" Metaphors

"Ghost" metaphors have shamed some egregious marketing practices and been the basis of some important scholarship.[19] Unfortunately, the critical weakness of the word "ghost" is that it steers attention to industry's role, and industry secrecy, and away from the multistakeholder responsibilities for mercantile literature and its misattribution. Ghostly practices are merely part of the overall activities and continuous with the subtler and less secretive ones I have described. By focusing on them, publication ethics has missed the bigger picture. Worse still, it has become bogged down in problems of definition and, in consequence, has been outflanked by commerce. For example, the standard definition of "ghostwriting" is manuscript composition by a writer who is not a named author.[20] By this definition, ghostwriting is widespread in industry publications, but marketers and journal editors have successfully promulgated an alternative in which articles are not considered ghostwritten if the writer's name and funding is mentioned—some would say buried—in the small print.[21] On this basis, industry may claim ghostwriting is not part of its modus operandi, and it is unfortunate that even some ethicists have been drawn into using this loaded formula.[22]

How, then, should these metaphors be used? In my view, the everyday definition of ghostwriting should be strictly adhered to and the industry-friendly rebranding firmly rejected. As for the term "ghost authorship," the standard meaning — namely, any contribution deserving author status that is not credited on the byline—remains valid, but the question of which contributions deserve authorship is difficult. The ICMJE authorship criteria are flawed, and studies of ghost authorship predicated upon them are correspondingly limited.[23] Future empirical studies should use a range of distinct metrics, and published literature should always discuss the problems of definition. Similar considerations apply to guest authorship—although, as I have discussed, this is not the chief problem surrounding the role of academics in commercial literature. Most academics probably deserve to be authors, and bylines are manipulated by excluding others who should be coauthors, such as commercial writers, or by massaging author order. The greater problems with pharma's academic authors are that they are replaceable and recruited for their names' sales value. Alternative terms such as "advocate," "selling," or, as I have used here, "disposable" author would better articulate these issues.

Finally, "ghost management" is a useful metaphor for criticizing the secretive aspects of commercial planning and development.[24] The value of "ghost management" is polemical, not analytical, and as such, it might be useful beyond publication ethics.

One might suggest, for instance, that the United States Grand Jury system is "ghost managed" by prosecutors. But "ghost management" does not provide a conceptual basis for understanding all publications-based marketing. It is preferable to describe industry literature as "commercially managed publications" or simply "commercial publications." These terms apply to all industry output rather than a secretive subset, cannot be negated by disclosure, expose the mercantile function of academic authors, and correctly imply that the fundamental issue with commercial

publications is, quite simply, commerce—irrespective of the degree of secrecy involved.

Integration, Not Subterfuge, as the Danger

The overenthusiastic promotion of ghost metaphors serves the popular narrative in which the primary threat posed by pharma to medicine is one of deception and external manipulation. This threat is indeed important, but it is not the foremost danger. The greatest threat is blending and assimilation, such that the distinction between the commercial and academic is by slow gradations ceasing to be apparent or even important within medical culture. This transformation in the quality of medical science and discourse is not being driven by deception or trickery so much as cultural and institutional proximity of commerce and academia, involving philanthropy, patronage, and most importantly, the increasingly routine nature of industry-academic research partnership.

The medical journal article should be a point of resistance and distinction between commerce and academia, but it operates instead as one of merger and ratification, its meticulous guidelines working not to differentiate but to bring the worlds of medicine and commerce more minutely together. As the distinction between the commercial and academic diminishes, marketing has progressively less need for ghostly subterfuge in communicating its propositions; the commercial-academic landscape is continuous. Contemporary industry literature positions academics, cor-

Many commercial publications are fashioned within a culture of open collaboration, where academic authors make substantial, independent contributions, pharmaceutical companies are showcased, and medicine's editorial standards assist the workings of commerce.

porations, journals, and readers side by side in the pursuit of truth: public, civilized, rational, and humane, it leads today's assimilated medicine naturally to the point of sale.

Let me then define contemporary advocacy-based marketing punctiliously, as *a practice in which content with potential commercial or promotional utility is planned, convened, funded, influenced or owned by a company, but communicated by, or disproportionately attributed to, the peers or opinion leaders of the intended customers.* Advocacy marketing thus defined is routine in medicine and its scholarly literature, and the chief policy conclusion of this essay is that it should be banned outright. This is a matter for academic medical institutions and societies as well as journals, and the first step to achieving it is to understand the nature of attribution. This concept has never been adequately understood by medicine's editors and is not even discussed in the ICMJE guidelines. Medicine's construction of authorship has long envisaged a "two-sided coin" of credit and responsibility,[25] and in thus focusing on the author has not adequately addressed the needs of the reader; but in any case, as I have shown here, attribution runs far wider than authorship and turns on what readers perceive as much as what is disclosed. If a project is instigated and funded by a company and its data are privately owned, then it is a commercial project, and by means both of authorship and other attributive devices, it should be presented clearly to readers *as* commercial, not the ambiguous, supposedly academic-led fare that is a staple of medicine's intellectual diet.

To ensure that readers perceive mercantile content for what it is, it would ideally be published separately from noncommercial research. Publishers could, for instance, restrict industry-funded content to new publications such as a "JAMA Commercial Medicine" or quarantine it in clearly labeled "Commercial Pages" within existing journals. Failing this, there should at least be conspicuous commercial attribution. Mercantile science should be welcomed with scholarly courtesy and respected on its merits but presented as commercial from the outset. Companies could, for instance, be identified in the titles of articles they finance ("A Pfizer Trial," for example) or listed as corporate coauthors. Abstracts should clearly state commercial finance, instigation, planning and data ownership, and identify the product the article promotes. Ideally, such measures would be introduced in a cross-media standard.[26] If every commercial article, web page, and lecture was introduced to its audience with stark labeling, this would encourage readers to think twice, expose the advocacy function of the academic authors, limit the unmarked seepage of marketing into medicine, and counter the creeping cultural merger of science and commerce. Differentiation can reverse integration.

In an ethics framed by the narrative of medicine's victimhood and the allure of ghostly explanations, medicine's journals have escaped adequate scrutiny, and the advocacy-based marketing they host has been insulated from reform. It is for journals to put these matters right and for ethicists to encourage them in the task. It is time to think more about the everyday mainstream of commercial publications, and less about ghosts. In words I came upon years ago, in my biologist's past, "as the road to hell is paved with good intentions, so the road to confusion is paved with good metaphors."[27]

Notes

1. C. Elliott, *White Coat, Black Hat: Adventures on the Dark Side of Medicine* (Boston: Beacon Press, 2010); D. Healy, *Pharmageddon* (Berkeley: University of California Press, 2013).

2. M. Angell, *The Truth about the Drug Companies: How They Deceive Us and What to Do about It* (New York: Random House, 2005); B. Goldacre, *Bad Pharma. How Drug Companies Mislead Doctors and Harm Patients* (London: Fourth Estate, 2012).

3. A. J. Fugh-Berman, "The Haunting of Medical Journals: How Ghostwriting Sold 'HRT,'" *PLoS Medicine* 7 (2010): e1000335; J. S. Ross et al., "Guest Authorship and Ghostwriting in Publications Related to Rofecoxib: A Case Study of Industry Documents from Rofecoxib Litigation," *Journal of the American Medical Association* 299 (2008): 1800-12; S. Ngai et al., "Haunted Manuscripts: Ghost Authorship in the Medical Literature," *Accountability in Research* 12 (2005): 103-14; *PLoS Medicine* editors, "Ghostwriting: The Dirty Little Secret of Medical Publishing That Just Got Bigger," *PLoS Medicine* 6 (2009): e1000156; S. Sismondo, "Ghost Management: How Much of the Medical Literature Is Shaped behind the Scenes by the Pharmaceutical Industry?," *PLoS Medicine* 4 (2007): e286; S. Sismondo and M. Doucet, "Publication Ethics and the Ghost Management of Medical Publication," *Bioethics* 24 (2010): 273-83; International Committee of Medical Journal Editors, "Recommendations for the Conduct, Reporting, Editing, and Publication of Scholarly Work in Medical Journals," July 2014, accessed February 2, 2015, at http://www.icmje.org/urm_main.html.

4. A. S. Relman, "The New Medical-Industrial Complex," *New England Journal of Medicine* 303 (1980): 963-70; R. Horton, "The Dawn of McScience," *New York Review of Books*, 51 (2004): 7-9; R. Smith, "Medical Journals Are an Extension of the Marketing Arm of Pharmaceutical Companies," *PLoS Medicine* 2 (2005): e138; T. Lemmens, "Leopards in the Temple: Restoring Scientific Integrity to the Commercialized Research Scene," *Journal of Law and Medical Ethics* 32 (2004): 641-57; Healy, *Pharmageddon*; Elliott, *White Coat, Black Hat*.

5. For a typical scientific discussion among academics concerning a commercial trial that coincidentally also failed, see R. S. Doody, M. Farlow, P. S. Aisen, and Alzheimer's Disease Cooperative Study Data Analysis and Publication Committee, "Phase 3 Trials of Solanezumab and Bapineuzumab for Alzheimer's Disease," *New England Journal of Medicine* 370 (2014): 1460.

6. Fugh-Berman, "The Haunting of Medical Journals"; Ross et al., "Guest Authorship and Ghostwriting in Publications Related to Rofecoxib"; Sismondo, "Ghost Management"; M. R. Wittek, M. J. Williams, and A. M. Carlson, "Evidence Development and Publication Planning: Strategic Process," *Current Medical Research and Opinion* 25 (2009): 2723-27; A. Matheson, "Corporate Science and the Husbandry of Scientific and Medical Knowledge by the Pharmaceutical Industry," *BioSocieties* 3 (2008): 355-82.

7. For an example, see Doody et al., "Phase 3 Trials."

8. Healy, *Pharmageddon*; Goldacre, *Bad Pharma*; J. Lexchin, "Those Who Have the Gold Make the Evidence: How the Pharmaceutical Industry Biases the Outcomes of Clinical Trials of Medications," *Science and Engineering Ethics* 18 (2012): 247-61; P. Gøtzsche, *Deadly Medicines and Organised Crime: How Big Pharma Has Corrupted Healthcare* (London: Radcliffe, 2013).

9. J. Hoekman et al., "The Geographical Distribution of Leadership in Globalized Clinical Trials," *PLoS One* 7 (2012): e45984.

10. D. Rennie, "Integrity in Scientific Publishing," *Health Services Research* 45 (2010): 885-96.

11. Little systematic empirical work on the attributional features of mainstream marketing has yet been published, although the features I have described are widely recognized and apparent in much industry literature. For a study of poor attribution in the *Lancet*, see A. Lundh, L. T. Krogsbøll, and P. C. Gøtzsche, "Sponsors' Participation in Conduct and Reporting of Industry Trials: A Descriptive Study," *Trials* 13 (2012): 146.

12. L. J. Hirsch, "Conflicts of Interest, Authorship, and Disclosures in Industry-Related Scientific Publications: The Tort Bar and Editorial Oversight of Medical Journals," *Mayo Clinic Proceedings* 84 (2009): 811-21.

13. G. Orwell, "Charles Dickens," in *All Art Is Propaganda*, compiled by G. Packer (New York: First Mariner Books, 2009), 1-62, at 36.

14. J. Leo, J. R. Lacasse, and A. N. Cimino, "Why Does Academic Medicine Allow Ghostwriting? A Prescription for Reform," *Society* 48 (2011): 371-75; A. Matheson, "How Industry Uses the ICMJE Guidelines to Manipulate Authorship—and How They Should be Revised," *PLoS Medicine* 8 (2011): e1001072.

15. C. Bombardier, et al., and VIGOR Study Group, "Comparison of Upper Gastrointestinal Toxicity of Rofecoxib and Naproxen in Patients with Rheumatoid Arthritis," *New England Journal of Medicine* 343 (2000): 1520-28.

16. Drug Industry Document Archive, Internal Merck documents on the VIGOR trial. For the evolution of company positioning in March 2000, see "Standby Statement—Vioxx and Cardiovascular Events in VIGOR," at http://dida.library.ucsf.edu/pdf/oxx12c10, and "VIGOR Version 6," at http://dida.library.ucsf.edu/pdf/oxx13w10. The journal manuscript was submitted by its academic lead author in May 2000; see cover letter at http://dida.library.ucsf.edu/pdf/oxx01w10. For a similar discussion of VIGOR, see A. Schafer, "The University as Corporate Handmaiden: Who're Ya Gonna Trust?," in *The Universities at Risk: How Politics, Special Interests, and Corporatization Threaten Academic Integrity*, ed. J. Turk (Toronto: James Lorimer and Co., 2008).

17. C. Bombardier et al., "Response to Expression of Concern regarding VIGOR Study," *New England Journal of Medicine* 354 (2006): 1196-99.

18. R. Smith, "Lapses at the New England Journal of Medicine," *Journal of the Royal Society of Medicine* 99 (2006): 380-2; H. M. Krumholz et al., "What Have We Learnt from Vioxx?," *British Medical Journal* 334 (2007): 120-3.

19. See, for instance, Fugh-Berman, "The Haunting of Medical Journals"; Ross et al., "Guest Authorship and Ghostwriting"; Sismondo, "Ghost Management"; L. B. McHenry and J. N. Jureidini, "Industry-Sponsored Ghostwriting in Clinical Trial Reporting: A Case Study," *Accountability in Research* 15 (2008): 152-67.

20. *Oxford Dictionaries* [online], s.v. "ghostwriter," accessed March 22, 2016, http://oxforddictionaries.com/definition/english/ghostwriter?q=ghostwriter; A. Jacobs et al. and European Medical Writers Association's Ghostwriting Task Force, "The Involvement of Professional Medical Writers in Medical Publications: Results of a Delphi Study," *Current Medical Research and Opinion* 21 (2005): 311-16.

21. C. Laine and C. D. Mulrow, "Exorcising Ghosts and Unwelcome Guests," *Annals of Internal Medicine* 143 (2005): 611-12; C. Graf et al., "Research Methods & Reporting: Good Publication Practice for Communicating Company Sponsored Medical Research: The GPP2 Guidelines," *British Medical Journal* 339 (2009): b4330.

22. For example, see X. Bosch, "Treat Ghostwriting as Misconduct," *Nature* 469 (2011): 472.

23. J. S. Wislar et al., "Honorary and Ghost Authorship in High Impact Biomedical Journals: A Cross Sectional Survey," *BMJ* 343 (2011): d6128.

24. Sismondo, "Ghost Management."

25. D. Rennie and A. Flanagin, "Authorship! Authorship! Guests, Ghosts, Grafters, and the Two-Sided Coin," *Journal of the American Medical Association* 271 (1994): 469-71.

26. Matheson, "How Industry Uses the ICMJE Guidelines to Manipulate Authorship—and How They Should Be Revised."

27. N. Macbeth, *Darwin Retried: An Appeal to Reason* (Boston: Harvard Common Press, 1971), 50.

5.6   Authorship Inflation in Medical Publications

Gaurie Tilak, Vinay Prasad, and Annupam B. Jena

Tilak, G, Prasad, V, Jena, AB. Authorship Inflation in Medical Publications. Inquiry: The Journal of Health Care Organization, Provision, and Financing 52, doi: https://doi.org/10.1177/0046958015598311 (2015).© The Author(s) 2015.

Reprinted with permission from Excellus Health Plan, Inc.

Research Letter

Authorship Inflation in Medical Publications

INQUIRY: The Journal of Health Care
Organization, Provision, and Financing
1–4
© The Author(s) 2015
Reprints and permissions:
sagepub.com/journalsPermissions.nav
DOI: 10.1177/0046958015598311
inq.sagepub.com
⑤SAGE

Gaurie Tilak, BA[1], Vinay Prasad, MD, MPH[2],
and Anupam B. Jena, MD, PhD[1]

Abstract

The number of authors per manuscript in peer-reviewed medical journals has increased substantially in the last several decades. Several reasons have been offered to explain this authorship growth, including increased researcher collaboration, honorary authorship driven by increased pressures for funding and promotion, the belief that including senior authors will facilitate publication, and the growing complexity of medical research. It is unknown, however, whether authorship has grown over time due to growing complexity of published academic articles, in which case growth could be warranted, or whether it has grown due to pressures of funding and academic promotion, which have created "authorship inflation." To answer this question, we analyzed data on authorship count, study type, and size of study population for the first 50 original articles published in each decade during 1960-2010 in 3 major medical journals. Within each type of study we considered (eg, randomized trials, observational studies, etc), average authorship rose more than 3-fold during this period. Similar growth persisted after adjustment for changes in study population sizes over time. Our findings suggest that increasing research complexity is an inadequate explanation for authorship growth. Instead, growth in authorship appears inflationary.

Keywords

authorship criteria

Introduction

The number of collaborators credited as study authors in peer-reviewed medical journals has increased substantially over time. As early as 1969, Diamond lamented an "explosion" in multi-authored original articles published in the *New England Journal of Medicine* between 1928 and 1968,[1] during which time single-author publications went from comprising the majority of original articles (78.4%) in 1928 to just a fraction (3.1%) in 1968. In the ensuing decades, several others have noted substantial growth in the number of study authors in medical publications.[2-4] Between 1980 and 2000, for example, the average number of authors per article published in 4 leading medical journals increased 53% (4.5-6.9).[3]

A number of factors have been offered to explain authorship growth, including increased researcher collaboration, honorary authorship (driven by increased pressures for funding and promotion), the belief that including senior authors will facilitate publication, and the growing complexity of medical research.[5-9] For example, in a prior survey of academic radiologists, the most common reason for authors to accept honorary authorship was to hasten promotion, and first authors reported giving honorary authorship to others out of obligation or for repayment.[10] Consistent with these data is survey evidence that the offering of honorary authorship is greatest in those with lower academic rank.[11] Not surprisingly,

based on these concerns, the rise in credited authors has led to efforts by the International Committee of Medical Journal Editors (ICMJE) and journal editors to redefine and clarify requirements for authorship.[6,12]

Growth in authorship counts over time may, however, also be a by-product of growing research complexity. Clinical trials have become larger and more complex, often involving multi-investigator/institutional collaborations. Observational studies too have become larger and more rigorous, requiring greater computational effort and analytic expertise. It is unknown, however, whether changes in research complexity, in particular shifts from observational studies toward clinical trials as well as increased complexity within study designs, can explain long-term increases in authorship numbers. Put differently, has authorship grown over time due to growing complexity of published academic articles, in which case growth would be warranted, or has it grown due to pressures of funding and academic promotion, which have created "authorship inflation?"

[1]Harvard Medical School, Boston, MA, USA
[2]National Institutes of Health, Bethesda, MD, USA

Corresponding Author:
Anupam B. Jena, Harvard Medical School, 180 Longwood Avenue, Boston, MA 02115, USA.
Email: jena@hcp.med.harvard.edu

Table 1. Characteristics of Study Types According to Year of Publishing.

Study type (n, % of total in year)	Year					
	1960	1970	1980	1990	2000	2010
Single-center RCT	2 (1.3)	9 (6.0)	11 (7.3)	15 (10.0)	21 (14.0)	12 (8.0)
Multi-center RCT	3 (2.0)	2 (1.3)	2 (1.3)	7 (4.7)	22 (14.7)	37 (24.7)
Observational study	145 (96.7)	137 (91.3)	132 (88.0)	119 (79.3)	96 (64.0)	80 (53.3)
Decision analysis/cost-effectiveness	0 (0)	0 (0)	2 (1.3)	7 (4.7)	8 (5.3)	5 (3.3)
Meta-analysis	0 (0)	2 (1.3)	3 (2)	2 (1.3)	3 (2.0)	16 (10.7)
Total	150	150	150	150	150	150

Note. RCT = randomized controlled trial.

Methods

We assembled data on authorship count, study type, and size of study population for the first 50 original articles published in each decade during 1960-2010 in the *Journal of the American Medical Association*, the *New England Journal of Medicine*, and the *British Medical Journal*. Studies were categorized as observational, single-center randomized controlled trial (RCT), multi-center RCT, meta-analysis, or cost-effectiveness/decision analysis. Studies with a group authorship name in the author byline were excluded. We computed the mean number of authors per article in each year. We accounted for changes over time in overall research complexity in two ways. First, we analyzed authorship growth *within* each study type. For example, demonstrating growth in authorship count within each study type could suggest a diffuse inflationary process such as growing pressure to publish and include honorary authors, or alternatively, it could suggest growing complexity within study types (eg, observational studies, meta-analyses, or cost-effectiveness analyses could simply be growing more complicated over time). To account for this second possibility, we used size of the study population (eg, the number of patients in a study) as a proxy for the complexity of research design for a given publication. We estimated publication-level linear regression models of authorship number as a function of publication year and study population size. We then reported trends in average authorship counts within each study type, adjusting for growing study population sizes over time.

Results

Study type changed dramatically over the period we examined; observational studies accounted for 96.7% (145/150) of studies in 1960, but only 53.3% (80/150) in 2010. By 2010, multi-center and single-center RCTs accounted for 8.0% and 24.7% of all studies, respectively (see Table 1). Within *each* study type, average authorship rose more than 3-fold and trends were unaffected by adjustment for changes in study population sizes (see Table 2). The increase was greatest in observational studies; for example, from 1960 to 2010, average authorship

in observational studies increased from 2.6 to 10.1 authors per study (unadjusted absolute increase 7.5, $P < .001$; adjusted absolute increase 7.4, $P < .001$). Restricted to a more recent time range from 1990 to 2010, increases in average authorship continued to be observed in multi-center RCTs, observational studies, and decision analysis/cost-effectiveness studies ($P < .01$ for average authorship in 2010 vs 1990, in each study type).

Discussion

Our findings suggest that credited authorship has grown significantly and likely reflects inflationary growth rather than growth warranted due to increasing research complexity. Within study types and adjusting for size of the study population in each publication, the average number of authors per publication in high-impact medical journals increased dramatically in the last 5 decades. For multi-center clinical trials in particular, it could be argued that participating physicians may only be able to enroll a few patients and thus larger modern trials may require more authors. Two things should be noted, however. First, our results do not validate this hypothesis, as authorship has grown even after adjustment for rising sizes of study populations. Second, and most importantly, simply recruiting patients to a trial does not constitute appropriate criteria for authorship, and is not recognized as criteria for authorship by the ICMJE.[13]

Although it is possible that adjusting for the size of the study population may not fully capture the growing complexity of randomized trials or observational studies, within studies of cost-effectiveness/decision analysis, the average number of authors also increased considerably, from 3.7 in 1990 and 9.6 in 2010. Put together, these findings raise the question of whether increasing research complexity and the shift toward clinical trials can substantively explain authorship inflation. Furthermore, one might contend that, if anything, the increasing importance and power of computerized data analysis would decrease the need for multiple authors in observational studies and cost-effectiveness/decision analyses. Instead, our results suggest precisely the opposite trend in medicine. Our findings therefore support the view that

Table 2. Trends in Authorship According to Study Design.

Study type	Mean no. of authors per article by year and change compared with the baseline year					
	1960	1970	1980	1990	2000	2010
Single-center RCT	3.5	3.3	4.8	11.3	7.0	9.3
Unadjusted difference compared with 1960 (*P* value)		−0.2 (.95)	1.3 (.63)	7.8 (.05)	3.5 (.18)	5.8 (.04)
Adjusted difference compared with 1960 (*P* value)		−0.1 (.96)	1.3 (.63)	5.0 (.05)	3.6 (.18)	5.8 (.03)
Multi-center RCT	5.3	4.5	6.0	8.3	9.1	14.0
Unadjusted difference compared with 1960 (*P* value)		−0.8 (.88)	0.7 (.54)	3.0 (.43)	3.8 (.32)	8.7 (.02)
Adjusted difference compared with 1960 (*P* value)		−0.6 (.92)	0.6 (.52)	2.7 (.59)	3.5 (.39)	8.4 (.03)
Observational study	2.6	3.3	3.9	5.6	7.1	10.1
Unadjusted difference compared with 1960 (*P* value)		0.7 (.17)	1.3 (.01)	3.0 (<.001)	4.5 (<.001)	7.5 (<.001)
Adjusted difference compared with 1960 (*P* value)		0.6 (.14)	1.2 (.01)	2.9 (<.001)	4.4 (<.001)	7.4 (<.001)
Decision analysis/cost-effectiveness	NA	NA	2.5	3.7	4.6	9.6
Unadjusted difference compared with 1980 (*P* value)				1.2 (.68)	2.1 (.48)	7.1 (.03)
Adjusted difference compared with 1980 (*P* value)				1.5 (.61)	2.4 (.43)	8.5 (.02)
Meta-analysis	NA	6.0	1.7	4.0	4.0	5.9
Unadjusted difference compared with 1970 (*P* value)			−4.3 (.17)	−2.0 (.55)	−2.0 (.55)	−0.1 (.96)
Adjusted difference compared with 1970 (*P* value)			−4.3 (.15)	−2.0 (.54)	−2.0 (.54)	−0.2 (.93)

Note. The table reports average unadjusted number of authors per article published in each decade from 1960 to 2010, by study type. It also reports unadjusted difference in the average number of authors per article between the baseline year (1960 in most instances) and subsequent years, as well as adjusted differences estimated from publication-level multivariate linear regression of the number of authors as a function of year indicator variables and sample size of each publication. NA implies no articles of a given study type existed in our sample in that year. RCT = randomized controlled trial.

authorship growth may be inflationary, a result of increased pressures for funding and promotion, as well as the perception that the inclusion of additional senior authors may hasten publication.[5-9]

There are limitations to our analysis. Most importantly, we cannot definitively conclude that the average contribution of authors to manuscripts has declined over time, as other confounding factors may have changed. For example, our approach may not fully account for other sources of increasing research complexity such as new analytic techniques (laboratory or statistical) or the growing need to recruit patients from multiple study sites. Our results may also underestimate authorship inflation in other journals with less stringent authorship requirements than the journals we considered. A small degree of authorship inflation may also simply reflect the desire of established researchers to involve students and trainees in small components of research, with the goal of promoting interest in research. This explanation, although still perhaps inconsistent with recognized authorship criteria, has different implications than authorship inflation for the sole purpose of promotion or obtaining funding.

In summary, the average number of authors per publication in leading medical journals has grown dramatically in the last five decades. Increasing effort required to analyze and publish research is unlikely to be an adequate explanation. Instead, authorship "inflation" due to increasing academic pressure to publish, combined with a relative paucity of incentives to authors to reduce multiple-authorship, appears more consistent with the observed data. Authorship

inflation has continued despite efforts of the ICMJE and journal editors to curb inappropriate authorship. Given the importance of authorship accountability, continued efforts should be made to address this issue.

Declaration of Conflicting Interests

The author(s) declared no potential conflicts of interest with respect to the research, authorship, and/or publication of this article.

Funding

The author(s) disclosed receipt of the following financial support for the research, authorship, and/or publication of this article: Funding was provided by the Office of the Director, National Institutes of Health (NIH Early Independence Award, grant 1DP5OD017897-01).

References

1. Diamond D. Multi-authorship explosion. *N Engl J Med.* 1969;280:1484-1485.
2. Sobal J, Ferentz KS. Abstract creep and author inflation. *N Engl J Med.* 1990;323:488-489.
3. Weeks WB, Wallace AE, Kimberly BC. Changes in authorship patterns in prestigious US medical journals. *Soc Sci Med.* 2004;59:1949-1954.
4. Levsky ME, Rosin A, Coon TP, Enslow WL, Miller MA. A descriptive analysis of authorship within medical journals, 1995-2005. *South Med J.* 2007;100:371-375.
5. Probyn LJ, Asch MR, Proto AV. The effect of changes in guidelines for authorship on current radiology publications. *Radiology.* 2000;215:615-616.

6. Rennie D, Yank V, Emanuel L. When authorship fails. A proposal to make contributors accountable. *JAMA*. 1997;278: 579-585.

7. Levsky ME, Rosin A, Coon TP, Enslow WL, Miller MA. A descriptive analysis of authorship within medical journals, 1995-2005. *South Med J*. 2007;100:371-375.

8. Rennie D, Flanagin A. Authorship! authorship! guests, ghosts, grafters, and the two-sided coin. *JAMA*. 1994;271:469-471.

9. Berquist TH. Authorship creep: do we need a new process. *Am J Roentgenol*. 2009;193:599-600.

10. Slone RM. Coauthors' contributions to major papers published in the AJR: frequency of undeserved coauthorship. *Am J Roentgenol*. 1996;167:571-579.

11. Eisenberg RL, Ngo L, Boiselle PM, Bankier AA. Honorary authorship in radiologic research articles: assessment of frequency and associated factors. *Radiology*. 2011;259:479-486.

12. Kassirer JP, Angell M. On authorship and acknowledgments. *N Engl J Med*. 1991;325:1510-1512.

13. Guidelines on authorship. International Committee of Medical Journal Editors. *Br Med J* (Clin Res Ed) 1985;291:722.

References

Kennedy M, Barnsteiner J, Daly J. Honorary and ghost authorship in nursing publications. J Nurs Scholarsh. 2014;46:416–22.

Matheson A. The ICMJE Recommendations and pharmaceutical marketing – strengths, weaknesses and the unsolved problem of attribution in publication ethics. BMC Med Ethics. 2016;17:20.

Oermann M, Conklin J, Nicholl L, Chinn P, Ashton K, Edie A, Amarasekara S, Budinger S. Study of predatory open access nursing journals. J Nurs Scholarsh. 2016;48:624–32.

Seeman J, House M. Authorship issues and conflict in the U.S. academic chemical community. Account Res. 2015;22:346–83.

Additional Suggested Reading

Carmichael K, Nolan S, Weston J, Smith C, Marson A. Assessment of the quality of harms reporting in non-randomised studies and randomised controlled studies of topiramate for the treatment of epilepsy using CONSORT criteria. Epilepsy Res. 2015;114:106–113.

Eriksson S, Helgesson G. The false academy: predatory publishing in science and bioethics. Med Health Care Philos. 2017;20:163–70.

Mentor-Mentee Responsibilities and Relationships

6

Arthur L. Caplan and Barbara K. Redman

Research training has historically followed an apprentice model, informal, minimally structured, and idiosyncratic. Adequate mentoring has been defined by the mentor and frequently derived from how the mentor has traditionally behaved with prior students. Mentees have sometimes been seen as simply ready labor for mentor projects.

More recently, mentoring in research is being defined as a skill set that should support mentee learning. Most research on this relationship has focused on student persistence and productivity in a course of study, not on learning research integrity or behaving with integrity. Overall, few metrics exist to assess the effectiveness of mentoring though some US federally funded training grants require a mentoring plan. Most research regulations, such as those for misconduct, do not mention mentor roles or responsibilities.

Many mentor-mentee relationships are highly positive partnerships that add benefit to both parties. Mentees bring new ideas; mentors help them to think independently, include mentees in professional networks, and foster their careers. Because this relationship has largely been minimally structured, it is important to agree on issues such as authorship, credit, access to and ownership of data, commitments for space, funding and workload, and to put these agreements in writing in a formal mentoring plan. Should a mentor or mentee move or become dissatisfied, it is important to also agree on how such situations will be managed.

Mentors can be very powerful, especially in historically hierarchical cultures in science where students may be expected to provide unquestioning loyalty to the mentor. In highly competitive environments, the needs of mentors and mentees can conflict, thus the importance of the written agreement of conditions for working together. Conflicts should be resolved by institutional officers such as department chairs or directors of graduate study.

The mentor-mentee relationship is a prime source of instruction about research integrity, learned through everyday interactions in the practice of science and is an essential experiential part of the responsible conduct of research (RCR). Mentees should feel free to ask mentors about their experience with misconduct, fraud, authorship, and related issues.

Advice: Carefully check out a proposed mentor, especially by talking with prior mentees about the quality of their experience. Many funders require a mentoring plan; ask for one even if your funder doesn't require it. Know the director of graduate study in your department, who should be checking on the quality of your experience with your mentor. Set regular meetings with your mentor asking for your work to be evaluated and to resolve any emerging issues. Harassment or bullying should not be tolerated and should be reported either to your schools HR department, director of graduate or professional studies, or both.

A. L. Caplan · B. K. Redman (✉)
New York University Langone Medical Center,
New York, NY, USA
e-mail: Arthur.Caplan@nyumc.org

© Springer International Publishing AG, part of Springer Nature 2018
A. L. Caplan, B. K. Redman (eds.), *Getting to Good*, https://doi.org/10.1007/978-3-319-51358-4_6

6.1   Closing the Barn Door: Coping with Findings of Research Misconduct by Trainees in the Biomedical Sciences

Barbara K. Redman and Arthur L. Caplan

Redman, B, Caplan, A. Closing the barn door: Coping with findings of research misconduct by trainees in the biomedical sciences. *Research Ethics* 11(3), 124–132 (2015). © The Author(s) 2015.

Article

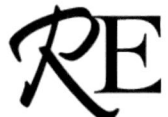

Research Ethics
2015, Vol. 11(3) 124–132
© The Author(s) 2015
Reprints and permissions:
sagepub.co.uk/journalsPermissions.nav
DOI: 10.1177/1747016115587157
rea.sagepub.com
$SAGE

Closing the barn door: Coping with findings of research misconduct by trainees in the biomedical sciences

Barbara K Redman
New York University Langone Medical Center, USA

Arthur L Caplan
New York University Langone Medical Center, USA

Abstract

The proportion of research misconduct cases among trainees in the biomedical sciences has risen, raising the question of why, and what are the responsibilities of research administrators and the research community to address this problem. Although there is no definitive research about causes, for trainees the relationship with a research mentor should play a major role in preventing actions that constitute research misconduct (fabrication, falsification and plagiarism). Examination of the limited literature and of the number of cases closed by the US Office of Research Integrity (ORI) between 2009 and 2013 raises questions about the mentor-student relationship and what it should be accomplishing. But many gaps in policy and its implementation inhibit this role. There is no acknowledgement of mentorship in federal regulations and research on how to teach research integrity is woefully underdeveloped, especially for international trainees. And some institutional research integrity officers may have had little preparation for the role.

Keywords
ethical review, graduate students, research misconduct

Corresponding author:

Barbara K Redman, Associate, Division of Medical Ethics, New York University Langone Medical Center, 227 East 30th Street, #753, New York, NY 10016, USA.
Email: br68@nyu.edu

Introduction

Cases of research misconduct (RM) continue unabated around the world. In the US, ORI reports new allegations rising from 86 in 1993 to 154 in 2012 (Office of Research Integrity [ORI], 2012). Others recently reported include lack of acknowledgement in the peer reviewed literature of findings by the FDA of fabricated and/or falsified data (Seife, 2015). The ongoing parade of misconduct raises questions about why researchers, students and staff falsify, fabricate and plagiarize and how these actions might be prevented. This paper suggests that re-examination of information about graduate students committing research misconduct is necessary. It also suggests actions that can be taken to ameliorate the situation.

In the years 2009 to 2013, 26 of the 56 cases of research misconduct reported in the US Office of Research Integrity (ORI) newsletter involved graduate trainees including postdocs and medical residents. This figure is up from 30% for cases between 1990 and 2004 (Wright et al., 2008).

For having intentionally fabricated and/or falsified data or plagiarized in Public Health Service (PHS)-supported research, these individuals entered into agreements to be excluded from serving in any advisory capacity to PHS and frequently to be excluded from contracting or subcontracting with an agency of the US government for a period of two to five years. Sixteen of the 26 were also required to have an ORI-approved plan for supervision of any subsequent PHS research prior to any future application submission. For 10 of the 16, their employing institutions had to certify to ORI that data provided by these individuals were legitimate.

These statistics raise several questions. Why are trainees such a large proportion of cases? Are they reported more frequently than are scientists in the professorial ranks? Is their misconduct related to immaturity in learning scientific norms or to pressures to succeed or both? Are their mentors lax in reviewing source data and setting standards? Wright et al. (2008) found these mentoring problems in three-fourths and two-thirds respectively of trainee cases closed by ORI prior to 2005.

Although there is no definitive research about the problem, research misconduct may occur because of: 1) sociopathology, 2) increasing pressure on researchers, 3) ignorance of research standards and ethical norms or some combination of these causes (Wright et al., 2008). Some argue misconduct is behavior confined to a few bad apples. An implicit assumption in the bad apple explanation is that sociopathology, or just not being able to "cut it", are the sources of the problem.

The research mentor-trainee relationship should moderate pressure and assure that research standards and ethical norms are taught and learned. But in the US federal research misconduct regulations there is no definition of the responsibilities of the research mentor and no requirement regarding mentoring (Wright et al.,

2008), leaving little direction for what actions and outcomes are expected of mentors. (Mentors are faculty supervisors employed by the university that will award the research degree and are assigned to guide graduate students through the research process. Other terms for this role may be used in other countries.) In addition, scholarship regarding researcher moral development or the efficacy of research integrity teaching is woefully underdeveloped (Evans, 2011).

Since 1989, NIH has required trainee instruction in responsible conduct of research (RCR). RCR training is required only of those supported on NIH training mechanisms. Even among top-funded US institutions, only half require RCR training of all students (Resnik and Dinse, 2012).

Despite this investment, little is known about what works (Mazmanian et al., 2014; Kalichman, 2013). A summary of the few available studies suggests that current RCR instruction is largely ineffective and in some cases may be harmful, deriving from student avoidance of ethical problems or overconfidence in their ability to handle them (Antes et al., 2009).

As a strategy for economic competitiveness, many countries are heavily investing in PhD education in science and technology (Mulvany, 2013). Among the large number of international trainees in the US, many are first introduced to research practice in their home countries and are bewildered by US expectations for RCR. These authors have also found international trainees to be less likely to accept US norms than are their US-trained counterparts. The normalcy of plagiarism in many international environments, vague policies about what constitutes plagiarism, and difficulty writing in English (Heitman and Litewka, 2011) may put them and their mentors at risk of misconduct.

In addition to the usual sanctions in a finding of research misconduct, ORI's requirements for supervision and in some instances certification of trainees' subsequent work are likely meant to provide them with guidance and oversight to develop the research skills and integrity they need. Current regulations target the actions of FFP after they occur, without regard for the developmental situation of trainees or the institutional environment in which they are operating. But this is "shutting the barn door after the horse is gone." A whistleblower, sometimes the mentor, has already reported evidence of fabrication and/or falsification or plagiarism. Federal misconduct regulations or institutions themselves ought to require some prospective monitoring of or outreach to trainees.

Trainees surely should expect to receive guidance and mentorship in practicing research ethics. If they are found to have "intentionally, knowingly or recklessly" (42 CFR, Part 93.104) committed research misconduct, it is reasonable to ask what went wrong in their development. Research administrators follow institutional policy for handling allegations and investigations. But policy as 42CFR, Part 90, section 93.300 does not address responsibilities that educational institutions assume for the development of the ethics of students.

Doctoral students

While PhD education should be the primary locus of socialization into research ethics, there is almost no literature about how successfully that is accomplished. A survey from Norway of PhD students in all of that country's medical faculties found that "10% did not find it inappropriate to report experimental data without having conducted the experiment; 38% did not find it inappropriate to try a variety of different methods of analysis to find a statistically significant result; 13% agreed that it is acceptable to selectively omit contradictory results to expedite publication; and 10% found it acceptable to falsify or fabricate data to expedite publication", although no participants reported they had fabricated, falsified or plagiarized data or publications (Hofmann et al., 2013: 1).

A smaller Swedish study found that students reported that they had experienced exploitation by being asked by their mentors to do work not related to their doctoral studies, abuse through public humiliation, and had their ideas and/or data misappropriated (Lofstrom and Pyhalto, 2014).

But perhaps the ultimate occurred with a group of doctoral students at the University of Wisconsin who reported their advisor for research misconduct, which she was found to have committed. One of those students describes the losses as including a mentor without a lab, many research projects never published, and students being advised to find a new laboratory home and start over on a new project. Those students now worry whether their roles as whistleblowers will affect their hireability (Allen and Dowell, 2013). Whistleblower protection policies assume threat to employment and do not address the educational impact on students when they act as whistleblowers. This must be explicitly addressed at institutions which host students. Also to be addressed is the university's responsibility in helping students in such a situation to finish a degree.

With one exception the PhD students in the current study, among those found to have committed research misconduct between 2009 and 2013, ceased publishing (as documented in Pub Med), although those found in later years of this period may yet regain the ability to publish. It's as if they simply vanished.

Postdocs

About half of biomedical postdoctoral fellows in the US are temporary residents, many of whom received PhD training outside the US (Ghaffarzadegan et al., 2014). Many are supported by research assistantships from NIH funds, which provide the institution with 50% indirects but on which they may not receive the documented formal and informal mentorship that is required of NIH-sponsored training grants, which yield 5% indirects. Such training grants require mentor plans and are judged by the quality of the mentor's training record and prior trainee outcomes (Rockey, 2014).

This constitutes a perverse incentive in US policy, largely benefiting senior researchers who depend on large numbers of graduate students and postdocs, well beyond the number who will find jobs (Stephan, 2012; Rockey, 2014). Indeed, a study of mentors affiliated with the Clinical and Translational Science Award (CTSA) program found 39% with four or more CTSA mentees, with most having additional non-CTSA mentees (Miyaoka et al., 2011), raising a question of mentor capacity.

Out of the 26 student cases settled by ORI between 2009 and 2013, 14 already held PhDs, and the misconduct was identified during the postdoctoral training (54% of student cases). One would expect such individuals to have been socialized to RCR during their PhD programs. Through publication records, four were verified as coming from a foreign country for a US postdoc and returning to their country of origin after the finding of misconduct (China, India, Japan), continuing to publish. Two others had been publishing from their country of origin prior to the US postdoc (China, Korea); recent publications show they are now working in US institutions. Japan also has suffered from multiple egregious cases of research misconduct, indicating a lack of research oversight and cultural reluctance to act on suspicions of peers (Agency for change, 2014; Normile, 2014). Many others could not be tracked because their publication records stopped or they could not be identified.

It is important to note that the major country supplying the US student or workforce in biology and other fields (17%) is China; the second is India (Franzon et al., 2012). Both countries have serious local problems with research misconduct. Conservative estimates indicate that a third of Chinese researchers have engaged in practices that include data fabrication and plagiarism (Cao, 2014). China has been very successful at recruiting overseas Chinese-born scientists back to their country of origin (Xie et al., 2014), raising the question of whether findings of RM in a US postdoc have any impact on a subsequent scientific career back in the homeland. India has no specific laws pertaining to scientific fraud. In a small study of medical colleges and hospitals, 56% of questionnaire respondents reported knowledge of alteration or fabrication of research data (Dhingra and Mishra, 2014). The rate reported largely in the US and UK summarized in a systematic review was 14% (Fanelli, 2009).

Role of the research administrator

Institutions receiving federal research funds must manage a number of regulatory requirements including protection of human and animal subjects, financial conflict of interest, biological risks. Among these regulations, in place since 1989, are those requiring assurance that policies and procedures are in place conforming to 42 CFR 93 to investigate allegations of research misconduct, defined as fabrication and/or falsification and/or plagiarism. The institutional official, the Research Integrity Officer (RIO), administers these policies and procedures.

Although every institution with an assurance of compliance must name a RIO, the role is not delineated in the federal regulations. Two studies have found that in the aggregate, preparation for the role is rare, most have handled few cases, and many RIOs report inconsistent legal and logistical support (Wright and Schneider, 2010). When compared with responses of expert RIOs to usual research misconduct situations (sequestering evidence, threat of retaliation, and coordination of responsibilities with the institutional review board), many RIOs did not demonstrate a high level of skill (Bonito et al., 2012).

What are our responsibilities as a research community?

It is clear that system-wide reforms are necessary. Leshner (2012) notes there is far too much variability in training for the 50,000 postdocs in the US. Calls a decade ago to establish standards, norms and expectations for mentors, mentees and their institutions have still not been addressed (Leshner, 2012). Alberts, Kirschner, Tilghman and Varmus (2014) note that the severe imbalance between limited funds available for research and the still-growing numbers of researchers and personnel in the scientific community in the US have created a hypercompetitive atmosphere, which can heavily influence the integrity of graduate students and postdocs. Devereaux (2014) describes the growing gap between scientific ideals and the institutional reward system (e.g. science asks for collaboration and openness but rewards competition and "getting there first"). Yet, despite a more perilous environment, next to nothing is known about how to educate to reduce misconduct.

Even in the absence of reforms in the broader governance of science, institutions can adopt policies aimed at preventing research misconduct among graduate students and can evaluate them to see if they are effective. First, accountable mentoring must be assured, undergirded by mandatory and effective RCR education tailored specifically to graduate students. Particular attention must be paid to at-risk non-English speaking groups and those from countries with research ethics standards discrepant from those expected in the host country.

Mentors should receive training for their roles and be expected to review source data and set standards (Wright et al., 2008), and these expectations should be built into the institution's code of conduct for faculty employment. Investigations of misconduct allegations against a student should require an accounting of the mentor's activities in carrying out these duties. And NIH policy should require all students supported by NIH grants (whether research or training grants) to be assigned an accountable mentor.

Students in training programs have described mentor pressure to behave unethically. A survey of the MD Anderson Cancer Center found a third of student respondents feeling pressure to prove the mentor's hypothesis, even if the trainee's data did not support it. Twenty percent of students reporting in this survey said they had been pressured to publish findings about which they had doubts (Mobley et al., 2013). And an Australian survey found student criticism that university academic integrity policy was not enforced (Mahmud and Bretag, 2014). These kinds of experiences/perceptions can undo any RCR program.

RCR education should incorporate these and other concerns of doctoral and postdoctoral students. Their roles as beginners make them vulnerable to uncertainties about correct courses of action in situations they will encounter and dubious about the consequences of acting on their judgments, especially against authority figures. And as a condition of accepting graduate students, including postdocs from non-English-speaking countries, institutions must seek to improve their writing of English manuscripts, to a documented standard of acceptability, and provide help in teaching how to express their ideas without being tempted to, or even out of respect, plagiarize. In general, guidance on effective research ethics for international trainees and US trainees in international research settings has been vague and irregular (Heitman and Litewka, 2011).

As typically conducted, much RCR is not especially effective. It is important for institutions to adopt models shown to be more effective to obtain the best outcomes for the investment. The most successful programs are case-based and interactive, requiring practice in identifying ethical issues and strategies for working through problems (Antes et al., 2010). Nedeker (2014) recommends actively engaging students with role-play, debate and use of authentic examples and formative evaluation during instruction. Mumford, Steele and Watts (2015) suggest evaluation of RCR programs in four areas: behavior, cognition, reaction and institutional outcomes, and review measures available to do so.

The scientific community and individual institutions are not doing what is needed to discourage misconduct among young investigators. Education and mentoring clearly have important roles to play but how and with what accountability remain unclear. What is clear is that focusing on punishment is not the best route to discourage unethical conduct.

Conclusion

Ongoing issues with research misconduct among trainees in the biomedical sciences require action by research training institutions and by the scientific community. The absence of federal regulations addressing responsible mentoring and lack of a research base for education in the responsible conduct of research constitute gaps in our knowledge. But development of best practices that are evidence-based can and should be undertaken by individual institutions and/or by consortia of research institutions. Accountable mentoring and effective RCR are basic. Graduate students operating in a hypercompetitive, hierarchical environment with a widening gap between scientific ideals and everyday practice are vulnerable. This is especially the case if they are not fluent in English and have been educated in a culture whose standards are not congruent with those in the host country.

The ultimate test of more rigorous standards will be a decrease in the percentage of research misconduct cases in students and their satisfaction that they have been supported in attaining scientific integrity.

Funding

This research received no specific grant from any funding agency in the public, commercial, or not-for-profit sectors.

References

Agency for change [editorial] (2014) *Nature* 509(7498), 30 April. Available at: http://www.nature.com/news/agency-for-change-1.15120 (accessed 8 May 2015).

Alberts B, Kirschner MW, Tilghman S and Varmus H (2014) Rescuing US biomedical research from its systemic flaws. *Proceedings of the National Academy of Science* 111(16): 5773–5777.

Allen M and Dowell R (2013) Retrospective reflections of a whistleblower: Opinions on misconduct responses. *Accountability in Research* 20: 339–348.

Antes AL, Murphy ST, Waples EP, Mumford MS, Brown RP, Connelly S and Davenport LB (2009) A meta-analysis of ethics instruction effectiveness in the sciences. *Ethics and Behavior* 19(5): 379–402.

Antes AL, Wang X, Mumford MD, Brown RP, Connelly S and Davenport LD (2010) Evaluating the effects that existing instruction on responsible conduct of research has on ethical decision making. *Academic Medicine* 85: 519–526.

Bonito AJ, Titus SL and Wright DE (2012) Assessing the preparedness of research integrity officers (RIOs) to appropriately handle possible research misconduct cases. *Science & Engineering Ethics* 18: 605–619.

Cao C (2014) The universal values of science and China's Nobel Prize pursuit. *Minerva* 52: 141–160.

Devereaux ML (2014) Rethinking the meaning of ethics in RCR education. *Journal of Microbiology & Biology Education* 15(2): 165–168.

Dhingra D and Mishra D (2014) Publication misconduct among medical professionals in India. *Indian Journal of Medical Ethics* 11: 104–107.

Evans L (2011) What research administrators need to know about researcher development: Towards a new conceptual model. *Journal of Research Administration* 42: 15–37.

Fanelli D (2009) How many scientists fabricate and falsify research? A systematic review and meta-analysis of survey data. *PLoS One* 4(5): e5738.

Franzon C, Scellato G and Stephan P (2012) Foreign-born scientists: Mobility patterns for 16 countries. *Nature Biotechnology* 30: 1250–1253.

Ghaffarzadegan N, Hawley J and Desai A (2014) Research workforce diversity: The case of balancing national versus international postdocs in US biomedical research. *Systems Research & Behavioral Science* 31: 301–315.

Heitman E and Litewka S (2011) International perspectives on plagiarism and considerations for teaching international trainees. *Urologic Oncology* 29: 104–108.

Hofmann B, Myhr AI and Holm S (2013) Scientific dishonesty: A nationwide survey of doctoral students in Norway. *BMC Medical Ethics* 14(3).

Kalichman M (2013) A brief history of RCR education. *Accountability in Research* 20: 380–394.

Leshner AI (2012) Standards for postdoc training. *Science* 336: 276.

Lofstrom E and Pyhalto K (2014) Ethical issues in doctoral supervision: The perspectives of PhD students in the natural and behavioral sciences. *Ethics & Behavior* 24(3): 195–214.

Mahmud S and Bretag T (2014) Integrity in postgraduate research: The student voice. *Science & Engineering Ethics*. Available at: http://link.springer.com/article/10.1007%2Fs11948-014-9616-y (accessed 8 May 2015).

Mazmanian PE, Coe AB, Evans JA, Longo DR and Wright BA (2014) Are researcher development interventions, alone or in any combination, effective in improving researcher behavior? A systematic review. *Evaluation and the Health Professions* 37: 114–139.

Miyaoka A, Spiegelman M, Paue K and Frechtling J (2011) Findings from the CTSA National Evaluation Education and Training Study. Westatt Reports.Westat, Rockville, MD.

Mobley A, Linder SK, Braever R, Ellis LM and Zwelling L (2013) A survey on data reproducibility in cancer medicine provides insight into our limited ability to translate findings from the laboratory to the clinic. *PLoS One* 8(5): e63221.

Mulvany MJ (2013) Biomedical PhD education: An international perspective. *Basic & Clinical Pharmacology & Technology* 112: 289–295.

Mumford MD, Steele L and Watts LL (2015) Evaluating ethics education programs: A multilevel approach. *Ethics & Behavior* 25: 37–60.

Nedeker C (2014) Smart teaching matters! Applying the research on learning to teaching RCR. *Journal of Microbiology & Biology Education* 15(2): 88–92.

Normile D (2014) Faulty drug trials tarnish Japan's clinical research. *Science* 345(6192): 17.

Office of Research Integrity Newsletter (2012) https://ori.hhs.gov/newsletters.

Resnik DB and Dinse GGE (2012) Do US research institutions meet or exceed federal requirements for instruction in responsible conduct of research? A national survey. *Academic Medicine* 87: 1237–1242.

Rockey SJ (2014) Mentorship matters for the biomedical workforce. *Nature Medicine* 20: 575.

Seife C (2015) Research misconduct identified by the US Food and Drug Administration: Out of sight, out of mind, out of the peer-reviewed literature. *JAMA Internal Medicine*. Available at: http://archinte.jamanetwork.com/article.aspx?articleid=2109855 (accessed 8 May 2015).

Stephan P (2012) Research efficiency: Perverse incentives. *Nature* 484: 29–31.

Wright DE and Schneider PF (2010) Training the research integrity officers (RIOs): The federally funded "RIO Boot Camps" backward design to train for the future. *Journal of Research Administration* 41(3): 99–117.

Wright DE, Titus SL and Cornelison JB (2008) Mentoring and research misconduct: An analysis of research mentoring in closed ORI cases. *Science & Engineering Ethics* 14: 323–336.

Xie Y, Zhang C and Lai Q (2014) China's rise as a major contributor to science and technology. *Proceedings of the National Academy of Science* 111(26): 9437–9442.

6.2 Mentoring and Research Misconduct: Analysis of Research Mentoring in Closed ORI Cases

David E. Wright, Sandra L. Titus, and Jered B. Cornelison

Wright, D, Titus, S. Mentoring and research misconduct: analysis of research mentoring in closed ORI cases. *Science & Engineering Ethics* 14(3), 323–336 (2006). © Springer Science+Business Media B.V. 2008. An imprint of Springer/ Nature.

Sci Eng Ethics (2008) 14:323–336
DOI 10.1007/s11948-008-9074-5

ORIGINAL PAPER

Mentoring and Research Misconduct: An Analysis of Research Mentoring in Closed ORI Cases

David E. Wright · Sandra L. Titus · Jered B. Cornelison

Received: 21 October 2007 / Accepted: 28 May 2008 / Published online: 10 July 2008
© Springer Science+Business Media B.V. 2008

Abstract   We are reporting on how involved the mentor was in promoting responsible research in cases of research misconduct. We reviewed the USPHS misconduct files of the Office of Research Integrity. These files are created by Institutions who prosecute a case of possible research misconduct; ORI has oversight review of these investigations. We explored the role of the mentor in the cases of trainee research misconduct on three specific behaviors that we believe mentors should perform with their trainee: (1) review source data, (2) teach specific research standards and (3) minimize stressful work situations. We found that almost three quarters of the mentors had not reviewed the source data and two thirds had not set standards. These two behaviors are positively correlated. We did not see convincing evidence in the records that mentors were causing stress, but it was apparent in the convicted trainees' confessions that over 50% experienced some kind of stress. Secondary data, while not created for this research purpose, allows us to look at concrete research behaviors that are otherwise not very researchable. We believe it is important for mentors and institutions to devote more attention to teaching

The views expressed herein represent those of the authors and do not necessarily represent the views of Michigan State University or the position of the Office of Research Integrity (ORI), the Department of Health and Human Services, or any component therein.

D. E. Wright
CARRS, Michigan State University, 135 Natural Resources Building, East Lansing, MI 48824, USA
e-mail: dewrite@msu.edu

S. L. Titus (✉)
Intramural Research, ORI, 1101 Wootton Parkway, Suite 750, Rockville, MD 20853, USA
e-mail: sandra.titus@hhs.gov

J. B. Cornelison
Department of Anthropology, Michigan State University, 204 Olds Hall, East Lansing, MI 48824, USA
e-mail: cornel24@msu.edu

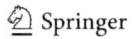 Springer

mentors about the process of education and their responsibilities in educating the next generation of scientists. This becomes a critical issue for large research groups who need to determine who is in charge educating, supervising and assuring data integrity.

Keywords   Research misconduct · Research mentoring · Supervision · Opportunity theory · Mentor · Trainee

Professor Eugene Braunwald, the head of the Cardiac Research Laboratory at Brigham & Women's Hospital, a teaching and research affiliate of Harvard Medical School, considered Dr. John Roland Darsee the most remarkable of the 130 fellows who had worked at the lab; he offered Dr. Darsee a faculty position at Harvard [1–3]. Indeed Dr. Darsee was to all appearances a rapidly rising star who, by 1981, had already published over 100 papers and abstracts—at Harvard (1979–1981) and in his previous position at Emory University (1974–1979). But then, fellow researchers who had suspected him of misconduct for some time observed him labeling the same data from one experiment "24 s," "72 h," "1 week," and "2 weeks," and reported him.

Dr. Darsee admitted to this instance of fabricating data, but claimed it was a unique error caused by extreme time-pressure. His mentors and the University were subsequently criticized as slow to realize the extent of the problem and to mount an effective investigation. When finally completed, however, formal investigation revealed the startling magnitude of Darsee's misconduct. Institutional and government investigators determined that he had "fabricated research publications beginning when he was a biology student at Notre Dame, continuing through his medical residency and cardiology fellowship at Emory University, and ending in Braunwald's Cardiology Lab at Harvard. More than 10 primary journal articles and more than 45 abstracts were retracted as a result of the investigations" [4].

The Darsee case challenged the widely shared beliefs that scientific research is honest and self-correcting with embarrassing questions about the diligence of his mentors and his co-authors. "A total of 47 medical researchers—24 from Emory and 23 from Harvard—coauthored Darsee's publications between 1978 and 1981" [5]. The Darsee case occurred at the beginning of the 1980s, the decade in which celebrated cases of research misconduct, a number involving trainees, came to national attention. Scrutiny by Congress followed scrutiny by the press, leading by the end of the decade to the promulgation of federal research misconduct regulations by both the Public Health Service, including the National Institutes of Health (PHS: 42 CFR 50, 1989; 42 CFR 93, 2005) and the National Science Foundation (NSF: 45 CFR 689, 1987, 1991, 2002). Created by the PHS regulation, the Office of Research Integrity (ORI)—originally the Office of Scientific Integrity (OSI)—has investigated or conducted oversight review of some 800 formal cases of alleged misconduct in research in 18 years since its inception. The Darsee case is not unique. Scores of ORI cases involve trainees who, while working under the supervision of mentors, have fabricated data—sometimes for extensive periods of

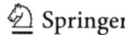

time. Most troubling, the pattern persists [6]. The research community has recognized this problem and responded with an effort to train young investigators in what has come to be called the *Responsible Conduct of Research* (RCR) [7]. However, cases of alleged research misconduct by trainees continue to confront us. How can trainees fabricate or falsify data, often extensively, without being detected by their mentors? What should be the level of responsibility borne by senior collaborators who participate in the submission of fraudulent trainee data for publication or for research grants?

Research Design and Methods

We decided to pursue these questions by investigating the role the mentor played in trainee research where the trainee—i.e., a graduate student a medical student or a postdoctoral fellow—was found responsible for misconduct. That is, we sought to learn whether deficient "mentoring" was a contributing factor in the misconduct. In the PHS regulation misconduct means "fabrication, falsification, or plagiarism in proposing, performing, or reviewing research, or in reporting research results."

In the biological or biomedical sciences which comprise most of these cases, the mentor is most likely to be the lab director, who has overall responsibility for the quality and integrity of the research in his or her lab/group and therefore has a personal stake in seeing that trainees understand the responsible conduct of research. Trainees are by definition supervised—with greater or lesser rigor. There is no federal definition, nor even a working definition in the sciences, that clearly specifies the responsibilities of this senior person. Nor is there any requirement regarding mentoring in the federal misconduct regulations. "Mentoring" is clearly a complex activity, but we sought to focus narrowly on the mentor–trainee relationship in the conduct of trainee research. Hence, we use the term mentor to refer to the person the institution identified as the responsible person's advisor. The trainee might also have other mentors, in addition to the formal one that the institution identified, however records did not indicate when or if that was the case.

In deciding what to measure, we began by asking, what would constitute clearly inadequate and deficient research mentoring. Thinking back to the Darsee case and other instances of well-publicized trainee misconduct, we believed it was clear that his mentors had not played an active role in the collaboration; further his co-authors had not appeared to have reviewed any of the source data on which their publications were based. Two of the authors of this paper, who have direct experience investigating allegations of research misconduct, also noted that trainees often reported that the relationship with their mentor was stressful. We hypothesized that we would see deficiencies in examining data and in setting standards; we further expected to see that trainees and others interviewed would indicate that there was a stressful working relationship between the mentor and trainee.

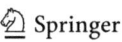 Springer

We decided to focus our research on the ORI cases of trainee misconduct. We reviewed all of the closed cases from the ORI files from 1990 to 2004 in which the accused was a trainee. These case files include the institution's documented record of its investigation (as required by the regulation) and the ORI oversight evaluation and its own analysis and separate finding of misconduct, if any. During this period ORI made a finding of misconduct in a total of 158 cases, with 30% of them involving these specific trainees (n = 45).

We began by reviewing a few case files to get a sense of the data we would find and then created our code so that we recorded evidence on the following questions: (1) Did the mentor review the source (raw) data produced by trainees? (2) Did the mentor set standards for conducting research, such as how to record and store data and see that trainees followed those standards? (3) Did the mentor create a stressful work environment? We conducted detailed reviews of cases in which a trainee was found guilty of misconduct. The case files identified the senior person who was responsible for the trainee. We read the records and took verbatim quotes regarding the mentor's conduct in working with the trainee for the three variables described above. In other words, we coded yes and no when we had substantive narrative to support the code.

These case files were created to document the institution's investigation and ORI's oversight review. Thus, they were not created to review the mentor's role in trainee research. A limitation of using these secondary data, therefore, is that the information we sought might not be present in some case files. Conversely, a strength of these data are that they allow an unobtrusive measurement based on the existing record which was not developed for the research purpose; therefore, there is less chance that the record will reflect a "desirable" response [8].

We recognize that not having a similar cohort of trainee–mentors where misconduct had not occurred certainly limits the interpretation of our findings. There are other limitations as well, discussed later in this paper. However, this is an exploratory study to see what we can learn about cases of misconduct and trainee–mentor relationships. We believe that focusing on the closed ORI cases of trainee misconduct will be useful in providing a description of critical mentor behaviors.

Demographics of Study Population

The sample is composed of 33 post docs, 10 graduate students and two additional trainees. Fifty-six percent (n = 19/34) were trained in the US. The next largest cohort of 35% (12/34) was trained in Asian countries. English was the first language for 58% (20/35) of the trainees. We determined from transcripts of interviews or written statements in the case files that English was not the first language for at least 43% (15/35) of the trainees (15); 22% (10/45) of the respondents could not be coded on this criterion due to insufficient evidence.

In all but three instances, these cases involved either or both fabrication and falsification. The trainee misconduct was discovered in various ways. In 39% (15/39) of cases misconduct was discovered because others could not replicate the

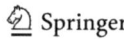 Springer

trainee's data. In 36% (14/39) of cases witnesses to an act or event reported the alleged trainee misconduct. And in another 25% (10/39) of the cases reports of misconduct were triggered by researchers who wanted to examine the source data and it could not be located by the respondent. There was inadequate information in the files to code six cases on this criterion. The trainee's research at issue was joint research with the faculty 79% (31/39) of the time; graduate students' fabrication or falsification always involved their dissertation and sometimes involved their advisor's research as well. Full professors were most likely to make the formal allegation (21/37) but informally the misconduct was often discovered by others in the research group who witnessed the act or who were attempting to replicate the findings. Technicians, students, post docs, assistant professors and associate professors also made complaints, and in eight cases there were multiple complainants.

The respondent eventually admitted to misconduct in 77% (33/43) of the cases. Seventy-three percent (33/45) of the trainee respondents signed a Voluntary Exclusion Agreement with ORI which generally precludes them from receiving federal funds for research for varying lengths of time ranging from 3 to 5 years. The finding of misconduct required retractions of published articles in 63% (26/41) of cases. Forty-one percent (15/37) of students were fired or dismissed from the university, and another 43% (16/37) of the respondents resigned. (We were unable to determine from the files what happened to the rest.) Only a few graduate students were allowed the opportunity to continue in graduate school, most often after taking some research ethics training that the university prescribed.

Findings: Examining Raw/Primary Data

We evaluated the record for information on whether the mentor regularly reviewed the research that was being conducted. Specifically, we coded whether the mentor had reviewed the trainee's raw data. Table 1 shows that in 12 of the cases mentors examined raw data; however in 32 cases mentors had not examined the raw data. When we adjusted this proportion by eliminating the cases we could not code, 73% of the mentors/PIs (32/44) had not looked at the raw data generated by their trainees. (We only had one case that could not be coded on this criterion).

Institutional Research Integrity Officers, Investigative Committees, and trainees themselves commented on the lack of attention by the mentor to the trainee's data.

Table 1 Mentor's role

Behavior	No	%	Adj% No	Yes	%	Adj% Yes	Unable to code
Did the mentor review raw data?	32	71	73	12	27	27	1
Did the mentor set standards?	21	47	62	13	29	38	11

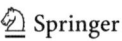 Springer

Deficient Review of Source Data

We have included illustrations from four different cases that focus on the deficient review of source data:

Trainee Statement

"The Mentor [M] indicated that he had not personally examined the lab notebooks, but that he had met with Trainee's [T] on a regular basis to discuss his work and had reviewed posters and manuscript drafts with him. He recalled that [T] had assured him that all the data included in the manuscript were verifiable. [M] noted that there was a close community of investigators in the [...] Center, with frequent meetings and discussion, but that it was not standard procedure for laboratory notebooks to be reviewed."

Trainee's Attorney Regarding the Lax Review of Primary Data

"His fabrications were not the result of careful planning but a frantic effort to appear to be productive. In fact, he did not even keep a lab notebook for a year and one half. If anyone in the lab had attempted to review his primary data, they would easily have been able to see that [T] was not producing any data." (T's lawyer, commenting on Inquiry Report)

ORI Report

Regarding oversight within the laboratory, there appeared to have been a lack of oversight as evidenced from the selection of raw Tracings appropriated for publication. DIO [ORI Division of Investigative Oversight] noted that "the coauthors had the opportunity to review a total of six versions of the questioned manuscript; at no time did any one of them observe errors or mistakes in the raw tracings, even though some had far greater experience with the [...] technique [than the T]."

Investigation Report

"[T] worked to a large extent in isolation, under quite distant supervision from [M] and without much collaborative interaction with other members of the lab. Indeed, our information is that [T] was routinely loath to give up his clones and reagents to other members of the lab for experiments he did not himself control. We consider this to be a relevant observation in the context of this report. We further consider it important that the supervision of [T] by his mentor seems to have been inadequate, at least in terms of the routine and regular examination of primary results, except at the very beginning of [the M's] tenure in [the] lab. Rather he simply accepted the processed data presented to him by his graduate student. Trust is, of course, absolutely intrinsic to and required for all scientific research, and no mentor, the committee members included, carefully inspects every primary experimental result from every graduate student and every postdoctoral fellow every day. We do, though, consider it highly unusual to essentially never see primary data, or even to ask for those data from time to time. Indeed we consider it astonishing

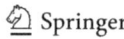

and, at very least, extremely poor practice for a thesis advisor. Concerning the question [with the hard data missing how can the committee determine if fabrication occurred] raised at the end of the previous paragraph our considered opinion is that this lack of direct, critical experimental supervision over the course of approximately three year's work would indeed allow the large scale fabrication of results that we suspect did, in fact, take place."

Setting Standards

We examined whether the mentor–trainee had a supervisory relationship in which information about standards (such as keeping a laboratory notebook) was conveyed. We coded comments made by the institution's investigative committee (usually the mentor's peers) or by the trainee on whether the mentor had specific rules or standards for collecting and maintaining data or other laboratory procedures.

Only 13 cases (38%) had mentors who supervised the trainee by setting standards. We found that 62% (21) appeared to have little awareness about the conduct of the research they were presumably supervising. We noted that when the mentor did not review the source documents there was a tendency for the mentor to have lax supervisory standards for conducting research—particularly standards on recording and reporting data. Inversely, 11 of the 13 cases that had a mentor who had examined raw data also provided contact and supervision with the trainee and had set standards for appropriate research behaviors.

Failure to Set Standards

The following passages from six institutional and ORI files, illustrate the failure of mentors to set supervisory standards:

Trainee Statement

She admitted to the actions that led to a finding of misconduct, but denied any intent to defraud—indeed she said she had been taught those techniques by her previous mentor, recorded them in her current lab book, and no current supervisor had asked her to change practice. [Paraphrase of a longer passage]

Trainee Statement

"There was a pervasive lack of integrity and disregard for rules in the lab. There was also a significant amount of scientific misguidance, especially in data analysis. Most of the people with prior lab experience found this disturbing and left the lab. I was not experienced enough to realize that what I was learning was incorrect."

Observation of Investigation Committee

"…it is also of significance that M did not begin the examination of the original data until after his return from Professional meeting (at which the data

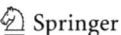 Springer

were presented in poster) in spite of the fact that he had been warned on at least two occasions about potential problems with the quality of T's data …M failed to establish proper practices for data management."

Observation of Investigation Committee

"Early in the course of the inquiry, it became known that [T] and others working under [M.s] supervision did not keep traditional laboratory notebooks."

Observation of Investigation Committee

The Investigation Committee, in response to what they found was a lack of appropriate oversight by the mentor, recommended that all graduate faculty members and graduate students be sent a copy of the NAS booklet, "Advisor, Teacher, Role Model, Friend" with a letter advising the faculty and students that scientific misconduct does occur, that improper mentoring can be a major contributing factor, and that lax oversight and/or supervision of experimental data recording also contributes to an environment that can lead to misconduct. [Paraphrasing Committee Report] The committee also noted that for misconduct to be committed over a long period of time, lax oversight mentoring was clearly implicated as well as poor communication between the trainee and mentor.

Observation of Investigation Committee and ORI

"There also were concerns about how data on research records were handled in the laboratory; each investigator used his own individual approach to record keeping. ORI noted that the direct oversight and supervision was the responsibility of the laboratory chief."

Attention to Stress

Stressful Work Environment

We examined the records for evidence that there were known stresses or conflicts between the trainee and the mentor and/or within the research group. While we found some comments about stress in the lab, we did not have enough data to code whether the mentor might be involved as a source of the stress or aware of its existence.

Ex Post Facto Analyses

We then reviewed the comments we had collected on stress and decided that we could examine, ex post facto, one pattern that emerged as we reviewed the files for comments on stress or stressors.

Twenty-four cases (53%) of trainee/respondents described their stress levels as a factor that caused or contributed to their misconduct. (We could not code this

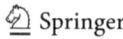

for 21 cases.) Fifteen of the 24 cases (62%) focused on statements that they fabricated or falsified data because they felt internal pressure to perform well. Nine respondents (38%) attributed their stress to specific time-related issues such as submitting a grant, publication or publication deadline, or to complete their dissertation requirements to begin a new job. While claiming stress as the cause of misconduct can be interpreted as the trainee's rationalization for his/her act, these responses are nevertheless worth attending to because many respondents clearly believed they were overwhelmed by stress. Further, if trainees were using stress as an "excuse" for their misconduct, one might expect that the majority would blame others—notably the mentor—for creating stressful working conditions. But this was not the case. There were only four instances where respondents cited unreasonable pressure from the mentor to get desired results or quick results, although some of these appear to be egregious as seen in the following example: "In 1993 [M] requested that members of the lab not take a summer vacation because it was important that we all work hard for his tenure." But the great majority of respondents did not complain about their relations with their mentor or others in their research group. We saw evidence in only four case files that there was a good deal of conflict between members of the group with their mentor. Instead, in testimony before investigative committees, in comments on investigative reports, and in admissions of misconduct, trainees most often reported self-generated stress, e.g. perfectionism, as the force that drove them to cheat. (We note, however, that in many cases the trainees seem to have been internalizing the expectations for productivity in the lab or in their institutions. In other words, external expectations seemed to lead to internal stress.) Whatever the etiology may be, stress does appear to be a significant factor that contributes to the likelihood that a trainee will commit misconduct.

Stress. The following examples illustrate trainee perspectives on stress:

From an Investigation Committee Report

The [T] stated that he was a perfectionist to a fault and when he failed to obtain results that he expected, he altered the data to correspond with what he expected the results to be. … He felt pressure to achieve perfection in the lab environment. He commented that the pressure was primarily internal, although he felt some external pressure to perform because [M] lab was so well respected by other researchers.

Trainee Testimony

"Even though I had already secured a position at [major university] and even though I had 18 publications, an NIH fellowship and several awards for my prior work, I have believed myself to be a complete failure as a scientist... Thus, I think that was going through my mind, has led me to believe that, if I could just show one piece of 'promising' data on a group meeting, my supervisor would let me continue working on the problem and produce real data that could be presented, published etc. … I am deeply ashamed …"

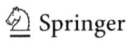 Springer

Trainee Letter of Admission

"There was much excitement over this [surprising and promising preliminary result] and I began to feel a self-imposed pressure to keep the positive data coming in. It was at this time that I began to substitute buffer for the control XXX. At the time I realized I was making a grave error in judgment, but as the excitement over the results grew and grew I felt more pressure to manipulate the system. At no time were any of the co-authors of the paper aware of my actions, nor could they have anticipated my behavior. Over time I lost more and more control and felt like I could not stop falsifying experiments.
I became worried…not being able to reproduce my earlier work. I placed a tremendous amount of pressure on my self to get my current data to confirm my earlier work. When my latter results did not support my previous work, I falsely informed [M] that there was consistency among all the data."

Institutional Awareness of Mentoring and Misconduct

When we began to review our notes we realized that institutions were beginning to ask the same question we were asking: Did the mentor contribute to the misconduct? Eighteen Investigative Committees addressed the issue of whether and how the mentor contributed to the problem. In only one instance, where the issue of mentoring arose in a misconduct investigation, did the committee assert that the mentor HAD NOT contributed to the misconduct. Yet, even here, the institution addressed the possibility.

The following four excerpts highlight the judgments that Investigative Committees made about the culpability or contributing negligence of the mentor/PI and their feeling that the graduate student deserved a second chance:

Investigation Report—Concluding Statement

"Although outright fraud can circumvent virtually any review process, we believe that every laboratory head must take the responsibility to ensure that procedures are in place in the laboratory so that the possibility of fraud is minimized. These include that (a) every manuscript receive adequate review by senior members of the laboratory, that the PI is directly informed of the resulting criticisms, and that the PI reviews the final manuscript before submission for responsiveness to all criticisms, and (b) every effort should be made to provide opportunities for each investigator to present primary unedited data to an appropriate group or subgroup of the laboratory for criticism and feedback."

Investigation Report

"Mentor/PIs should provide a more formal process of initial training for their graduate students as they join a research project. This should include coverage of IRB regulations and the responsibility inherent in maintaining the integrity of research. The Board also recommends that [M/PI] should have more contact

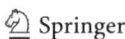

with the graduate students throughout the research project ... [T] should contact his academic advisor and with that advisor develop a mentoring plan."

Investigation Report

"The committee believes that it is a good practice for the mentor to examine the primary laboratory notebooks for a student conducting his/her Ph.D. thesis research in the mentor's laboratory. More than just checking the validity of results, it helps the mentor better understand some of the details and nuances of the work which will help with both the thesis and the publications. The committee recognizes that this practice currently varies widely from scientist to scientist. The committee recommends that the University consider establishing a set of recommendations which might be called "Good Laboratory Practice Guidelines" which would be applicable to the mentoring situation."

Investigation Report

"The committee concluded that [M] should have been more directly involved in the critical analysis of data and results in published works. Greater diligence in overseeing the work of [T], who alone appeared to have committed the fraudulent acts, was particularly called for because of [T's] lack of scientific training."

We believe the opinions and statements made by institutions thru their investigative committee provide further support to our observations on how deficient behaviors on the part of the mentor have been a major contributing factor.

Limitations of Data

These data provide information on instances of misconduct by trainees that is usually not available to scholars: institutional investigation reports (and related documents such as correspondence among administrators, and between administrators and the respondent and complainant), as well as ORI analyses of institutional investigation; testimony and letters from the respondent and other witnesses (including administrators) regarding why the misconduct may have occurred, about the quality of the mentoring relationship and collegial relationships in the research group. At the same time there are limitations to these data beyond those discussed in the introduction:

- The data are from instances where trainee misconduct were found and therefore can tell us nothing about the benchmark of normal or exemplary mentor–trainee relationships.
- Data from the potentially valuable subset of cases where trainee misconduct was alleged but not found are unavailable because many of these cases, when concluded at the assessment or inquiry stages, are not required by the regulation to be submitted to ORI and are kept confidential by institutions.
- Case files that are thorough in documenting and analyzing trainee misconduct may not address issues of mentoring and, indeed, they are not required to do so under the regulation.

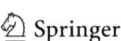 Springer

- In some instances we have had to infer information about the mentor–trainee relationship by comments (e.g. by institutional administrators) in institutional case files.
- Admissions of misconduct and other explanations of conduct by respondents are post hoc and may be self-justifications or crafted to secure lenient treatment.
- As with all descriptive research, our findings do not clearly show a cause and effect structure. Hence other things could be causing the research misconduct and not be related to the mentor.
- The projects are all in biomedical or behavioral research funded by PHS, and therefore represent only a portion, albeit a very large one, of the research universe.
- The term mentor is an ambiguous term and there is no agreed upon definition. We have no way to assure that ALL those identified in the case files believed they were the mentor. What we do know is that the institution in all cases believed the person identified was the person who had some oversight responsibility for the trainee.

Conclusions and Recommendations

We suspect that many mentors avoid thinking about whether they have a role in preventing research misconduct. They are busy conducting research themselves and in many instances have had little formal education on educating trainees to conduct research. Indeed, in a large study of 2,000 laboratory directors, the investigators found that only 33% of the directors said that they had had a mentor who prepared them very well to be a good mentor to those that they supervise today. In this same study the directors indicated that they supervised on average 4.7 individuals in their group [9].

Further evidence on how mentors may have difficulty providing adequate mentoring comes from the research of Martinson et al. They have reported that 27% of their sample of NIH funded scientists indicated "inadequate record keeping related to research projects" [10]. If mentors aren't keeping good records of their own research, would we expect them to be engaging in adequate monitoring of their trainees' research? In another study by this team, we learn that 56% of 3,257 researchers admit to cutting corners; one component of this composite variable included "inadequate monitoring of research projects because of work overload" [11].

Adams and Pimple highlight another avenue on promoting integrity and preventing research misconduct [12]. They posit that responsible conduct of research (RCR) education must focus not only on the development of the researcher's [in this case the trainee's] ethical awareness—the ability to evaluate dilemmas, discuss value choices and develop the self control to resist unethical solutions to research problems—but also on issues of "opportunity." Norms and expectations are transmitted by mentors and by team members. Where there is the absence of capable supervision and the lack of informal social interaction the normative pressure to follow the group's standards can erode. This can allow the trainee to have opportunities to fabricate data to impress others, to get ahead, or to meet a deadline. If trainees work alone, they can easily hide their behavior. If they know how to use sophisticated equipment that few others use, then they can falsify their data. We believe that prevention of research misconduct is most likely to be

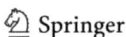

assured when there is involvement by the mentor to enforce research standards as well as pressure from the research group to conform to the group's rules.

If we are striving to build a culture of integrity, it becomes very important to examine how to address the fact that mentors feel less than well qualified to know how to mentor. With the growing trend to larger research groups, one can see that mentoring for the responsible conduct or research is likely to become an even more complex phenomena. Institutional leaders need to become involved in working with researchers in their institution to build programs that teach mentors how to mentor.

If the mentors had been more diligent in setting and monitoring appropriate research standards, in reviewing trainee raw data, in establishing a supportive work environment, and increasing their support and vigilance at times of high trainee stress, would the incidence of research misconduct in these cases have been reduced? This is an exceedingly difficult question to answer. No one knows what causes misconduct. Speculation in the literature and among those who handle allegations of misconduct include the following potential causes: (a) sociopathology; (b) increasing pressure on researchers—especially those trying to secure tenure or continuing employment—to publish and secure grants; (c) arrogance—already knowing the right answer without bothering to do the experiment; (d) ignorance of research standards and ethical norms in research, i.e. poor mentoring. These proposed causes are, of course, not mutually exclusive. We did not look for, nor do we have a definitive answer on what caused the actual misconduct for the cases we reviewed. We believe that the cases we examined illustrate all the potential causes listed above.

In summary, our findings suggest that there are straight-forward, concrete steps mentors could take that might reduce the incidence of trainee misconduct, or limit its seriousness or impact: (1) regular review of trainee raw data, (2) standard-setting, enforcement of standards, and (3) attention to trainee stress levels—all primary elements of supervision. Every mentor should, in our opinion, articulate and implement appropriate standards and rules for his or her research group for how to collect, record and maintain data; for when and how key experiments are to be replicated before data are submitted in manuscripts and grant applications; for who is responsible for assuring and documenting compliance with regulatory obligations (e.g. laboratory animal care, handling of hazardous materials); and for authorship practices. While we did not find evidence that the mentors caused stress, we did find trainees talking about their stresses in a manner that was believable. We think it would be prudent for mentors to realize that trainees are trying to produce research and learn new skills and that it would be an exceptional trainee who did not feel some stress at some time in the process.

Surprisingly, in doing our literature review we found that there appear to be no agreed upon standards or best practices in the research community recommending that mentors or lab directors review trainee raw data at regular intervals, whereas there should be.

Mentor review of raw data would certainly allow for its early detection when some misconduct did occur, but in addition it would create a powerful preventive strategy by reducing the opportunity for traniee misconduct. Regular mentor review of raw data presumes that the trainees record and manage their data in appropriate fashion in the first place. But in the cases we reviewed there was a troublingly high

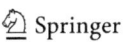 Springer

incidence of missing data or of no lab books at all (even in the laboratories of renowned scientists).

The National Academy's call for responsible research occurred almost 20 years ago [13]. Have we heeded the call? Institutions, perhaps through peer review of mentoring practices, should assure that research standards are implemented and enforced. Some exemplary laboratories distribute their standards, rules and procedures in a booklet during orientation for each new member of the research group and ask each new member to sign a statement that they understand and will abide by those rules. Where agreed-upon standards and best practices do not exist we hope the research community, particularly those charged with research mentoring, will take up these issues and adopt standards.

Acknowledgements   We would like to thank the following colleagues for reading and commenting on earlier versions of this paper: Prof. Douglas Adams, University of Arkansas; Dean Karen Klomparens, Michigan State University; Dr. Larry Rhoades, ORI.

References

1. Greenberg Daniel, S. (1983). How scientists get away with cheating. *Journal of Commerce and Commercial*, (357), 4A.
2. Judson, H. F. (2004). *The great betrayal* (pp. 112–122, 144–146). New York: Harcourt, Inc.
3. Wallis, C. (1983). Fraud in a Harvard Lab. *Time, 121*(Feb 28), 49.
4. Columbia University, (n.d.). RCR: Research misconduct. 3. John Darsee and Robert Slutsky. http://ccnmtl.Columbia.edu/projects/rcr/rcr_misconduct/foundation/index.html.#1_B_3. Accessed 15 Apr 2008.
5. Murray, M. (1987). A long-disputed paper goes to press. *Science News, 131*, 52. doi:10.2307/3971418.
6. *Federal Register* notices are posted when a case of misconduct occurs. The following cases are considered major by ORI: Rosner (NIH, 1992), Tracy (University of Southern California, 2002), Muenchen (University of Michigan, 2002), Simmons (University of Texas Southwest Medical Campus, 2000), Lin (Medical University of South Carolina, 2001), and Hajra (University of Michigan, 1997). These can be found at http://ori.dhhs.gov/. Accessed 8 June 2008.
7. National Academy of Sciences. (2002). *Scientific research: Creating an environment that promotes responsible conduct.* Washington: National Academy Press.
8. Webb, E. J., Campbell, D. T., Schwartz, R. D., & Sechrest, L. (2000). Unobtrusive measures; revised edition. Sage Publications Inc.
9. Rodbard, D. Survey of research integrity measures utilized in biomedical research laboratories, report prepared for ORI, 2003. http://ori.dhhs.gov/documents/research/intergity_measures_final_report_11_07_03.pdf. Accessed 8 June 2008.
10. Martinson, B. C., Anderson, M. S., & Devries, R. (2005). Scientists behaving badly. *Nature, 435*(7043), 737–738. doi:10.1038/435737a.
11. Anderson, M. S., Horn, A. S., Risbey, K. R., Ronning, E. A., De Vries, R., & Martinson, B. C. (2007). What do mentoring and training in the responsible conduct of research have to do with scientists' misbehavior? Findings from a national survey of NIH-funded scientists. *Academic Medicine, 82*(9), 853–860. doi:10.1097/ACM.0b013e31812f764c.
12. Adams, D., & Pimple, K. D. (2005). Research misconduct and crime lessons from criminal science on preventing misconduct and promoting integrity. *Accountability in Research, 12*, 225–240. doi: 10.1080/08989620500217495.
13. National Academy of Sciences. (1989, 1995 2nd ed.). *Responsible conduct of research: On being a scientist.* Washington: National Academy Press.

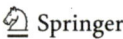

6.3   Mentorship Matters
for the Biomedical Workforce

Sally J. Rockey

Rockey, SJ. Mentorship matters for the biomedical work-force. *Nature Medicine* 20(6), 575 (2014). © 2014 Nature America, Inc. All rights reserved. And imprint of SpringerNature.

Mentorship matters for the biomedical workforce

Sally J Rockey

The mentorship of early-career scientists is necessary to their individual career success and the future of the biomedical research enterprise as a whole. Recently launched NIH programs and tools aim to facilitate this important type of training.

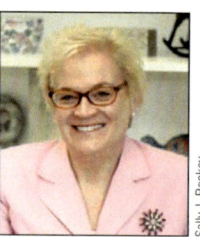

As scientists, we have the opportunity to make new discoveries that contribute to fundamental knowledge and improve people's health and quality of life through our research. But we also influence lives by fostering the careers of the less experienced investigators with whom we interact on a daily basis. We shape their professional development by mentoring them on how to be productive researchers who contribute to both science and the community.

Being a mentor goes beyond supervising lab projects and teaching sound experimental design. It includes training less experienced investigators how to conduct research ethically and with integrity. It includes advising on potential career paths, providing networking and collaboration opportunities and helping new researchers navigate the research funding process. Seasoned scientists can attest that breadth of knowledge is just as important as depth, and they can encourage mentees to develop a range of professional skill sets.

Biomedical research needs scientists who can effectively translate and communicate its intricacies and value to many stakeholders, such as journalists, advocates, members of industry, policy makers and the general public. Good mentors transfer these skills to their mentees. We can show young investigators how valuable they are to the future of science. They are the next generation of great ideas, further propelling us toward our goal of advancing the scientific enterprise and improving health.

In the last decade, more graduate students and postdoctoral fellows are supported by research grants, not just career- or training-focused awards. In 2011, 65% of full-time graduate students supported by the US National Institutes of Health (NIH) received funding from research assistantships, compared to 60% in 2001. This speaks to the evolving landscape of biomedical workforce support and the need to reaffirm the importance of both formal and informal mentorship, as students and postdocs on research grants may not receive the formal mentorship that is part of NIH-sponsored training programs.

The NIH's extramural and intramural programs have long recognized the importance of mentorship in research training. The agency offers mentored career ('K') awards for research career development under the guidance of an experienced mentor or mentoring team. For these and most pre- and post-doctoral fellowship ('F') awards, mentors provide a statement of support in the application that describes their mentoring plans and provide progress report updates throughout the duration of the award. Similarly, the NIH's institutional training ('T') review criteria ensure that reviewers will consider both the training records of the proposed mentors and historical trainee outcomes.

The NIH has a robust intramural research training program where trainees at all levels—from high school students through postdoctoral and clinical fellow—come to the NIH to pursue research and seek research mentors. The training resources, such as videos and panel discussion webcasts, are also available to those outside of the NIH. Among the diverse career-related topics they cover are mentorship and how to choose mentors.

In 2012, a working group of the NIH Advisory Council to the Director examined ways to support a sustainable and diverse biomedical workforce. The group discussed the need for strong mentorship and appreciation of the diversity of scientific career options that trainees may choose. In response

to these recommendations, the NIH launched several new programs and policy changes to further enhance training of future scientists.

One of these is the Broadening Experiences in Scientific Training (BEST) award program started last year by the NIH to help institutions develop programs to expose trainees—both graduate students and postdocs—to the multitude of career paths utilizing PhD training. Programs such as this intend to create a culture change by enhancing appreciation for different scientific career options and diversifying the training experiences of graduate students and postdocs. Through the BEST program, trainees are connected to mentors in research-related fields and participate in much-needed opportunities for professional growth.

Another new program aims to enhance diversity within the biomedical workforce specifically through mentorship. The NIH-supported National Research Mentoring Network will engage individuals from many research disciplines to serve as mentors and link them to mentees who are at a wide array of career stages, ranging from undergrads to early-career faculty members. It will also provide training for mentors and networking and professional opportunities for mentees.

NIH-wide initiatives are complemented by programs developed by NIH institutes and centers. For example, the National Institute of General Medical Sciences recently announced Innovative Programs to Enhance Research Training (IPERT) to encourage creative new educational activities for students, postdocs and early-career faculty. IPERT focuses on courses for skills development such as problem solving and leadership, structured mentoring activities to promote career planning, and outreach programs such as evidence-based science education.

The NIH is facilitating mentorship by promoting individual development plans, or IDPs, which it encourages institutions to begin reporting in progress reports submitted this October and going forward. An IDP is a living document that maps out approaches for developing skills that help an individual identify and achieve short- and long-term career goals. The IDP process can facilitate communication between faculty mentors and trainees. We have encouraged grantee organizations to develop an institutional policy requiring an IDP for graduate students and postdocs supported by *any* NIH grant, not just training grants and fellowships. Many academic institutions already use IDPs, and the NIH is cognizant of administrative burdens on scientists and research administrators, so it allows flexibility for grantee institutions to choose the IDP format that is the best fit for their community. IDPs will be meaningful only if mentors and mentees make full use of their potential as career development tools. I hope our grantees join as full partners in this effort.

The training of the biomedical workforce has always been an integral part of the NIH mission, and through its infrastructure of funding opportunities and other initiatives, the agency hopes to champion a culture of mentorship in the research community. It takes just one good mentor to influence the career of a new investigator; it takes a robust culture of mentorship across the research community to strengthen, sustain and diversify the entire biomedical research enterprise.

Sally J. Rockey is deputy director for extramural research at the National Institutes of Health, Bethesda, Maryland, USA.

6.4   Professional Responsibility

C. K. Gunsalus

Gunsalus, CK. Professional responsibility. *Inside Higher Education,* May 14, 2013.

Reprinted with permission from Inside Higher Ed.

Professional Responsibility

| Teaching ethics should be part of the job of all faculty members in all disciplines, writes C.K. Gunsalus.

By C.K. Gunsalus   // May 14, 2013

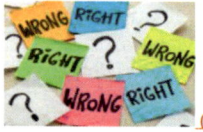

(https://www.insidehighered.com/sites/default/server_files/styles/large/public/media/iStock_000017356047XSmall.jpg?
itok=m6fWWJy4)

People who hire and supervise others in the real world are desperate to hire people — our graduates — who have the "whole package": substantive knowledge plus "soft" skills (basic responsibility, working well with others, ethics, etc.) that contribute to success in the world of work. You might argue that teaching those skills isn't our problem because we're providing educational foundations for professional knowledge. Or that we can hardly be held responsible for failings of families and society, which ought to be the ones instilling work ethic and manners and common sense.

Still, didn't we open this can of worms ourselves when we started arguing that colleges and universities are engines of economic development and that government should keep (or go back to) investing in education because it creates a knowledgeable workforce? When employers complain about what they perceive as a lazy and entitled attitude among young workers, and we see an apparently never-ending stream of ethics scandals, maybe there's another way to think about this that is directly congruent with our mission and, furthermore, falls directly within our expertise: embedding ethics and concepts of professional responsibility throughout our curriculums and courses.

If you think about it, doing so is a positive and preventive approach to what many perceive as an epidemic of cheating. There is research suggesting (http://http://www.swarthmore.edu/Documents/academics/economics/Dee/w15672.pdf) that an educational approach can be an effective strategy, and if enough faculty members purposefully and thoughtfully incorporate ethical connections into classes, it will help those among our students who mean well and want to follow the rules. If we can help those students to find a voice and provide positive examples, we gain, too.

Over the years, I've heard countless arguments about why faculty cannot or do not include ethics in their courses, or add courses about professional responsibility to their disciplines. The curriculum is too full already, and besides, you cannot teach people not to lie and cheat if they didn't learn that in their families. The objections I hear go further, though, and betray a serious discomfort, fear even, about teaching "ethics": I don't want to have to talk about deontology (I don't like Kant or haven't read it and don't want to); it's too hard or too subjective; I'm not qualified; someone else can handle it (bosses, the research compliance people, someone across the street, whatever). Ethics is boring and dry. I don't know enough and don't have time to go learn another field while I'm working on getting promoted/getting the next grant/serving on too many committees. What if someone asks a question and I don't know the answer? What if I look stupid? I might come off as judgmental or not judgmental enough. A required event is going to get really bad student evaluations.

We Can All Teach This Stuff, and We Should

As higher education experiences disruptive transformation through the changing economics of what we do, price pressures and technological upending, homing in on what we uniquely do is likely to be part of our path to the future. What is more central to that than helping students explore questions about and learn to use responsibly the knowledge we are conveying? The responsibilities of professionals — researchers, scientists, scholars, teachers — are deeply personal ones, and too important to leave to others outside our disciplines to teach. Outsourcing shortchanges our students and ourselves.

If you think matters of professional responsibility in your discipline matter, if you care about accountability and transparency and fairness and rigor, you can and should teach ethics in your field, whether that's a course or workshop that meets the requirements for responsible conduct of research education or topics that you integrate into your substantive classes — or both.

There are good reasons to teach in courses that are not about ethics, and it needn't be daunting or hard. There are some straightforward ways to do it and as a practicing professional in your field (they pay you to do what you do at work, right?), you can and you should. Here's how.

1. Think and talk about your mistakes. Who hasn't made a mistake at work? A big one? An embarrassing one? One you still cringe thinking about? What did you learn from those mistakes? If you've thought about it over the years, can you talk about it, obviously not naming names if that would violate confidences or confidentiality requirements?

Have you ever looked back on something that seemed perfectly reasonable at the time, and with the value of hindsight, thought "How could I have been such an idiot?" Or, been sitting with someone who's making a huge mistake and thought "no, no, no!"

If you can find a way to talk about those moments and the lessons you took away from them, your students will learn. Talking calmly and clearly about mistakes you have made will shape them as professionals and as people — and not so coincidentally, the world you are going to live in when they take over. (Another plus: modeling how you deal with hard stuff, and showing that life and careers rarely go in a clean, clear forward path without setbacks will be memorable and they will like you all the more for it.)

2. Articulate one of the lessons that govern your professional life. Where and when did you learn about the value of boundaries and when to refer students to other resources rather than trying to help them yourself? That it's easier to start out relatively strictly in a course and relax the rules as you go than vice versa? That's a lesson that extrapolates to a lot of other contexts. How did you learn to set the ground rules for talking to reporters about your work or setting boundaries when acting as a consultant or expert witness? When have you made a hard choice about a professional topic that you found challenging? If the lesson is connected to a mistake, it will be even more gripping to your class.

If you ask the students make a connection to the topic you're teaching that day, you will likely be surprised and pleased with what emerges. And even if your examples are all from your life in academe, the examples will likely have relevant lessons for students looking at other careers.

3. Talk with students about ethical dilemmas or hard moments they've faced (or will face). For years, I've asked students to write a short (200 word) description of an ethical dilemma they have faced. (This is an assignment idea from Harris Sondak of the University of Utah, a friend of a friend who was kind enough to talk with me about his teaching techniques and syllabus when I first started teaching ethics in a business school.) Not only does this essay get students thinking about these issues in their own lives, properly managed it creates a wonderful set of discussion topics.

Even if you don't ask students to do exactly that, or if you adapt and ask them to write about ethical applications of your topic or questions they have, it will tell you a lot about where the students are. In the dilemmas I've gotten over the years, the same issues come up over and over again: bosses who put pressure on workers to cut corners to meet deadlines. Perverse incentives in reward systems. Peer pressure. Temptation and rationalization in the face of a desire to succeed. You know, all those human frailties that come up when you work with other people.

And not one of those is hard to connect to the kinds of problems our students will face in what they do after college or grad school. Believe me, they are all cued into power imbalances, fairness, and how to navigate difficult situations. Connect it to how you use what you're teaching, even if you only do that once in a while, even if it's only talking about your policy for awarding grades, and you'll be contributing to their development in a broader way.

Students who've never held a job have faced dilemmas in school, like a friend who asked for help with an assignment when it was against the rules to collaborate. That situation is relevant to most every class and a great place to use it is it when you're discussing the syllabus, especially if that's all you do on your first day (contrary to advice offered here (https://www.insidehighered.com/blogs/first-day-class-rituals)).

If you're nervous about flying blind, take a look at the range of ethics resources, including "two-minute challenge" (2MC) collection on Ethics CORE (http://www.NationalEthicsCenter.org) . What's a 2MC? It's a problem that you cannot necessarily resolve in two minutes, but comes up and you may need to respond to it in two minutes — or less. It's the kind of problem that comes up all the time in professional life and you need to be prepared to handle. Use the same simple framework for structuring discussion of your own or other ethical dilemmas.

Don't come prepared with the "answer," and do come prepared to point out that you already know what you would do in hard situations (mostly), and that you won't be going to work with them, so it's THEIR answers that matter the most. If you are going to opine or editorialize, do it only after they've all had their say. Prepare a few questions to keep the discussion going, using the framework as your basis for that.

If you do that, based on real problems people (in the room sometimes!) have faced, you'll be doing some of the most important things that emerging research on efficacy in ethics education suggest: using short examples that carry emotional punch because they happened to real people. Modeling a way to talk about them. Helping to analyze them by practicing. Over and over. (If any of them are musicians or athletes, ask them to talk about the value of practicing scales or free throws for a useful analogy.)

You'll be helping your students to anticipate consequences of various actions. Apply labels to what the problems are (deception, temptation, rationalization, slippery slope problems…).

Or pick articles out of the newspaper or journals in your field about someone who's crossed the line. If you cannot find something, go to Ethics CORE and look at the recent news feed. There won't be a shortage of examples. Look for the videos. Try out some of the role plays there. Read my most recent book and use some of those examples.

what's right and what's wrong. How you act on it. What you're willing to sacrifice for your principles. (Are they really principles if you're not willing to sacrifice for them?)

You are a practicing professional. Who better than you to teach your students about professional ethics in your field?

Bio

C.K. Gunsalus is the director of the National Center for Professional and Research Ethics, professor emerita of business, and research professor at the Coordinated Sciences Laboratory at the University of Illinois at Urbana-Champaign. She is the author of The Young Professional's Survival Guide (http://www.hup.harvard.edu/catalog.php?isbn=9780674049444) *(Harvard University Press).*

Read more by C.K. Gunsalus

jump to comments (#comment-target)

(/print/views/2013/05/14/essay-
responsibility-teach-ethics?
width=775&height=500&iframe=true)

Get our Daily News Update
(/newsletter/signup)

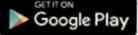

(https://play.google.com/store/apps/details?
id=com.insidehighered)

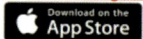

(https://itunes.apple.com/us/app/inside-
higher-ed/id401721294?mt=8)

site&utm_content=sidebar-link&utm_campaign=jobs)

Hide comments

6.5   All You Need is Mentorship

Robert A. Weinberg, Maya Schuldiner, Hong Wu, Beth
Stevens, Jens Nielsen, P. Robin Hiesinger, and Bassem
A. Hassan

All you need is mentorship. *Cell* 10, 1092–1093 (2016).
© 2016 Elsevier Inc.

Reprinted with permission from Elsevier.

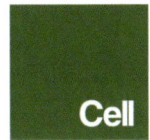

Leading Edge

Voices

All You Need Is Mentorship

The Importance of Scientific Taste

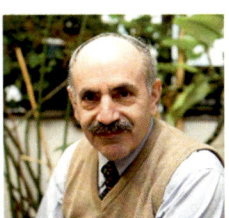

Robert A. Weinberg
Whitehead Institute/MIT

I find it humbling to confess that most of the truly original ideas that have driven my research group's agenda over four decades of time have come, not from my own brain, but instead from the minds of my trainees, both graduate students and post-docs. This on its own might explain why I, rather selfishly, have given them long leashes, allowing them to strike out on their own and craft their own research trajectories.

But there has also been a slightly more altruistic agenda: recently arrived trainees often assume that mastery of a set of experimental strategies and a familiarity with the relevant scientific literature should represent the core of their training. I, in stark contrast, have always viewed my own job quite differently, hoping to train my mentees to think independently, to think critically about their own work and that of others and, most importantly, to develop a sense of which problems are important conceptually and which are, in one way or another, trivial and not worth their time. Developing this last element in the cognitive toolkit is ultimately the most challenging one for many, who would rather direct their experimental agenda toward problems that are sure to yield abundant data rather than those that actually matter. In a time when generating large datasets and mastering novel, elegant technologies has become progressively easier, the temptations increase inexorably to embrace what is new rather than what is truly important in remodeling our conceptual understanding. If I, as a mentor, can imbue my trainees with this last skill—a taste for important problems—I view their experience with me as a major success!

A Passion for Mentoring

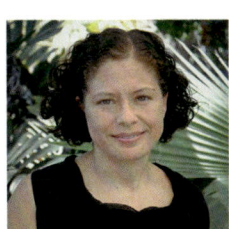

Maya Schuldiner
Weizmann Institute of Science

The biology textbooks that I read as a student described scientists that made great discoveries and changed the world. I decided to become a scientist myself because I wanted to be just like them. However, through the years, I started seeing that although I liked making discoveries, there was, in fact, something that I loved much more. As I started mentoring my very own PhD students I realized that, for me, the best thing about doing science is not the process of discovery itself but rather the process of mentoring other people on the path to discovery.

I love my students. I care about their success and spend time thinking about their needs and about ways to help them grow and flourish. An important part of mentoring, for me, is being someone that they can relate to and not someone that they must look up to. I try to convey to my students that I am not so different than them—I am mostly more experienced.

One important aspect for me is mentoring women to succeed in combining family with a career. Having three children, I know that it is not easy but it is doable. Together with my friends Prof. Nirit Dudovich and Prof. Michal Sharon, we have created a workshop to help women who wish to combine the two to acquire these skills.

I think that much of my scientific success comes from my dedication to my students and to mentoring because I have an amazing team. I will probably never change the world but I am touching the lives of my students. And they might very well change the world. Or their students.

Pay It Forward

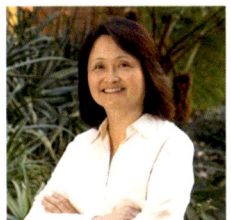

Hong Wu
Peking University

Both my graduate and postdoctoral advisers have been key in my growth as a scientist. With them, I learned to identify and focus on the big questions, while taking risks to explore uncharted frontiers. Importantly, they also taught me to stay critical to myself. As both labs were rather large in size, I had the privilege to interact with many scientists working on a myriad of scientific questions. This "environmental mentorship" has contributed tremendously to widen my knowledge and horizons. In my eyes, effective mentorship depends on the quality of both the direct mentors, as well as the scientific environment they offer.

I have used these lessons as a foundation for my mentorship style, while adding my own touch. I talk to every student and postdoctoral fellow who applies to my lab about my expectations and mentorship goals—they should become independent scientists, not my spare hands. Therefore, they must lead their own projects and follow their own interests. I also emphasize that willingness to accept criticism is instrumental for success and that professional criticism should not be taken personally.

After returning to China, I realized that, in contrast to labs in the United States, there is a general lack of senior scientists and postdoctoral fellows in Chinese labs. With inadequate "environmental mentorship," direct interactions between mentors and trainees become even more important. Unfortunately, graduate students in Chinese research labs are regarded as the primary force of productivity but are often overlooked as the future leaders in the field. A training program on effective mentorship is therefore desperately needed in China—by teaching the value of good mentorship to our current independent scientists, we will be able to positively impact all generations to come.

1092 Cell *164*, March 10, 2016 ©2016 Elsevier Inc.

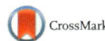

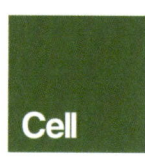

Mentorship Is a Two-Way Street

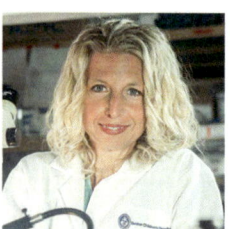

Beth Stevens
Boston Children's Hospital

A Journey of Equals

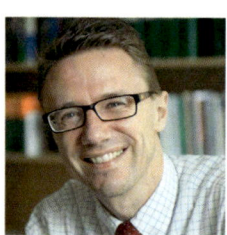

Jens Nielsen
Chalmers University of Technology

The Tightrope of Mentorship!

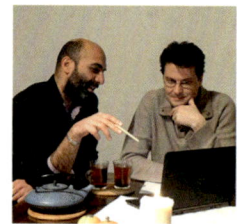

P. Robin Hiesinger[1] and Bassem A. Hassan[2]
[1]Free University Berlin; [2]VIB/KU LEUVEN/ICM

Mentors shape who we are as scientists and as future mentors. At every critical step in my scientific journey, I can look back and see the more senior scientist who helped me, whether it was challenging me on my critical thinking, inspiring me to tackle big problems, or reminding me that I needed to ask questions when attending meetings to learn how to become a part of the conversation. The importance of mentors is undeniable.

What is perhaps less well appreciated is that mentorship is a two-way street. The mentee needs to take responsibility and action to capture the attention of potential mentors. Just as other aspects of science are intensely competitive, so too is the competition for the time and interest of more senior scientists. How does a trainee or a junior faculty stand out in a sea of talented and driven young scientists? The student who often captures my attention is not necessarily the one who has a *Cell* paper in press (though that sure helps!) but is the person who consistently asks great questions, engages in interesting discussions, shows they care about the field and where it is headed, and works very hard. As we move up in science, all of us have a responsibility to not just help young scientists become good scientists but to create opportunities for them to shine and show their true potential. So next time you spot an impressive trainee with a fire in their belly, seek them out and engage them. You won't regret it. That conversation could be hugely impactful for both of you.

Throughout my career, my mentoring philosophy has always been based on trust and enthusiasm. Young talented people who want to work in science and engineering should be inspired through enthusiasm. They should be encouraged to embrace all opportunities and to tackle big problems, while pursuing their aspirations for carrying out research that may impact society. Basically, I tell them from the beginning that we should learn new things together and that my primary role as their mentor is not only to help when problems arise or they need to make complicated decisions but also to challenge them so they understand and identify the important questions we should be focusing on. This is a process that involves keeping my trainees up to date on the current status of the research field and aware of the relevance of their own work. Additionally, I include them in publications as early as possible and connect them to the industry and their international peers at conferences and meetings. I generally tend to give an overall direction for a project and let the young researchers (including the PhD students) influence the path of their project, including the choice of methodologies and scientific hypotheses. I see my role to advise, guide, and encourage them during that journey, but I insist the journey to be discussed equally between the mentor and the student in order to foster their independence and creative thinking. In practice, based on my initial ideas and introduction, I expect them to propose which directions they prefer to take, how and why, in a dialogue where we define the problem and the projects together. My knowledge and experience are crucial in this step since I have a better overview about the relevance or technical limitations that a young researcher may not be aware of. However, if they insist on certain paths that I believe may be problematic, but strongly believe in their hypothesis, I let them test their ideas and will support them fully in their endeavor, hoping that, in that case, I am wrong and they are right, and that way we may end up discovering something really exciting!

Both mentoring and being mentored can be hard. One, because it involves people! Two, because it requires compromises between two people with partially divergent interests in the context of a hierarchical relationship. A one-sided benefit is a failure; a two-sided benefit is the goal of successful mentorship. Whenever different personalities are involved, sharing and promoting positive experiences may be more helpful than general advice. Our experience is one of an unusually generous mentorship from our common postdoctoral mentor. Based on this experience, we learned to appreciate open, and sometimes uncompromising, two-way communication. Mentors should be clear about expectations and "mentees" clear about goals. Students and postdocs are not just employees. They work on their own projects and on their own future. Mentors need to recognize their intellectual independence, for instance by allowing them to independently publish or act as corresponding authors on work to which the mentor did not directly contribute intellectually.

Scientific research is not a classical business and the rules and jargon of business management should have little place in the laboratory. Mentors and their mentees are colleagues and partners in a creative enterprise that seeks to solve the mysteries of the universe. When it comes to the business side, when we needed it, we were given the opportunity not only to learn the skills of transforming experimental data into publishable papers and fundable grants but also the right to take projects with us without fear of competition. This is an experience worth sharing.

Scientists often are fiercely independent and ambitious people working in a competitive environment. This makes one size fits all solutions unlikely to be successful. But, if there is one key experience we would like to share, it is this: dare to be open with each other about your thoughts, doubts, and plans. You might not always get what you want, but more often than not, you'll get what you need!

Additional Suggested Reading

McGee R. Biomedical workforce diversity: the context for mentoring to develop talents and foster success within the 'pipeline'. AIDS Behav. 2016;20(Supplement):231–7. (*Describes necessity of mentoring diverse trainees in order to solve a particular clinical/research problem.*)

Plagiarism

7

Arthur L. Caplan and Barbara K. Redman

Plagiarism is using someone else's text, ideas or results, without attribution, implying they are your own. While this can occur accidentally, plagiarism is done with an intent to deceive. The aim is the acquisition of scientific credit, publication credit, and ultimately to garner prestige and promotion. Self-plagiarism, the reuse of ideas and text from one's own previous work, if referenced, is usually not a problem, especially if it appears in the materials and methods section of a series of papers reporting on a program of research. The antidote to plagiarism is citing sources and listing references. When you are not sure, cite.

Estimates of the frequency of plagiarism in the published literature found that nearly 20% of retractions (Amos 2014) and of manuscript submissions (Higgins et al. 2016) involve plagiarism. In both cases, the percentage was much higher in countries where English was not an official language.

A different perspective may be found in literature on teaching second-language writing. Instead of being seen as rule violation, plagiarism can be seen as a stage of language development – student knowledge of citing conventions, skills in using source material, an example of different styles of textual practices across academic disciplines, or having been immersed in an educational system that emphasizes memorization and rote learning (Pecorari and Petric 2014). But culture is not an excuse. Adherence to international standards as set by peer-reviewed journals must be followed.

Screening for plagiarism is now routine in many journals and should be utilized before paper submission. This practice protects authors and journals (Shafer 2016). Electronic tools measuring plagiarism can also be used by students to protect their own work or themselves against allegations of unauthorized use of text/ideas. While there is not agreement about an acceptable threshold for the amount of text/ideas used from another author or source automated programs can detect suspicious cases. Plagiarism is intellectual theft and departments and institutions must treat it as such.

Research integrity requires that credit for scientific work be honestly earned; plagiarism violates that norm. The degree of pain and loss experienced by an author who was plagiarized by a reviewer of his submitted manuscript can be found in "Dear Plagiarist". In his case, the journal editor took the appropriate action as did the editor in which the plagiarized paper had been published as it was retracted. It is less clear that the plagiarist's institution took appropriate action against the plagiarist.

Advice: Access to plagiarism-detection software (libraries likely have it) will allow you to check your own manuscripts to see if they cross a threshold that may be considered plagiarism. It will also allow you to check if someone else is plagiarizing your work. If you believe something has been plagiarized in a published work, report it to the editor or publisher of the work.

A. L. Caplan · B. K. Redman (✉)
New York University Langone Medical Center,
New York, NY, USA
e-mail: Arthur.Caplan@nyumc.org

© Springer International Publishing AG, part of Springer Nature 2018
A. L. Caplan, B. K. Redman (eds.), *Getting to Good*, https://doi.org/10.1007/978-3-319-51358-4_7

7.1   Plagiarism in Research

Gert Helgesson and Stefan Eriksson

Helgesson, G, Eriksson, S. Plagiarism in research. *Medicine Health Care and Philosophy* 18, 91–101 (2015). Springer Science+Business Media Dordrecht 2014. An imprint of SpringerNature.

Med Health Care and Philos (2015) 18:91–101
DOI 10.1007/s11019-014-9583-8

SCIENTIFIC CONTRIBUTION

Plagiarism in research

Gert Helgesson · Stefan Eriksson

Published online: 4 July 2014
© Springer Science+Business Media Dordrecht 2014

Abstract Plagiarism is a major problem for research. There are, however, divergent views on how to define plagiarism and on what makes plagiarism reprehensible. In this paper we explicate the concept of "plagiarism" and discuss plagiarism normatively in relation to research. We suggest that plagiarism should be understood as "someone using someone else's intellectual product (such as texts, ideas, or results), thereby implying that it is their own" and argue that this is an adequate and fruitful definition. We discuss a number of circumstances that make plagiarism more or less grave and the plagiariser more or less blameworthy. As a result of our normative analysis, we suggest that what makes plagiarism reprehensible as such is that it distorts scientific credit. In addition, intentional plagiarism involves dishonesty. There are, furthermore, a number of potentially negative consequences of plagiarism.

Keywords Fabrication · Intellectual contribution · Plagiarism · Scientific misconduct · Software · Scientific credit

Introduction

Plagiarism is a well-known and growing issue in the academic world. It is estimated to make up a substantial part of

G. Helgesson (✉)
Department of Learning, Informatics, Management and Ethics, Stockholm Centre for Healthcare Ethics, Karolinska Institutet, 171 77 Stockholm, Sweden
e-mail: gert.helgesson@ki.se

S. Eriksson
Centre for Research Ethics and Bioethics, Uppsala University, Uppsala, Sweden

the total number of serious deviations from good research practice (Titus et al. 2008; Vitse and Poland 2012). For some journals it is indeed a serious problem, with up to a third of the published papers containing plagiarism (Zhang 2010; Baždaric et al. 2012; Butler 2010). Given that plagiarism is perceived as a considerable problem for the research community, spelling out in some detail what is to count as plagiarism becomes a matter of pressing concern. The technical development of software for detecting plagiarism also raises questions: What degree of overlapping constitutes plagiarism, and is overlapping all that matters?

Clarifying what constitutes plagiarism is one thing, and making clear what is wrong with it is another, although the two are interrelated. Are all forms of plagiarism equally bad? Are there perhaps even legitimate ways to plagiarise? If so, what makes plagiarism wrong?

In this paper we will mainly do two things. First, we will explicate the concept of "plagiarism", i.e. present an analysis of the concept aimed at further clarifying it. This means that we will look at previous uses of the term and through critical analysis come up with what we take to be an improved definition. While many organizations and research ethical guidelines present their definitions of "plagiarism", little work has so far been done in explaining and justifying the chosen definitions. Here we hope to make an important contribution. The point of the definition that we present is not to identify the essence or 'real nature' of plagiarism (we doubt that there is such a thing), but rather to extract one that is useful for the purpose of clarifying normative issues related to plagiarism, while being true to common uses of the term. Second, we will discuss plagiarism normatively, by taking a closer look at different aspects of it. We restrict our analysis to the context of research, since plagiarism in the arts, for instance, raise a partly different set of issues, and include partly different normative intuitions, which would require a separate analysis.

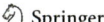 Springer

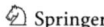

In order to evaluate an explication of "plagiarism" in relation to the present purpose, we first need to identify a set of conditions for adequacy. Although we will not systematically test suggested definitions against these conditions, they show what requirements our definition is intended, and believed, to meet to a reasonable extent.

Conditions of adequacy

The conditions of adequacy should identify relevant restrictions on any suggested definition for the definition to be reasonably adequate for the intended purpose in the intended context. Partly different criteria may become relevant depending on the intended use of the definition. We suggest, inspired by Brülde and Tengland (2003), that the following criteria for adequacy are relevant to a definition of "plagiarism" for our intended use:

- *Fitting language use*: The definition should not deviate too much from established language use, which is to say that it should catch basic semantic intuitions and should be able to handle paradigmatic cases—if acts that are usually considered to be instances of plagiarism are rarely taken to be so by your definition, then it fulfils this criterion poorly. The greater the number of such cases it covers, the better. However, it goes without saying that if there is no uniform language use, a logically consistent definition cannot cover all uses.
- *Precision*: The greater the precision of the definition, the better it is. Ideally, for each case the definition should settle whether or not it is a case of plagiarism.
- *Reliability (intersubjectivity)*: The definition is reliable if different users of it pass the same judgment on specific cases ("If plagiarism is defined as so-and-so, then this is (or is not) a case of plagiarism"). If a definition is reliable, then it produces the same outcome regardless of who is using it, which means that there is intersubjectivity in the use.
- *Theoretical fruitfulness*: The definition is more theoretically fruitful if it is better at distinguishing things that may be important to keep apart; it is better the greater the "job" it can do. For example, it is more theoretically fruitful if it can help to explain claims about plagiarism, such as why some instances count as plagiarism (or why some aspects are relevant for settling the issue) whilst others do not.
- *Relevance for normative purposes*: The definition should as far as possible identify as plagiarism those events that one would like to single out as morally problematic in this regard.
- *Simplicity*: The general idea that it is preferable for a definition to be homogeneous and ad hoc-free.

What is plagiarism?

Since it is important to determine what constitutes misconduct in scientific writing, and "plagiarism" is a much used concept in discussions of scientific misconduct, one could perhaps expect agreement and a fairly high level of precision regarding what constitutes plagiarism. However, while there is agreement about paradigmatic cases of plagiarism, there is less agreement regarding how plagiarism should be defined. In fact, the issue is rarely discussed in detail.

When the concept is explained in a recent newsletter from the US Office of Research Integrity, it looks deceptively simple: "It involves stealing someone else's work and lying about it afterward" (Sox 2012). Others prefer to speak of "copying" part of someone else's published work and using it without showing that it is borrowed from someone else. In the Longman Contemporary English Advanced Learner's Dictionary, the act of plagiarism is defined as "when someone uses another person's words, ideas, or work and pretends they are their own".

In the scholarly definitions, the more technical notions of "appropriation" and "credit" are central: "Plagiarism is the appropriation of other people's material without giving proper credit" (The European Code of Conduct for Research Integrity); "Plagiarism is the appropriation of another person's ideas, processes, results, or words without giving appropriate credit" (US Federal Policy on Research Misconduct). So the basic ideas seem to be that someone deliberately takes someone else's work, whether in the form of an idea, a method, data, results, or text, and presents it as their own instead of giving credit to the person whose ideas, results, or words it is. This is mirrored in the definition given by Merriam-Webster: "to steal and pass off (the ideas or words of another) as one's own: use (another's production) without crediting the source".

Two components of plagiarism

Common to these definitions is that plagiarism is composed of two parts: (1) to appropriate the work of someone else and (2) passing it off as one's own by not giving proper credit.

Let us first ask what it means to appropriate someone else's work. In some definitions, plagiarism is characterised as stealing. However, if plagiarism by definition concerns stealing, then it is not theft in the traditional sense of taking a thing, where if person A takes it from person B, then B will no longer have it. What is appropriated in such instances of plagiarism is *intellectual* property, as when people download copyright-protected films or music from the Internet. Thus, to the extent that plagiarism is theft, it is stealing someone else's intellectual work by copying.

Related to research papers, it is about copying another's text, tables, graphs, or pictures into one's own paper without having permission to do so (and with certain pretence, a point we shall be returning to presently).

We are, however, disinclined to include stealing in our definition. Although one may steal intellectual as well as non-intellectual property, and even talk about "theft of the recognition due to the original contributor" (Rathod 2012), talking about plagiarism as stealing is nevertheless misguided, at least as part of a definition. This is so because using someone else's text, say, and passing it off as one's own can be done regardless of whether one steals the text or not. One can do it by finding the text in a journal or book or by using an unpublished paper—or by stealing it from someone's computer or drawer. Thus, it seems that stealing is not a constituent part of plagiarising. In fact, you plagiarise a text even if it was willingly handed to you by a research acquaintance—if your use of it implies that it was you who created it. However, plagiarism does not preclude that the text presented as one's own has been literally stolen from someone else; you may steal a manuscript in order to plagiarise it (just as you may steal it in order to keep it without showing it to anyone). If you do, that means that you pass off the stolen manuscript as your own.

It may still be argued that there is a sense of "stealing" that concerns appropriating someone else's intellectual work and passing it off as one's own. In this sense you may steal someone's song if you play it and claim to have composed it yourself. This seems to mean that there is a sense of "stealing" that is equivalent to "plagiarising". If so, this second understanding of "stealing", which is distinct from the one discussed above, cannot contribute anything to a definition of "plagiarism". The conclusion remains: stealing, or theft, cannot be used as part of the definition of "plagiarism".

"To appropriate" does not have to imply stealing. It could also mean, for instance, acquire, borrow, take, or expropriate. We nevertheless suggest that "appropriate" should be avoided, just because it is such an ambiguous term and therefore would introduce obscurity in the definition. We instead suggest that "use" is employed.

It seems, then, that it is the second part of the definition that will distinguish cases of plagiarism from acceptable cases of using the results of another's intellectual effort. The second alleged aspect or component of plagiarism is passing it off as one's own. This can be done with or without the approval of the person or persons being plagiarised, so it is not about whether or not the re-use has the author's approval, but about what impression is given by that use. Using someone else's work and being dishonest or otherwise misleading about where it comes from seems to be what makes the act an act of plagiarism. But dishonest or misleading in a special way: If person A uses a passage

from a text by B but claims that it was written by C, then, even though it is an incorrect claim, it is not plagiarism, but simply incorrect referring (if intentional, it is a kind of fraudulent behaviour). It is when A claims (explicitly or implicitly) to have written the passage him- or herself that it becomes plagiarism. This was brought out in the definition provided by Merriam-Webster above: it is when we *pass something off as our own*, although it isn't, that we plagiarise. This seems to be the core of plagiarism.

An intellectual product of one's own

It is no accident that plagiarism is discussed in relation to research, although it is also clearly relevant in relation to music, literature, art, and design, since it relates to using the product of someone else's *intellectual work* while passing it off as one's own. Note that there is no reason to restrict the use of the term to published work, since you may use someone else's work while passing it off as your own even if it is not published. For instance, you may do it by first stealing the manuscript from the author, by using passages from an unpublished manuscript circulated at a seminar, or by using ideas communicated at a lecture.

What if a person does not go to the trouble of writing up a paper in which the results of others' intellectual efforts are used with the pretence of being the person's own; what if the person simply makes the wrongful claim that "this is my work"? Would that also be plagiarism? Example: A scientific paper in astrophysics is published in a renowned journal by a group of researchers. Researcher Ynotme, not part of the group, then goes public falsely claiming that the published results are hers. Would she thereby be plagiarising? Our explication so far leans towards the view that plagiarism concerns *a product of one's own*, containing the appropriation of the intellectual work of someone else. We believe that it would be constructive to claim that plagiarism consists not only in passing someone else's work or intellectual product off as one's own, but also in using it *as a product of one's own*. Going for this position, falsely claiming a work of another's to be one's own would not be plagiarism, but would count as a false accusation of plagiarism and theft.

Our definition of "to plagiarise" would, thus, at this stage be: to *use* someone else's intellectual product while passing it off as one's own, where "use" is meant to indicate that it is made part, or the whole, of a product of one's own. However, although quite a few attempts at a definition of "plagiarism" include elements such as lying or pretending it is one's own intellectual work, others rather describe the second part of the definition in terms of not giving the proper or appropriate credit. While the first set of expressions—lying, stealing, and pretending—implies *intention*, the second set is neutral in this regard.

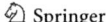

While ordinary language use of "plagiarism" certainly allows for the act of plagiarising being intentional, it seems as clear that plagiarism does not necessarily involve an intention to deceive. We therefore would like to suggest a definition that does not require intention. The notion of "passing something off" also seems to imply intention, and therefore ought preferably to be avoided. A slightly modified definition, where we define "plagiarism" rather than "to plagiarise", would therefore read: *Plagiarism = an instance of someone using someone else's work, thereby implying that it is their own.*

Plagiarising ideas? Plagiarising work?

What, then, counts as an intellectual product? The standard case of plagiarism is the use of someone else's text. We have seen that Merriam-Webster mentions "words or ideas", while Longman talks of "words, ideas, or work". Is it reasonable to say that ideas can be plagiarised—and what about work? Let us look at ideas first.

It seems that one can talk about plagiarising ideas just as well as one can talk about plagiarising research results or text, since ideas are obvious examples of results of intellectual work. If someone uses another's idea and implies that it is an idea of their own, that someone is plagiarising. True, it must be admitted that it may often be much more difficult to verify that an idea has been plagiarised compared to research results or text. Ideas are not always documented, but might be presented at conferences or in personal conversation, etc. The difficulty pertains both to finding out about the plagiarism and to making a convincing case for idea plagiarism to have taken place. There is no clever software to discern this, nor is it easily proven that an idea is not independently arrived at. These difficulties are, however, practical; they do not change the fact that ideas can be plagiarised.

Some might be reluctant on ideological grounds to accept that ideas can be plagiarised. They might think that ideas should be free and not be the intellectual property of anyone. However, our position is agnostic on this ideological debate since the definition does not rely on notions of stealing intellectual property. Freedom of ideas is compatible with the view that you are plagiarising if you use someone else's idea while implying that it is your own.

What, then, about plagiarising work? As previously noted, plagiarism in relation to work must concern intellectual work. In this context, the term "work" has two distinct senses: a product based on intellectual labour or that labour itself. When someone is plagiarising a text presenting research results, thereby implying that they are presenting their own results, then that person also implies that they have done the work leading up to the results. In that sense you can say that the person is also plagiarising

the work put into it. By plagiarising someone's idea, you, by the same token, make implicit claims about the work leading up to that idea.

But it is hard to see that it makes sense to talk about plagiarising work (labour) directly. Let us look at an example: Say that Mr A visits Ms B and sees a beautiful chair that Ms B has made to her own design. Mr A goes home, builds an identical chair, and claims when friends ask that it is of his own design. When it comes to the chair, it is clear that it is the idea of making the chair just like that, i.e. the design, and not the work of making the chair (which he in fact did), that is plagiarised. Plagiarising work means plagiarising ideas relating to how to do the work, the results of work, or the documentation of how the work was performed, not the labour itself—the latter would be to *repeat* the work, not to plagiarise it.[1] We therefore choose not to talk about work, but instead of an intellectual product being plagiarised. So, our definition will be the following.

> Plagiarism = *def.* an instance of someone using someone else's intellectual product (such as texts, ideas, or results), thereby implying that it is their own.

Demarcations: self-plagiarism et cetera

Plagiarism being part of the standard definition of research misconduct, and therefore often regulated, allegations of plagiarism are more likely to be investigated than many other potential instances of deviations from good research practice. If it can be shown that other problematic behaviours can be covered by the definition of plagiarism, this will help make them eligible for investigation. Anekwe has in this way suggested that honorary authorship and ghost-writing[2] are instances of plagiarism, since these practices entail claiming merit for work done by others, even if those others condone the act (Anekwe 2010). It follows from our definition that we can agree with his conclusion.

It has become increasingly common to discuss so-called self-plagiarism as a special case of plagiarism (Roig 2006; Brogan 1992; Samuelson 1994). Perhaps this is prompted by a similar wish to include such behaviour in what can be

---

[1] Only if the result of intellectual work is a novel idea about a way to process a certain task (a method) will it be possible to plagiarise by *repeating the processes* and not disclosing where the idea of doing it like *that* originated. Which is to say that (the idea of) a method may be plagiarised by using it and not disclosing that someone else came up with it, thereby implying that you invented it yourself.

[2] It is, of course, not the writing that constitutes plagiarism in the context of ghost-writing, but the claim to have written or co-authored a text completely written by others.

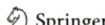

reported and investigated. However, there is a considerable difference between plagiarism and self-plagiarism, in that plagiarism involves presenting the results of someone else's intellectual efforts as one's own (as is reflected in the different definitions discussed above), while self-plagiarism does not involve the work of others but is restricted to the reuse of one's own material. Similarly, if considered in the light of our explication of plagiarism, self-plagiarism clearly cannot be described as "using someone else's intellectual product, thereby implying that it is one's own". Therefore one might argue that self-plagiarism is a contradiction in terms, and thus a confusing way of raising the problem of redundantly overlapping publication (Bruton 2014 with many references).

Still, there are similarities between plagiarism and cases described as self-plagiarism. Both usually involve redundant publication—in both cases, new efforts and findings are quite often implied when in fact previous research has just been republished, with the consequence that scientific credit is obtained twice (or more) for something that deserves credit once only. Perhaps this is the greatest perceived similarity: in both plagiarism and so-called self-plagiarism, researchers are acquiring undeserved credit for research. Inspired by this, one might be inclined to suggest a definition that differs from the ones discussed above, stressing the "undeserved credit" aspect, such as: Plagiarism = *def.* an instance of someone's acquiring undeserved scientific credit, either by using someone else's intellectual product, thereby implying that it is one's own, or by presenting one's own previously recognized work as new.

However, this definition has some important weaknesses compared to the one we propose. First, it deviates from the vast majority of definitions of plagiarism, since it doesn't require that *someone else's* intellectual product is involved. Thus, it fits established language use poorly. Furthermore, it makes plagiarism hinge on whether or not undeserved scientific credit was in fact acquired, which is irrelevant in ordinary language use—it is still plagiarism, even if the submitted paper containing unacknowledged copied material does not get published. One might try to counter this weakness by adding "or trying to acquire" after "someone's acquiring". But that trick does not work; because it may be an act of plagiarism even though the plagiarizer does not succeed in acquiring undeserved credit, nor tries to do so (he may not know that the cut-and-paste method is unacceptable). Neither *acquiring undeserved scientific credit* nor *trying to do so* is a necessary component of plagiarism. The basic error in this attempt at a definition is that it puts focus on the wrong thing, namely on the *effect*, or the intended effect, of doing something rather than on the very act that the definition concerns. This will no doubt have implications for the theoretical fruitfulness of the

definition, as well as for its relevance for normative purposes. Furthermore, although of lesser importance, by containing two distinct components, this definition is not as simple as the one we propose. This lack of simplicity means that in many situations it will be unclear what happened when we learn that "P plagiarised", since it may be either that P used someone else's intellectual product or reused his/her own. For clarity, it is preferable, all else equal, that definitions do not have the form "A is defined as this *or* that".

In many research areas papers are co-written. If one of the authors reuses text without proper notification, thereby implying that what is written is his/her own, then this is primarily a case of plagiarism, not self-plagiarism, because here we have an individual claiming by implication to be the sole author of that which is the result of an intellectual effort also made by others.

It can be helpful to distinguish plagiarism from duplicate publication, text recycling, salami slicing, and copyright infringement (Bruton 2014; Roig 2006). While we define plagiarism as "using someone else's intellectual product, thereby implying that it is one's own", self-plagiarism is sometimes better described as duplicate publication. Duplicate publication concerns publication of whole articles or texts (or sets of data or results) more than once without proper notification of this fact. When the "self-plagiariser" uses shorter passages of texts (or some figures, etc.) in repeated instances, we prefer to speak of inappropriate recycling of material. When the same study or set of experiments is dispensed in small chunks in different papers just to increase the number of publications, we have what is commonly known as "salami slicing".

Plagiarising someone else's intellectual product is not the same thing as infringing on someone's copyright. This follows clearly from our definition. The results of intellectual endeavour can be plagiarised without intellectual property claims being involved; for instance, it is perfectly possible to pass off as one's own a text of unknown origin from the dim and distant past. It is also possible to infringe someone's copyright without plagiarising. To publish an illustration owned by others or a passage of text that contains a large number of words might, proper referencing notwithstanding, be an infringement if in fact you need the owner's permission to publish. A further difference is that ideas can only be protected by copyright if given a tangible form (if they are written out) while they can be plagiarised even if only communicated orally. Yet another is that copyright protects the economic interests of the copyright holder while a do-not-plagiarise principle protects due recognition. To sum up, these instances of improper handling of material can co-exist in the same act and occur separately (they neither imply nor rule out each other).

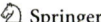 Springer

Irrelevant aspects

It is sometimes asked whether certain aspects other than the ones discussed above are relevant in determining whether or not a certain act is an instance of plagiarism:

- the scientific merit to be gained from the publication
- the locus of the plagiarism (for instance, a published paper, a student essay, a summary of a doctoral thesis, or an oral presentation at a seminar)
- who is plagiarised
- the intended audience or purpose of the plagiarising work as compared to the original

One idea that we have encountered is that something that would be considered plagiarism if appearing in a published scientific paper may not be considered plagiarism if, for instance, appearing in a report ordered by a public authority or in a student paper not intended for publication. However, the locus of the plagiarising work or how conducive it is to career promotion is irrelevant to whether it is plagiarism, although that may be relevant to an evaluation of how serious the misconduct is; for instance, one may argue that the greater the research merit of a paper containing plagiarism, the more serious it might be considered, analogously to how theft may be considered more serious the more money that is stolen.

If something is to be considered plagiarism or not is also independent of who is plagiarised. For instance, it makes no difference if the person plagiarised is considered insignificant. It is also irrelevant to the evaluation of whether or not there is plagiarism if the plagiarised and plagiarising texts are used for different purposes, have different intended readers, or are of very different dimensions. It is still plagiarism if someone copies something from a short research paper and includes it in an extensive book. Whether or not the plagiarised text was published in an indexed, peer-reviewed journal is equally irrelevant.

Plagiarisers sometimes defend their actions by referring to cultural differences in the attitudes towards the work of others, and especially work of authorities (Sun 2012; Chandrasoma et al. 2004; DeVoss and Rosati 2002). They refer to an attitude that, out of respect, one must not meddle with the thoughts of great thinkers by re-writing their work—it should be left as it is. If such an attitude of respect, or even reverence, also exists in relation to research, this is at variance with the scientific ethos that is assumed all over the world: there should be no exemptions for local idiosyncrasies. However, using quotations to a reasonable degree is in accordance with good scientific practice as long as quotation marks or indentations with correct references are used.

It has happened that researchers with insufficient skills in the English language have been encouraged by their supervisors or colleagues to use another paper as a template and change data in order to include their own results instead of those in the template, with a considerable text overlap as a consequence (Couzin-Frankel and Grom 2009). Regardless of what the underlying explanations are, they have no bearing on whether or not a certain act is an act of plagiarism.

Does size matter? Or only originality?

Plagiarism can be more or less extensive, ranging from whole chapters of books, or entire academic papers, to shorter passages. Is there a lower limit to what counts as plagiarism? If so, when does it cease to be plagiarism—is it if it falls short of a certain number of copied words in a line or of a certain percentage of overlapping text in an essay, or does it depend on something else, such as the quality of that which is reused without notification?

We will argue that to the extent that quantity matters, it depends on whether quantity has an impact on quality. This is to say that quantity matters only indirectly, while quality matters directly (i.e. as such). Plagiarism may consist in very short passages of text. In principle, it may consist in one word or expression only. But that would have to be a very special, novel word or expression creatively used, e.g. for naming a new concept, perhaps something that throws new light on an area of interest. It would also have to be a situation where the plagiariser, by plagiarising, gives the impression that s/he invented the concept.

Using ordinary words like "and", "it", or "are" can never, as such, constitute plagiarism. Nor can the use of series of words, or sentences, which are so ordinary that they cannot meaningfully be ascribed to anyone. Examples: "He saw me", "Open the door", or "I am tired and need some sleep." Due to their commonness, they belong to a common pool of expressions and sentences to which no one has an intellectual claim. If a number of people independently have "created" the same expressions, these expressions *ipso facto* lose their exclusivity. Such word combinations *cannot* be plagiarised (or so we would like to argue) because they cannot be considered to have been taken from someone else (in particular). This means that there is no case of plagiarism if such sentences have been copied and pasted from another text without (ordinarily due) notification. The Committee on Publication Ethics (COPE) gives the example of "smokers with chronic obstructive pulmonary disease" being used in science as a standard phrase, having more than 58,000 hits on Google (Wager 2011). Other examples are "The questionnaire was distributed to a random selection of…", "Statistical analysis was conducted using SPSS …", and "The study was granted ethical approval by the ethical review board in …".

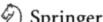

It is our firm belief that researchers can produce many more examples of this kind from their respective fields.

However, one reservation is called for. If a sufficient number of ordinary sentences not really belonging to anyone are put after each other in exactly the same way as by another author, then this may again be considered to be plagiarism. The longer passage may uniquely be attributed to a particular author, even though the individual sentences cannot.

Nor is it plagiarism to refer to others' results by stating numbers, like percentages, that express the results, without putting them between quotation marks. The same goes if someone, with references, states analysis categories identified in someone else's qualitative study. This is so because, in the case of the numbers and categories, adding quotation marks does not make things any clearer. If there is any reason to believe that some readers will hesitate about whether you named the qualitative categories yourself, while you intended to state them literally from the cited paper, then you might need to be more explicit about this or add quotation marks after all.

To summarise, we claim that plagiarism (in principle) can consist in as little as one word, while there are many standard sentences describing research methods that will not be plagiarism even if, in fact, copied from someone else. This is to say that the unmarked reuse of some very short passages might be plagiarism, even though the reuse of other equally short passages would not. The conclusion to draw from this is that plagiarism has to do with quality rather than quantity—or, more precisely, with what is unique rather than so common that it cannot be attributed to anyone.

Plagiarism and probabilities

When it comes to investigating accusations of plagiarism, failing direct proof, the investigation will have to rest on probabilities. The longer and the more unique the identical passage, the greater the likelihood of its having been plagiarised. Still, if fairly ordinary passages or sentences, which are not common enough to be considered as not belonging to anyone, are in fact copied from someone else without use of quotation marks, then they *are* plagiarised, even if, for lack of further evidence, they will be considered by an investigator as not plagiarised. The criterion for plagiarism does not involve probabilities. Probabilities become relevant as part of a decision method when trying to settle whether or not an act of plagiarism has been committed. Also, if exactly the same, non-trivial sentence is written independently by two different authors, then there is no plagiarism involved, even if it will seem unlikely to an investigator that it was not. It does not become plagiarism because it seems to be plagiarism.

It is important to notice that software used to identify plagiarism—like iThenticate, Viper, and Turnitin (Khan 2011)—only detects text similarity. Such software can certainly be of help in detecting potential cases of plagiarism, but does not, of itself, identify plagiarism. In most cases, a proportion of overlapping text, expressed in a certain percentage, is insufficient to settle whether or not plagiarism is present. If you have 100 % overlap, then you know. You can also strongly suspect plagiarism if you find an overlap exceeding, say, 70 % for the entire text. But using a certain percentage over an entire paper, as some scientific journal editors do, seems to be a shaky foundation for deciding whether or not to investigate plagiarism. For instance, for a four-page paper a completely copied half-page would render a 12.5 % rate for the entire paper. To copy a third of a page word for word in a four-page paper, which in most cases would suffice for a convincing case of plagiarism, would render an overall overlapping rate of only 8.33 %. Clearly, then, you cannot use an arbitrary cut-off point of say, 20 %, because that would potentially miss many an instance of plagiarism.

Furthermore, this software can only help to identify plagiarism of text or numbers, whereas it is useless if instead what is plagiarised is ideas. It is also sensitive to language, which means that it does not detect plagiarism resulting from, say, taking a text written in English and using it, translated, in a text in German or French.

The normative status of plagiarism

It is part and parcel of good research practice to know the difference between plagiarism and established rules for citations and quotations. But judging the normative status of different cases of plagiarism is another issue. While some will constitute major cases of misconduct, others may be considered minor deviations from good research practice. While copying half a research article into one's own paper would be serious misconduct, copying 5–10 average-length and spread-out sentences of limited importance in a five-page paper is perhaps not. Yet another issue (left aside in this paper) is what policies are reasonable to adopt at universities and research institutes.

Before discussing what makes some forms of plagiarism worse than others, we should say something about what makes plagiarism bad to begin with. Plagiarism is one of the "core" instances of research misconduct, the other two being fabrication and falsification. "Fabrication" concerns making up research results instead of actually producing them by doing research. "Falsification" concerns tampering with research results, research methods, or data analysis. Common to both is that the researchers are misleading about what they have accomplished—they

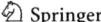 Springer

pretend to have done the research, to have reached the presented results, to have used the correct methods and procedures, or to have applied appropriate analyses in the way described. Fabrication and falsification are directly detrimental to science, with the indirect effect that researchers may prosper from publications based on these kinds of fraud.

Plagiarism is commonly held to be reprehensible because it makes publications (etc.) misleading regarding who deserves credit for the intellectual work done—thus, it is unjust. It is also common to refer to the very act itself, declaring it to be an instance of cheating and betraying, both reprehensible acts. Some also point to the person plagiarising, maintaining that an additional wrongness of plagiarism lies in the fact that it makes the person a cheat and an impostor. These remarks, however, are restricted to intentional plagiarism. Plagiarism may, further, have unjust consequences by affecting who gets good grades, academic positions, and research funding.

In addition, plagiarism of data or results distorts the scientific record by giving a misleading account of research accomplishments. What is presented as new collections of data or as new results is not—instead it is a reiteration of what has already been done. Thereby it also distorts meta-analyses.

Let us now ask what aspects affect the normative status of a case of plagiarism. There is no direct connection between what aspects are relevant to determine whether or not something *is* plagiarism and what aspects are relevant to a specific normative judgment of an instance of plagiarism. For instance, aspects that are relevant when determining whether or not something is plagiarism may have nothing to add when it comes to evaluating gravity, as might sometimes be the case when regarding the originality versus ordinariness of passages appropriated in material of one's own. Other aspects are irrelevant when determining whether or not it is a case of plagiarism, but may be relevant when determining the seriousness of the plagiarism, such as whether or not the plagiarism was intended or the scientific merit value of the publication or presentation containing plagiarism. So what aspects affect the normative status of a case of plagiarism? Candidates include:

- the value of that which is appropriated
- the manner in which the plagiarism is performed
- the degree of harm to the plagiarised person(s)
- the degree of personal gain to the offender(s)
- whether the plagiarism is intentional or not

Before going any further, we should first note that one may distinguish between what makes plagiarism worse *qua* plagiarism (roughly points 1 and 2), what makes an action involving plagiarism worse on the whole (points 3 and 4), and what makes the plagiariser more or less blameworthy (point 5).

Intentional or unintentional?

To begin with the last point, a case of plagiarism is judged differently depending on whether or not the offender did it on purpose, just as other intentional wrongdoings are considered more blameworthy than unintentional ones. Sloppy quotation practices, or ignorance, are not as blameworthy as intentional fraud. If someone falls prey to *cryptomnesia*, i.e. unconscious plagiarism that happens when you remember the idea but not that you got it from someone (Roig 2006), they might to a certain extent be excused. However, one might argue that the very plagiarism is equally bad whether intended or not, while it is more reprehensible to plagiarise intentionally than otherwise.

Even though a case of plagiarism is judged differently depending on whether the offender did it on purpose or not, one may also be held responsible for one's ignorance. Good research practice involves knowing where to draw the line between acceptable and unacceptable behaviours relating to research, such as the unacceptability of fabricating or tampering with data or results. That it is unacceptable to cut and paste from other people's published work, without stating the source and showing exactly what passages are quoted, is part of that required knowledge of good research practice. If one has not been taught this, part of the blame for plagiarism must fall on one's teachers and supervisors. Excuses nevertheless cannot eliminate the fact that disrespecting standard rules of quotation is a deviation from good practice. Someone who is plagiarising is always blameworthy, to the extent that readers thereby are misled about who deserves credit for the work.[3] Still, those who mislead intentionally are more blameworthy.

Wrong as such and bad consequences

Let us return to the previous points. While the first two points concern the disvalue of plagiarism as such, the other two points concern the consequences of plagiarism. A case of plagiarism might be considered graver if the material plagiarised had the potential for greatly benefitting the originator economically or by having great impact. For example, a plagiarising publication can rule out the possibility of obtaining a patent. Conversely, we would perhaps think it worse to build a whole well-renowned career upon plagiarising others, than to plagiarise in a way that never brought any particular advantages.

---

[3] It should be noted that it does not have to be the authors' fault that a paper is misleading about who deserves credit. Leonard Fleck has brought to our attention instances of journals, unbeknown to the authors, having mistakenly removed references or quotation marks in the text, causing the text to give the impression that some phrases quoted from others are the authors' own.

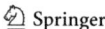

As can be seen in these examples, what harm is caused to the plagiarised person(s) and what the offenders gain in a specific case depends not only on the characteristics of the specific plagiarism as such but also on things that lie beyond that (such as the reception of the alleged work, or the legal consequences of making ideas public). Depending on these "external" circumstances, the harm or benefit may be limited or great. This supports the idea that it is meaningful to distinguish between judging the plagiarism *qua* plagiarism and judging the act of plagiarism and its consequences as a whole.

What, then, makes plagiarism *qua* plagiarism more or less reprehensible? First, it normally makes a moral difference what is plagiarised: is it an idea, or research data or results, or is it rather useful phrases or background descriptions? Plagiarism of research results, and also discussion, is seen by many as considerably worse than plagiarism from the introduction or methods sections. One rationale for this view is that plagiarism of data or results involves fabrication (the offender gives the impression of presenting new data/results while this in fact is not the case). This means that plagiarism of data or results is worse than simple textual plagiarism because it also involves something else that is bad (fabrication).

Second, plagiarism of data/results may be considered worse as plagiarism because it involves something more novel, more creative, and thus scientifically more valuable than background and methods sections normally do; plagiarism of the latter often only involves free-riding on the labour and phrasing skills of others. There may, of course, be exceptions to this rule: the background section may present previous research endeavours in a new and eye-opening way likely to revolutionise future research; and the methods sections of methodological papers do indeed tend to contain their most novel and creative work. Regardless of where the main merits of a paper are located, plagiarism of those parts is more reprehensible than plagiarism of less important parts. To sum up, the greater the value of that which is plagiarised, the graver the plagiarism. The value we have in mind stems from the novelty and potential of affecting knowledge development within the specific field. Arguably these are also the aspects that are most likely to affect the scientific credit to be gained from the publication (regardless of whether it is the original or the plagiarising piece).

Lastly, the very act of plagiarism might be perceived differently according to the manner in which it was performed. If someone has a reference to where the material has been lifted but neglects to use proper quotation marks, it might be a sign of not having the *intention* to deceive, and we therefore find the act less reprehensible. But the *very act* also seems less objectionable in this example, since at least some merit is given to the original source and because readers are able to check the source, which they

otherwise wouldn't. How you do it thus plays a part in evaluating the seriousness of the offence of plagiarism.

Pre-comprehension and being misleading

Within some research fields in medicine and the natural sciences, it seems to be quite common when writing up a paper to state certain key passages by recognised authorities, particularly in the methods section, with references but without showing that it is a literal quotation. It also seems common to recycle text literally from methods sections of one's previous papers without quoting. This practice is sometimes taken so far as to use whole sections verbatim over and over again without proper citation practices being followed. For example, research groups may write up what they believe to be the perfect method section, and then it is a given that this section is used in any paper originating from the group. Those who are used to this argue that everyone knows about it and that the practice therefore is not misleading.[4] One might, of course, question this; for instance, when papers are attracting a wider audience, these readers cannot be expected to know of the particular authoritative text sections taken for granted by the insiders.

It would, of course, be easy to change the practice, if there is such, and abide by standard rules for quotations, for instance, by adding quotation marks to the quoted passages. But is it reprehensible to leave them out? What position one takes on this issue may have to do with academic background. In areas where the written word is central and where researchers are used to considering the entire paper as the results of the research, people will not be inclined to take quotation rules lightly, while there seems to be a partly different attitude within medicine and the natural sciences, where what is considered to be the research results is that which you find in the results section of the paper, primarily in the tables or expressed in mathematical form. The discussion section is then usually also considered to contain material that is clearly the researchers' own contribution, while little sentimentality or personal strings are felt regarding background and methods sections (unless it is a methodological paper).

One could point out that it would be a disservice to science to change the description of a commonly used method every time a publication is prepared, just to avoid charges of plagiarism, if doing so results in a less comprehensible text. So if everyone knows of this practice, more is gained by reproducing the methods section

---

[4] Our claims here regarding practices are based on anecdotic evidence only. However, based on our teaching about 500 doctoral students per year, and having heard this frequently in class, we believe this to be fairly common, or at least far from unique.

verbatim than what is lost. Still, why not do this *and* follow proper citation practices?

This example illustrates that whether certain behaviours are misleading or not partly depends on the pre-comprehension of those receiving the message. What you ought to do, then, is dependent upon what the pre-comprehension actually is, or what it reasonably can be expected to be.

We noted above that some non-native speakers of English defend their actions by reference to their using others' papers as templates, and we said that this response has no bearing on whether their acts are plagiarism or not. Might this line of reasoning regarding pre-comprehension be used in defence? In 2007, a letter to the editor appeared in Nature that defended this practice both by downplaying the importance of anything but the results and by reference to the commonness of this practice. The author of the letter also suggested that when borrowing sentences makes a non-essential section better, this should not be considered plagiarism in a normative sense (Yilmaz 2007), a statement which some scientists seem to agree with (Pecorari 2012).

There are several possible responses to this. One is that if someone else's text is used as a template without the fact being duly noted, then this will very likely constitute plagiarism. Unless there is an open agreement beforehand that certain texts are free to use as templates, the practice is reprehensible. Another response is that if scientists do not have a working skill in English, then it would be better if they wrote their papers in their native language and had them translated by professional translators.

There are some other important things to note as well, to which we now turn.

Copyright and the risk of getting reported

Even if the use of certain key passages by recognised authorities without following established general referencing practices is recognised as good research practice in a certain context, there are two circumstances that argue strongly for a cautious approach to such a practice. They both point out that the suggested practice only "works" as long as you do not get exposed to the wider research society practising it. First, to reuse, for instance, a widely known methods section might not fool anyone in the field about its origin, but it might still be wronging the publishing houses involved. The copyright in the original text is likely to be owned by someone, and if someone else uses the text without proper referencing then that person will be infringing the copyright. Also, the publisher of the text will expect all material to be original unless the contrary is explicitly stated or shown. If the author or authors are not open about this, the publisher will be deceived. Second, to have sections imported from other sources without proper

references and quotations is to invite accusations of research misconduct from those who spot the practice and are willing to cause harm to those doing it. We thus advise against this practice on these grounds.

Conclusions

We suggest that plagiarism should be understood as "using someone else's intellectual product (such as texts, ideas, or results), thereby implying that it is their own". This may be done intentionally or unintentionally. This fits the use of the term in ordinary language fairly well, while at the same time being sufficiently precise. Arguably it is reliable by being simple and easily comprehensible. We suggest that our discussion supports the view that the definition is theoretically fruitful and highly relevant for normative purposes. As a result of our normative analysis, we suggest that what makes plagiarism reprehensible is that it involves an unfair acquisition of scientific credit. In addition, intentional plagiarism involves dishonesty. In plagiarism of data or results, fabrication is also implied.

Acknowledgments We would like to thank the participants at seminars at Stockholm Centre for Healthcare Ethics, Centre for Research Ethics and Bioethics at Uppsala University, and at the International Bioethics retreat in Paris 2013 for valuable suggestions and constructive criticism of earlier versions of this paper.

References

Anekwe, T.D. 2010. Profits and plagiarism: The case of medical ghostwriting. *Bioethics* 24(6): 267–272.

Baždarić, K., L. Bilić-Zulle, G. Brumini, and M. Petrovečki. 2012. Prevalence of plagiarism in recent submissions to the Croatian Medical Journal. *Science and Engineering Ethics* 18: 223–239.

Brogan, M. 1992. Recycling ideas. *College and Research Libraries* 52(5): 453–464.

Bruton, S.V. 2014. Self-plagiarism and textual recycling: Legitimate forms of research misconduct. *Accountability in Research: Policies and Quality Assurance* 21(3): 176–197.

Brülde, B., and P.-A. Tengland. 2003. *Hälsa och sjukdom: en begreppslig utredning (Health and disease: A conceptual inquiry)*. Lund: Studentlitteratur.

Butler, D. 2010. Journals step up plagiarism policing. *Nature* 466(7303): 167.

Chandrasoma, R., C. Thompson, and A. Pennycook. 2004. Beyond plagiarism: Transgressive and nontransgressive intertextuality. *Journal of Language, Identity and Education* 3(3): 171–193.

Couzin-Frankel, J., and J. Grom. 2009. Plagiarism sleuths. *Science* 324(5930): 1004–1007.

DeVoss, D., and A.C. Rosati. 2002. "It wasn't me, was it?" Plagiarism and the web. *Computers and Composition* 19: 191–203.

Khan, B.A. 2011. Plagiarism: An academic theft. *International Journal of Pharmaceutical Investigation* 1(4): 255.

Pecorari, D. 2012. Textual plagiarism: How should it be regarded? *Office of Research Integrity Newsletter* 20(3): 3,10.

Rathod, S.D. 2012. Plagiarism: the human solution. *Office of Research Integrity Newsletter* 20(3): 1,7.

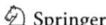

Roig, M. 2006. Avoiding plagiarism, self-plagiarism, and other questionable writing practices: A guide to ethical writing. Office of Research Integrity 2006. www.cse.msu.edu/~alexliu/plagiarism.pdf.

Samuelson, P. 1994. Self-plagiarism or fair use. *Communications of the ACM* 37(8): 21–25.

Sox, H. C. 2012. Plagiarism in the digital age. *Office of Research Integrity Newsletter* 20(3): 1,6.

Sun, Y.C. 2012. Does text readability matter? A study of paraphrasing and plagiarism in English as a foreign language writing context. *The Asia-Pacific Education Researcher* 21(2): 296–306.

Titus, S.L., J.A. Wells, and L.J. Rhoades. 2008. Repairing research integrity. *Nature* 453(7198): 980–982.

Vitse, C.L., and G.A. Poland. 2012. Plagiarism, self-plagiarism, scientific misconduct and VACCINE: Protecting the science and the public. *Vaccine* 30(50): 7131–7133. doi:10.1016/j.vaccine.2012.08.053.

Wager, L. 2011. How should editors respond to plagiarism? COPE discussion paper. 26th April, 2011. http://publicationethics.org/files/Discussion%20document.pdf.

Yilmaz, I. 2007. Plagiarism? No, we're just borrowing better English. *Nature* 449(7163): 658.

Zhang, Y. 2010. Chinese journal finds 31% of submissions plagiarized. *Nature* 467(7312): 153.

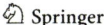

7.2 Text-Based Plagiarism in Scientific Publishing: Issues, Developments and Education

Yongyan Li

Li, Y. Text-based plagiarism in scientific publishing: Issues, developments and education. *Science & Engineering Ethics* 19, 1241–1254 (2013). © The Author(s) 2012.

Sci Eng Ethics (2013) 19:1241–1254
DOI 10.1007/s11948-012-9367-6

ORIGINAL PAPER

Text-Based Plagiarism in Scientific Publishing: Issues, Developments and Education

Yongyan Li

Received: 25 January 2012 / Accepted: 12 April 2012 / Published online: 26 April 2012
© The Author(s) 2012. This article is published with open access at Springerlink.com

Abstract Text-based plagiarism, or copying language from sources, has recently become an issue of growing concern in scientific publishing. Use of CrossCheck (a computational text-matching tool) by journals has sometimes exposed an unexpected amount of textual similarity between submissions and databases of scholarly literature. In this paper I provide an overview of the relevant literature, to examine how journal gatekeepers perceive textual appropriation, and how automated plagiarism-screening tools have been developed to detect text matching, with the technique now available for self-check of manuscripts before submission; I also discuss issues around English as an additional language (EAL) authors and in particular EAL novices being the typical offenders of textual borrowing. The final section of the paper proposes a few educational directions to take in tackling text-based plagiarism, highlighting the roles of the publishing industry, senior authors and English for academic purposes professionals.

Keywords Text-based plagiarism · Automated text-matching · English as an additional language (EAL) authors · Novice scientists

Introduction

A potential distinction between the borrowing of ideas and the borrowing of text in scientific writing is suggested by such terms as *semantic reuse* vs. *textual reuse* (Collberg and Kobourov 2005), and *plagiarism of ideas* vs. *plagiarism of text* (Vessal and Habibzadeh 2007). The distinction between the two scenarios highlights a need to treat the two differently, as recently emphasized by Bouville (2008). Nevertheless, such a distinction does not justify either of the two scenarios: it is

Y. Li (✉)
Faculty of Education, University of Hong Kong, Pokfulam Road, Hong Kong, China
e-mail: yongyan@hku.hk

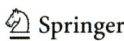 Springer

generally agreed that borrowing of ideas or else borrowing of text (with the implication that proper acknowledgement is lacking) is wrong.

Plagiarism in the sense of stealing ideas continues to be fought against as with other forms of research misconduct (e.g., fraud and duplication); meanwhile, reusing words from published papers, or "the misappropriation of language from other authors," has recently been raised as a "quite significant trend" by some editors of scientific journals (Williams 2007, p. 2535; see also "It's a steal," 2007; Kara Mosher, cited in Perry 2010; Zhang 2010a). Although the papers found guilty of such practice may have "unique data results" (Kara Mosher, cited in Perry 2010), their reuse of "basic textual wording" (Kara Mosher, cited in Perry 2010) or of "eloquent phrases, sentences or even whole paragraphs" from published texts is considered by journal editors a questionable or even "morally wrong" practice (Williams 2007, p. 2535).

The primary purpose of this paper is to provide an overview of some issues and developments concerning the tackling of the phenomenon of textual borrowing, or text-based plagiarism (Li 2012a), in scientific publishing, with the hope of inspiring concerted efforts on the part of the publishing industry, senior authors, and English for Academic Purposes (EAP) professionals to educate authors, perhaps especially novice English as an Additional Language (EAL) authors, against unwarranted textual appropriation. In the following I will begin by discussing the development of automated anti-plagiarism check, and then examine gatekeepers' stance on textual copying. This is followed by a look into the question of whether textual copying may be justifiable in some cases and a focus on EAL authors, in particular novices, as the typical culprit of textual appropriation. Then I will examine the use of pre-submission text-screening, before proposing a few areas where educational actions can be taken.

Automated Text-Matching Screening

Automated text-matching detection in the publishing industry is a later development compared with the use of the technology in universities for checking student assignments. To trace its development in recent years, a Self-Plagiarism Detection Tool (SPlaT), produced at the University of Arizona, was applied to computer science articles to search for self-plagiarism (Collberg and Kobourov 2005); this was followed by software developed at Cornell University, which trawled papers lodged in arXiv, a preprint server that collected mostly physics papers (Sorokina et al. 2006). Out of more than 0.28 million of arXiv articles combed at the time of the study, 677 pairs of papers were found to have "at least four sentences sharing uncommon 7-grams" (common 7-grams such as *can be expressed in terms of the* were excluded) (Sorokina et al. 2006, p. 1073). These 677 pairs, or 1,086 unique articles, included cases of one paper copying from multiple sources and one source copied by more than one paper (Sorokina et al. 2006, p. 1073). Human inspection of 20 of the 677 pairs excluded four "innocent mistakes" and found three cases of almost complete duplications, with the rest showing text matching in parts of a paper, such as in the introduction section (Giles 2006, p. 524). In a later study

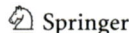 Springer

conducted by some researchers based at the University of Texas Southwestern Medical Center, survey of the abstracts in MEDLINE (a biomedical citation index of titles and abstracts) using a search engine called eTBLAST generated a large number of potential duplicates (Errami and Garner 2008) and by October 2008, 75,000 highly similar abstracts had been identified (Butler 2008).

Meanwhile, after years of preparation, CrossRef, a non-profit membership association of publishers, joined hands with iParadigms, the software company that also produced Turnitin (educational text-matching software now widely used in universities), to launch CrossCheck, an anti-plagiarism program powered by iThenticate (iParadigms's corporate text-matching software). Similar to the working principle of Turnitin, CrossCheck works on the basis of a continuously expanding database of scholarly full-text literature, and a text-similarity analyzer (the web-based iThenticate tool) which compares an authored work against the database. CrossCheck exposes both "very blatant unethical cases of plagiarism" as well as language reuse of various degrees of severity (Butler 2010, p. 167). The program has so far been put to test by such major publishers as Elsevier, Springer, Taylor and Francis, Wiley-Blackwell, and the Nature Publishing Group (Butler 2010; Colón 2008; Hu 2010; "Plagiarism pinioned," 2010), and has been widely hailed as a valuable text screening tool.

To determine the nature of the offence would necessitate manual check, which was reportedly incorporated into the research using SPlaT (Collberg and Kobourov 2005), as well as the survey study of MEDLINE (Long et al. 2009) and arXiv (Sorokina et al. 2006); apparently it is now also a regular part of journals' screening process using CrossCheck (e.g., Zhang 2010b). As a recent editorial carried in *Nature* pointed out, "plagiarism-detection software is an aid to, not a substitute for, human judgement" ("Plagiarism pinioned," 2010, p. 160). The same editorial went on to state:

> One rule of thumb used by Nature journals and others in considering an article's degree of similarity to past articles – in particular, for small amounts of self-plagiarism in review articles – is whether the paper is otherwise of sufficient originality and interest. ("Plagiarism pinioned," 2010, p. 160)

Statements like this issued by journals may help to settle some uncertainty among scientist authors. However, it may still be suggested that such indication of the possible use of human assessment over "originality and interest" in addition to the text-matching check does not itself provide guidance to scientists as to what levels or scenarios of textual copying are not acceptable, e.g., requiring rephrasing before peer review, or simply leading to rejection.

Gatekeepers' Stance on Text-Based Plagiarism[1]

Notably, the quotation above, by emphasizing the importance of using human judgement, indicates a context-sensitive approach to plagiarism. For instance, the

---

[1] Here "gatekeepers" is used to generically refer to the personalities and organizations in the publishing industry that are involved in laying down protocols and assessing the merits of a manuscript on its course of seeking publication.

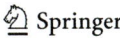

same editorial put forward a "mitigating" scenario of language reuse that may be relevant to EAL scientists: "All plagiarism can also involve honest errors or mitigating circumstances, such as a scientist with a poor command of English paraphrasing some sentences of the introduction from similar work."[2] ("Plagiarism pinioned," 2010, p. 160)

Textual copying in the introduction section of a research article does seem to be a common feature of language reuse detected in EAL authors' papers (Brumfiel 2007; Lin et al. 2011; Sorokina et al. 2006). Paul Ginsparg, a Cornell University professor on the research team that developed software to investigate duplications in arXiv (i.e., Sorokina et al. 2006), reportedly "thinks that although such practices are ethically questionable, it is inappropriate to be overly draconian" (Brumfiel 2007, p. 8). Such a mitigating stance, of course, does not imply that textual borrowing, such as that in the introduction of an article, is positively regarded. Indeed, as cited earlier, David Williams, the editor-in-chief of *Biomaterials*, suggested that such practices are simply "morally wrong" (Williams 2007, p. 2535). Similar reservation or clear opposition to textual copying, in any section of an article, is generally expressed by editors, editorial managers, or researchers of scientific texts (see Brumfiel 2007; Butler 2010; Eckel 2010; Lin et al. 2011; Schilperoort 1995; Zhang 2010b).

The Committee on Publication Ethics (COPE), "a forum for editors and publishers of peer-reviewed journals to discuss all aspects of publication ethics" (http://www.publicationethics.org), has published two flowcharts, on *What to do if you suspect plagiarism* with *(a) Suspected plagiarism in a submitted manuscript* and *(b) Suspected plagiarism in a published article* respectively (COPE 2008). Both flowcharts distinguish between "clear plagiarism" ("unattributed use of large portions of text and/or data, presented as if they were by the plagiarist") and "minor copying of short phrases." The instructions over the latter ("minor copying of short phrases") which indicate a lesser degree of severity of copying as compared with the former, are noteworthy. Specifically, within scenario (a), an arrow (indicating steps of actions to take) leads from "Minor copying of short phrases only (e.g. in discussion of research paper from non-native language speaker)//No misattribution of data" to "Contact author in neutral terms/expressing disappointment/explaining journal's position//Ask author to rephrase copied phrases or include as direct quotations with references//Proceed with review".[3] And within scenario (b), an arrow leads from "Minor copying of short phrases only (e.g. in discussion of research paper)//No misattribution of data" to "Contact author in neutral terms/expressing disappointment/explaining journal's position//Discuss publishing correction giving reference to original paper(s) if this has been omitted" and then to "Inform reader (and plagiarized author(s) if different) of journal's actions". It is thus clear that COPE upholds a high standard: that even "minor copying of short phrases" such as that "in discussion of research paper from non-native language speaker" is not

---

[2] The word "paraphrase" in this quote does not seem to be in the sense of the word as commonly understood, for instance, by EAP professionals. Instead, the word here seems to be equivalent to *patchwriting* (Howard 1995).

[3] It should be noted that to "include as direct quotation with references" is not a common practice in science and engineering research texts, compared with the case in humanities and social science texts.

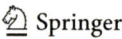 Springer

acceptable, from the point of view of COPE, and by extension, from the point of view of the international publishers and journals that subscribe to the tenets of COPE.

In short, to journal gatekeepers, textual borrowing "in discussion of research paper" (COPE 2008) or in the introduction section (Paul Ginsparg, cited in Brumfiel 2007), despite being "mitigating circumstances" if a relatively small amount of borrowing is involved ("Plagiarism pinioned," 2010), is not acceptable in either submissions or published papers.

Rewriting, Rather Than Reusing, Almost Under All Circumstances

A scenario where unattributed language reuse (i.e., with a high level of similarity between two texts) seems acceptable to some journal editors, concerns the description of highly standard experimental or statistical procedures in the methods section (Lin et al. 2011, p. 5). For example, Catriona Fennell, director of journal services at Elsevier, commented: "There are only so many different ways you can describe how to run a gel" (Butler 2010, p. 167).[4] Yet a controversial scenario is where a researcher does a series of studies, with a shared research background and following some shared, self-developed (original), experimental procedure. The researcher might thus argue that because of the parallel nature of the studies, text similarity between the separate papers in the methods section cannot be avoided (Brumfiel 2007). Changjie Hu, publishing manager at Wiley-Blackwell, has described such a case with a journal within his remit of management, and noted that after the editor of the journal had communicated with the author concerned and learned about the background for the similarity between the submitted paper and the author's previous paper, "the editor asked the author to add the relevant explanation and references, and agreed to send the manuscript out for review" (Hu 2010). It was not clear whether the referees later approved the text similarity in the methods section in this case, but evidence of journal gatekeepers supporting this kind of textual overlap seems lacking in the literature. At the same time, publishing a series of similar articles (presumably reporting a series of similar studies) has been widely condemned as misconduct. For example, Paul M. Evans, former Vice-President of Elsevier's Science and Technology Department in China, and currently managing director at Sage Publications Asia Pacific, talked of the need to prevent "salami" style publishing (i.e., cutting one study into thin pieces to be published separately) (Evans 2004: Evans and Huke 2011). Arnout Jacobs, manager of publishing development at Elsevier, likewise pointed out in an interview with *Keji Shibao* [Science News] in China (Wang 2008): "it is a nuisance for journal editors when researchers publish a series of highly similar papers. Often, these papers could easily be rewritten as one single excellent paper." (cited in Zhang 2010b, p. 11).

Where entirely different studies, rather than similar studies, are reported, how about reusing methodological descriptions from one's own previous paper, or a

---

[4] However, some would point out that such standard procedures can just be indicated with a citation rather than being repeated (Swales 1990, pp. 166–167).

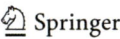 Springer

previous paper of one's own research group, or someone else's paper? Some EAL authors (including novices) seem to think this is a good strategy (as reported in Flowerdew and Li 2007; Li 2007; and Zhang 2010b). Yet again, this is not approved by experienced EAL scientist writers (Dubois 1988) or journal editors ("Plagiarism pinioned," 2010). Using CrossCheck to screen submissions to the China-based SCI journal, *Journal of Zhejiang University-Science (JZUS)*, Yuehong Zhang (Journal Director of *JZUS*) found "Direct copying of Methods section, with new data inserted" to be "a particularly common phenomenon in biomedical papers" (Zhang 2010b, p. 11). She emphasized:

> In principle we believe that, although much research refers to or repeats others' successful methods in testing new materials and discussing new results, the authors should use their own language to describe and summarize their methods and ideas. (Zhang, 2010b, p. 11)

Inexperienced EAL Authors as the Typical Culprit of Textual Borrowing

The use of computational originality-verification tools have helped to bring to the fore the typical culprit of textual copying: EAL scientists who may have difficulty in English or who have had limited experience in English writing (Brumfiel 2007; Butler 2008; "It's a steal," 2007; Lin et al. 2011; Sorokina et al. 2006). Defending their language reuse, some EAL scientists argued that they were "just borrowing better English" (Yilmaz 2007, p. 658) because "he or she is disinclined to sacrifice quality and accuracy for want of linguistic expertise" (Vessal and Habibzadeh 2007, p. 641). They pointed out that theirs is not plagiarism, and in scientific writing it is the reported science, not words, that count (for a reasoned discussion of the issue, see Bouville 2008). The following argument is typical (see also Zeng 2010):

> Borrowing sentences in the part of a paper that simply helps to better introduce the problem should not be seen as plagiarism. Even if our introductions are not entirely original, our results are – and these are the most important part of any scientific paper. (Yilmaz, 2007, p. 658)

Speaking of textual borrowing in the introduction section, the same author pointed out this is for facilitating the publication of a paper so that their research would gain visibility (Yilmaz 2007, p. 658). Other EAL scientists who also held a textual-copying-is-harmless view suggested that "Rules of the game of scientific publishing," being "set by native English-speakers," "greatly disadvantage authors whose first language is not English" (Vessal and Habibzadeh 2007, p. 641); as the game is not "fair play," reviewers and editors should "ignore such *faux pas*, since we are not sure that they would fare any better if they were to write a similar article in their own second language" (Vessal and Habibzadeh 2007, p. 641).

By contrast, yet other EAL scientists have expressed strong opposition to such laisse-faire approach to textual copying, echoing the gatekeepers' stance discussed above. The following quote from a Chinese scientist's blog is illustrative (see also Afifi 2007):

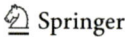 Springer

If you can not work out a new narration when writing a paper, your paper is perhaps limited in its academic value and contribution. A paper of real innovation is necessarily a result of someone's word-for-word contemplation. Some friends think, since I was following a line of research in the literature, but provided new results from a different perspective, can't I reproduce something from the literature in the introduction and literature review? Yes you can, but that way you put yourself in the position of a low-level scientist. (Yuan, 2010; my translation from Chinese).

If this Chinese scientist blogger was discussing a high versus a low standard for oneself in scientific writing which would reflect one's attitude toward textual borrowing, indeed research has revealed that duplications (encompassing textual borrowing) tend to appear in low-profile journals (Brumfiel 2007; Long et al. 2009). To cite a contrasting example, journals published by the Nature Publishing Group have detected through CrossCheck "only trace levels of plagiarism in research articles," "often in only the supplementary methods" ("Plagiarism pinioned," 2010, p. 160).

Why are EAL authors often the culprit of text-based plagiarism? Some EAL authors have cited the difficulty with English and unwillingness to sacrifice the accuracy of meaning (against a need to get published for their research to gain visibility) to justify their language reuse, as noted above. Gatekeepers tend to acknowledge the language barrier as a cause, but they have also cited culture and insufficient ethics education as contributing factors (Brumfiel 2007; Butler 2008; Errami and Garner 2008; Zhang 2010a). Errami and Garner (2008), for instance, commenting on their estimate that MEDLINE holds duplications produced by scientists in China and Japan at a level well exceeding what would be proportionate to the number of the two countries' publications in the database, suggested, "Perhaps the complexity of translation between different scripts [implying a language barrier—the present author's note], differences in ethics training and cultural norms contribute to elevated duplication rates in these two countries" (p. 398). In addition, pressure of publication in EAL countries has also been cited as a contributing factor (Brumfiel 2007; Perry 2010; Qiu 2010).

EAL Novice Scientists as Offenders of Textual Borrowing

Research in language education has reported differences between expert and novice writers in their attitude toward textual borrowing (Dong 1996; Flowerdew and Li 2007; Pecorari 2003). Automated screening of arXiv reveals that "while prominent (highly cited) authors are frequently victimized, they do not appear to reuse text from others" (Sorokina et al. 2006, p. 1075). Meanwhile, it is noticeable that novice/junior EAL scientists have been the key offenders in a number of reported cases of plagiarism, or extensive textual copying, if the involved novice authors' defence that they reported original research results is accepted (see Brumfiel 2007, for a report of Turkish doctoral students of physics being charged with plagiarism, from a study of arXiv; and see Li and Xiong 1996 for description of a case involving junior Chinese scientist authors).

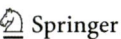 Springer

Participation of novice/junior EAL scientists, typically doctoral science students, in scientific publication has been widely reported (Li 2006, 2007; Blakeslee 1997; Florence and Yore 2004; Gosden 1995; Swales 1990). The involvement of novice scientists in the English publication arena has, to take the prominent case of China as an example, grown with the expansion of enrollment at the graduate (especially doctoral) level in the country's higher education sector, and with the increasing entrenchment of English (international) publication as a graduation requirement in many universities (see Cargill et al. 2012). The graduation pressure, language barrier, confusion over what constitutes plagiarism, inadequate vigilance against plagiarism in previous and current education, and even laziness, are likely to combine to lead to a high level of textual copying in the novices' texts. The view that "culture" has motivated plagiarism (according to some gatekeepers, as noted above) is probably not convincing in discussing the problem of plagiarism in this context, despite its apparent appeal (see also e.g., Chandrasoma et al. 2004; Li 2012a).

Where there is a lack of monitoring by experienced senior writers, textual borrowing may carry into submissions and even published papers, though CrossCheck now potentially forestalls this. A different scenario, where the senior experienced author plays a dominant role in the process of writing for publication, seems ideal insofar as eliminating textual appropriation is concerned (Li 2012b). However, in such cases how much a novice learns in terms of the need and strategies for such elimination, is questionable, because the process of eradicating the novice's textual copying in his/her preliminary text is actually embedded in the reiterative rhetorical construction of a paper, in which the novice has had little participation (Li 2012b).

Pre-Submission Text-Screening for Eliminating Textual Borrowing

A recent initiative by iParadigms, the company that provided software technology for both Turnitin and CrossCheck, is to extend the iThenticate solution (the text-matching software that CrossCheck relies on) to serve individual authors and researchers (research.ithenticate.com). The idea is to allow individuals to screen their work against a massive live database of scholarly literature before submission ("iThenticate introduces," 2011). "Within seconds, iThenticate produces a report that highlights content matches and provides links to significant text found within iThenticate's databases." ("iThenticate introduces," 2011)

While the value of this new initiative seems obvious, a potential concern, as teachers may have by allowing students access to Turnitin (Emerson 2008), may be: does individual authors' access to such tools facilitate "smarter plagiarism" ("Use of anti-plagiarism software," 2011)? This concern was expressed by Geoffrey Bilder, director of strategic initiatives at CrossRef, when CrossCheck was being piloted in 2007 before its formal launching in 2008. Projecting the prospect of authors running an automated check of their papers prior to submission, the director said this would give honest authors a chance to root out inadvertent verbatim cut and paste; yet the downside could be "It might just force people to become more sophisticated plagiarists" (cited in Butler 2007, p. 633). Such smart plagiarism will

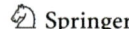 Springer

pose a challenge to automated detection. Indeed, in a *Nature* report featuring the technology that searched through arXiv for duplications (Sorokina et al. 2006), it was noted that "the software is unable to pick up 'intelligent plagiarism', where material copied from another author is reworded." (Giles 2006, p. 525) From the point of view of helping authors to get rid of inadvertent, relatively minor extent of textual borrowing in a manuscript, this pre-submission text-screening scheme will certainly be valuable. Yet ill-intentioned cheating by re-wording long stretches of text (i.e., without proper attribution of the sources) to circumvent detection remains likely.

Both pre-submission automated checking by the authors themselves and post-submission vetting by the journals are ad hoc mechanisms, in the sense that they are about checking a paper after it has been written. Even so, the current (still growing) integration of originality-verifying software into the scholarly publication process is sure to alert research writers to the issue of plagiarism, including text-based plagiarism, so that they are more vigilant *during* the composing process.

Addressing Text-Based Plagiarism Through Education

In the foregoing sections I reviewed issues and developments concerning the occurrence and handling of text-based plagiarism in scientific publication. In this section I will make proposals with an educational intent, highlighting the roles of three parties: the publishing industry, senior authors (by which I refer in particular to disciplinary advisors at the graduate level), and EAP professionals.

An Explicit Guide Teaching About Text-Based Plagiarism Is Needed in the Scientific Publishing Industry

Scientific journals have constantly maintained a firm policy against plagiarism, as can be seen in the numerous editorials carried in a wide range of journals and conveying a message of zero-tolerance on plagiarism. However, distinction between the stealing of science and the copying of language, as explicitly stated in editorials or by individual editors, has been quite recent. The foregoing sections of the present paper have shown that text-based plagiarism is a valid notion in the world of scientific publication and it is an issue worthy of wider discussion. In addition to the use of CrossCheck, the publishing industry—COPE, publishers, and individual journals—should perhaps provide on the Web a downloadable handbook, which spells out guidelines dedicated to illuminating and exemplifying what is text-based plagiarism, the forms it takes, and how to avoid it in varied scenarios. It can be noted that scientific academia has no lack of handbooks on ethics, such as *On being a scientist: Responsible conduct in research* (Committee on Science, Engineering, and Public Policy, National Academy of Sciences, National Academy of Engineering, and Institute of Medicine 1995), and *Publishing ethics resource kit* (n.d.), just to name two. Yet it seems text-based plagiarism needs to be separately addressed, in the level of detail and depth it deserves, for dispelling various misconceptions that scientist authors (especially novices) may have concerning

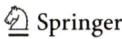 Springer

language reuse, and for providing a valuable reference in the ethics education and English enhancement training for these authors. It is worth noting that an in-depth analysis of text similarity in scientific writing is in the plan of a team of recent recipients (and the first Chinese recipients) of the COPE grant for publication ethics research. Yuehong Zhang, who leads the China-based SCI publication *Journal of Zhejiang University-Science* (noted earlier), with her editorial research team, has won COPE's December 2010 grant, to work on their project *CrossCheck guidance: An analysis of typical cases of plagiarism in different disciplines*. A major target of the project is to produce a handbook listing the "typical cases of plagiarism in different disciplines" based on investigations using CrossCheck ("COPE grant awarded," 2011, p. 3). Such a handbook is likely to become a profoundly valuable reference for scientific writing and publishing.

Where a journal has a mentorship scheme supporting EAL or inexperienced authors (e.g., Mišak et al. 2005) (though this seems extremely rare), even with the absence of a comprehensive guide geared to teaching about text-based plagiarism, some illustrative guidance should still be a valuable component of the mentoring mechanism.

Senior Authors Should Take Responsibility in Educating Novices

David Williams, editor-in-chief of *Biomaterials* quoted earlier, on observing "in several of the cases [of text-based plagiarism] that have come to light, these authors [senior authors] have graciously admitted that they did not diligently read the final version that was submitted," proposed that "the ultimate responsibility does lie with the senior authors" (Williams 2007, p. 2535). Similarly, the *Nature* editorial, also cited above, ends by stating the following: "It is crucial that research organizations in all countries, and particularly the mentors of young researchers, instil in their scientists the accepted norms of the international scientific community when it comes to plagiarism and publication ethics." ("Plagiarism pinioned," 2010, p. 160) In addition, the flowcharts of COPE, excerpted above, clearly indicate the responsibility of senior authors in helping to guard against unwarranted language reuse in submissions.

Senior authors' awareness of the issue will be reflected in their teaching of novices. Web-based, easily accessible, and user-friendly materials, such as the COPE flowcharts (and promisingly the handbook that Yuehong Zhang's research group aims to produce in the near future), are potentially valuable teaching materials, both for supervisors' self-education (see Hamp-Lyons 2011) and for mentoring novices against text-based plagiarism. At the end of a previous section of this paper ("EAL Novice Scientists as Offenders of Textual Borrowing"), I referred to a scenario where a senior experienced author may play a dominant role in the writing for publication process, by rewriting novices' initial drafts of research papers; I suggested that the extent of novices' learning regarding the eradication of textual copying may be limited, with their lack of substantial participation in the rhetorical construction process of a paper (see also Li 2012b). Although it is likely that such division of labor between a supervisor and novices is effective in a local context, by facilitating a research group's efficient publication of papers, it does also seem to

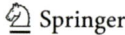 Springer

depend on the novices as well as the supervisor to make a difference, without diminishing the research group's track record of publication, to enhance the novices' participation in the process of writing for publication (as for instance, described in Florence and Yore 2004 and Li 2006). Disciplinary supervisors' conscientious effort to engage novices in a program of hands-on writing practice whereby they receive enough exposure to and have sufficient practice in research writing will be crucial for facilitating the novices' learning to write without text-based plagiarism.

English for Academic Purposes Professionals May Utilize a Wide Range of Teaching Resources

The issue of text-based plagiarism in scientific publishing intimately bears upon the stakeholders that EAP professionals commonly work with, i.e., authors who use English as an additional language, including novice EAL scientists. EAP practitioners, perhaps especially those working with EAL students, have extensively addressed the issue of how to help novices to avoid text-based plagiarism in disciplinary writing (e.g., Abasi and Akbari 2008; Barks and Watts 2001; Krishnan and Kathpalia 2002; Tardy 2009), more recently with particular recourse to specialized corpora of disciplinary texts which have facilitated educating EAL novices on learning to use recurrent language (e.g., Bianchi and Pazzaglia 2007; Lee and Swales 2006; Simpson-Vlach and Ellis 2010). In addition to incorporating the immensely valuable corpus-based strategies, a wide range of resources can also be integrated into the EAP instruction. These include, firstly, relevant views of gatekeepers and supervisors (as found, for instance, in Dong 1996; Li 2012b; Williams 2007), and secondly, currently available user-friendly resources such as the COPE flowcharts and relevant sections in *On being a scientist: Responsible conduct in research*, and *Publishing ethics resource kit* (both noted above). In addition, a case study approach centering around discussions of publicized cases of plagiarism, especially where the accused authors argued that they had reported original research (such as the cases reported in Brumfiel 2007; Li and Xiong 1996), seems potentially productive (Myers 1998). Furthermore, recent developments in the use of CrossCheck by journals and the possibility of a pre-submission check can be explored with their learning implications pursued. With EAL students, the influence of previous education and the native culture can be discussed and debated; and where the teaching takes place in an English as a Foreign Language (EFL) context, local Web-based discussions of the issue of plagiarism, reports of plagiarism cases in the media, and ethical codes for research conduct issued at local universities, all make valuable teaching resources. Apart from engaging novices in activities that may be developed from using these open resources, guided examination by students of their own texts and their supervisors' revisions, as well as of source use in journal articles (and for possible comparative findings, using low-profile and high-profile journals), can create an enlightening learning experience. By raising students' rhetorical awareness about writing from sources, EAP practitioners will also be indirectly facilitating novices' participation in the process of writing for publication, which in turn is likely to strengthen their ability to produce texts unique to the presentation of their own research.

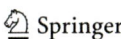 Springer

In short, the publishing industry, senior authors, and EAP professionals need to collaborate in the educational undertaking of addressing the problem of text-based plagiarism and promoting healthy scholarly publishing.

References

Abasi, A. R., & Akbari, N. (2008). Are we encouraging patchwriting? Reconsidering the role of the pedagogical context in ESL student writers' transgressive intertextuality. *English for Specific Purposes, 27*(3), 267–284.

Afifi, M. (2007). Plagiarism is not fair play. *The Lancet, 369*, 1428.

Barks, D., & Watts, P. (2001). Textual borrowing strategies for graduate-level ESL writers. In D. Belcher & A. Hirvela (Eds.), *Linking literacies: Perspectives on L2 reading-writing connections* (pp. 246–267). Ann Arbor: University of Michigan Press.

Bianchi, F., & Pazzaglia, R. (2007). Student writing of research articles in a foreign language: Metacognition and corpora. In R. Facchinetti (Ed.), *Corpus linguistics 25 years on* (pp. 259–287). Amsterdam & New York: Rodopi.

Blakeslee, A. M. (1997). Activity, context, interaction, and authority: Learning to write scientific papers in situ. *Journal of Business and Technical Communication, 11*(2), 125–169.

Bouville, M. (2008). Plagiarism: Words and Ideas. *Science and Engineering Ethics, 14*, 311–322. doi: 10.1007/s11948-008-9057-6.

Brumfiel, G. (2007). Turkish physicists face accusations of plagiarism. *Nature, 449*, 8.

Butler, D. (2007). Copycat trap. *Nature, 448*, 633.

Butler, D. (2008). Entire-paper plagiarism caught by software. *Nature, 455*, 715.

Butler, D. (2010). Journals step up plagiarism policing. *Nature, 466*, 167.

Cargill, M., O'Connor, P., & Li, Y. (2012). Educating Chinese scientists to write for international journals: Addressing the divide between science and technology education and English language teaching. *English for Specific Purposes, 31*, 60–69.

Chandrasoma, R., Thompson, C., & Pennycook, A. (2004). Beyond plagiarism: Transgressive and nontransgressive intertextuality. *Journal of Language, Identity, and Education, 3*, 171–193.

Collberg, C., & Kobourov, S. (2005). Self-plagiarism in computer science. *Communications of the ACM, 48*(4), 88–94.

Colón, R. (2008). New editorial enhancements for Springer journals: COPE and CrossCheck. Retrieved from http://www.springer.com/authors/author+zone?SGWID=0-168002-12-563000-0. Accessed 13 July 2011.

Committee on Science, Engineering, and Public Policy, National Academy of Sciences, National Academy of Engineering, and Institute of Medicine. (1995). *On being a scientist: Responsible conduct in research* (2nd ed.). Retrieved from http://www.reflexives-lpr.org/webadmin/documents/On_being_a_scientist.pdf. Accessed 10 June 2011.

COPE (Committee on Publication Ethics). (2008). *What to do if you suspect plagiarism*. Retrieved from http://www.publicationethics.org Accessed 5 May 2010.

COPE grant awarded for first time to recipients from China. (2011). *Ethical Editing*. Spring 2011, 3.

Dong, Y. R. (1996). Learning how to use citations for knowledge transformation: Non-native doctoral students' dissertation writing in science. *Research in the Teaching of English, 30*, 428–457.

Dubois, B. L. (1988). Citation in biomedical journal articles. *English for Specific Purposes, 7*, 181–193.

Eckel, E. J. (2010). Textual appropriation in engineering Master's theses: A preliminary study. *Science and Engineering Ethics*. doi:10.1007/s11948-010-9214-6.

Emerson, L. (2008). Plagiarism, a Turnitin trial, and an experience of cultural disorientation. In C. Eisner & M. Vicinus (Eds.), *Originality, imitation, and plagiarism: Teaching writing in the digital age* (pp. 183–194). Ann Arbor: University of Michigan Press.

Errami, M., & Garner, H. (2008). A tale of two citations. *Nature, 451*, 397–399.

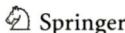

Evans, P. M. (2004). *The publishing cycle, Greater China developments, copyright and publishing etiquette*. Seminar. Run Run Shaw Library, City University of Hong Kong, Hong Kong, December 2004.

Evans, P. M., & Huke, D. (2011). *A guide from SAGE Publications on writing papers for journals—The publisher's perspective*. Roundtable on Academic Writing, School of Humanities & Social Sciences, Nanyang Technological University, Singapore, December 1–2, 2011.

Florence, M., & Yore, L. (2004). Learning to write like a scientist. Coauthoring as an enculturation task. *Journal of Research on Science Teaching, 41*(6), 637–668.

Flowerdew, J., & Li, Y. (2007). Plagiarism and second language writing in an electronic age. *Annual Review of Applied Linguistics, 27*, 161–183.

Giles, J. (2006). Preprint analysis quantifies scientific plagiarism. *Nature, 444*, 524–525.

Gosden, H. (1995). Success in research article writing and revision: A social constructionist perspective. *English for Specific Purpose, 14*, 35–57.

Hamp-Lyons, L. (2011). English for academic purposes: 2011 and beyond. *Journal of English for Academic Purposes, 10*, 2–4.

Howard, R. M. (1995). Plagiarisms, authorships, and the academic death penalty. *College English, 57*(7), 788–806.

Hu, C. (2010, September 14). Fan piaoqie ruanjian CrossCheck gongzuo yuanli jianjie [A brief introduction of anti-plagiarism software CrossCheck] [Web log comment]. Retrieved from http://blog.sciencenet.cn/home.php?mod=space&uid=204729&do=blog&id=362797. Accessed 15 June 2011.

iThenticate introduces new plagiarism detection service for individual authors and researchers (2011, January 18). Retrieved from http://turnitin.com/static/aboutus/newsroom.php. Accessed 15 June 2011.

It's a steal. (2007). *New Scientist, 193*(2597), 7.

Krishnan, L. A., & Kathpalia, S. S. (2002). Literature reviews in student project reports. *IEEE Transactions of Professional Communication, 45*(3), 187–197.

Lee, D., & Swales, J. (2006). A corpus-based EAP course for NNS doctoral students: Moving from available specialized corpora to self-compiled corpora. *English for Specific Purposes, 25*, 56–75.

Li, Y. (2006). A doctoral student of physics writing for international publication: A sociopolitically-oriented case study. *English for Specific Purposes, 25*, 456–478.

Li, Y. (2007). Apprentice scholarly writing in a *community of practice*: An "intraview" of an NNES graduate student writing a research article. *TESOL Quarterly, 41*(1), 55–79.

Li, Y. (2012a). Text-based plagiarism in scientific writing: What Chinese supervisors think about copying and how to reduce it in students' writing. *Science and Engineering Ethics*. doi:10.1007/s11948-011-9342-7.

Li, Y. (2012b). "I have no time to find out where the sentences came from; I just rebuild them": A biochemistry professor eliminating novices' textual borrowing. *Journal of Second Language Writing, 21*, 59–70.

Li, X., & Xiong, L. (1996). Chinese researchers debate rash of plagiarism cases. *Science, 274*, 337–338.

Lin, H., Jia, X., Zhang, Y., Zhang, C., Jin, M., Zhang, X., et al. (2011). Zhongshi xueshu lunli shi qikan bianji yiburongci de zeren—*Zhejiang Daxue Xuebao* (yingwenban) chutan CrossCheck de gongzuo moshi he guifan biaozhun [Guarantee academic originality: Duty of journal editors—Workflow and analysis with Crosscheck of Journal of Zhejiang University—Science (A/B/C). *Zhongguo Keji Qikan Yanjiu [Chinese Journal of Scientific and Technical Periodical], 22*(3), 328–333.

Long, T. C., Errami, M., George, A. C., Sun, Z., & Garner, H. R. (2009). Responding to possible plagiarism. *Science, 323*, 1293–1294.

Mišak, A., Marušić, M., & Marušić, A. (2005). Manuscript editing as a way of teaching academic writing: Experience from a small scientific journal. *Journal of Second Language Writing, 14*, 122–131.

Myers, S. (1998). Questioning author(ity): ESL/EFL, science, and teaching about plagiarism. *TESL-EJ, 3*(2), 1–20.

Pecorari, D. (2003). Good and original: Plagiarism and patchwriting in academic second-language writing. *Journal of Second Language Writing, 12*, 317–345.

Perry, J. (2010, October 27). *Plagiarism in China [Web log comment]*. Retrieved from http://www.ithenticate.com/blog/bid/52953/Plagiarism-in-China. Accessed 10 June 2011.

Plagiarism pinioned. (2010). [Editorial]. *Nature, 466*, 159–160.

Publishing ethics resource kit. (n.d). Retrieved from http://www.elsevier.com/wps/find/editorshome.editors/Introduction. Accessed 10 June 2011

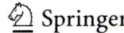 Springer

Qiu, J. (2010). Publish or perish in China. *Nature, 463,* 142–143.

Schilperoort, R. A. (1995). Editorial. *Plant Molecular Biology, 28,* v.

Simpson-Vlach, R., & Ellis, N. C. (2010). An academic formulas list: New methods in phraseology research. *Applied Linguistics, 31*(4), 487–512.

Sorokina, D., Gehrke, J., Warner, S., & Ginsparg, P. (2006). *Plagiarism detection in arXiv.* Paper presented at the Sixth International Conference on Data Mining, Hong Kong.

Swales, J. M. (1990). *Genre analysis: English in academic and research settings.* Cambridge: Cambridge University Press.

Tardy, C. M. (2009). *Building genre knowledge.* West Lafayette, IN: Parlor Press.

Use of anti-plagiarism software sparks controversy. (2011, January 17). *China Daily.* Retrieved from http://www.chinadaily.com.cn/china/2011-01/17/content_11869018.htm. Accessed 12 July 2011.

Vessal, K., & Habibzadeh, F. (2007). Rules of the game of scientific writing: Fair play and plagiarism. *The Lancet, 369,* 641.

Wang, D. (2008). Xueshu qizha'an pingfa, xueshu qikan ruhe yingfu [How academic journals respond to the frequent occurrence of academic dishonesty]. Retrieved from http://www.cas.cn/jzd/jlt/jrdhp/200804/t20080402_1688476.shtml. Accessed 15 June 2011.

Williams, D. (2007). Plagiarism and redundancy [Editorial]. *Biomaterials, 28,* 2535.

Yilmaz, I. (2007). Plagiarism? No, we're just borrowing better English. *Nature, 449,* 658.

Yuan, X. (2010, September). Guanyu chaoxi [About plagiarism] [Web log]. Retrieved from http://bbs.sciencenet.cn/home.php?mod=space&uid=103568&do=blog&id=426420. Accessed 15 June 2011.

Zeng, Q. (2010, September 15). Chaoxi jiduanhua fan shenme zui le! [What's wrong with copying several passages!] [Web log comment]. Retrieved from http://blog.sciencenet.cn/home.php?mod=space&uid=281238&do=blog&id=363183. Accessed 10 June 2011.

Zhang, Y. (2010a). Chinese journal finds 31% of submissions plagiarized. *Nature, 467,* 271.

Zhang, Y. (2010b). CrossCheck: An effective tool for detecting plagiarism. *Learned Publishing, 23*(1), 9–14.

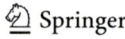

7.3 Avoiding Plagiarism, Self-Plagiarism, and Other Questionable Writing Practices: A Guide to Ethical Writing

Miguel Roig

Roig M. Avoiding plagiarism, self-plagiarism, and other questionable writing practices: A guide to ethical writing. US Office of Research Integrity.

1

Avoiding plagiarism, self-plagiarism, and other questionable writing practices: A guide to ethical writing
Miguel Roig, Ph.D.

Created in 2003

First revision, 2006

Second revision, 2015

Please send any questions, comments, or suggestions to Miguel Roig, Ph.D
(roigm@stjohns.edu)

PREFACE

In recognizing the importance of educating aspiring scientists in the responsible conduct of research (RCR), the Office of Research Integrity (ORI) began sponsoring the creation of instructional resources to address this pressing need in 2002. The present guide on avoiding plagiarism and other inappropriate writing practices was created to help students, as well as professionals, identify and prevent such malpractices and to develop an awareness of ethical writing and authorship. This guide is one of the many products stemming from ORI's effort to promote the RCR.

Many other writing guides are available to assist scientists in preparing their research reports for publication in scholarly and scientific outlets. Some of these resources focus on matters of scientific style and are written for those who are completing theses and/or dissertations. Other guides target professionals and focus on topics, such as the traditional Introduction, Methods, Results, [and] Discussion (IMRAD) journal article and submission process, along with other elements of scientific publishing. Few writing guides, however, focus solely on issues related to responsible writing, an area that continues to receive increasing attention in part because of rapid changes occurring in science dissemination and globalization within the last few decades. The latter factor has resulted in the addition of increasing numbers of researchers whose primary language is not English, the *lingua franca* of science, who must struggle to function in a highly competitive research climate. The changes in science publishing that have taken place in recent years (e.g., open access movement) have also resulted in many more outlets for the publication of scientific research. At the same time, the emergence of so-called "predatory publishers" is thought to have also contributed to a decline in the quality of science that ultimately becomes part of the scientific record (Beal 2013; Clark & Smith, 2015). Because these and related factors are likely associated with questionable writing and authorship practices, ORI felt that an updated and more detailed treatment of the issues covered in the two previous versions of this guide was necessary. Thus, the current version is herein presented.

INTRODUCTION

Scientific writing can be a cognitively demanding and arduous process, for it simultaneously demands exceptional degrees of clarity and conciseness, two elements that often clash with each other. In addition, accuracy and transparency, fundamental aspects of the scientific enterprise are also critical components of scientific writing. Good

2

scientific writing must be characterized by clear expression, conciseness, accuracy, and perhaps most importantly, honesty. Unfortunately, modern scientific research often takes place within all sorts of constraints and competing pressures. As a result, a portion of the scientific literature, whether generated by students of science or by seasoned professionals, is likely to be deficient in one or more of the above components.

Insufficient clarity or lack of conciseness is typically unintentional and relatively easy to remedy by standard educational and/or editorial steps. Lapses in the accuracy of what is reported (e.g., faulty observations, incorrect interpretation of results) are also assumed to be most often unintentional in nature. Yet such lapses, even if unintentional, can have significant negative consequences if not corrected. Intentional lapses in research integrity represent the most serious threat to the scientific enterprise, for such misconduct runs contrary to the principal goal of science, which is the search for truth.

In scientific writing, plagiarism is perhaps the most serious and the most widely recognized ethical lapse. It can occur in many forms and some of the more subtle instances, while arguably unethical in nature, may not rise to the level of research misconduct by federal agencies such as the National Science Foundation (NSF) or the Office of Research Integrity (ORI). On the other hand, minor plagiarism may still result in serious negative consequences for the perpetrator as per institutional policies, those of professional associations *or* those of the publishers where the plagiarized material appears. Because members of the scientific community are held, or should be held, to the highest standards of excellence, they are expected to uphold those high standards across all facets of their scientific work. Consequently, they must be aware of, and actively avoid, all questionable research practices, including writing practices that might be considered ethically problematic. A relatively common example of the latter occurs when authors report and discuss the results of their research only in the context of literature that is supportive of their conclusions, but ignore literature that clearly runs contrary to their findings.

On ethical writing

A general principle underlying ethical writing is the notion that the written work of an author, be it a manuscript for a magazine or scientific journal, a research paper submitted for a course, or a grant proposal submitted to a funding agency, represents an implicit contract between the author of that work and his/her readers. Accordingly, the reader assumes that the author is the sole originator of the written work and that any material, text, data, or ideas borrowed from others is clearly identified as such by established scholarly conventions, such as footnotes, block-indented text, and quotations marks. The reader also assumes that all information conveyed therein is accurately represented to the best of the author's abilities. In sum, as Kolin (2015) points out, "Ethical writing is clear, accurate, fair, and honest" (p. 29) and its promotion conveys to readers a commitment to ethical practice in other aspects of the author's work.

As is the case with most other human activities, inadvertent errors may occur in the process of writing that end up violating the spirit of the contract. For example, in proposing a new idea or presenting new data, an author may sincerely consider a certain line of evidence as unimportant or irrelevant, and thus ignore other existing data or evidence that fail to support, or outright contradict, his/her own ideas. In other cases, an author may fail to give credit to a unique theoretical position or a fundamental methodological step that is necessary for an experiment to work as described. An example of the latter situation that eventually led to a correction of a published article (i.e., Anastasia, Deinhardt, Chao, Will, Irmady, Lee,

3

Hempstead, & Bracken, 2014) is described by Marcus (2014). Judging by some of the reader commentary appearing in various emerging outlets, such as PubPeer and Retraction Watch,, these types of oversights occur relatively frequently in the sciences, particularly when dealing with controversial topics.

Other errors include situations in which an idea claimed to be completely original by its author/s may have actually been articulated earlier by someone else. Such "rediscovery" of ideas is a relatively well-known phenomenon in the sciences, often occurring within a relatively close timeframe. In some cases, these "new" discoveries are completely independent in that it is possible for the new proponents to appear to have no knowledge of the original discovery. In other instances, it is possible for the new proponents to have been actually exposed to these ideas at some point but to have genuinely forgotten. A recent example of a rediscovery of an old phenomenon occurred when Dieter, Hu, Knill, Blake, and Tadin (2013) claimed to have discovered that moving one's hand from side to side in front of one's covered eyes causes visual sensations of motion. However, as a subsequent correction points out (Dieter, et al., 2014), these authors were apparently unaware that reports of this phenomenon had been published earlier, starting with the work of Hofstetter (1970) and followed by the work of Brosgole & Neylon (1973) and Brosgole & Roig (1983). The latter study reported at least one experiment with similar methodology and results as one of those reported later by Dieter, et al. Cognitive psychologists have provided considerable evidence for the existence of cryptomnesia, or unconscious plagiarism, which refers to the notion that individuals previously exposed to others' ideas will often remember the idea, but not its source, and mistakenly misattribute the idea to them (see Brown & Murphy, 1989; Brown & Halliday, 1991; Marsh & Bower, 1993). Unfortunately, it is often difficult to establish whether prior exposure to ideas has occurred.

Other unintentional errors occur, such as when authors borrow heavily from a source and, in careless oversight, fail to fully credit the source. These and other types of inadvertent lapses are thought to occur with some frequency in the sciences. Unfortunately, in some cases, such lapses are thought to be intentional and therefore constitute instances of unethical writing and quite possibly constitute research misconduct. Without a doubt, plagiarism is the most widely recognized and one of the most serious violations of the contract between the reader and the writer. Moreover, plagiarism is one of the three major types of scientific misconduct as defined by the Public Health Service, the other two being falsification and fabrication (U. S. Public Health Service, 1989). Most often, individuals found to have committed substantial plagiarism pay a steep price. Plagiarists have been demoted, dismissed from their schools, from their jobs, and their degrees and honors have been rescinded as a result of their misdeeds (Standler, 2000). Let us take a closer look at this type of misconduct.

PLAGIARISM

"Taking over the ideas, methods, or written words of another, without acknowledgment and with the intention that they be taken as the work of the deceiver." American Association of University Professors (September/October,1989).

As the above quotation shows, plagiarism has been traditionally defined as the taking of words, images, processes, structure and design elements, ideas, etc. of others and presenting them as one's own. It is often associated with phrases such as kidnapping of words, kidnapping of ideas, fraud, and literary theft. Plagiarism can manifest itself in a

4

variety of ways and is not just confined to student papers or published articles or books. For example, consider a scientist who makes a presentation at a conference and discusses at length an idea or concept that had already been proposed by someone else yet not considered common knowledge. During his presentation, he fails to fully acknowledge the specific source of the idea and, consequently, misleads the audience into believing that he was the originator of that idea. This, too, may constitute an instance of plagiarism. The fact is that plagiarism manifests itself in a variety of situations and the following examples are just a small sample of the many ways in which it occurs and of the types of consequences that can follow as a result.

- A historian resigns from the Pulitzer board after allegations that she had appropriated text from other sources in one of her books.
- A writer for a newspaper who was found to have plagiarized material for some of his articles ended up resigning his position.
- A biochemist resigns from a prestigious clinic after accusations that a book he wrote contained appropriated portions of text from a National Academy of Sciences report.
- A famous musician is found guilty of unconscious plagiarism by including elements of another musical group's previously recorded song in one of his new songs which then becomes a hit. The musician is forced to pay compensation for the infraction.
- A college president is forced to resign after allegations that he failed to attribute the source of material that was part of a college convocation speech.
- A U.S. Senator has his Master's degree rescinded after findings of plagiarism in one of this academic papers; he withdraws from the Senate race.
- An education minister resigns her government position after a university rescinds her doctoral degree for plagiarism.
- A psychologist has his doctoral degree rescinded after the university finds that portions of his doctoral dissertation had been plagiarized.

In sum, plagiarism can be a very serious form of ethical misconduct. For this reason, the concept of plagiarism is universally addressed in all scholarly, artistic, and scientific disciplines. In the humanities and the sciences, for example, a plethora of writing guides for students and professionals exist to provide guidance to authors on discipline-specific procedures for acknowledging the contributions of others.

While instruction on proper attribution, a key concept in avoiding plagiarism, is almost always provided, coverage of this important topic often fails to go beyond the most common forms: plagiarism of ideas and plagiarism of text.

Plagiarism of ideas

Appropriating someone else's idea (e.g., an explanation, a theory, a conclusion, a hypothesis, a metaphor) in whole or in part, or with superficial modifications without giving credit to its originator.

In the sciences, as in most other scholarly endeavors, ethical writing demands that any ideas, data, and conclusions borrowed from others and used as the foundation of one's own contributions to the literature, be properly acknowledged. The specific manner in which we make such acknowledgement may vary depending on the context

5

and even on the discipline, but it often takes the form of either a footnote or a reference citation.

Acknowledging the source of our ideas

Just about every scholarly or scientific paper contains several footnotes or references documenting the source of the facts, ideas, or evidence used in support of arguments, hypotheses, etc. In some cases, as in those papers that review the literature in a specific area of research, the reference section listing the sources cited in the paper can be quite extensive, sometimes taking up more than a third of the published article (see, for example, Logan, Walker, Cole, & Leukefeld, 2002). Most often, the contributions we rely upon come from the published work or personal observations of other scientists or scholars. On occasion, however, we may derive an important insight about a phenomenon or process that we are studying, through a casual interaction with an individual not at all connected with scholarly or scientific work. But, even in such cases, we still have a moral obligation to credit the source of our ideas. A good illustrative example of the latter point was reported by Alan Gilchrist in a 1979 *Scientific American* article on color perception. In a section of the article which describes the perception of rooms uniformly painted in one color, Gilchrist states: "We now have a promising lead to how the visual system determines the shade of gray in these rooms, although we do not yet have a complete explanation. (John Robinson helped me develop this lead.)" (p. 122; Gilchrist, 1979). The reader might assume that Mr. Robinson is another scientist working in the field of visual perception, or perhaps an academic colleague or an advanced graduate student of Gilchrist's. Not so. John Robinson was a local plumber and an acquaintance of Gilchrist in the town where the author spent his summers. During a casual discussion between Gilchrist and Robinson over the former's work, Robinson provided insights into the problem that Gilchrist had been working on that were sufficiently important to the development of his theory of lightness perception that Gilchrist felt ethically obligated to credit Robinson's contribution.

Unconscious plagiarism of ideas. Even the most ethical authors can fall prey to the inadvertent appropriation of others' ideas, concepts, or metaphors. Here we are again referring to the phenomenon of unconscious plagiarism (i.e,. cryptomnesia), which, as noted earlier, takes place when an author generates an idea that s/he believes to be original, but which in reality had been encountered at an earlier time. Given the free and frequent exchange of ideas in science and other scholarly disciplines, it is not unreasonable to expect instances in which earlier exposure to an idea that lies dormant in someone's unconscious emerges into consciousness at a later point, but in a context different from the one in which the idea had originally occurred. Presumably, this is exactly what happened in the case of former Beatle George Harrison, whose song "My Sweet Lord" was found to have musical elements of the song "He's So Fine," which had been released years earlier by The Chiffons (see Bright Tunes Music Corp. v. Harrisongs Music, Ltd., 1976). One has to wonder how many other John Robinsons, as well as other accomplished scientists, scholars, and artists, now forgotten, contributed original ideas without acknowledgement.

Some instances of misappropriation of ideas suggest intentionality on the part of the perpetrators. For example, according to Resnik (e.g., Shamoo and Resnik, 2009; Resnik 2012), many instances exist in which professors take ideas from their students but fail to give them credit for their contributions. Ferguson (2014) describes a case of this type in which a mathematics paper published in 2013 was retracted the following year

6

because it been determined that the work had been largely derived from a student's Master's thesis without any acknowledged of her contributions.

In other cases the misappropriation of an idea can be a subtle process. Consider the famous case of Albert Schatz who, as a graduate student working under Selman Waksman at Rutgers, discovered the antibiotic streptomycin. Even though the first publications describing his discovery identified Schatz as primary author (Martin, 1997), it was Wakman who, over a period of time, began to take sole credit for the discovery, ultimately earning him the Nobel prize in 1952 (see, for example, Shatz, 1993; Mistiaen, 2002 for a fuller description of this case).

The confidential peer review process is thought to be a common source of plagiarism. Consider the scenario where the offender is a journal or conference referee, or a member of a review panel for a funding agency. He reads a paper or a grant proposal describing a promising new methodology in an area of research directly related to his own work. The grant fails to get funded based perhaps on his negative evaluation of the protocol. He then goes back to his lab and prepares a grant proposal using the methodology stolen from the proposal that he refereed earlier and submits his proposal to a different granting agency. Cases similar to the above scenario have been documented in the research misconduct literature (see Price, 2006)

Most of us would deem the behavior depicted in the above scenario as downright despicable. Unfortunately, similar situations have occurred. In fact, elements of the above scenario are based on actual cases of scientific misconduct investigated by ORI. The notion that the peer review context appears to be sufficiently susceptible to the appropriation of ideas was likely the impetus behind the 1999 Federal Office of Science and Technology Policy's expansion of their definition of plagiarism, which states:

> **"Plagiarism is the appropriation of another person's ideas, processes, results, or words without giving appropriate credit, including those obtained through confidential review of others' research proposals and manuscripts."** (Office of Science and Technology Policy, 1999).

And, even small-scale plagiarism of ideas may lead to very negative consequences. (See, for example, Abbott, 2009).

Guideline 1: An ethical writer ALWAYS acknowledges the contributions of others to his/her work.

Plagiarism of text

Copying a portion of text from another source without giving appropriate credit to its author.

When it comes to using others' word-for-word (i.e., verbatim) text in our writing the universally accepted rule is to enclose that information in quotations and to indicate the specific source of that text. When quoting text from other sources, a writer must provide a reference citation and, depending on the style manual that guides the work (e.g., Turabian, American Psychological Association [APA], American Medical Association [AMA]), the page number indicating where the quoted text is located in the original.

Although the use of direct quotes appears to be uncommon in biomedical literature, in some instances it may be warranted. The material quoted earlier from Gilchrist (1979) serves as a good example of when to use quotations. Some writing style manuals require that larger portions of text that are borrowed be block-indented. For example quoting directly from Iverson, et al (2007; p. 361):

> **Block Quotations.** – If material quoted from texts or speeches is longer than 4 typewritten lines. The material should be set off in a block, i.e., in reduced type and without the quotation mark. Paragraph indents are generally not used unless the quoted material is known to begin a paragraph. Space is often added both above and below these longer quotations.

Although the evidence indicates that most authors, including college students, are aware of rules regarding the use of quotation marks, plagiarism of text is probably the most common type of plagiarism. For example, some authors seem to believe that as long as a citation is provided, it is acceptable to use verbatim text from another source without needing to enclose the borrowed material in quotation marks (Julliard, 1993). However, plagiarism of text can occur in a variety of forms. The following review will familiarize the reader with the various subtle forms of plagiarism of text.

Guideline 2: Any verbatim text taken from another source must be enclosed in quotation marks and be accompanied by a citation to indicate its origin.

Let's consider the following variety:

> *Copying portions of text from one or more sources, inserting and/or deleting some of the words, or substituting some words with synonyms, but never giving credit to its author nor enclosing the verbatim material in quotation marks.*

The above form of plagiarism is relatively well known and has been given names, such as patchwriting (Howard, 1999) and paraphragiarism (Levin & Marshall, 1993). Iverson, et al. (2007) in the American Medical Association's Manual of Style identify this type of unethical writing practice as mosaic plagiarism and they define it as follows:

> "Mosaic: Borrowing the ideas and opinions from an original source and a few verbatim words or phrases without crediting the original author. In this case, the plagiarist intertwines his or her own ideas and opinions with those of the original author, creating a 'confused plagiarized mass'" (p. 158).

Another, more blatant form which may also fall under the more general category of plagiarism of ideas occurs when an author takes a portion of text from another source, thoroughly paraphrases it, but never gives credit to its author. Consistent with the first guideline, we must be careful to indicate which ideas/material in our writing have been derived from which source.

Inappropriate paraphrasing

> *Taking portions of text from one or more sources, crediting the author/s, but only*

8

making 'cosmetic' changes to the borrowed material, such as changing one or two words, simply rearranging the order, voice (i.e., active vs. passive) and/or tense of the sentences is NOT paraphrasing.

Inappropriate paraphrasing is perhaps the most common form of plagiarism and, at the same time, the most controversial. This is because the criteria for what constitutes proper paraphrasing differ between individuals, even within the same discipline (Roig, 2001). We will discuss these issues shortly, but first let's consider the process of paraphrasing.

Paraphrasing and summarizing

Scholarly writing, including scientific writing, often involves **paraphrasing** and **summarizing** others' work. For example, in the introduction of a traditional IMRAD paper it is customary to provide a brief and concise review of the pertinent literature. Such a review is accomplished by the cogent synthesis of relevant theoretical and empirical studies that form the background and rationale for the hypotheses being tested or for the main thesis of the paper being written. Such reviews call for the synthesis (i.e., summarizing) of relatively large amounts of information.

Guideline 3: When we summarize others' work, we use our own words to condense and convey others' contributions in a shorter version of the original.

At other times, and for a variety of reasons, we may wish to restate in detail and in our own words a certain portion of another author's writing. In this case, we must rely on the process of paraphrasing. Unlike a summary, which results in a substantially shorter textual product, a paraphrase usually results in writing of roughly equivalent textual length as the original, but, of course, with different words and sentence structure. Whether paraphrasing or summarizing others' work, we must always provide proper credit.

Guideline 4: When paraphrasing others' work, not only must we use our own words, but we must also use our own syntactical structure.

Guideline 5: Whether we are paraphrasing or summarizing we must always identify the source of our information.

Paraphrasing and plagiarism: what the writing guides say

Although virtually all professional and student writing guides, including those in the sciences, provide specific instructions on the proper use of quotation marks, references, etc., some fail to offer specific details on proper paraphrasing. With some exceptions, writing guides that provide instructions for proper paraphrasing and for avoiding plagiarism tend to subscribe to a "conservative" approach to paraphrasing. That is, these guides often suggest that when paraphrasing, an author must substantially modify the original material. Consider the following examples of paraphrasing guidelines:

"**Don't plagiarize**. Express your own thoughts in your own words…. Note, too, that simply changing a few words here and there, or changing the order of a few words in a sentence or paragraph, is still plagiarism. Plagiarism is one of the most serious crimes in academia." (Pechenik, 2001; p.10).

"You paraphrase appropriately when you represent an idea in your own words more clearly and pointedly than the source does. But readers will think that you plagiarize if they can match your words and phrasing with those of your source." (Booth, Colomb, & Williams, 2008; p. 194).

Guideline 6: When paraphrasing and/or summarizing others' work we must ensure that we are reproducing the exact meaning of the other author's ideas or facts and that we are doing so using our own words and sentence structure.

Examples of paraphrasing: good and bad

The ethical writer takes great care to insure that any paraphrased text is sufficiently modified so as to be judged as new writing. Let's consider various paraphrased versions of the following material on the electrochemical properties of neurons (taken from Martini & Bartholomew, 1997). In acknowledging the source, we will use the footnote method commonly used in the biomedical sciences. The actual reference would appear in the reference section of the paper.

"**Because the intracellular concentration of potassium ions is relatively high, potassium ions tend to diffuse out of the cell. This movement is driven by the concentration gradient for potassium ions. Similarly, the concentration gradient for sodium ions tends to promote their movement into the cell. However, the cell membrane is significantly more permeable to potassium ions than to sodium ions. As a result, potassium ions diffuse out of the cell faster than sodium ions enter the cytoplasm. The cell therefore experiences a net loss of positive charges, and as a result the interior of the cell membrane contains an excess of negative charges, primarily from negatively charged proteins.**"[1] (p. 204).

Here is an <u>Appropriate Paraphrase</u> of the above material:

A textbook of anatomy and physiology[1] reports that the concentration of potassium ions inside of the cell is relatively high and, consequently, some potassium tends to escape out of the cell. Just the opposite occurs with sodium ions. Their concentration outside of the cell causes sodium ions to cross the membrane into the cell, but they do so at a slower rate. According to these authors, this is because the permeability of the cell membrane is such that it favors the movement of potassium relative to sodium ions.

10

Because the rate of crossing for potassium ions that exit the cell is higher
than that for sodium ions that enter the cell, the inside portion of the cell is
left with an overload of negatively charged particles, namely, proteins that
contain a negative charge.

Notice that, in addition to thoroughly changing much of the language and some of
the structure of the original paragraph, the paraphrase also indicates, as per guideline 5,
that the ideas contained in the rewritten version were taken from another source. When we
paraphrase and/or summarize others' work we must also give them due credit, a rule not
always applied by inexperienced writers.

Let's suppose that instead of paraphrasing, we decide to summarize the above
paragraph from Martini and Bartholomew. Here is one summarized version of that
paragraph:

The interior of a cell maintains a negative charge because more potassium
ions exit the cell relative to sodium ions that enter it, leaving an over
abundance of negatively charged protein inside of the cell.[1]

In their attempts at paraphrasing, some authors commit "near plagiarism" (or
plagiarism, depending on who is doing the judging) because they fail to sufficiently
modify the original text and, thus, produce an inappropriately paraphrased version.
Depending on the extent of modifications to the original, the amount of text involved, and
the unique perspective of the reader about what constitutes ethical scholarship,
inappropriate paraphrasing may constitute an instance of plagiarism. For example, the
following versions of the Martini and Bartholomew paragraph inappropriately
paraphrased-and can thus be classified as plagiarized.

Inappropriate paraphrase (version 1):

Because the intracellular concentration of potassium ions is _ high,
potassium ions tend to diffuse out of the cell. This movement
is triggered by the concentration gradient for potassium ions.
Similarly, the concentration gradient for sodium ions tends to
promote their movement into the cell. However, the cell membrane
is much more permeable to potassium ions than to it is to sodium
ions. As a result, potassium ions diffuse out of the cell more
rapidly than sodium ions enter the cytoplasm. The cell therefore
experiences a _ loss of positive charges, and as a result the interior
of the cell membrane contains a surplus of negative charges,
primarily from negatively charged proteins.[1] (p. 204).

A comparison between the original version of the Martini and Bartholomew
paragraph to the 'rewritten' version above reveals that the rewritten version is a mere copy
of the original. The few modifications that were made are superficial, consisting merely of
a couple of word deletions, substitutions, and additions. Even though the writer has
credited Martini and Bartholomew's ideas by the insertion of a reference note ([1]), most of
the words and structure of the original paragraph are preserved in the rewritten version
and the paragraph is, therefore, considered plagiarism. In other words, making only
cosmetic modifications to others' writing misleads the reader as to who the true author of
the original writing really is.

11

Inappropriate paraphrase (version 2):

> The concentration gradient for sodium (Na) ions tends to promote their movement into the cell. Similarly, the high intracellular concentration of potassium (K) ions is relatively high resulting in K's tendency to diffuse out of the cell. Because the cell membrane is significantly more permeable to K than to Na, K diffuses out of the cell faster than Na enters the cytoplasm. The cell therefore experiences a net loss of positive charges and, as a result the interior of the cell membrane now has an excess of negative charges, primarily from negatively charged proteins.[1] (p. 204).

At first glance this second 'rewritten' version may look as if it has been significantly modified from the original but, in reality, the changes made are only superficial and the resulting paraphrase is not all that different from original. In this particular instance, the writer has made a seemingly disingenuous change by substituting the names of the atoms with their chemical symbols (e.g., sodium = Na). In addition, the order of the first two sentences was changed giving the appearance of a substantial modification. As in the previous version, however, the language and much of the rest of structure is still too close to the original.

Again, it must be emphasized that when we paraphrase we must make every effort to restate the ideas in our own voice. Obviously, certain key terms, such as specific cellular structures (e.g., membrane) and molecules (e.g., sodium) cannot be changed. This will be often the case with precise terminology of a scientific nature for which there are no adequate substitutes. Here is another properly paraphrased version:

Appropriate paraphrase (version 2):

> The relatively high concentration gradient of sodium ions outside of the cell causes them to enter into the cell's cytoplasm. In a similar fashion, the interior concentration gradient of potassium ions is also high and, therefore, potassium ions tend to scatter out of the cell through the cell's membrane. But, a notable feature of this process is that Potassium ions tend to leave the cell faster than sodium ions enter the cytoplasm. This is because of the nature of the cell membrane's permeability, which allows potassium ions to cross much more freely than sodium ions. The end result is that the interior of the cell membrane's loss of positive charges results in a greater proportion of negative charges and these are made up mostly of proteins that have acquired a negative charge.[1]

Paraphrasing highly technical language

Taking a paragraph, or for that matter, even a unique sentence from another source, and using it in our own writing without enclosing the material in quotations constitutes plagiarism. Similarly, inappropriate paraphrasing may also be classified as plagiarism.

The available evidence indicates that one of the reasons writers misappropriate text is because they may be unfamiliar with the concepts and/or language with which s/he is working. The ability to properly paraphrase technical text depends in large part on an author's conceptual understanding of the material and his/her mastery and command of the

12

language and of her knowledge of, and ability, to convey discipline-specific expressions typically used to describe relevant phenomena, laboratory processes and procedures, etc. Accordingly, it is relatively easy to thoroughly paraphrase others' work when we have a full grasp of the issues and of the language involved. For example, studies show that when asked to paraphrase a short paragraph, students (Roig, 1999; Walker, 2008) as well as university professors (Roig 2001) are more likely to appropriate and, therefore, plagiarize text when the original material to be paraphrased is made up of technical language likely to be unfamiliar to them, than when the topic is a familiar one and the original is written in plain language.

Obviously, inexperienced writers (e.g., students) have the greatest difficulty paraphrasing the advanced technical text often found in the primary scientific literature. In an effort to introduce them to primary sources of information in a given discipline, college students are often required to write a research paper from articles published in professional journals. For those students who must complete this type of assignment for the first time, and, in particular for foreign students whose primary language is not English, writing a research paper can be a daunting task. This is because scholarly prose: 1) can be very intricate, 2) adheres to unique stylistic conventions (e.g., use of the passive voice in the biomedical sciences), and 3) relies heavily on jargon and unusual expressions that novice writers have yet to master. Consequently, students need to create an acceptable academic product that is not only grammatically correct, but also demonstrates knowledge of the concepts discussed. These circumstances force many such students to rely on close paraphrases of the original text. Unfortunately, such writing can result in a charge of plagiarism.

Guideline 7: In order to be able to make the types of substantial modifications to the original text that result in a proper paraphrase, one must have a thorough command of the language and a good understanding of the ideas and terminology being used.

An analogous situation can occur at the professional level when authors see the need to paraphrase a complex process or methodology. As indicated earlier, traditional scholarly conventions provide us with the option to re-use any material by enclosing it in quotation marks or by block-quoting it (i.e., indenting the material within both margins) with some type of indication (e.g., a footnote) as to its origin. Therefore, if the text is so technical that it would be very difficult or nearly impossible to modify substantially without altering its meaning, then perhaps it would be best to leave it in the original author's wording, enclose it in quotation marks (or block-quote it), and include a citation. However, unlike literature or philosophy, quoting in certain disciplines (e.g., biomedical sciences) is not encouraged (see Pechnick, 2001). One would be hard pressed to find an entire sentence quoted, let alone a short paragraph, in the pages of prestigious biomedical journals (e.g., *Nature, Science, New England Journal of Medicine*).

In sum, the reality is that in many instances, scientific prose and diction can be very difficult to paraphrase. To illustrate the difficulties inherent in paraphrasing highly technical language, let's consider the following paragraph from a report recently published in *Science* (Lunyak, et al., 2002).

"Mammalian histone lysine methyltransferase, suppressor of variegation 39H1 (SUV39H1), initiates silencing with selective methylation on Lys^9 of histone H3, thus creating a high-affinity binding

13

site for HP1. When an antibody to endogenous SUV39H1 was used for immunoprecipitation, MeCP2 was effectively coimmunoprecipitated; conversely, αHA antibodies to HA-tagged MeCP2 could immunoprecipitate SUV39H1 (Fig. 2G)."[2] (p. 1748)

Here is an attempt at paraphrasing the above material:

The H3 methyltransferase SUV39H1 mediates gene silencing of neuronal genes in Rat-1 fibroblasts by methylating lysine 9 of histone H3, thus creating a binding site for the heterochromatin protein HP1 and subsequent formation of a chromatin complex involving multiple silencing factors including the methyl-CpG- binding protein MeCP2 and SUV39H1 itself (Lunyak, et al., 2002).[1]

Unlike the previous examples of appropriate paraphrasing, the above example does not embody as many textual modifications. In order for the exact meaning of the original *Science* paragraph to be preserved in the present case, many of the same terms must be left intact in the paraphrased version. Although synonyms for some of the words may be available, their use in the specific context of the original paragraph is simply not appropriate. For example, take the word *affinity,* which is defined as "that force by which a substance chooses or elects to unite with one substance rather than with another" (Dorland, 2000) or, in its more recent edition, "a special attraction for a specific element, organ or structure" (Dorland, 2011). *Roget's Thesaurus* (Moorhead, 2002) lists the following synonyms for *affinity: liking, attraction, relations, similarity.* Although it might be possible to rewrite the first sentence using the synonym *"attraction,"* this alternative fails to capture the precise meaning conveyed by the original sentence, given how the term is used in this area of biomedical research. The word *affinity* has a very specific denotation in the context in which is being used in the *Science* paragraph and it is the only practical and meaningful alternative available. The same can be said for other words that might have synonyms (e.g., binding, silencing, site). Other terms, such as *methylation* and *antibodies* are unique and do not have synonyms. In sum, most of the rest of the technical terms (e.g., immunoprecipitation, endogenous, coimmunoprecipitated) and expressions (e.g., HA-tagged, high-affinity, mammalian histone lysing methyltransferase) in the above paragraph are extremely difficult, if not impossible, to substitute without altering the intended meaning of the paragraph. As a result, a properly paraphrased version such as the one offered above will share many common elements with the original and thus, applying the strict definitions of paraphrasing provided by some writing guides might render the above paraphrase as a borderline, or an outright, case of plagiarism.

It may be worth noting that the "correct paraphrase" version of the Lunyak, et al (2002) paragraph that had been included in the previous version of this guide and which is reproduced immediately below had been written by a nonspecialist in that field and contained a subtle misinterpretation of the processes described in the original material paragraph:

A high affinity binding site for HP1 can be produced by silencing Lys[9] of histone H3 by methylation with mammalian histone lysine methyltransferase, a suppressor of variegation 39H1 (SUV39H1). MeCP2 can be immunoprecipitated with antibodies prepared against endogenous SUV39H1; on the other hand, immunoprecipitation of SUB39H1 resulted from aHA antibodies to HA-tagged MeCP2. [2]

---

[1] Paraphrased version prepared by John Rodgers.

14

Such subtle misrepresentations illustrates the fact that highly technical descriptions of a methodology, phenomena, etc., can be extremely difficult to properly paraphrase and, to do so, a writer mush have a thorough conceptual understanding of the concepts and processes being described. It is perhaps for this reason that ORI's definition of plagiarism (Office of Research Integrity, 1994) provides the following caveat:

> "ORI generally does not pursue the limited use of identical or nearly-identical phrases which describe a commonly-used methodology or previous research because ORI does not consider such use as substantially misleading to the reader or of great significance."

All of the above considerations serve to illustrate the reason why an operational definition of proper paraphrasing/plagiarism (i.e., how many consecutive words taken from the original constitutes plagiarism) is impractical, not to mention the fact that there are certain stock phrases, perhaps even entire sentences that occur with some frequency in unrelated journal articles (e.g., "the results obtained do not support the hypothesis"). Nevertheless, and in spite of the above clarification provided by ORI, a responsible writer has an ethical responsibility to readers and to the author/s from whom s/he is borrowing, to always respect and acknowledge their intellectual content.

Plagiarism and common knowledge

As noted above, we always must give proper credit to those whose ideas and facts we are using. One general exception to this principle occurs when the ideas we are discussing represent "common knowledge.". If the specific facts and figures we are discussing are assumed to be known by the readership, then one need not provide a citation. For example, suppose you are an American student writing a paper on the history of the United States for a college course. In your paper, you mention the fact that George Washington was the first president of the United States and that the Declaration of Independence was signed in the year 1776. Must you provide a citation for that pair of facts? Most likely not, as these are facts commonly known by average American high school and college students. The general expectation is that "everybody knows that". However, suppose that in the same paper you must identify the 23rd president, his running mate, and the main platform under which they were running for office, plus the year they both assumed power. Should such material be considered common knowledge? The answer is probably no, for it is doubtful that the average American student would readily know those facts without needing to consult an authoritative source (I had to look up the answers).

But, the question of what constitutes common knowledge is a little more complicated. Let's take another example. Imagine that we are writing a paper and we need to discuss the movement of sodium and potassium ions across a cell's membrane as described by the Martini and Bartholomew paragraph above. Surely, those ideas are not common knowledge amongst college students and if they were expected to use those concepts in a paper they would be expected to provide a citation. However, let's suppose that the individual writing the paper was a seasoned neuroscientist and that she intended to submit her paper for publication to a professional journal. Would the author need to provide a citation for that material? Not necessarily. Although for the non-scientist the description of the concentration gradients of sodium and potassium ions inside neurons may look sufficiently complex and unfamiliar, the material is considered common

15

knowledge amongst neuroscientists. It would, indeed, be shocking to find a neuroscientist or biomedical researcher who was not familiar with those fundamental concepts.

In sum, the question of whether the information we write about constitutes common knowledge is not easily answerable and depends on several factors, such as who the author is, who the readers are, and the expectations of each of these groups. Given these considerations, we recommend that authors abide by the following guideline:

Guideline 8: When in doubt as to whether a concept or fact is common knowledge, provide a citation.

Plagiarism and authorship disputes

Consider the following scenario. Two researchers who have collaborated on various projects in the past have jointly published a number of papers. Three quarters into the writing of the manuscript from their most recent joint project, the researchers experience a profound difference of opinion regarding the direction of the current project and the incident leads to the eventual break-up of their research collaboration. Soon after, one of the researchers moves to another institution in another country and begins to pursue a different line of research. A year later, the remaining researcher decides to finish writing the remaining quarter of the manuscript and submits it for publication with his name as sole author. By appropriating the joint manuscript and submitting it under his name, has this other researcher committed plagiarism?

Before attempting to answer this question, let's consider another scenario. A graduate student working under her mentor's supervision makes an interesting discovery as part of her doctoral thesis work. Before she is ready to publish her thesis, however, her mentor feels that the discovery merits immediate publication and decides to report her data, along with other data he had collected from other graduate fellows working in his lab, in a journal article. The mentor does not list the graduate student's name as a co-author nor is there a byline in the article indicating the extent of her contribution under the pretext that the student's contribution in and of itself was not sufficient to merit authorship.

In the above scenarios, it should be clear that the intellectual property of one individual has been misappropriated. Denial of earned authorship represents an ethical breach that many individuals and institutional policies, including that of the National Science Foundation, would consider an instance of plagiarism. However, not everyone agrees that these types of cases are plagiarism and, therefore, research misconduct. For example, ORI classifies these problems as **authorship disputes** and not within their definition of research misconduct. The involved parties can avoid these and other troublesome situations, such as disputes regarding the order of authorship of a paper, by discussing and agreeing on a plan **before** work on a project commences (see section on authorship).

An interesting fact of our work as scientists is that our research and writing may be simultaneously governed by more than one set of policies. For example, and especially in North America, the institution at which we work will likely have a research misconduct policy, the organization that funds our work may have its own misconduct policy, and so might the professional organizations to which we belong. In most instances, those policies will be similar across the various domains of coverage (e.g., plagiarism, authorship, data

16

sharing). However, there may also be subtle differences in how specific situations might be interpreted. For example, authorship resulting from students' doctoral work can differ across disciplines (e.g., psychology vs. biomedicine) and also across countries within a single discipline (see Australian Psychological Association). Similarly, authorship disputes may be classified as instances of plagiarism by one misconduct policy, but not by another policy. As result of these differences a problematic research behavior, such as certain instances of plagiarism, may be viewed as misconduct by an institution, but not by the funding agency.

As this document illustrates, plagiarism can manifest itself in a variety of situations and these can range in degree of seriousness. Although coverage has been provided for the most common forms, there are surely many other scenarios that represent instances of this type of misconduct. In the next section our attention is turned to the problem of self-plagiarism.

SELF-PLAGIARISM
(This section of the module has been substantially modified from its earlier version)

Given that plagiarism is often conceptualized as theft, the notion of self-plagiarism does not seem to make much sense. After all, is it possible to steal from oneself? In fact, Hexam (1999) has pointed out that it is, indeed, possible to steal from oneself as when one engages in embezzlement or insurance fraud. However, when applied to research and scholarship, self-plagiarism refers to authors who reuse their own previously disseminated content and pass it off as a "new" product without letting the reader know that this material has appeared previously. According to Hexam, "… the essence of self- plagiarism is [that] the author attempts to deceive the reader." Let us remember that the concept of ethical writing, upon which the present instructional resource is grounded on, entails an implicit contract between reader and writer whereby the reader assumes, unless otherwise noted, that the material was written by the individual/s listed as authors, and that it is new and is accurate to the best of the author's abilities. As such, self-plagiarism misleads the reader about the novelty of the material. In this section we review some of the most common instances of self-plagiarism and provide guidelines to avoid these pitfalls.

Self-plagiarism is often described in the context of several distinct practices in which some or all elements of a previous publication (e.g., text, data, and images) are reused in a new publication with ambiguous acknowledgement or no acknowledgement at all as to their prior dissemination. Perhaps the most blatant of these practices occurs when a previously published paper is later published again with very little or no modification. However, less blatant forms of duplication exist and these are sometimes classified with various labels, such as redundant, dual or overlapping publication. In examining these types of malpractices, the reader should keep in mind that the various forms of self-plagiarism are best thought as laying in a continuum in which the extent and the type of duplication can vary from substantial to minor, as does their potentially serious effects on the integrity of the scientific record.

A common practice for authors of trade books is to send their manuscript to several publishers. However, for authors of scientific or scholarly papers the acceptable practice is to submit their paper for publication to a single journal. Of course, an author may submit the same paper or a revised version of it to another journal, but only if it is determined that the journal to which it was first submitted has declined to publish it. Only under specific circumstances (see below) would it be acceptable for a paper published in one journal to appear in another journal.

17

In spite of these universally accepted practices, redundant publication[1] continues to be a problem in the biomedical sciences. For example, in one editorial, Schein (2001) describes the results of a study he and a colleague carried out which found that 92 out of 660 studies taken from 3 major surgical journals were actual cases of redundant publication. The rate of duplication in the rest of the biomedical literature has been estimated to be between 10% to 20% (Jefferson, 1998), though one review of the literature suggests the more conservative figure of approximately 10% (Steneck, 2000). However, the true rate may depend on the discipline and even the journal and more recent studies in individual biomedical journals do show rates ranging from as low as just over 1% in one journal to as high as 28% in another (see Kim, Bae, Hahm, & Cho, 2014) The current situation has become serious enough that biomedical journal editors consider redundancy and duplication one of the top areas of concern (Wager, Fiack, Graf, Robinson, & Rowlands, 2009) and it is the second highest cause for articles to be retracted from the literature between the years 2007 and 2011 (Fang, Steen, & Casadevall, 2012). Many biomedical journals now have explicit policies clarifying their opposition to multiple submissions of the same paper. Some journals even request that authors who submit a manuscript for publication must also submit previously published papers or those that are currently under review that are related to the topic of the manuscript under consideration. This requirement has been implemented to allow editors to determine whether the extent of overlap between such papers warrants the publication of yet another similar paper. If, in the opinion of the editor, the extent of overlap were substantial, the paper would likely not be published.

Duplicate (dual) publication

A sizable portion of scientific and scholarly research is carried out by individuals working in academic or research institutions where advancement structures continue to rely on the presentation and subsequent publication of research in peer-reviewed journals. Because the number and the quality of publications continue to be the most important criteria for gaining tenure and/or promotion, the more publications authored by a researcher, the better his/her chances of earning a promotion or tenure. As can be expected, and in the context of decreasing or, at best, stagnant funding for research, the current reward system produces a tremendous amount of pressure for scientists to generate as many publications as possible. Unfortunately, some of the most serious negative consequences of the present system, aside from fabrication, falsification and outright plagiarism, are the problems of duplicate publication and of other forms of redundancy. In the sciences, duplicate publication generally refers to the practice of submitting a paper with identical or near identical content to more than one journal, without alerting the editors or readers to the existence of its earlier published version. The new publication may be exactly the same (e.g., identical title, content, and author list) or differ only slightly from the original by, for example, changes to the title (see, for example, Attoui, Kherici, and Kherici-Bousnoubra, 2014), abstract, and/or order of the authors. Papers representing instances of duplicate publication almost always contain identical or nearly identical text and/or data relative to the earlier published version. More problematic instances of duplicate publication occur when various components of a paper change (e.g., title, authorship), but the underlying data remain the same, making duplication more difficult to uncover.

Duplicate publication in the academic context: 'Double-dipping'. Duplicate publication has a direct counterpart in the area of academic dishonesty. In the US it is commonly referred to as 'double dipping'. It occurs when a student submits a whole paper, or a substantial portion of a paper that had been previously submitted and graded in another course to fulfill a

18

requirement of a new course. Many college undergraduates and even some instructors are not aware that this type of practice is a serious academic offense (Hallupa & Bolliger, 2013). Of course, as is the case with duplicate publication, submitting the same paper or a large portion of a paper, to two different courses is entirely acceptable if the student sought permission from the instructors of both courses and they both agreed to the arrangement. However, some institutions may have specific policies prohibiting this practice under most circumstances.

Instances in which dual publication may be acceptable. Some authors who submit the same article to more than one journal rationalize their behavior by explaining that each journal has its own independent readership and that their duplicate paper would be of interest to each set of readers who would probably not otherwise be aware of the other publication. Indeed, there may be circumstances that justify the dual publication of a paper. For example, duplicate publication may be acceptable when an article published in one language is translated into a different language and published in a different journal. However, and consistent with existing guidelines, in all cases where the same paper is published in different journals, whether it is a translated version or the same identical paper, editors of both journals would have to agree to this arrangement and the new version must clearly indicate that it is a duplicate of an existing version. In addition other important conditions must be met and the interested reader should consult sources, such as ICMJE (2014) or Iverson et al. (2007). Similarly, any documentation in which authors list their publications as evidence of their research productivity (e.g., personal vita, ResearchGate), authors would be expected to identify both papers as being identical.

Redundancy, publication overlap and other forms of duplication

 Although the prevalence of blatant duplicate publications varies across disciplines, its overall prevalence is relatively low (see Larivière & Gingras, 2010) and their impact on the integrity of science is likely minor, particularly in instances when the published papers are truly identical (i.e., same title, abstract, author list). However, other forms of duplication exist and these are often classified with terms such as redundant publication or overlapping publication (see p 148 of Iverson, et al., 2007 for additional descriptive terms). As indicated earlier, these types of self-plagiarism are more prevalent and likely more detrimental to science because they involve the dissemination of earlier published data that are presented as new data, thereby skewing the scientific record. Bruton (2014) and others (e.g., von Elm, Poglia, Walder & Tramer, 2004) have discussed various other types of duplication. Below are some of the most common forms.

 Data aggregation/augmentation. In this type of duplication, data that have already been published are published again with some additional new data (see Smolčić & Bilić-Zulle, 2013. The resulting representation of the aggregated data is likely to be conceptually consistent with the original data set, but it will have different numerical outcomes (i.e., means and standard deviations), figures, and graphs (see Bonnell, Hafner, Hersam, Kotov, Buriak, Hammond, Javey, Nordlander, Parak, Schaak, Wee, Weiss, Rogach, Stevens & Willson, 2012 for an example). This type of publication is highly problematic when the author presents the data in a way that misleads the reader into believing that the entire data set is independently derived from the data that had been originally published. That is, the reader is never informed that a portion of the data being described had already been published or perhaps the presentation is ambiguous enough for the reader to be unable to discern the true nature of the data.

 Data disaggregation. As the label suggests, data disaggregation occurs when data from a previously published study are published again minus some data points and with no

19

indication or, at best, ambiguous indication as to their relationship to the originally published paper. The new study may consist of the original data set minus a few data points now considered outliers, or perhaps data points at both ends of their range that happen to lie outside a newly established criterion for inclusion in the new analyses, or perhaps some other procedure that results in the exclusion of some of the data points appearing in the original study. As with data augmentation, the new publication with the disaggregated data will contain different numerical outcomes (i.e., means and standard deviations), figures, and graphs, however, the underlying data are largely the same as the previously published data, but are presented in a way that misleads the reader into interpreting the 'new' data as having been independently collected.

Data segmentation. Also known as Salami Publication or Least Publishable Unit, data segmentation is a practice that is often subsumed under the heading of self-plagiarism, but which, technically is not necessarily a form of duplication or of redundancy as Bruton, 2014 has correctly pointed out. It is usually mentioned in the context of self-plagiarism because the practice often does include a substantial amount of text overlap and possibly some data as well, with earlier publications by the same author/s. Consider the examples provided by Kassirer and Angell (1995), former editors of *The New England Journal of Medicine*:

> "Several months ago, for example, we received a manuscript describing a controlled intervention in a birthing center. The authors sent the results on the mothers to us, and the results on the infants to another journal. The two outcomes would have more appropriately been reported together. We also received a manuscript on a molecular marker as a prognostic tool for a type of cancer; another journal was sent the results of a second marker from the same pathological specimens. Combining the two sets of data clearly would have added meaning to the findings." (p. 450).

In some cases, the segmenting of a large study into two or more publications may, in fact, be the most meaningful approach to reporting the results of that research. Longitudinal studies are an example of this type of situation. However, dividing a study into smaller segments must always be done with full transparency, showing exactly how the data being reported in the later publication are related to the earlier publication. An often stated rationale used by some authors for not disclosing the relationship between related publications or for other forms of covert overlap between publications is that both reports are prepared and submitted simultaneously to different journals (see, for example, Katsnelson, 2015). However, this should not be considered an acceptable excuse for not disclosing any overlap between studies, especially to the editors of the journals. Authors should describe how the study data being described are related to a larger project. They can always provide a footnote, author note or some other indication that manuscripts describing the other portions of the data set are in preparation or under consideration, etc., which ever the case may be. The important point is that readers need to be made aware that the data being reported were collected in the context of a larger study. As with other forms of redundancy and actual duplication, salami slicing can lead to a distortion of the literature by leading unsuspecting readers to believe that data presented in each salami slice (i.e., journal article) are independently derived from a different data collection effort or subject sample.

Guideline 9: Authors of complex studies should heed the advice previously put forth by Angell & Relman (1989). If the results of a single complex study are best presented as a 'cohesive' single whole, they should not be partitioned into individual papers.

20

Furthermore, if there is any doubt as to whether a paper submitted for publication represents fragmented data, authors should enclose other papers (published or unpublished) that might be part of the paper under consideration (Kassirer & Angell, 1995).

Other forms of redundancy with or without text or data duplication.

Reanalysis of the same data. There may be occasions in which previously published data can be analyzed using a novel technique not available at the time of publication. Or perhaps the authors thought of a new way to analyze the data using an existing technique. Both of these scenarios and still others perhaps may warrant a re-examination of the data. However, it should be obvious that authors need to be fully transparent with their readers by indicating the fact that earlier analyses of the data have already been published.

Same data; different conclusions. von Elm, et al, (2004) describe have described various other forms of redundancy. For example, a related practice occurs when authors publish the same data, with a somewhat different textual slant within the body of the paper and, again, with ambiguous or non existent acknowledgment of the earlier publication. Such redundant papers may contain a slightly different interpretation of the data or the introduction to the paper may be described in a somewhat different theoretical, empirical, or perhaps subject sample context. Sometimes, additional data or somewhat different analyses of the same, previously published data are reported in the redundant paper.

Why duplication and other forms of redundancy must be avoided

The fact of the matter is that all the above malpractices in which readers are fully informed or are outright misled about the provenance of the data are frowned upon by most scientific journals (see Kassirer & Angell, 1995) and most of the major scientific writing guides caution against them (e.g., Iverson, et al., 2007).

The apparent glut of quality scientific journals notwithstanding, a paper that appears in two different journals unbeknownst to readers and editors may have robbed other authors of the opportunity to publish their worthwhile original work. In addition, while a paper can always benefit from additional critical peer review, journal referees often must volunteer their valuable time to review others' work in the service of science and scholarship. Refereeing what turns out to be a duplicate or redundant publication places undue time and limited resource constraints on the editorial and peer review system. More importantly and particularly in the sciences, is the fact that covert dual/redundant publications likely result in readers being misled as to the true nature of a given phenomenon or process. For example, an author who wishes to study the significance of an experimental effect or phenomenon using sophisticated statistical techniques, such as meta-analysis, will likely overestimate or perhaps underestimate the magnitude or reliability of an effect if the same experiment were to be counted twice. Consider the following anecdote reported by Wheeler (1989):

"In one such instance, a description of a serious adverse pulmonary effect associated with a new drug used to treat cardiovascular patients was published twice, five months apart in different journals. Although the authors were different, they wrote from the same medical school about patients that appear identical. Any researcher counting the incidence of complications associated with this drug from the published literature could easily be misled into concluding that the incidence is

21

higher than it really is." (p.1).

Redundant publication practices can distort the conclusions of literature reviews if the various segments of a salami publication or the augmented data that represent data from the same subject sample, are included in a meta analysis under the assumption that all of the data are derived from independent samples (Tramer, Reynolds, Moore, and McQuay, 1997) and evidence indicates that some meta-analytic studies have been contaminated by duplicate data (Choi, Song, Ock, Kim, Lee, Chang, & Kim, 2014). For this reason, all forms of covert data reuse can have serious negative consequences for the integrity of the scientific database. In certain key areas of biomedical and social science research the consequences of duplicated data can result in wrong health policy recommendations that could place the public at risk.

Guideline 10: Authors who submit a manuscript for publication containing previously disseminated data, reviews, conclusions, etc., must clearly indicate to the editors and readers the nature of the previous dissemination. The provenance of data must never be in doubt.

Text recycling from an author's previously disseminated work

Authors who engage in programmatic research often end up writing a series of related papers each of which describes individual empirical investigations that use similar or nearly identical methodologies. The background literature pertinent to one paper may be largely applicable to the other papers on the same subject. Thus, it is possible for some authors to have to generate two or more papers describing truly independent studies that contain identical or very similar methodologies, background literature, and discussion elements. The pressure to publish felt by most researchers, together with the ease with which entire blocks of text can be transferred from one document to another one, present unique challenges to those authors who recognize that substantial text reuse is highly problematic. The allure to reuse previously disseminated, well-written text can be particularly difficult to resist for authors who are not dominant in English, especially for those who have traditionally relied on the practice of reusing smaller snippets of text out of pure necessity (see Flowerdew and Li, 2007). Regrettably, instances do occur in the scientific literature of published empirical investigations that are subsequently retracted for self-plagiarism of text because much of the paper is taken verbatim from a previously published one by the same author (see Marcus, 2010, for an example).

Just as there is no consensus or official guidance on the extent to which text must be modified to qualify as an appropriate paraphrase, there is also no consensus as to how much text an author may recycle from his/her previous writings. It should be evident, however, that from the perspective of the reader-writer contract, the recycling of one's own previously disseminated content is not consistent with the principles of ethical writing. Thus, an overview of the more common situations in which recycling is likely to occur is worth examining.

Situations in which recycling previously disseminated textual content may be acceptable.

22

As with redundant publication, certain situations exist under which text recycling may be deemed acceptable even if, on the surface, it would seemingly violate the spirit of the reader-writer contract. For example, before engaging in the actual research project, authors will need to prepare protocols (e.g., IRB protocol, trial registration applications), that describe in detail the background of the research, purpose, scope, expected results, etc. The convenience of recycling from these documents (e.g., Institutional Review Board (IRB) applications, Animal Care and Use Committee applications, internal grant applications) or other forms of unpublished 'internal' documents is obvious. Given the limited dissemination of these documents, the fact that they are not copyrighted or published, it should be acceptable to reuse their content in subsequent presentations/publications targeted for wider dissemination (e.g., conference presentations, published papers). Of course, there may be exceptions, such as when the original documents are written for a private entity which may have claims of ownership of any material generated by the author. In these cases permission to subsequently publish portions of such material must be obtained. Another problematic situation occurs when the text in question was the result of a collaborative effort between multiple individuals. Although reuse of certain methodological material (see section below on boilerplate language) and related content may be acceptable across various subsequent published papers, reuse of other content from these documents in more than one paper is less clear and possibly not consistent with the reader-writer contract. Be that as it may, any reuse of limited-circulation internal-type documents (e.g., IRB protocols) should, when applicable, have the approval of the institution under which they were generated and also of any co-authors of the original documents.

Recycling boilerplate language. Boilerplate language is most often associated with the legal profession and it refers to portions of text that are routinely reused in legal documents that convey a specific, standard meaning. In the sciences, the term "boilerplate language" has been used in recent decades to describe analogous standard language usually, but not always, of a technical nature. For example, language from the operating instructions of scientific equipment may be adopted by authors in their description of the technical aspects of an instrument and/or procedures associated with the proper use of that instrument. Similarly, laboratories working in a difficult research problem may develop a set of precise descriptions of highly complex processes and/or procedures that may be equally applicable, perhaps with minor modifications, across many different experiments. Thus, in certain journal articles produced by the same or even different groups of author-investigators, it is possible to find portions of identical so-called boilerplate text in sections that describe these same complex processes or procedures. However, and especially in the absence of any other duplication, such reused text should be deemed acceptable and be interpreted as standard, boilerplate, language. Other instances of boilerplate language that describe the nature of an institution's research facilities, laboratory, or computing equipment may be offered by, for example, an institutions' grant offices about for purposes of assisting their staff in preparing their grant applications.

Recycling methods and other sections from our previously published papers. In writing methodology sections of empirical papers, one of the goals of authors is to provide all the necessary details so that an independent researcher can replicate the study. These sections are often highly technical and, consequently, can be very laborious to produce given the need for exceptional clarity and precision. Given these considerations, the question arises as to the acceptability of recycling entire methods sections or large portions of these sections with only the necessary modifications to reflect the new conditions being studied (except for an attempt at replication, it is probably rare for the exact same method to be repeated from one related experiment to the next). A similar situation occurs when we summarize others' work in literature reviews, arguably a less complex writing task relative to writing a methods section. Of course, if an author were to adhere to formal rules of scholarship and to the implicit contract between reader and writer embodied in the concept of ethical writing, s/he would need to put any verbatim text from the method section in quotation marks and appropriately paraphrase any other recycled text that is not placed in quotations. But, as stated earlier, the use of quoted material is seldom practiced in IMRD papers in the sciences.

Unfortunately, as shown by a recent review of journal editorials on the subject of plagiarism and self-plagiarism, there seems to be no clear consensus on this matter (Roig, 2014). For example, some journals may allow the reuse of text from literature reviews and methods sections (e.g., Kohler, 2012). Others will allow reuse of methods sections only (Shafer, 2011), while others Swaan (2010) do not permit any text reuse. One potential danger in copy pasting earlier used methods sections lies in the possibility of including material that is not relevant. For example, in a section titled "Avoidable errors in manuscripts" Biros (2000), a former editor-in-chief of *Academic Emergency Medicine* writes:

> "Methods are reported that were not actually used. [This] most frequently occurs when an author has published similar methods previously and has devised a template for the methods which is used from paper to paper. Reproducing the template exactly is self-plagiarism and can be misleading if the template is not updated to reflect the current research project." (p. 3).

In addition to self-plagiarism, the reuse of large portions of text from previously published papers may be problematic for other reasons. One reason for avoiding copy-pasting content between papers concerns the possibility of introducing material that is not relevant to the current manuscript. For example, a study by Hammond, Helbig, Benson and Brahtwaite-Sketoe (2003) revealed that copy-pasting in the context of medical records resulted in errors, some of which were deemed potentially unsafe for patients. Surely, an analogous situation can occur when authors copy-paste from their previously published papers (or from others' papers!). Evidence suggests that this malpractice continues to be a problem (O'Reilly, 2013). The other reason why reusing text from one publication to another may be problematic is best illustrated in the following scenario: an author takes a substantial amount of text from one of her papers that had been published in a journal owned by one publisher and recycles that text in a paper that will now be published by a journal owned by a different publisher. In this situation, the author may be violating copyright rules. Thus, Biros (2000) also cautions that:

> "Many authors do not understand the implications of signing the copyright release form. In essence, this transfers ownership of the paper and all of its contents from the author to the publisher. Subsequent papers written by the same author therefore must be careful not to reproduce in any way material that has previously been published, even if it is written by them. Such copying constitutes self-plagiarism." (p. 4).

Again, the question of reusing segments from previously published work becomes a bit more complicated when the original work was multi-authored and there is no agreement as to who might reuse such work if reuse is permitted. In these types of situations the potential for an accusation of plagiarism by a co-author who does not approve of the reuse could easily develop.

24

On the other hand, there is a very good argument to allow liberal reuse of previously published methodologies. As discussed earlier, methods sections often include very intricately complex descriptions of procedures and processes that are laden with unique terminology and phraseology for which there are no acceptable equivalents (e.g., *Mammalian histone lysine methyltransferase, suppressor of variegation 39H1 (SUV39H1)*. Even when major textual modifications to these sections are possible, a change in the language can run the risk of slightly altering the intended meaning of what is being described and such an outcome is a highly undesirable in the sciences. Thus authors should be allowed some latitude in terms of the extent to which they should modify portions of text when paraphrasing material from methodology sections that is highly technical in nature, even if the material is derived from other sources. In this context, it is worth keeping in mind the following segment from ORI's definition of plagiarism (Office of Research Integrity, 1994):

"ORI generally does not pursue the limited use of identical or nearly-identical phrases which describe a commonly-used methodology or previous research because ORI does not consider such use as substantially misleading to the reader or of great significance".

Guideline 11: While there are some situations where text recycling is an acceptable practice, it may not be so in other situations. Authors are urged to adhere to the spirit of ethical writing and avoid reusing their own previously published text, unless it is done in a manner that alerts readers about the reuse or one that is consistent with standard scholarly conventions (e.g., by using of quotations and proper paraphrasing).

There are benefits to the limited reuse of textual material from methods sections. However, substantial text recycling of most other parts of a typical journal article and particularly when carried out by native writers of English, suggest a certain degree of scholarly laziness. At worst, these practices, particularly when they involve the presentation of previously published data that is presented as new data, can result in serious consequences to the scholarly and scientific literature, to public health, and even to the perpetrator if the trespass is serious enough to warrant a charge of research misconduct. Authors are well advised to carefully review the editorial guidelines of journals to which they submit their manuscripts, as well as their disciplines' codes of ethics. More importantly, scientists and scholars need to be reminded that they are always held to the highest standards of ethical conduct and need to be 100% transparent with their readers.

Self-plagiarism within and across various other dissemination domains

The material reviewed above raises some questions about the appropriateness of content reuse in other domains of research and scholarship. The discussion below addresses some of the more common situations where reuse should be carefully reconsidered.

From conference to conference. In most disciplines, presenting one's work at conferences has been a long-standing tradition in scholarly and scientific work. Audiences are exposed to the latest ideas/data on a given topic and, in turn, authors gain valuable feedback on their

25

work, which allows them to further refine their ideas, thereby maximizing their chances of getting their work published in a peer-reviewed journal. In some disciplines, such as political science, the presentation of the same paper in multiple conferences has become a more common practice (Dometrius, 2008) and this development has been a source of concern for some in that discipline about possible skewed perceptions of authors' productivity for some in that discipline (e.g., Sigelman, 2008), though not for others (e.g., Cooper & Jacoby, 2008; Schneider & Jacoby, 2008). No doubt similar questions have been raised by members of other scientific disciplines. But, as with matters related to self-plagiarism where there can be wide differences of opinion, it is likely that academics are equally split with respect to the appropriateness of recycling conference papers.

 A number of factors ought to be considered when deciding to recycle a conference paper and the type of presentation made (e.g., invited address, symposium, panel discussion, traditional paper) and the context in which the presentation is made may determine the acceptability of recycling a paper. For example, in any discipline renowned subject-matter experts are routinely invited by universities, professional organizations (i.e., conferences) or by other entities to present their research. In these situations there should be no particular assumption of novelty on the part of the audience about the content of the presentation. Nonetheless, and consistent with the theme of this module, it would be highly recommended for presenters to indicate to their audience at the beginning of each event whether the presentation is new or a revised version of an earlier presentation.

 For traditional conference submissions, an important consideration is whether the organization sponsoring the meeting only accepts original presentations. Determining whether a presentation is original is not always easy because of the possibility that an original presentation may also contain previously disseminated data, text and/or figures. As might be done with papers submitted to journals, authors of papers that may contain some previously presented content should inquire with the conference organizers whether their presentation is sufficiently original to warrant submission. For example, when a previously presented paper is disseminated at a different conference and retains the same title and authorship, audience members who happened to have heard the first version are more likely to recognize that the same material, with perhaps some revisions, is being presented again and can decide whether to attend or not. Certainly, in situations where conference activity is taken into account as a measure of research productivity, members of promotion and/or tenure committees should be readily able to discern that individual's true level of productivity when the same presentation is listed separately, but maintains the same identical title, authorship, and text. On the other hand, questions can arise when authors change the title and/or authorship of a presentation without making additional substantive changes to the actual paper. Although audience members who heard the first presentation in a previous conference might recognize the author, the presence of a different title may lead them to mistakenly believe that the new presentation is substantially different from the earlier one when, in fact, it is not. The same will apply to members of promotion and tenure review committees who review the author's curriculum vitae. Because members of such committees might not have the time to carefully examine each presentation listed, a mere change in titles may mislead them into believing that the various presentations with different titles are independent products, suggesting that the author is much more productive than s/he truly is. For these reasons, it is important for authors to alert audience members and those reviewing the author's curriculum vitae, as to whether each presentation may be a revised version of an earlier presentation, a brand new presentation or a combination of the two, especially if there are changes to the title, abstract or authorship. Again, in principle, these issues are applicable to all academic researchers, for not only must data always be clearly conveyed as either new or previously disseminated, but data collection in some disciplines can be an arduous and

26

time-consuming task that can take many weeks or months. Thus, if members of promotion and tenure committees from countries where conference presentations are used as evidence of research productivity interpret a recycled paper as presenting new data, whether the paper is a conference presentation or a journal article, such a misinterpretation will give a mistaken impression that the author is much more productive than s/he truly is.

  A related issue concerns the subsequent publication as conference proceedings of conference presentations. Given the emphasis on characteristics, such as clarity, thoroughness, completeness, etc., in scientific writing, there should never be any confusion as to the provenance of the data so that audience members or readers of proceedings can properly assimilate the results of that research. Failure to interpret new data as previously disseminated could conceivably lead to a misrepresentation of the exact scientific status of an effect/phenomenon. Therefore, as with instances of recycled data in published papers, presenting previously disseminated data in conferences as new data, may, under certain conditions, be analogous to fabricating data, a serious form of research misconduct.

GUIDELINE 12: In the domain of conferences and similar audio-visual presentations of their work, authors should practice the same principles of transparency with their audiences.

From conference to journal article/book. After delivering a conference paper and perhaps based on the audience's feedback, authors will often prepare a formal paper to be submitted for publication to a journal or perhaps an edited book. This practice is a long-standing tradition and has generally been always acceptable. However, recent trends in the publication of conference proceedings call for caution in subsequent submissions to journals and/or books. For example, in cases where abridged versions of the paper or even the preliminary papers themselves are copyrighted and subsequently published as proceedings by the sponsoring organization, authors should inquire as to whether these organizations permit republication of their materials. Likewise, and in the case in which published proceedings exist and subsequent publication of the paper is allowed by the publisher of the proceedings, authors submitting a paper for publication must first alert the editor about the existence of the earlier published version of the paper. In addition, readers must also be informed about the prior version and such communication can be easily accomplished through an author note or analogous mechanism. Keep in mind that different journals have different criteria for publishing earlier presented work that later appears in proceedings in either electronic or print form. Some editors will consider the expanded publication of an earlier published proceedings abridged paper or long abstract as a case of redundancy. In some such cases, the expanded published version of the paper may be retracted as occurred in a recent case described by Vasconcelos and Roig (2015).

From journal article to journal article or from journal article to book. Instances have occurred in which authors of, say, review papers, whether these reviews appear in a journal article or in a book, misappropriate significant portions of material without enclosing such material in quotation marks and providing a citation, or without giving any indication as to the material's true origin. This practice, of course, represents an instance of plagiarism. However, what if the reused material is derived from the author/s' previously published articles or books? Such practices are ethically inappropriate even if the author him/herself owns the copyright to the previously published material. Again, the important consideration here is the failure to inform the author that the material has appeared elsewhere. Of course, one should be free to reuse with proper attribution and quotation one's earlier work. But, even here there may be proprietary issues if the author does not hold the copyright to his/her

27

earlier work. Some publishers have strict guidelines as to how much material one may quote from with attribution. For example, consider the American Psychological Association's position on this matter (*Publication Manual of the American Psychological Association*, 2010, p. 173):

> APA policy permits author to use, with some exceptions, a maximum of three figures or tables from a journal article or book chapter, single text extracts of fewer than 400 words, or a series of text extracts that total fewer than 800 words without requesting formal permission from APA. It is important to check with the publisher or copyright owner regarding specific requirements for permission to quote from or adapt copyrighted material.

From dissertation to journal article/book and vice versa. It is common for authors of theses and dissertations to subsequently publish their thesis or dissertation work in journal articles or books. This practice has been traditionally acceptable even when the thesis or dissertation has already been submitted to an electronic repository such as ProQuest's UMI® (Ramirez, Dalton, McMillan, Read, and Seamans, 2013). Nevertheless it is important for authors to check with the publisher to whom they intend to submit their work. If acceptable, authors must nevertheless include a note in the journal article or book indicating that the work is based on the author's thesis or dissertation work. In cases where the dissertation work leads to two or more articles, authors must ensure that each article also mentions that the work described in the paper is part of a larger work published elsewhere. Authors must also have a legitimate rationale for publishing the papers separately, lest there be a charge of salami publishing. A related question is whether authors may reuse smaller portions of their thesis or dissertation work in an article or book. Again, this is perfectly acceptable as long as the author provides a full citation and uses quotation marks. Should there be an objection to the use of quotation marks an author can always alert the reader by prefacing the material with a statement such as, "As I described in my doctoral thesis, which I reproduce here verbatim….".

In some academic programs, the tradition has been for the doctoral student to first publish an article or two and then to reformat the published work and submit it as a dissertation. In some cases, research that has already been published outside of the immediate academic department where work for the degree is being carried out may be an acceptable fulfillment of the requirements of the dissertation. Such cases may be somewhat complicated if the outside work was carried out in collaboration with others, which may make it difficult to estimate the exact contribution of the student working for the degree. Obviously, the doctoral student must disclose in full the extent of his/her contribution to the published work.

Grant proposals

The ability to obtain external funding to carry out one's research is increasingly a requirement for hiring, promotion, and tenure in some disciplines. For many scholars and scientists already working within a "publish-or-perish" climate, writing grant proposals is an additional challenge to survival within the profession. Given these pressures, many authors elect to use shortcuts by reusing previously disseminated content in their funding applications in an effort to save time and effort. For example, an internal study of 8,000 funded grant applications to the US National Science Foundation (NSF), uncovered plagiarism in about 1% to 1.5% of those applications (Mervis, 2013). More recently, Garner, McIver, and Waitzkin, (2013) analyzed over 800,000 grant application summaries to 5 major funding agencies and, using a conservative measure of analysis, uncovered a total of 167 duplicates.

28

With a more liberal approach, these authors reported that as many as 12,441 pairs may have included some degree of duplication. Needless to say, recycling content from others' work without permission and/or acknowledgement, including funded or unfunded grant proposals constitutes plagiarism, a type of research misconduct. But, what about recycling content in grant applications from our own previously disseminated work, including previously submitted funding requests?

Recycling from grant proposal to grant proposal. It is not uncommon for researchers working on a complex problem to prepare separate funding proposals on various separate but related components of the phenomena being studied. Such proposals will likely have identical or nearly identical common literature review, methodology and materials, and perhaps still other elements of a previously submitted application. In addition, funding applications are also increasingly multi-authored. In these and other situations, questions may arise as to whether an author can simply reuse portions of text from one proposal in which s/he is principal investigator or co-investigator to another proposal. From the perspective of the reader-writer contract, such reuse is probably acceptable, given the nature of the written product: the application itself is not published and the scope of dissemination of its contents is limited. However, authors must remember that some funding agencies may have specific parameters for the reuse of content from earlier submitted grant proposals to the same agency, whether these earlier proposals have been funded or not. (Obviously, one may reuse the entire contents of an unfunded grant application in a new grant application that is targeted to another funding agency). For example, in the United States, a grant that is not funded after the first submission to the National Institutes of Health (NIH) may be resubmitted with revisions. The reuse of content from the older application to the newer application does not come into question as the situation is analogous to revising a textbook. However, if the second time it is submitted the proposal is not funded, it may not be resubmitted again to that agency. Thus, the question arises as to whether an applicant may reuse substantial portions of the unfunded proposal for a "new" proposal to the same agency. Of course, a grant applicant may submit, as new, a proposal related to the earlier problem for which funding had been sought and denied, but this must be done such that the project investigates a substantially new, albeit, related problem or perhaps studies the old problem using a different methodology. With this in mind, there would be no harm in reusing portions of, say, literature reviews and perhaps even some methodology. However, the applicant must ensure that the focus of the investigation is different from the previously unfunded submission. Alternatively, the applicant may submit a proposal about a related idea and may consider reusing relevant material from the older unfunded proposal or from another related proposal that had been previously funded. In such cases, the applicant should check with the relevant agency for their guidelines regarding reuse and the criteria for determining whether the new submission to that agency constitutes a new proposal or a revised version of an earlier one. Given the current science funding climate in the US and elsewhere, the question of what constitutes a new proposal vs. a revised one is not an easy one to answer. For example, the NIH has some very specific requirements about these matters with which applicants must become familiar (see http://grants.nih.gov/grants/policy/resubmission_q&a.htm). Nonetheless, if material is being reused from a previous application, whether funded or unfunded, nothing prevents the applicant from adhering to the spirit of the reader-writer contract and alerting the reader about the extent of the reuse. This is especially relevant given the possibility that some of the referees reviewing the new grant proposal may have reviewed the old proposal. In that respect, and at a time of increasing emphasis on transparency in all aspects of scientific work, it would be prudent to ensure such transparency in funding applications. Therefore, a footnote or some other mechanism could easily be used to indicate which portions of the review, methodology, etc., are derived from a previously submitted application.

Recycling from grant proposal to published paper*.* Because the readership of a grant proposal is relatively small, the reuse of content from a grant proposal to a published paper probably does not violate the spirit of the reader-writer contract as there is an expectation that such reuse routinely takes place. The same can probably be said for recycling from other non-publishable documents, such as research ethics board applications (i.e., Institutional Review Boards). The principle may also apply to *recycling from same-authored-published-papers-to-grants*. There could conceivably be copyright infringement if the author does not own the copyright to the work from which s/he wants to recycle content. However, as grant proposals are not normally published and only disseminated in limited fashion, it is difficult to imagine that reuse of copyrighted content in a grant proposal would be problematic, especially if such content also contains revisions, even if only minor ones. Two other important factors merit consideration: 1) whether content from the grant that had been recycled from a copyrighted paper is reused in a later paper whose copyright is owned by a different publisher and 2) whether the material being recycled was co-authored by others. If the latter, then written permission for reusing co-authored content might need to be sought and such permission would need to include authorship clarification of the new output that will contain the reused previously co-authored material.

Readers who are experienced grant writers will readily recognize that there are many other possible scenarios related to reuse in the context of grant applications. In thinking about each possible scenario, it may be worth keeping in mind the assumption of novelty in the reader-writer contract. Thus, as indicated above, and in the service of ethical transparency and depending on the particular scenario, an author may wish to consider the appropriateness of including a simple note that alerts the readers as to the nature and extent of any content that has been reused.

GUIDELINE 13: In addition to standard practices of ethical scholarship, authors must be mindful of readers' expectations, applicable issues related to intellectual content rights (i.e., copyright), and, especially, the need to always be transparent in our work when reusing material across the various dissemination domains.

Copyright Law

This document has mentioned copyright at various points throughout. Because some instances of plagiarism and self-plagiarism (e.g., redundant publication) have the potential for violating copyright law, the following section is devoted to a brief review of the concept of copyright.

Copyright law is based on Article 1, sec. 8, cl. 8 of the United States Constitution, the purpose of which is "to promote the progress of science and useful arts, by securing for limited times to authors and inventors the exclusive right to their respective writings and discoveries." Once owners of an artistic (e.g., song, lyrics, films) or an intellectual work (e.g., book, article) copyright a product, they have the exclusive right to publish, reproduce, sell, distribute, or modify those products. For authors who wish to have their papers published in traditional journals, the typical arrangement is for the copyright of the author's work to be transferred to the publisher of the journal. The journal can then reproduce and distribute the author's work legally. An increasing number of journals now

30

allow the author to maintain ownership of their work, but both entities sign an agreement specifying the journals' right to publish and re-use the author's material. In the case of "Open Access" journals (freely available to the public without expectation of payment), the author agrees to allow for the free dissemination of his/her works without prior permission.

  With some exceptions, the unauthorized use of copyrighted work violates copyright law and represents copyright infringement. Exceptions to copyright infringement fall under the doctrine of "Fair Use" of copyright law and represent instances in which the activity is largely for nonprofit educational, scholarship, or research purposes (see US Copyright Office, 1996). For example, in some situations, a student or individual researcher may make a copy of a journal article or book chapter for his/her own personal use without asking permission. Likewise, an author describing the results of a published study may take a couple of lines of data from a table from a journal article, include a citation, and reproduce it in his/her paper. The American Medical Association's *Manual of Style* (Iverson, et al., 2007) provides additional examples of instances of "fair use."

Copyright Infringement, fair use, and plagiarism

  The use of relatively short direct quotes from a published work does not usually require permission from the copyright holder as it typically falls under the "fair use" provision. However, extensive quoting of text from a copyrighted source can constitute copyright infringement, whether the appropriated text is properly enclosed in quotation marks or correctly paraphrased, even if a citation is provided according to established scholarly conventions. Obviously, the same applies if the material is plagiarized outright. Moreover, the reader should note that intellectual or artistic work does not need to be published in order to be copyrighted. In fact, the moment the work becomes final it is automatically copyrighted. Thus, instances of plagiarism, whether from a published article or even an unpublished manuscript, can also constitute copyright infringement, though, of course, copyright infringement does not always constitute plagiarism. For example, if I were to quote extensively and with proper citation beyond the limit dictated by the publisher of the work from which I quoted, I would be in violation of that publisher's copyright, but the infraction would not constitute plagiarism as I am letting the reader know, by my use of quotations and a citation, that the material being used is not mine.

Iverson, et al., (2007) cautions the reader that the amount of text that can be taken from a copyrighted source without permission depends on its proportion to the entire work. However, the reader should also note that some publishers, such as the APA, have established word limits for borrowing text. Given the above considerations, it should then be clear that extensive plagiarism and self-plagiarism may also qualify as copyright infringement because the copyright of the plagiarized or self-plagiarized content may be held by the publisher; not by the author. This would certainly be the case if the original article were published in a journal owned by one publisher and the second article were to appear in a journal owned by a different publisher both of which require that authors transfer the copyright of their papers to the publishers. One should note that not all publishers require that authors transfer their copyright to them.

Guideline 14: Because some instances of plagiarism, self-plagiarism, and even some writing practices that might otherwise be acceptable (e.g., extensive paraphrasing or quoting of key elements of a book) can constitute copyright infringement, authors are strongly encouraged to become familiar with basic elements of copyright law.

Cultural-linguistic considerations of plagiarism and self-plagiarism

Plagiarism amongst non English-speaking students has been, in part, attributed to a variety of cultural factors, including their different conceptions of intellectual property, originality and attribution. For example, students from some Asian countries presumably follow ancient traditions of memorizing and copying texts from original sources out of respect for the authority those individuals represent (see Pecorari, 2013, p. 110) and they do so without attribution under the assumption that the reader will already be familiar with the provenance of the material (Bloch 2012, p. 14). Certainly, earlier research suggested that some Asian students may not even be familiar with the concept of plagiarism (see, for example, Decker, 1993), but more recent evidence does suggest that even if they are familiar with the concept, plagiarism may simply be ignored by teachers because such behavior does not seem to be a matter of concern to them (see, for example, Moon 2002). To be fair, such lax attitude toward plagiarism on the part of teaching staff and of students is not confined to Asian nations. Heitman and Litewka (2011), point out how students in Eastern European nations (see Magnus, Polteroich and Danilov, 2002; Pupovac, Bilic-Zulle & Petrovecki, 2008) and also Middle East, Latin America, India, and Africa are much more tolerant about issues of misconduct than some Western European nations or the United States (see Vasconcelos, Leta, and Costa, 2009). On the other hand, many of these attitudes may be slowly changing as individual nations and even entire regions attempt to become more competitive in an increasingly global market. For example, Chinese-English bilingual education is growing rapidly in China (Hu, 2008) and, invariably, such instruction will likely lead to wider exposure and familiarity with Western scholarly traditions, including issues related to plagiarism and proper attribution of sources. Other emerging economies (i.e., Brazil) are similarly making great strides toward curbing both, academic and research misconduct (Vasconcelos, et al, 2009).

In addition to cultural variables, Heitman and Litewa (2011) identify two other major factors that predispose some non English speaking individuals to plagiarize: 1) The acceptability of plagiarism in their home environments and 2) vague or non-existent policies on this and related subjects.

With respect to the second point, it should be noted that in most Western, English-speaking nations, secondary, and tertiary academic institutions familiarize students with issues of academic integrity, and plagiarism in particular, via a number of mechanisms, such as in-class verbal admonitions, written academic integrity policies, student honor codes, and similar guidance. Yet, studies repeatedly show that many students from these same nations, including those from North America, admit to plagiarizing at all educational levels, i.e., graduate and professional schools, even though they likely know what plagiarism is and are well-aware that it is wrong. Similarly, most Western academic institutions, funding agencies, professional associations, etc., have written policies in place that identify plagiarism as a form of research misconduct. Yet, plagiarism is one of the most frequent areas of concern for journal editors (Wager, et al., 2009) with a third of retracted journal articles being due to plagiarism or self-plagiarism (Fang, et al., 2012). Some of these retracted papers are from native English-speaking authors who work at Western institutions with strong misconduct

32

policies.

The academic dishonesty literature can help inform us about factors that can influence whether students will plagiarize. For example, according to Donald McCabe, perhaps the most widely published researcher in this area, one of most important predictors of whether students will cheat is their perception of whether others will do so (McCabe, Treviño, & Butterfield, 2002). Thus, and consistent with Heitman and Litewa's (2011) observation, if there is a perception that others plagiarize and/or that this misbehavior will be tolerated, students are more likely to engage in it, especially if they believe that doing so does not lead to any negative consequences.

Admittedly, some of the evidence does suggest that many native English-speaking students (McGowan & Lightbody, 2008; Power, 2009; Roig, 1997; 1999) and even some professionals (Julliard, 1994; Roig, 2001) are simply not familiar with the nuances of appropriate scholarship. In addition, the evidence also suggests that an important factor that leads writers to misappropriate long strings of text from sources is a combination of uniqueness of the terminology used, etc. (cite sources). To this point, Pecorari (2013) writes: "Most people, from undergraduates in their first term to senior and frequently published scholars, find academic writing challenging because of the high degree of accuracy and precision of expression it requires" (p. 113). It makes sense, then, to suspect that a major factor in the incidence of plagiarism by non-native writers of English lies in these writers' difficulties managing the production of mechanically sound, appropriate grade-level prose in their acquired second language. Consider what is involved in being able to write correctly in a second language: one must be able to memorize the meaning of thousands of words and learn the syntactical rules for combining those words to form grammatically correct sentences. The ease of acquisition will depend on many factors, such as the age and the context in which the second language is acquired, and the educational and linguistic background of the individual. For example, it is probably much easier for someone whose native language uses an European alphabet system than, say, someone who uses an Arabic or Asian system with little to no prior exposure to English. In addition to learning a new language, there is the added step of needing to learn the language (e.g., terminology, technical expressions) of the discipline being studied. Thus, in the context of the sciences, learning to write proper English is not enough. Additionally, the student needs to then learn the unique vocabulary and expressions of the specific discipline in which s/he operates, including the additional requirements for utmost clarity and conciseness demanded by scientific writing.

The "rules" of scholarly-scientific English have a long-standing tradition and are unlikely to change in order to accommodate the needs of non native English writers. However, considering the fact that some native speakers of English will take years to master the production of good scientific writing, it is important for all of us to have some appreciation of how much more difficult it is for most non-native writers of English, who often lack many of the resources available to native speakers, to master this important task. Thus, in the words of Pennycook (1996), "... we need to be flexible, not dogmatic, about where we draw boundaries between acceptable and unacceptable textual borrowings." It is, therefore, essential for all of us to take all of the above considerations into account in judging ethical writing lapses of these linguistic groups.

THE LESSER CRIMES OF WRITING:
OTHER QUESTIONABLE WRITING PRACTICES

33

Zigmond and Fischer (2002) have called attention to what they refer as the "misdemeanors" of science: ethically inappropriate practices in the conduct of scientific research. These authors explain that, whereas fabrication, falsification, and plagiarism are considered to be the "high crimes" of science, many other questionable practices frequently take place and that these lesser crimes should command more attention. Evidence for their position was verified in a study by Martison et al., (2005) who reported have shown that 33% of US scientists surveyed admitted to engage in some form of questionable research practices. Some examples of common misdemeanors are, neglecting to indicate one's source of funding, failing to identify possible conflicts of interest, and establishing honorary authorship (assigning authorship to an individual whose contributions to the work do not earn him/her such status).

We can apply the high crimes vs. misdemeanors classification in the area of writing. In our previous discussion of plagiarism and self-plagiarism, we described a variety of practices, some of which would undoubtedly be classified as high crimes (e.g., appropriating the ideas or data of someone else without attribution), while others would fall under the misdemeanor category (e.g., inadequate paraphrasing and substantial text recycling). In this section, we turn our attention to other questionable practices that violate the spirit of ethical writing and that mostly fall under Zigmond & Fischer's (2002) misdemeanor category.

ETHICALLY QUESTIONABLE CITATION PRACTICES

Citations and References

Citations are the notations in the text of a paper that identify the source and/or evidence for our claims and for related research and theories mentioned in the paper. Depending on the style of writing being used these are typically represented as numbers in parentheses or in superscript (e.g., AMA) or as last names with dates (e.g., APA). The list of references is always found at the end of a paper and these contain the full bibliographic information and/or sufficient detail for readers to track down copies of these works (e.g., names of the authors, titles of articles or books, journal title, volume number, pagination and year of publication, Digital Object Identifier [DOI] and Uniform Resource Locator [URL] if required).

Carelessness in citing sources

References play a crucial role in scholarly and scientific writing for they allow the reader to explore in more detail a given line of thinking or evidence. For these reasons, it is important that authors strive for accuracy when listing references in manuscripts. Unfortunately, it appears that some authors do not always give the proper level of attention to citations and reference sections. In fact, the available evidence suggests that a disproportionate number of errors occur in reference sections even in some of the most prestigious biomedical journals (e.g., Siebers and Holt, 2000). Moreover, with the advent of online-only journals and digital stand-alone documents, the temporary nature of some of these works is an emerging problem. That is, a document may be located in one digital domain, only to change domains later and have a different URL. A case in point is this very resource. Originally, the first version of this document resided in a St. John's University domain address and later migrated to an ORI domain. Often, in situations like this, the source can be located with relatively little effort. However, other digital documents may disappear altogether and can no longer be easily obtained. When a

34

reference that is used as supporting evidence cannot be accessed, its absence can raise questions about, and/or weakens, the validity of claims that rest upon it.

The importance of citing the original observation

Another area of concern is the failure to cite the author who first reports the phenomenon being studied. Apparently, some authors instead cite later studies that better substantiate the original observation. Often, this outcome is a result of our attempts at being concise or perhaps a journal's limitation on the numbers of references that can be included in an article. Admittedly, some discoveries and their originators are so well-known that they are treated as common knowledge within the immediate domain-specific research community. However, in cases in which the pertinent information may not be generally known, it is important to acknowledge and credit the original discovery. As Zigmond and Fischer (2002) note, failure to cite the original report denies the individual who made the initial discovery his/her due credit.

GUIDELINE 15: Authors are strongly urged to double-check their citations. Specifically, authors should always ensure that each reference notation appearing in the body of the manuscript corresponds to the correct citation listed in the reference section and vice versa and that each source listed in the reference section has been cited at some point in the manuscript. In addition, authors should also ensure that all elements of a citation (e.g., spelling of authors' names, volume number of journal, pagination) are derived directly from the original paper, rather than from a citation that appears on a secondary source. Finally, when appropriate, authors should ensure that credit is given to those authors who first reported the phenomenon being studied.

Inappropriate Manipulation of References

In a later section I discuss the tendency on the part of some authors to provide what others view as a biased review of the relevant literature. That is, in placing their data or theory in the context of existing relevant work, authors sometimes cite only references that are favorable to their position. However, consistent with the basic tenets of ethical writing and scientific objectivity, we have a responsibility to cite all relevant material, even work that may contradict our own position. Failure to do so compromises our professional obligation to remain unbiased and is antithetical to the primary mission of a scientist's search for truth.

Citation Stuffing. Another inappropriate use of references occurs when authors intentionally cite their own work, regardless of its relevance, in an attempt to manipulate their own articles' impact factor. Although several criticisms of this measure have emerged over the years (Khaled, 2015; Rossner, Van Epps, & Hill, 2007), the impact factor, which takes into account how often articles published in those journals are cited, continues to be used as a measure of importance and prestige by journals. Likewise, a measure of the number of times a journal article is cited in other articles can also be used as an estimation of its importance in an individuals' tenure and review decisions, thus the tendency of some authors to weave into their paper references of their own prior work that may be of limited relevance to the actual topic of the paper.

A related matter involves the inappropriate inclusion of references that are authored by individuals thought to be likely peer reviewers of the article in question, the thought being that a reviewer will be more likely to give a favorable review to a paper that cites his or her own work than to one that does not.

Finally, there is some evidence that editors of some journals sometimes insist that authors include references from their journal for the mere purpose of enhancing that journal's impact factor (Wilhite & Fong, 2012). Authors should attempt to resist such requests unless the editors' or reviewers' recommendations are genuinely relevant to their paper.

GUIDELINE 16: The references used in a paper should only be those that are directly related to its contents. The intentional inclusion of references of questionable relevance for purposes such as manipulating a journal's or a paper's impact factor or a paper's chances of acceptance, is an unacceptable practice.

Relying on an abstract or a preliminary version of a paper while citing the published version. At the beginning of this instructional resource we identified clarity, conciseness, accuracy, and integrity as essential elements of scientific writing. Unfortunately, the latter two concepts are sometimes overlooked with certain citation practices. Consider what can happen in the following scenario. A researcher needs to conduct a literature review for a manuscript that she will be submitting for publication to a biomedical journal. A literature search yields several useful abstracts and the researcher proceeds to track down the various journal articles. Unfortunately, one key article is not available online. It is not carried by her institution's library, nor is it available at nearby libraries as it has been published as a technical report in an obscure nontraditional journal with limited circulation. Pressed for time, the researcher decides, instead, to rely on material from the abstract for the literature review and includes the journal article citation in the reference section. However, nowhere in the paper does she reveal that she relied on the abstract and not on the actual journal article.

Another variation of this problem occurs when the researcher cites the published version of the paper, but actually relies on the contents of an earlier version that was published in the proceedings of a conference, or the preliminary version that had been distributed at the conference presentation itself or a pre-print server. These behaviors violate the requisites of accuracy and integrity.

The main problem with relying on versions other than the published paper is that elements of these earlier versions may be different from their counterparts in the published version of the paper. Such changes are typically the result of the peer review process, editorial changes, or errors that are spotted and corrected by the author between the time the paper is presented at a conference and the time that it is subsequently published. In some cases, the published version will contain additional data and/or interpretations that are substantially different or perhaps even contrary to those of earlier versions. For example, a conference paper describing experimental data may, in its published form, contain additional data from a new experimental condition or new statistical analyses that were carried out in response to referees' suggestions. Data from

36

the new condition can place the earlier data in a new perspective possibly leading to somewhat different interpretations. With respect to abstracts, relying on such summaries can be problematic because abstracts typically may not provide sufficient details about the paper's relevance (i.e., Taylor, 2002). In addition, because of their condensed form, abstracts cannot provide essential details about a study's methodology, and results. Moreover, it should be noted that in some databases there may be instances in which individuals other than the author/s of the journal article write the article's abstract. As a result, subtle misrepresentations are likely more common with these abstracts. Writing guidelines, such as the *Uniform Requirements for Manuscripts Submitted to Biomedical Journals,* discourage the use of abstracts as references.

Lastly, given the rise in retractions and corrections, authors must ensure that the evidence cited is up-to-date. Regrettably, a significant number of retracted papers continue to be cited in the literature (see Ferguson, 2015). In addition, the large number of corrections, errata, etc., issued each year suggests that a substantial number of uncorrected results and/or interpretations are being cited as legitimate evidence and both of these outcomes contribute to the further contamination of the scientific record.

GUIDELINE 17: Always cite the actual worked that is consulted. When the published paper cannot be obtained, cite the specific version of the material being used whether it is conference presentation, abstract, or an unpublished manuscript. Ensure that the cited work has not been subsequently corrected or retracted.

Citing sources that were not read or thoroughly understood. The practice of relying on a published paper's abstract to describe its contents also fits in the present category. However, there are other scenarios that better illustrate the practice of citing papers that were either poorly understood or perhaps not even read by the author citing them. Below are a couple of examples:

Consider an investigator who is in the process of writing the results of a series of studies he conducted. In his search for background literature relevant to his work, he finds one particular journal article whose introduction cites a number of other works that seem very relevant to his own paper. Although he recognizes most of the references cited, there are a couple of papers that he is not familiar with and, for a variety of reasons, he cannot obtain copies of them at this point. Given the context of the published paper's description of these two other papers that are unfamiliar to him, our author decides to include them in his own review of the literature by paraphrasing the relevant portions of the published paper's introduction that summarize the contributions of these two unfamiliar (to him) papers. He then includes these papers as references in his manuscript's reference section, along with that of the journal article from which he derived the information. Finally, although our author cites the published article in at least one other context, he does not indicate that this article had served as the source of the information from the two other papers, which he had never read.

By not revealing the true source of the paraphrased content from these two papers, the reader is deceived by falsely assuming that the brief summary of these two papers was based on the author's reading of them. Technically, this type of transgression could conceivably qualify as a form of plagiarism because the author has paraphrased a summary of another's work, but attributed his summary to the author of the journal article. Of course, a formal charge of plagiarism would depend on a number of variables, such as the amount of paraphrasing that took place without proper attribution, the significance or uniqueness of the material involved, etc.

This type of deceptive citation practice can also be risky because of the possibility that other key aspects of the papers cited (but which were not read) do not quite support the offending author's thesis. Therefore, there may be significant lapses in his rationale for the study. Inexperienced students sometimes use this short-cut when given the task of reviewing the literature on a given topic. In their search for relevant literature, they may come upon a published paper that reviews roughly the same literature that the student has been tasked to summarize. In an effort to optimize his time, and given the great cognitive effort needed to read, assimilate, and synthesize the literature into a coherent summary, some students will rely primarily on the published review and paraphrase its contents in such a deceptive manner as to give the appearance that he has read and summarized the research. To maintain the deception, the student will include in his/her paper's reference section many of the sources cited in the published review, including perhaps the article from which all of the material was taken. Again, this strategy misleads the reader (i.e., the professor) into assuming that the student has actually read all of the papers cited in his/her review when, in fact, he has not. Ironically, these transgressions are typically uncovered, not only because the students' paraphrases are often too close to the original, thus betraying the students' less sophisticated writing, but also because at least some of the papers cited are perhaps known to their professor to only be tangentially supportive of the students' main thesis. Other clues in the quality of the writing often point to the deception that the student did not really review the pertinent literature.

The reader should note, however, that there might be instances in which the practice of citing sources that were not read may be acceptable. For example, an author may simply wish to point out a well-known discovery or theory and provide the reader with the original citation. When this is done without misleading the reader into believing that the author read the paper detailing the discovery and is thoroughly acquainted with its contents, then no real harm is done. For example, in a paper on intelligence testing I may want to refer the reader to the psychometric properties of the X test and write: "for a review of validity of reliability of X test see reference Y". Although I am clearly aware that reference Y reviews validity and reliability for various intelligence tests, including test X, my citation of this work does not imply that I have read and processed its contents. I am merely aware that relevant material may be found in that reference and point the reader to it. However, if in a different paper I were to write that "Smith (1879) studied the effects of X on Y and concluded that X is as important as Z and both are critical causal variables in the incidence of Y" such a statement strongly suggests that my summary of the study is, in fact, based on my reading of that paper.

GUIDELINE 18: Generally, when describing others' work, do not cite an original paper if you are only relying on a secondary summary of that paper. Doing so is a deceptive practice, reflects poor scholarly standards, and can lead to a flawed description of the work described.

Some writing manuals have spelled out specific conventions to deal with a situation when an important paper relevant to one's manuscript contains a reference that we would like to cite, but is not available to us. One such writing manual, is the current edition of the *Style Manual of the American Psychological Association* (American

38

Psychological Association, 2010) which offers a simple strategy for authors who need to cite a source that is not available to them, but that is contained within another source (as described earlier). Let's say that our author had read about the work of Smith from a paper published in 1999 in an article authored by Rodriguez that was published in 2015. According to the APA Manual the author can use this material by stating as follows: "According to Smith (1999; as cited in Rodriguez, 2015) an important variable ..." The reader may have noticed that I have already relied on this strategy elsewhere in this instructional resource.

There is at least one other inappropriate citation practice that merits mentioning. Consider the situation in which a "landmark" paper, whose contributions are relatively well known, needs to be cited in a manuscript. The author, a senior researcher with a lengthy publication record cannot readily find a copy of the paper, but he knows that he has read it at least once, back in his graduate school days, and has cited it before, as he is very familiar with it. In summarizing the contents of this landmark paper, the author relies on his recollection of its contents based on his prior reading of the paper and on summaries published by others. After all, this is a paper that is widely known throughout the discipline. The problem with the above situation is that there is a strong possibility that our recollection of subtle details about a paper read at a much earlier time is probably less than optimal. In addition, even though we may have read about those same details via secondary sources, these may have inadvertently slanted or distorted important details of the work, particularly if the material in question is of a controversial nature. Even if the material is accurately described elsewhere, the different contexts in which it is read may lead to differences in how that material is encoded in our minds which, therefore, could lead to difference in how certain elements are recalled. Taken together, these factors can ultimately result in the dissemination of faulty information.

An excellent example of this type of problem within the social sciences concerns current descriptions of a famous demonstration carried out by psychologists John B. Watson and Rosalie Rayner (1920) in which an infant known as "Little Albert" was conditioned to fear a rat. Watson and Rayner's demonstration with Little Albert is cited in a large proportion of introductory psychology textbooks and in many other textbooks within that discipline and beyond (e.g., education, nursing). However, according to Paul and Blumenthal (1989), investigators have pointed out a number of serious flaws in this classic demonstration and have shown how, over the years, various elements of the demonstration have become distorted. For example, some descriptions of Little Albert indicate that Watson & Rayner used a white rabbit rather than a white rat. In explaining the continued presence of this classic demonstration in textbooks without mention of the flaws, Paul and Blumenthal state:

> "Textbook authors are under considerable pressure to keep their references current. An author who cites older works will often be instructed by manuscript reviewers and editors to consult the current literature. Most surely do. But from the evidence of the texts, others simply update their citations or lists of 'suggestion for further reading.' As a result, references in introductory textbooks sometimes bear little relationship to authors' substantive discussions. Indeed, citation may directly contradict claims asserted in the text." (p. 551).

Interestingly, factual errors, albeit mostly minor in scope, concerning the story of Little Albert continue to be found in introductory texts that cover this material (Harris, 2011).

GUIDELINE 19: If an author must rely on a secondary source (e.g., textbook) to describe the contents of a primary source (e.g., an empirical journal article), s/he should consult writing manuals used in her discipline to follow the proper convention to do so. Above all, always indicate to the reader the actual source of the information being reported.

Borrowing extensively from a source but only acknowledging a small portion of what is borrowed. When we write a review of the literature in the biological and social sciences we often summarize the ideas or data of each source we consult. Such summaries can range from one or more sentences to perhaps to two or more paragraphs. Of course, we must also include citations within these summaries to alert the reader as to the source of the material we are presenting. Thus, a typical review of the literature is sprinkled with many citations. There are instances, however, when an author might need to draw heavily from a single source. In these cases, acknowledging the source of the material can be challenging for some inexperienced writers. For example, in some cases inexperienced writers will add the same citation liberally in several places within the summarized text to ensure that the material is properly credited. However, this technique looks awkward, which is why readers will typically not see the same reference appear every few sentences throughout the paragraph or paragraphs in which the same work is being discussed. Experienced writers avoid the overuse of the same citation by providing only one or two citations strategically placed throughout the portion of text derived from that single source, and by carefully crafting the writing to indicate to the reader that the ideas expressed are not the author's. For example, one can name the authors (e.g., "According to so-and-so …"; "These authors also suggest …"; "Their study also revealed …"). Some authors, however, are not as consistently conscientious about crediting their sources and will sometimes inadvertently intersperse their ideas with those of the secondary source. The result is that the reader is uncertain where the contributions of the source end and those of the manuscript's author begin (see Iverson, et al., 2007, p. 158). In the event that the resulting text leads the reader to identify the borrowed ideas as belonging to the manuscript's author, the author faces the risk of being accused of plagiarism.

GUIDELINE 20: When borrowing heavily from a source, authors should always craft their writing in a way that makes clear to readers which ideas/data are their own and which are derived from sources being consulted.

ENSURING RESPONSIBLE WRITING PRACTICES

Responsible science and scholarship entail the highest degree of objectivity in reporting the results of our research. Most authors will make every effort to describe their observations without exaggerating the importance of the findings or overstating their conclusions, sometimes with the assistance of the journal referees. However, lapses in objectivity when presenting research to a general audience have been noted in journal articles (see Cummings & Rivara, 2012) and, especially in institutional press releases that

40

are later used by science writers to describe the latest research findings. For example, Woloshin and Schwartz (2002) have carried out an analysis of press releases and reported that such documents often fail to emphasize the limitations of the studies. These authors noted that "[d]ata are often presented using formats that may exaggerate the perceived importance of findings." Their results are noteworthy because, in some cases, study authors are consulted during the editorial stages of producing a press release. The hype surrounding scientific findings, particularly those related to health and technology, can inflate public expectations about new treatment possibilities and other technological advances. Thus, we face a real risk of further erosion in the public's trust in science if the promises of these findings fall short (Master and Resnik, 2011)

Selective reporting of literature, One of the main purposes of reviewing the relevant literature and citing others' work is to provide empirical and/or theoretical support for one's thesis, be it a paper for a course we are taking, a grant application, a doctoral dissertation, or a paper targeted for publication in a scientific journal. The literature review provides readers with the proper context to understand a proposed study or theory by informing them of important issues, such as the current state of knowledge on the topic, the type of methodologies being used in the area, the theoretical underpinnings of the research, and the significance of the problem. Depending on the type of manuscript under development, the literature review will be either comprehensive (e.g., doctoral dissertation, review article) or very succinct (e.g., journal article). The latter situation presents a unique challenge because even though the cost of online publication is relatively inexpensive, print journal space can still be expensive forcing authors to be concise in their writing (thus the move toward online supplemental material).

For aspiring scholars and scientists, the classroom represents the training ground for future professionals. As a result, professors tailor the requirements for academic papers assigned in many graduate and advanced undergraduate courses to those demanded by scholarly journals (see for example, Salazar, 1993). These constraints sometimes present a real challenge for authors, who must always make an effort to simplify their literature reviews and only include a concise summary of highly relevant papers.

Obviously, literature cited in support of our hypotheses must be grounded in sound arguments, tight research methodologies, and flawless data. Citing references known to be methodologically or logically deficient in support of our work is ethically problematic, particularly if we fail to mention these shortcomings. Likewise, if in our search for relevant literature we become aware of important relevant evidence that runs contrary to our data or point of view, we have an ethical obligation to cite such evidence, either in the introduction or the discussion section of our paper. We must not do this dismissively, but in an unbiased manner. Of course, there are situations in which the extent of our examination of the literature is limited by publishing concerns specific to the type of articles proposed (e.g., short communication, brief report, letter to the editor). Space limitations in such contexts may render it impractical to provide adequate coverage of relevant literature, let alone contrary evidence.

The main purpose of an introductory section of a manuscript is to describe the problem being investigated and the relevant research/and or scholarship on the subject. Based on the rapid pace at which some areas in science and scholarship continue to grow, authors are not always able to cite all of the relevant literature, either because of space constraints or their inability to simply keep up with the burgeoning literature. On the other hand, some authors will deliberately leave out pertinent literature, for a variety of reasons. Thus a perusal of scholarly journals that accept letters to the editor as commentaries to recently published articles will reveal instances in which such seemingly intentional writing lapses are fairly common (see Goodman, 1998; Perkin, 1999; Nathan, 1994).

GUIDELINE 21: When appropriate, authors have an ethical responsibility to report evidence that runs contrary to their point of view. In addition, evidence that we use in support of our position must be methodologically sound. When citing supporting studies that suffer from methodological, statistical, or other types of shortcomings, such flaws must be pointed out to the reader.

Selective reporting of methodology. Replication of others' research is one of the hallmarks of the scientific enterprise. As such, scientists and scholars have a professional obligation to inform others about the specific procedures used in their research. This information is found in the methods section of a research paper, the purpose of which is to provide other researchers with sufficient details about the study so that anyone who wishes to verify the results will have the necessary information to do so. In the methods section we identify the subjects of our study (e.g., select clinical population, specific species of animals) and provide important details about characteristics of the sample, such as how subjects were recruited, that are relevant to the variables that are being manipulated and measured.

The Methods section also contains description of instrumentation or other observational and measuring techniques that are used to obtain the outcomes reported. Whether data were collected using sophisticated instrumentation, such as a positron emission tomography or via a simple paper-and-pencil questionnaire, scientists must describe these materials with sufficient detail to allow others to carry out the study and verify the results.

Perhaps the most important part of a Methods section is the description of the actual procedure used to carry out the study. Here, investigators must explain in clear language the series of steps used to establish, observe, and/or manipulate all relevant variables. They must offer a complete description of the testing conditions and all of the other necessary details that would allow an independent investigator to carry out the exact same study again. Admittedly, some studies may include several highly complex components that are carried out by different members of a research team. Nonetheless, it is essential that all key details and steps be described in this section in a most clear manner. The inadvertent omission or ambiguous presentation of a single step or piece of information may doom to failure the replication efforts of other researchers, thus needlessly wasting valuable time and resources. Obviously, a more serious offense occurs when an author intentionally leaves out an important detail about the procedure or fails to report a crucial event that altered the conditions of the study. There may be several reasons why some authors will knowingly leave important details out of a research report (e.g., assumed irrelevance, perceived minimal impact). Perhaps an extraneous variable was inadvertently introduced late into the study while it was still in progress leading to biased results. Thus, for the sake of expediency, rather than discarding the biased results and starting all over again, the investigator may inappropriately leave that major detail out of the report. The important point here is that authors have an ethical obligation to describe all of the important aspects of the research conducted, even if some of those details reflect poorly on the abilities of any member of the research team.

42

Because of the concern that some investigators may at times omit important details of the methodology used, guidelines have been formulated to help authors write better research reports. For example, for reports describing randomized control trials authors are advised to consult Moher, Schultz, and Altman's (2001) Consort statement, which is a set of guidelines designed to improve the quality of such reports.

GUIDELINE 22: Authors have an ethical obligation to report all aspects of the study that may impact the replicability of their research by independent observers.

Selective reporting of results. Designing an empirical study takes planning and careful consideration of existing theory and research in the area under investigation. When testing for simple causal relationships, it should be relatively easy to predict the specific outcome when producing a change in the causal variable. Most modern scientific investigations, however, are far from simple- they often involve several variables all of which interact in ways that are sometimes difficult, if not impossible, to predict. One positive feature of complex studies is that they can yield many interesting outcomes, though some of these outcomes may end up being irrelevant or even contrary to our expectations. When the latter happens, there may be a temptation to try different statistical analyses and select the one that best fits our hypothesized results (e.g., using a less powerful statistical test, removing outliers). Another temptation is to simply not report null results or only report those statistically significant results that are consistent with our hypotheses. Other techniques, such as the manipulation of graphs, have been used to subtly change, and therefore distort, the visual presentation of results in a way that make them more consistent with our expected findings. Such practices are almost always fundamentally deceptive and are contrary to the basic scholarly-scientific mission of searching for truth. However, there are instances in which practices, such as the removal of outliers, are acceptable, but only when the author follows established procedures, informs readers of these actions, and provides a cogent rationale for carrying them out.

GUIDELINE 23: Researchers have an ethical responsibility to report the results of their studies according to their a priori plans. Any post hoc manipulations that may alter the results initially obtained, such as the elimination of outliers or the use of alternative statistical techniques, must be clearly described along with an acceptable rationale for using such techniques.

AUTHORSHIP ISSUES AND CONFLICTS OF INTEREST

An instructional resource on scholarly and scientific writing would not be complete without some discussion of conflicts of interest and authorship issues. We now turn our attention to these matters.

Advances in biotechnology, communication, instrumentation, and computing have allowed scientists to investigate increasingly complex problems. It is not uncommon these days for large-scale investigations to be carried out by teams of scientists from various institutions sometimes spanning two or more continents. Groups and individual contributors may work on the same or different key aspects of a project and these collaborations will invariably result in multiple-authored publications. Unfortunately, some of these collaborative efforts have given rise to disputes about authorship issues. The most frequent disputes center around the following questions: 1) Which members of a research team merit authorship? 2) Who is designated as senior or corresponding author of the resulting journal article? And 3) How should the rest of the authorship order be determined?

Given that authorship, particularly the designation of senior author of a paper in scientific and scholarly publications plays such a prominent role in the current merit system, it is extremely important to have sound criteria for establishing authorship. For example, in writing about these issues, Steinbok (1995) questions whether various situational roles in biomedical research merit authorship. He writes: "Should the head of the department automatically be an author? Should the various clinicians involved in the care of the patients who are subjects of a paper automatically be authors? What about the person who goes through a set of charts and puts information into a database? What about the statistician who analyzes the data?" (p. 324). Others have raised questions related to the current trend for graduate and undergraduate students to be directly involved in research and in the authoring of papers.

Fortunately, individuals and a number of professional societies have proposed relevant guidelines in this area (e.g., ICMJE and other references in a later section). Although these sets of guidelines have similar criteria for authorship, there is sufficient overlap to offer readers a certain number of sensible recommendations. In considering these guidelines, readers are advised to consult their professional associations for any specific authorship guidance that these entities may have developed. Readers are also advised to consult the institutions with which they are affiliated, as well as the individual journals to which they intend to submit a manuscript.

Deciding on authorship. Whether students or professionals, individuals collaborating on a research project should discuss authorship issues, such as who will be designated as senior author, the order of other authors, and any other individual acknowledgements for other contributions, before initiating work on the project. All parties should familiarize themselves with authorship guidelines suggested by their respective disciplines. In the absence of such guidelines, prospective authors should follow the guidelines of the International Committee of Medical Journal Editors. Any agreement reached regarding authorship should, ideally, be recorded in writing and should outline the formula used for determining who the senior author should be while also establishing the authorship order for the rest of the investigators involved in the project. The agreement should be sufficiently flexible to accommodate changes that may arise while the project is in progress (e.g., an individual not initially designated as author ends up making substantive contributions that earn her authorship in the paper, or an individual previously designated as author fails to carry out the designated duties, making his/her contributions not sufficiently or importantly enough to merit authorship).

GUIDELINE 24: Authorship determination should be discussed prior to commencing research collaboration and should be based on established guidelines, such as those of the International Committee of Medical Journal Editors.

Establishing authorship. Generally, and as per the guidelines of the International

44

Committee of Medical Journal Editors, only individuals who make substantive intellectual contributions to the project should be listed as authors and the order of authorship should be based on the degree of importance of each author's contribution to the project. The latter may be difficult to establish in disciplines such as genomics where teams of several dozen, hundreds, or perhaps several thousand contributors (i.e., particle physics), may be authors in a single paper (see Castelvecchi, 2015). Authorship usually entails the ability to publicly take responsibility for the contents of the project (e.g., being sufficiently knowledgeable about the project to be able to present it in a formal forum). What determines whether a contribution is substantive or not is a matter of debate and, technically, it should not matter whether the aim of the collaboration is an internal technical report, a conference presentation, or an article targeted for refereed journal. Generally, examples of substantive contributions include, but are not limited to, aiding in the conceptualization of the hypotheses, designing the methodology of the investigation and significantly contributing to the writing the manuscript. "Menial" activities, such as entering information in a database or merely collecting actual data (e.g., running subjects, collecting specimens, distributing and collecting questionnaires) are not, by themselves, sufficient grounds for authorship, but should be acknowledged in a footnote. In addition, "honorary" or "courtesy" authorship assigned on the basis of some leadership position (e.g., such as being head of the department where the research is carried out) must also be avoided.

GUIDELINE 25: Only those individuals who have made substantive contributions to a project merit authorship in a paper.

Authorship in faculty-student collaborations. Undergraduates, and certainly graduate students, are increasingly involved in research collaboration with their faculty. Along with high grade point averages and scores on standardized testing, undergraduate research experiences are one of the most valued criteria for advanced graduate training. As a result, an increasing number of undergraduates are becoming involved in research and even authoring journal articles. Their participation in the research process raises the question as to whether current authorship guidelines that have been designed for professionals should be equally applicable to students. Fine and Kurdek (1993) who have written on these issues, offer the following sensible remarks

> "To be included as an author on a scholarly publication, a student should, in a cumulative sense, make a professional contribution that is creative and intellectual in nature, that is integral to completion of the paper, and that requires an overarching perspective of the project. Examples of professional contributions include developing the research design, writing portions of the manuscript, integrating diverse theoretical perspectives, developing new conceptual models, designing assessments, contributing to data analysis decision and interpreting results …" (p. 1145).

Faculty mentors may view the above guidelines for students as rather harsh. However, consider part of the rationale for these authors' position that awarding authorship to an undeserving student is unethical:

> "First, a publication on one's record that is not legitimately earned may falsely represent the individual's scholarly expertise. Second, if because he or she is now a published author, the student is perceived as being more skilled than a peer who is not published, the student is given an unfair advantage professionally. Finally, if the student is perceived to have a level of competence that he or she does not actually have, he or she will be expected to accomplish tasks that may be outside

45

the student's range of expertise" (p. 1143).

On the other hand, there is evidence suggesting that students' earned authorship credit is sometimes underrepresented or outright denied by supervising faculty (Swazey, Anderson, & Lewis, 1993; Tarnow, 1999). Clearly, such outcomes are highly unethical as they rob the deserving student of their due credit.

GUIDELINE 26: Faculty-student collaborations should follow the same criteria to establish authorship. Mentors must exercise great care to neither award authorship to students whose contributions do not merit it, nor to deny authorship and due credit to the work of students.

Ghost Authorship. Ghost authorship occurs when a written work fails to identify individuals who made significant contributions to the research and writing of that work. Although in recent times this unethical practice is typically associated with the pharmaceutical and biomedical device industry, the term is also applicable in a number of other contexts. For example, in academic contexts, it is widely recognized as cheating to have someone other than the named student author write a paper that is then submitted as the student's own. Perhaps with some exceptions (e.g., speech writers), ghost authorship is ethically unacceptable because the reader is mislead as to the actual contributions made by the named author.

Academic Ghost Authorship. A not uncommon form of academic dishonesty that has probably always existed is to have someone else other than the student (e.g., a friend or relative), complete an assignment or write a paper. Several Internet sites now exist that, in addition to making available copies of papers that have already been written, also provide custom-written papers, including doctoral theses. The customer (i.e., student) specifies the topic and other requirements for the paper and, for a fee, a staff writer for the service will supply the custom-written product. Anecdotal evidence suggests that these practices are not all that uncommon, particularly for those students with the financial means to hire these ghost authors. For an eye-opening account of how this practice works even before the proliferation of on-line paper mill sites, I refer the reader to Whitherspoon's (1995) personal account as a ghostwriter. More recent accounts of this emerging industry are provided by Dante (2010) and Shahghasemi and Akhavan (2015).

Situations in which authors, whether students or professionals, find themselves in need of extensive external assistance with their writing can also raise some interesting ethical dilemmas. For example, consider the doctoral candidate who, because of limited writing skills and/or considerable financial resources, relies heavily on an individual or editorial service resulting in someone other than the doctoral candidate making substantial editorial changes to the writing of the thesis. Such a situation may be acceptable as long as the author of the thesis indicates in a byline or acknowledgement section the full extent of others' assistance. This, however, is not always done. One of the reasons is that such acknowledgement would obviously reflect negatively on the author by possibly suggesting that s/he might not have the necessary skills expected of a doctoral candidate. By mischaracterizing or by failing to acknowledge altogether the high level of assistance received, students falsely portray a level of academic competence that they either do not have or did not practice. In instances in which doctoral students anticipate relying on external assistance to help with the writing of a thesis or even term paper, it is strongly recommended that they confer with their thesis committee, supervisor, or professor to determine the

46

accepted parameters of such assistance and to fully disclose the nature of the assistance received.

Professional Ghost Authorship. In the literary world ghost authorship is most often associated with celebrity-authored works in which a celebrity, together with a skilled writer, produce written products, such as an autobiography or a memoir. Although much of the writing may be done by the ghost writer whose contributions may not always be acknowledged and, consequently, in those instances the reader is misled into believing that the celebrity is the sole author of the work.

In the biomedical sciences ghost writing has become particularly problematic (see Ngai, Gold, Gill, & Rochon, 2005). For example, in a typical scenario, a pharmaceutical or medical device company will hire an outside researcher with known expertise in the company's line of products (e.g., antidepressants) to write a "balanced" review of their product. To facilitate the write-up of the paper, the company furnishes the expert with a draft of the paper that had already been prepared by a ghost author employed by the company. And, as it often happens with industry-sponsored research, the resulting paper ends up portraying the product in a more favorable light than in reality it might deserve (Bekelman, Li, & Gross, 2003). It is important to highlight the distinction between ghost writers and medical writers. As Woolley (2008) points out, medical writers are professionals who assist researchers in the preparation of manuscripts. They abide by a professional code of ethics that includes full disclosure in the publication as to the medical writer's involvement and funding source (see American Medical Writers Association, 2008; or the ethical guidelines of the European Medical Writers Association, Jacobs & Wager, 2005).

The extent of ghost contributions can range from the initial draft framing of a manuscript to the complete or nearly complete write-up of the paper. In addition to the obscuring of the true authorship of these works, the extent to which the writing encourages bias toward a particular product or point of view emerges as a concern. In the past few years, several articles and editorials have condemned the practice as ethically questionable (e.g., The PLoS Medicine Editors, 2009; Sismondo & Doucet, 2010). The World Association of Medical Editors (2005) has produced a position statement, which considers ghost authorship dishonest and unacceptable.

GUIDELINE 27: Academic or professional ghost authorship in the sciences is ethically unacceptable.

A brief overview on Conflict of Interests

When an investigator's relationship to an organization affects, or gives the appearance of affecting, his/her objectivity in the conduct of scholarly or scientific research, a conflict of interest is said to occur. The relationship does not have to be a personal nor a financial one. For example, a conflict of interest could arise when a family member of a researcher is associated with an organization whose product the researcher is in the process of evaluating. Does the family member's association with the organization compromise his ability to carry out the evaluation objectively? Perhaps. Let's consider another example. Imagine an investigator who has been conducting basic science on the various processes involved in the release of certain neurotransmitters and whose work has been steadily funded by the maker of one of the most popular antidepressants. Now imagine a new situation where the research carried out by that investigator naturally leads him to study the efficacy of that same antidepressant while being funded by the company that manufactures it. In conducting the research, is that investigator's objectivity affected by his long-standing relationship to the drug company? Perhaps ….

Naturally, some conflicts of interest are unavoidable and having a conflict of interest is not in itself unethical. However, industry has played an increasing role in sponsoring research that bears on commercial applications, leading to a focus on how such sponsorship affects the research process and outcomes. The situation appears to be particularly serious in the realm of pharmaceutical research. For example, Stelfox, Chua, O'Rourke, and Detsky (1998) collected a sample of published reports (e.g., studies, letters to the editor) on the safety of calcium channel blockers, drugs used to treat cardiovascular disease, and correlated the authors' conclusions about their efficacy with whether or not the investigators had received financial support from companies that manufacture those types of drugs. The results revealed a strong association between conclusions that were supportive of the drugs and prior financial support from companies that were associated with those types of drugs. Other studies have similarly shown these types of troubling relationships (e.g., Lexchin, Bero. Djulbegovic, & Clark, 2003; Lundh, Sismondo, Lexchin, Busuioc, & Bero, 2012).

To ameliorate the situation, research institutions, professional societies, and an increasing number of journals have formulated guidelines for dealing with potential conflicts of interest. Essentially, most of these guidelines require authors to disclose such conflicts either in the cover letter to the editor of the journal to which an investigator submits a manuscript and/or ideally in a footnote on the manuscript itself. For additional guidance on this important topic, the reader should consult the various resources offered by ORI, https://ori.hhs.gov/conflicts-interest-and-commitment.

GUIDELINE 28: Authors must become aware of possible conflicts of interest in their own research and to make every effort to disclose those situations (e.g., stock ownership, consulting agreements to the sponsoring organization) that may pose actual or potential conflicts of interest.

48

Acknowledgements

I wish to thank the following individuals and organizations for their support in developing this project. Marisela Torres assisted me in locating some of the material used as background for the first edition of this resource. Michael Balas, Alice Powers, and Jay Zimmerman reviewed the examples of paraphrases. Maryellen Reardon read early drafts of the various sections of the first edition of the resource and provided valuable feedback on them. Stephen Black, Eugen Tarnow, and many others have also provided valuable feedback on initial web version of the instructional resource. I have also benefited from discussions on plagiarism and on other matters related to publication ethics that have appeared in forums such as the World Association of Medical Editors (WAME) forum and RetractionWatch.com, as well as from private discussions with many individuals, such as Mary Ellen Kerans, Elizabeth Wager Karen Shashok and John Rodgers. I am, of course, indebted to the Office of Research Integrity, for providing initial funding for this project as well as for the current revision. The support of St. John's University is also gratefully acknowledged with special thanks to Betty Farbman formerly of the Office of Grants and Sponsored Research at St. John's.

49

Paraphrasing/Plagiarism Exercise

Earlier, when we covered paraphrasing and plagiarism, we offered various examples of properly paraphrased and plagiarized text. Because inappropriate paraphrasing appears to be one of the most common forms of plagiarism it is important that contributors to the scientific literature become sensitive to this problem and integrate proper paraphrasing practices in their writing. To that effect, an exercise has been developed for the purpose of offering instruction on acceptable paraphrasing strategies.

For this exercise, the reader is asked to imagine the following scenario: you are working on a manuscript in which you review published studies on the colony raiding behavior of fire ants, *S. invicta*. One of the journal articles you are reading for your review contains a short paragraph that you deem very important and thus, you decide that you want to include the information in your manuscript. Here is the paragraph:

> *This study examines whether workers of S. invicta are able to assist their mothers in colony usurpations. First we tested whether [queens] of S. invicta are better able to usurp colonies to which their daughters have moved. Second, we tested whether the effect of daughters on usurpation success is due to familiarity with the queen or to genetic relatedness. Aggressive behavior during these usurpation attempts was observed to determine if the presence of familiar or related workers influenced the aggressive response toward either the resident queen or the queen attempting usurpation.[1]*

.[1]Balas M, Adams ES, 1996.Intraspecific usurpation of incipient fire ant colonies. Behav Ecol 8:99-103.

You could copy the above paragraph verbatim, enclose it in quotation marks, and include it in your manuscript. But while the use of quoted text is fairly common practice in certain disciplines within the humanities, the practice is typically shunned by most authors and editors of biomedical journals. Another option would be for you to summarize the important points of the above paragraph by condensing it into one or two shorter sentences that fully capture the essence of the ideas being conveyed. However, let's assume that your intention is to paraphrase the entire paragraph, thereby preserving all of the information contained in the paragraph. How would you paraphrase the paragraph without committing plagiarism and in a manner that is consistent with the principles of ethical writing?

For the first part of this exercise, please paraphrase the above paragraph to the best of your ability. Take your time and use whatever resources you deem necessary (e.g., dictionary, thesaurus). Before commencing, keep in mind that when paraphrasing you must substantially modify the original text while preserving the exact meaning of the ideas conveyed in the original paragraph. You should note that when faced with the task of paraphrasing text, many individuals often complain that the reason their paraphrases are too close to the original is because there are only a limited number of ways that one can express the same thought. Although this may be true to some extent when the original text is comprised of highly technical language, such as the paragraph on mammalian histone lysine methyltransferase used earlier in our discussion of plagiarism, it is not true for most other writing. It is certainly not true for the sample paragraph on fire ants that we have selected.

You should also remember that your paraphrase must also indicate the source of the

50

original material. This is typically done with either a footnote or with some form of parenthetical notation indicating the source of the original. For example, in the style suggested by the American Psychological Association, you might insert the following at the end of your paraphrase: (Balas and Adams, 1996). For this exercise, please assume that your paraphrase contains the proper reference notation indicating the source of the material. You should also assume that a full citation has been placed in the reference section of your paper.

Use the space below to paraphrase the paragraph:

The second part of the exercise will help you to determine whether your rewritten version of the paragraph meets the requirements of an appropriate paraphrase. For this portion of the exercise, you are to place yourself in the same scenario as described above: That you are writing a paper on the ecology and behavior of fire ants and that you discover a paragraph that you wish to paraphrase in your paper.

Below you will find several rewritten versions of the original paragraph. Please examine each version and determine whether it has been properly paraphrased or whether it constitutes an instance of potential plagiarism. As you consider each rewritten version, please assume that you have already incorporated it into your manuscript and that you are now reviewing that section of your paper for accuracy and proper scholarship. Immediately after you select your answer you will be given feedback as to the correctness of your responses.

ORIGINAL PARAGRAPH

> *"This study examines whether workers of S. invicta are able to assist their mothers in colony usurpations. First we tested whether [queens] of S. invicta are better able to usurp colonies to which their daughters have moved. Second, we tested whether the effect of daughters on usurpation success is due to familiarity with the queen or to genetic relatedness. Aggressive behavior during these usurpation attempts was observed to determine if the presence of familiar or related workers influenced the aggressive response toward either the resident queen or the queen attempting usurpation."*

REWRITTEN VERSION 1:

A study was conducted to examine whether workers of *S. invicta* can assist their mothers in colony usurpations. The first hypothesis tested was whether queens of *S. invicta* are better able to usurp colonies to which their daughters have moved. For the second

<u>hypothesis, the researchers tested</u> whether the effect of daughters on usurpation success <u>is</u> <u>due to familiarity with the queen or to genetic relatedness.</u> <u>The researchers observed</u> aggressive behavior during these usurpation attempts to determine if the presence of familiar or related workers influenced the aggressive response toward either the resident queen or the queen attempting usurpation.

Please indicate whether the above paragraph is:
1. Properly paraphrased.
2. Definitely plagiarized.
3. Cannot determine.

FEEDBACK: This rewritten version is definitely plagiarized. The author has merely added or substituted a few words at the beginning of each sentence, and copied verbatim the remainder of the sentences. Notice that although none of the sentences in the rewritten paragraph are identical to their counterparts in the original, the rewritten version is still deemed as an instance of plagiarism because the author has simply appropriated too many phrases from the original. Thus, the attempted paraphrase falls way short of the requirement for the original text to be thoroughly modified. This is a clear-cut case of plagiarism. See the following tables for comparisons between the original paragraph and its rewritten counterpart.

ORIGINAL VERSION	PLAGIARIZED VERSION
"This study examines whether workers of S. invicta are able to assist their mothers in colony usurpations. First we tested whether [queens] of S. invicta are better able to usurp colonies to which their daughters have moved. Second, we tested whether the effect of daughters on usurpation success is due to familiarity with the queen or to genetic relatedness. Aggressive behavior during these usurpation attempts was observed to determine if the presence of familiar or related workers influenced the aggressive response toward either the resident queen or the queen attempting usurpation."	A study was conducted to *examine whether workers of S. invicta can assist their mothers in colony usurpations.* The first hypothesis tested was *whether queens of S. invicta are better able to usurp colonies to which their daughters have moved.* For the second hypothesis, the researchers *tested whether the effect of daughters on usurpation success is due to familiarity with the queen or to genetic relatedness.* The researchers observed *aggressive behavior during these usurpation attempts to determine if the presence of familiar or related workers influenced the aggressive response toward either the resident queen or the queen attempting usurpation.*

52

* Red colored, underlined strings of text indicate that they have been taken verbatim from the original paragraph.

* Blue highlighted text indicates that it has been appropriated from the original paragraph with a change in the order of the words or phrases.

ORIGINAL PARAGRAPH

"This study examines whether workers of S. invicta are able to assist their mothers in colony usurpations. First we tested whether [queens] of S. invicta are better able to usurp colonies to which their daughters have moved. Second, we tested whether the effect of daughters on usurpation success is due to familiarity with the queen or to genetic relatedness. Aggressive behavior during these usurpation attempts was observed to determine if the presence of familiar or related workers influenced the aggressive response toward either the resident queen or the queen attempting usurpation."

REWRITTEN VERSION 2

53

An investigation was carried out to examine whether workers of *S. invicta* can assist their mothers in colony usurpations. The first hypothesis tested was whether queens of *S. invicta* are better able to usurp colonies to which their daughters have moved. The second hypothesis tested whether the effect of daughters on usurpation success is due to familiarity with the queen or to genetic relatedness. Aggressiveness during these usurpation attempts was measured to determine if the presence of familiar or related workers influenced the aggressive response toward either the resident queen or the queen attempting usurpation.

Please indicate whether the above paragraph is:
1. Properly paraphrased.
2. Definitely plagiarized.
3. Cannot determine.

FEEDBACK: The author has not truly paraphrased the original paragraph. As with the first rewritten version, only a few words have been substituted, deleted, or added, leaving the rest of the sentences in the new paragraph virtually unchanged. Once again, too many of the phrases that make up the original paragraph are reproduced in the rewritten version. The author has simply failed to modify the original material sufficiently. For these reasons, the current rewritten version is considered an instance of definite plagiarism.

ORIGINAL VERSION	PLAGIARIZED VERSION
"This study examines whether workers of S. invicta are able to assist their mothers in colony usurpations. First we tested whether [queens] of S. invicta are better able to usurp colonies to which their daughters have moved. Second, we tested whether the effect of daughters on usurpation success is due to familiarity with the queen or to genetic relatedness. Aggressive behavior during these usurpation attempts was observed to determine if the presence of familiar or related workers influenced the aggressive response toward either the resident queen or the queen attempting usurpation."	An investigation was carried out to examine whether workers of S. invicta can assist their mothers in colony usurpations. The first hypothesis tested was whether queens of S. invicta are better able to usurp colonies to which their daughters have moved. The second hypothesis tested whether the effect of daughters on usurpation success is due to familiarity with the queen or to genetic relatedness. Aggressiveness during these usurpation attempts was mesured to determine if the presence of familiar or related workers influenced the aggressive response toward either the resident queen or the queen attempting ussurpation

* Red colored, underlined strings of text indicate that they have been taken verbatim from the original paragraph.

54

ORIGINAL PARAGRAPH

> *"This study examines whether workers of S. invicta are able to assist their mothers in colony usurpations. First we tested whether [queens] of S. invicta are better able to usurp colonies to which their daughters have moved. Second, we tested whether the effect of daughters on usurpation success is due to familiarity with the queen or to genetic relatedness. Aggressive behavior during these usurpation attempts was observed to determine if the presence of familiar or related workers influenced the aggressive response toward either the resident queen or the queen attempting usurpation."*

REWRITTEN VERSION 3

<u>To determine whether workers of *S. invicta* can assist their mothers in colony usurpations,</u> <u>two researchers have conducted a study in which the following hypotheses were tested:</u> First, they wanted to see whether queens of *S. invicta* are better able to usurp colonies to <u>which their daughters have moved.</u> Second, they tested whether the effect of daughters on <u>usurpation success is due to familiarity with the queen or to genetic relatedness.</u> The ants' <u>aggressive behavior during these usurpation attempts was observed to determine if the presence of related or familiar workers influenced the aggressive response toward either</u> the resident queen or the queen attempting a colonytake- over.

Please indicate whether the above paragraph is:

1. Properly paraphrased.
2. Definitely plagiarized.
3. Cannot determine.

FEEDBACK: The first sentence of the rewritten version is probably an acceptable paraphrase of the first sentence in the original paragraph. However, with the exception of a minor transposition of words in the last sentence, the rest of the sentences have only been superficially changed by the addition or substitution of a few words at the beginning of each sentence. The remaining phrases in these sentences have not changed. As with the previous example, none of the sentences in the rewritten paragraph are totally identical to their counterparts in the original. Because there is still a significant amount of verbatim material taken from the original, the rewritten version would still be deemed as an example of plagiarism.

ORIGINAL VERSION VERSION

PLAGIARIZED

"This study examines whether workers of S. invicta are able to assist their mothers in colony usurpations. First we tested whether [queens] of S. invicta are better able to usurp colonies to which their daughters have moved. Second, we tested whether the effect of daughters on usurpation success is due to familiarity with the queen or to genetic relatedness. Aggressive behavior during these usurpation attempts was observed to determine if the presence of familiar or related workers influenced the aggressive response toward either the resident queen or the queen attempting usurpation."

* Red colored, underlined strings of text indicate that they have been taken verbatim from the original paragraph.

* Blue highlighted text indicates that it has been appropriated from the original paragraph with a change in the order of the words or phrases.

ORIGINAL PARAGRAPH

> *"This study examines whether workers of S. invicta are able to assist their mothers in colony usurpations. First we tested whether [queens] of S. invicta are better able to usurp colonies to which their daughters have moved. Second, we tested whether the effect of daughters on usurpation success is due to familiarity with the queen or to genetic relatedness. Aggressive behavior during these usurpation attempts was observed to determine if the presence of familiar or related workers influenced the aggressive response toward either the resident queen or the queen attempting usurpation."*

REWRITTEN VERSION 4

To determine whether workers of *S. invicta* can assist their mothers in colony usurpations, a study was conducted in which the following variables were investigated: First, *S. invicta* queens' hypothesized ability to usurp colonies to which their daughters have moved was examined. The second hypothesis tested whether the effect of daughters on usurpation success is due to familiarity with the queen or to genetic relatedness. During these usurpation attempts aggressive behavior was observed to determine if the presence of familiar or related workers influenced aggression toward either the resident queen or the queen attempting colony usurpation.

Please indicate whether the above paragraph is:

1. Properly paraphrased.
2. Definitely plagiarized.
3. Cannot determine.

FEEDBACK: In this version the first two paraphrased sentences appear to have undergone moderate modifications. However, the second two sentences have not been adequately paraphrased. As with previous versions, the third sentence was changed by a mere substitution of the first two of three words and the fourth sentence has not been changed at all making these two sentences plagiarized versions of the original. Because the first two sentences were not sufficiently modified and because the last two sentences contain only minimal changes, this rewritten version of the original paragraph is still considered as a case of plagiarism.

ORIGINAL VERSION

"This study examines whether workers of S. invicta are able to assist their mothers in colony usurpations. First we tested whether [queens] of S. invicta are better able to usurp colonies to which their daughters have moved. Second, we tested whether the effect of daughters on usurpation success is due to familiarity with the queen or to genetic relatedness. Aggressive behavior during these usurpation attempts was observed to determine if the presence of familiar or related workers influenced the aggressive response toward either the resident queen or the queen attempting usurpation."

PLAGIARIZED VERSION

To determine whether workers of S. invicta can assist their mothers in colony usurpations, a study was conducted in which the following variables were investigated: First, S. invicta queens' hypothesized ability to usurp colonies to which their daughters have moved was examined. The second hypothesis tested whether the effect of daughters on usurpation success is due to familiarity with the queen or to genetic relatedness. During these usurpation attempts aggressive behavior was observed to determine if the presence of familiar or related workers influenced aggression toward either the resident queen or the queen attempting colony usurpation.

58

* Red colored, underlined strings of text indicate that they have been taken verbatim from the original paragraph.

* Blue highlighted text indicates that it has been appropriated from the original paragraph with a change in the order of the words or phrases.

ORIGINAL PARAGRAPH

> *"This study examines whether workers of S. invicta are able to assist their mothers in colony usurpations. First we tested whether [queens] of S. invicta are better able to usurp colonies to which their daughters have moved. Second, we tested whether the effect of daughters on usurpation success is due to familiarity with the queen or to genetic relatedness. Aggressive behavior during these usurpation attempts was observed to determine if the presence of familiar or related workers influenced the aggressive response toward either the resident queen or the queen attempting usurpation "*

REWRITTEN VERSION 5

An investigation was carried out to determine whether S. invicta mothers are helped by their worker offspring during colony usurpations. The study's focus of investigation was the question of whether colony take-over by S. invicta queens is more effective when their daughters first invade the colonies. One hypothesis concerned the extent to which daughters' familiarity with the queen, or their genetic similarity to her, affects successful colony take-over. During attempts at taking over another colony, behavioral observations were made of usurping workers that were either familiar or genetically related to the queens to see if these variables were related to aggressive behavior toward the resident or the invading queen.

Please indicate whether the above paragraph is:
1. Properly paraphrased.
2. Definitely plagiarized.
3. Cannot determine.

FEEDBACK: Although some of the terms from the original paragraph have been retained in the rewritten version, the current paraphrased version has been sufficiently modified from the original and is, therefore, classified as having been correctly paraphrased.

ORIGINAL VERSION

"This study examines whether workers of S. invicta are able to assist their mothers in colony usurpations. First we tested whether [queens] of S. invicta are better able to usurp colonies to which their daughters have moved. Second, we tested whether the effect of daughters on usurpation success is due to familiarity with the queen or to genetic relatedness. Aggressive behavior during these usurpation attempts was observed to determine if the presence of familiar or related workers influenced the aggressive response toward either the resident queen or the queen attempting usurpation."

PLAGIARIZED VERSION

An investigation was carried out to determine whether S. invicta mothers are helped by their worker offspring during colony usurpations. The study's focus of investigation was the question of whether colony take-over by S. invicta queens is more effective when their daughters first invade the colonies. One hypothesis concerned the extent to which daughters' familiarity with the queen, or their genetic similarity to her, affects successful colony take-over. During attempts at taking over another colony, behavioral observations were made of usurping workers that were either familiar or genetically related to the queens to see if these variables were related to aggressive behavior toward the resident or the invading queen.

60

* Red colored, underlined strings of text indicate that they have been taken verbatim from the original paragraph.

* Blue highlighted text indicates that it has been appropriated from the original paragraph with a change in the order of the words or phrases.

ORIGINAL PARAGRAPH

> *"This study examines whether workers of S. invicta are able to assist their mothers in colony usurpations. First we tested whether [queens] of S. invicta are better able to usurp colonies to which their daughters have moved. Second, we tested whether the effect of daughters on usurpation success is due to familiarity with the queen or to genetic relatedness. Aggressive behavior during these usurpation attempts was observed to determine if the presence of familiar or related workers influenced the aggressive response toward either the resident queen or the queen attempting usurpation."*

REWRITTEN VERSION 6

Balas and Adams carried out an investigation to determine whether S. invicta mothers are helped by their worker offspring during colony take-overs. These authors asked whether colony take-over by S. invicta queens is more effective when their daughters first invade the colonies. A second hypothesis concerned the extent to which daughters' familiarity with the queen, or their genetic similarity to her, affects successful colony take-over.
During these occupation attempts, aggressive behavior of usurping workers that were either familiar or genetically related was observed to see if these variables mediated aggressive behavior toward the invading or the resident queen.

Please indicate whether the above paragraph is:

1. Properly paraphrased.
2. Definitely plagiarized.
3. Cannot determine.

FEEDBACK: If you selected "properly paraphrased", you are correct. Although as in the earlier example (No. 5) the structure of the paragraph (i.e., order of the sentences) has been preserved, the present rewritten paragraph represents a thoroughly modified version of the original. The reader is reminded; however, that in some disciplines, particularly within the humanities, a proper paraphrase entails a change in the overall structure of the paragraph as well as a change in the wording. Given, that scientific writing is sometimes multidisciplinary in scope, authors should make every effort to be thoroughly acquainted with the rules of scholarship encompassing the readership of their work.

ORIGINAL VERSION

"This study examines whether workers of S. invicta are able to assist their mothers in colony usurpations. First we tested whether [queens] of S. invicta are better able to usurp colonies to which their daughters have moved. Second, we tested whether the effect of daughters on usurpation success is due to familiarity with the queen or to genetic relatedness. Aggressive behavior during these usurpation attempts was observed to determine if the presence of familiar or related workers influenced the aggressive response toward either the resident queen or the queen attempting usurpation."

PLAGIARIZED VERSION

Balas and Adams carried out an investigation to determine whether S. invicta mothers are helped by their worker offspring during colony take-overs. These authors asked whether colony take-over by S. invicta queens is more effective when their daughters first invade the colonies. A second hypothesis concerned the extent to which daughters' familiarity with the queen, or their genetic similarity to her, affects successful colony take-over. During these occupation attempts, aggressive behavior of usurping workers that were either familiar or genetically related was observed to see if these variables mediated aggressive behavior toward the invading or the resident queen.

62

* Red colored, underlined strings of text indicate that they have been taken verbatim from the original paragraph.

* Blue highlighted text indicates that it has been appropriated from the original paragraph with a change in the order of the words or phrases.

References

Abbott, A. (2009). Editor retracts sperm-creation paper. *Nature, July 30, available at* http://www.nature.com/news/2009/090730/full/ news.2009.753.html.

Altman D. G., Schulz K. F., & Moher D., for the CONSORT Group (2001). The revised CONSORT statement for reporting randomized trials: explanation and Elaboration. *Journal of the American Medical Association, 285,* 1987-1991. Retrieved August 14th, 2006 from http://www.consort-statement.org/Statement/jama.pdf

American Association of University Professors (September/October, 1989). "Statement on Plagiarism." *Academe, 75,* 5, 47-48.

American Medical Writers Association (2008). *AMWA code of Ethics,* http://www.amwa.org/amwa_ethics.

American Psychological Association (2010). Publication Manual of the American Psychological Association (6th ed.). Washington, DC: American Psychological Association.

Anastasia, A., Deinhardt, K., Chao, M. V., Will, N. E., Irmady, K., Lee, F. S., Hempstead, B. L., & Bracken C. (2014). Corrigendum: Val66Met polymorphism of BDNF alters prodomain structure to induce neuronal growth cone retraction. *Nature Communications 4, 2490,* http://www.nature.com/ncomms/2014/140408/ncomms4564/pdf/ncomms4564.pdf

Angell, M. and A.S. Relman (1989). Redundant publication. *New England Journal of Medicine, 320,* 1212-14.

Attoui, B., Kherici, N, and Kherici-Bousnoubra, H. (2014). Use of a new method for determining the vulnerability and risk of pollution of major groundwater reservoirs in the region of Annaba–Bouteldja (NE Algeria). *Environmental Earth Science, 72(3),* 891-903. (Retraction published 2015, *Environmental Earth Sciences, 73,* p. 4396).

Beall, J. (2013). Medical Publishing Triage – Chronicling Predatory Open Access Publishers *Annals of Medicine and Surgery. 2(2),* 47–49.

Bekelman, J. E., Li, Y., & Gross, C. P. (2003), Scope and impact of financial conflicts of interest in biomedical research. *Journal of the American Medical Association, 289(4),* 454-65.

Biros, M. H. (2000). Advice to Authors: Getting Published in *Academic Emergency Medicine*. Retrieved March 6, 2003 from http://www.saem.org/inform/aempub.htm.

Bloch J. (2012). Plagiarism, intellectual property and the teaching of L2 writing. Bristol, UK: Multilingual Matters.

Bonnell, D. A., Hafner, J. H., Hersam, M. C., Kotov., N. A., Buriak, J. M., Hammond, P. T., Javey, A., Nordlander, P., Parak, W. J., Schaak, R. E., Wee, A. T., Weiss, P. S., Rogach, A. L., Stevens, M. M., & Willson, C. G. (2012). Recycling is not always good: The Dangers of self-plagiarism. *ACS Nano, 6,* 1–4.

64

Booth, W. C., Colomb, G. G., & Williams, J. M. (2008). *The craft of research*. Chicago: The University of Chicago Press.

Bright Tunes Music Corp. v. Harrisongs Music, Ltd. (1976). 420 F.Supp. 177 (S.D.N.Y).

Brosgole, L. & Neylon, A. (1973). Kinetic visual imagery. *Perceptual and Motor Skills, 37*, 423-425.

Brosgole, L., & Roig, M. (1983). On the mechanisms underlying kinetic visual imagery: I. The role of eye movements and reafferent stimulation. Journal of Mental Imagery, 7(2), 57-66.

Brown, A. S., & Halliday, H. E. (1991). Cryptomnesia and source memory difficulties. *American Journal of Psychology, 104*, 475–490.

Bruton, S. V. (2014). Self-plagiarism and textual recycling: legitimate forms of research misconduct. *Accountability in Research, 21*, 176-197.

Brown, A. S., & Murphy, D. R. (1989). Cryptomnesia: Delineating inadvertent plagiarism. *Journal of Experimental Psychology: Learning, Memory, and Cognition, 15*, 432–442.

Castelvecchi, D. (2015). Physics paper sets record with more than 5,000 authors. *Nature*, May 15, Available at http://www.nature.com/news/physics-paper-sets-record-with-more-than-5-000-authors-1.17567.

Clark, J. & Smith, R. (2015). Firm action needed on predatory journals. *British Medical Journal, 350*, https://nursingeditors.files.wordpress.com/2014/11/bmj-h210-full-1.pdf.

Choi, W.-S., Song, S.-W., Ock, S.-M., Kim, C.-M., Lee, J.-B, Chang, W.-J., & Kim, S.-H. (2014). Duplicate publication of articles used in meta-analysis in Korea. *SpringerPlus, 3, 182*, 1-6.

Cooper, C. A. (2008). Reassessing Conference Goals and Outcomes: A Defense of Presenting Similar Papers at Multiple Conferences. *PS: Political Science and Politics 41(2)*, 293-296.

Cummings, P., & Rivara, F. P. (2012). Spin and boasting in research articles. *Archives of Pediatric Adolescent Medicine, 166*, 1099–1100.

Dante, E. (2010). The Shadow Scholar. *The Chronicle of Higher Education*, Available at http://chronicle.com/article/The-Shadow-Scholar/125329/

Deckert, G. D. (1993). A pedagogical response to learned plagiarism among tertiarylevel ESL students. *Journal of Second Language Writing, 2*, 94-104.

Dieter, K.C., Hu, B., Knill, D.C., Blake, R. & Tadin, D. (2013). Kinesthesis can make an invisible hand visible. Psychological Science, 23, 1013-1017.

Dieter, K.C., Hu, B., Knill, D.C., Blake, R. & Tadin, D. (2014). Corrigendum: Kinesthesis can make an invisible hand visible. Psychological Science, 25(3), 842.

65

Dometrius, N. C. (2008). Academic Double-Dipping: Professional Profit or Loss? *PS: Political Science & Politics, 41:2 (April)*, 289-92

Dorland, W. A. N. (2000). *Dorland's illustrated medical dictionary, 29th edition.* Philadelphia: W. B. Saunders.

Dorland, W. A. N. (2011). *Dorland's illustrated medical dictionary.* Elevier Saunders.

Fang, F. C, Steen, R. G., & Casadevall, A. (2012). Misconduct accounts for the majority of retracted scientific publications. *Proceedings of the National Academies of Science U. S. A. 109*, 17028–17033.

Ferguson, C. (2015). More evidence scientists continue to cite retracted papers, http://retractionwatch.com/2015/02/18/evidence-scientists-continue-cite-retracted-papers/. Accessed July 28th, 2015.

Ferguson, C. (2014). Student denied credit, math article retracted. Retraction Watch http://retractionwatch.com/2014/10/28/student-denied-credit-math-article-retracted/. Accessed April 10, 2015.

Fine, M. A. and Kurdek, L. A. (1993). Reflections on determining authorship credit and authorship order on faculty-student collaborations. *American Psychologist, 48*, 1141-1147.

Flowerdew, J., & Li, Y. (2007). Language re-use among Chinese apprentice scientists writing for publication. *Applied Linguistics, 28(3)*, 440-465.

Garner, H. R., McIver, L. J., & Waitzkin, M. B. (2013). Research funding: Same work, twice the money? *Nature, 493*, 599-601.

Gilchrist, A. (1979). The perception of surface blacks and whites. *Scientific American, 24*, 88-97.

Goodman, N. (1998). Paper failed to mention earlier review (letter). *British Medical Journal, 317*, 884.

Halupa, C. & Bolliger, D. U. (2013). Faculty perceptions of student self-plagiarism: An exploratory multi-university study, *Journal of Academic Ethics, 11(4)*, 297-310.

Hammond, K. W., Helbig, S. T., Benson, C. C., & Brathwaite-Sketoe, B. M. (2003). Are electronic medical records trustworthy? Observations on copying, pasting and duplications. *AMIA Annual Symposium Proceedings*, 269-273.

Harris, B. (2011). Letting go of Little Albert: Disciplinary memory, history, and the uses of myth. *Journal of the History of the Behavioral Sciences, 47*, 1–17.

Heitman, E., and S. Litewka. (2011). International perspectives on plagiarism and considerations for teaching international trainees. *Urologic Oncology, 29*, 104–108.

Hexham, I. (1999). *The plague of plagiarism.* Department of Religious Studies. The University of Calgary. Retrieved March 15, 2003 from http://c.faculty.umkc.edu/cowande/plague.htm#self.

66

Hoffstetter, H. W. (1970), Some observations on phantom visual imagery. *American Journal of Optometry and Archives of American Academy of Optometry, 47,* 361-366.

Howard, R. M. (1999). The new abolitionism comes to plagiarism. In L. Buranen, L. & M. Roy (Eds.) *Perspectives on plagiarism and intellectual property in a postmodern world.* N.Y.: State University of New York.

Hu, G. (2008). The misleading academic discourse on Chinese-English bilingual education in China. *Review of Educational Research, 78(2),* 195-231.

Iverson, C, et al. (2007). *American Medical Association Manual of Style. A Guide for Authors and Editors, 10th ed.* Oxford. .

International Committee of Medial Journal Editors (2014). *Uniform Requirements for Manuscript Submitted to Biomedical Journals.* http://www.icmje.org/.

Jacobs, A. & Wager, E. (2005). European Medical Writers Association (ENWA) guidelines on the role of medical writers in developing peer-reviewed publication. *Current medical Research Opinion, 21,* 317-322.

Jefferson, T. (1998). Redundant publication in biomedical sciences: Scientific Misconduct or necessity? *Science and Engineering Ethics, 4,* 135-140.

Julliard, K. (1993). Perceptions of plagiarism in the use of other authors' language. *Family Medicine. 26,* 356–360.

Kassirer, J. P. & Angell, M. (1995). Redundant publication: A reminder. *The New England Journal of Medicine, 333,* 449-450. Retrieved, March 7, 2003 from http://content.nejm.org/cgi/content/full/333/7/449.

Katsnelson, A. (2015). Cancer paper pulled due to "identical text" from one published 6 days prior; author objects. *Retraction Watch.* Available at http://retractionwatch.com/2015/06/12/cancer-paper-pulled-due-to-identical-text-from-one-published-6-days-prior-author-objects/

Khaled. K. (2015). The disaster of the impact factor. *Science and Engineering Ethics 21 (1),* 139–142.

Kim, S. Y, Bae, C-W, Hahm, C. K, & Cho, H. M. (2014). Duplicate publication rate decline in Korean medical journals. *Journal of Korean Medical Science. 29(2),* 172-175.

Kohler, C. S. (2012). Publications Policy Committee of the American Diabetes Association. Updates to policies and procedures related to potential scientific and academic misconduct in the journals of the American Diabetes Association. *Diabetes, 61,* 38–39.

Kolin, F. C. (2013). *Successful Writing at Work, 10th Edition.* Cengage Learning.

67

Larivière, V. & Gingras, Y. (2010). On the prevalence and scientific impact of duplicate publications in different scientific fields (1980-2007). *Journal of Documentation, 66(2)*, 179-190.

Levin, J. R. & Marhsall, H. (1993). Publishing in the Journal of Educational Psychology: Reflections at midstream (Editorial). *Journal of Educational Psychology, 85*, 3-6.

Lexchin, J., Bero, L. A, Djulbegovic, B., & Clark, O. (2003). Pharmaceutical industry sponsorship and research outcome and quality: Systematic review. *British Medical Journal, 326(7400)*, 1167-1170

Logan, T. K., Walker, R., Cole, J., & Leukefeld, C. (2002). Victimization and substance abuse among women: Contributing factors, interventions, and implications. *Review of General Psychology, 6*, 325-397.

Lundh, A., Sismondo, S., Lexchin, J., Busuioc, O. A., & Bero, L. (2012). Industry sponsorship and research outcome. *Cochrane Database Systematic Reviews. 12:MR000033.*

Lunyak, V., et al., (2002). Corepressor-dependent silencing of chromosomal regions encoding neuronal genes. *Science, 298*, 1747-1756.

Magnus, J. R., Polterovich, V. M., Danilov, D.L. & Savvateev (2002). Tolerance of cheating: an analysis across countries. *The Journal of Economic Education, 33(2),* 125-135.

Marcus, A. (2010). Redundancy, redux: Anesthesia journal retracts obesity paper in self-plagiarism case. http://retractionwatch.com/2010/08/04/redundancy-redux-anesthesia-journal-retracts-obesity-paper-in-self-plagiarism-case/

Marcus, A. (2014). Lack of citation prompts correction in Nature journal. http://retractionwatch.com/2014/04/10/lack-of-citation-prompts-correction-in-nature-journal/

Marsh, R. L., & Bower, G. H. (1993). Eliciting cryptomnesia: Unconscious plagiarism in a puzzle task. *Journal of Experimental Psychology: Learning, Memory, and Cognition, 19,* 673–688.

Martin, B. (1997). Credit where credit is due. *Campus Review, 7,* 11. Retrieved February 3rd, 2003 from http://www.uow.edu.au/arts/sts/bmartin/pubs/plagiarismfraud.html.

Martini, F. H., & Bartholomew, M. S. (1997). *Essentials of Anatomy and Physiology.* Upper Saddle River, NJ: Prentice Hall.

Martinson, B. C., Anderson, M. S., & de Vries, R. (2005). Scientists behaving badly. *Nature, 435*, 737-738.

Master, Z. & Resnik, D. B. (2013). Hype and Public Trust in Science. *Science and Engineering Ethics, 19(2)*, 321-335.

Mervis, J. (2013). NSF Audit of Successful Proposals Finds Numerous Cases of Alleged Plagiarism. *ScienceInsider, March 8th,* http://news.sciencemag.org/2013/03/nsf-audit-successful-proposals-finds-numerous-cases-alleged-plagiarism.

68

McCabe, D. L., Treviño, L. K., & Butterfield, K. D. (2002). Honor codes and other contextual influences on academic integrity: A replication and extension of modified honor code settings. *Research in Higher Education, 43,* 357–378.

McGowan, S. & Lightbody, M. (2008). Enhancing students' understanding of plagiarism within a discipline context. *Accounting Education: an international journal, 17,* 273-290.

Mistiaen, V. (2002). Time and the great healer. *The Guardian,* November 2. Retrieved February 19th, 2006 from http://www.guardian.co.uk/weekend/story/0,3605,823114,00.html.

Morehead, P. D. (2002). *The New American Roget's College Thesaurus in Dictionary Form,* 3rd ed., Signet Press: Seattle.

Nathan, M. H. (1994). Variations of plagiarism (letter). *American Journal of Roentgenology, 163,* 727.

Ngai, S., Gold, J. L., Gill, S. S., & Rochon, P. A. (2005). Haunted manuscripts: ghost authorship in the medical literature. *Accountability in Research, 12,* 103-114

Office of Research Integrity (1994): Working definition of plagiarism. Office of Research Integrity Newsletter 3(1). http://ori.dhhs.gov/html/misconduct/plagiarism.asp.

Office of Science and Technology Policy (1999). *Research Misconduct – A New Definition and New Procedures for Federal Research Agencies.* Retrieved August 14th, 2006 from http://clinton3.nara.gov/WH/EOP/OSTP/html/misconduct.html.

O'Reilly, K. (2013). EHRs: 'Sloppy and paste' endures despite patient safety risk. American Medical News, February 4, http://www.amednews.com/article/20130204/profession/130209993/2/

Paul, D. B. and Blumenthal, A. L. (1989). On the trail of Little Albert. *Psychological Record, 39,* 547-553.

Pechnick, J. A. (2009). *A short guide to writing about biology,* 7th Edition. New York: Longman Publishing Group.

Pecorari, D. (2013). *Teaching to avoid plagiarism.* Open University Press.

Pennycook, A. (1996). Borrowing others' words: text, ownership, memory, and plagiarism. *TESOL Quarterly 30(2),* 201-230.

Perkin, M. (1999). References were misinterpreted. *British Medical Journal, 318,* 1288.

Power, L. G. (2009). University students' perceptions of plagiarism. *The Journal of Higher Education, 80,* 643-662.

Price, A. (2006). Cases of plagiarism handled by the United States Office of Research Integrity 1992-2005. *Plagiary: Cross Disciplinary Studies in Plagiarism, Fabrication, and Falsification, 1(1),* 1-11. Available at http://www.plagiary.org.

Pupovac, V, Bilić-Zulle, L., & Petrovečki, M. (2008). On academic plagiarism in Europe: An analytical approach based on four studies. *Digithumn, 10*,14–17, http://www/uoc.edu/digithum/10/dt/eng/pupovac_bilic-zulle_Petrovecki.pdf.

Ramirez, M., Dalton, J. T. McMillan, G, Read, M and Seamans, N. H. (2013). Do Open Access Electronic Theses and Dissertations Diminish Publishing Opportunities in the Social Sciences and Humanities? Findings from a 2011 Survey of Academic Publishers" College & Research Libraries 74(4), 368-380. Available at: http://works.bepress.com/marisa_ramirez/25

Resnik, D. B. (2012). Plagiarism: Words and ideas. *Accountability in Research, 19,* 269–272.

Roig, M. (1997). Can undergraduate students determine whether text has been plagiarized? *The Psychological Record, 47(1),* 113-122.

Roig, M. (1999). When college students' attempts at paraphrasing become instances of potential plagiarism. *Psychological Reports, 84(3),* 973-982.

Roig, M. (2001). Plagiarism and paraphrasing criteria of college and university   professors. *Ethics and Behavior 11(3),* 307–323.

Roig, M. (2005). Re-using text from one's own previously published papers: An exploratory study of potential self-plagiarism. *Psychological Reports, 97,* 43-49

Roig, M. (2014). Journal editorials on plagiarism: What is the message? *European Science Editing, 40,* 58-59.

Rossner, M., Van Epps, H., & Hill, E. (2007). Show me the data. *Journal of Cell Biology, 179 (6),* 1091–1092.

Salazar, M. K. (1993). Using the words and works of others: A commentary. *Journal of the American Association of Occupational Health, 41,* 46-49.

Schatz, A. (1993). The true story of the discovery of streptomycin. *Actinomycetes, 4,* 27-39.

Schein, M. (2001). Redundant publications: From self-plagiarism to "Salami-Slicing". *New Surgery, 1,* 139-140.

Schneider, S. K. & Jacoby, W. G. (2008). Are Repeated Conference Papers Really a Problem? *PS: Political Science and Politics 41(2),* 307-308.

Shafer, S. L. (2011). You will be caught. *Anesthesia and Analgesia, 112(3),* 491-493.

Shahghasemi, E. & Akhavan, M. (2015). Confessions of academic ghost authors: The Iranian experience, *SageOpen*. Available at http://sgo.sagepub.com/content/5/1/2158244015572262.full-text.pdf+html.

Shamoo, A. S. & Resnik, D. B. (2009). *Responsible Conduct of Research*. New York: Oxford University Press.

70

Siebers, R. and Holt, S. (2000). Accuracy of references in five leading medical journals (letter). *The Lancet, 356*, 1445. Retrieved June 15th, 2006 from http://www.thelancet.com/journals/lancet/article/PIIS0140673605740903/fulltext

Sigelman, L. (2008). Multiple Presentations of "the Same" Paper: A Skeptical View. *PS: Political Science and Politics 41(2)*, 305-306.

Sismondo, S. & Doucet, M. (2010) Publication ethics and the ghost management of medical publication. *Bioethics, 24,* 273-283.

Smolčić, V. S. & Bilić-Zulle, L. (2013). How do we handle self-plagiarism in submitted manuscripts? *Biochemia Medica, 23(2)*, 150–153.

Standler, R. B. (2000). *Plagiarism in Colleges in USA.* Retrieved February 17th, 2003 from http://www.rbs2.com/plag.htm.

Steinbok, P. (1995). Ethical considerations relating to writing a medical scientific paper for publication. *Child's Nervous System, 11,* 323-328.

Stelfox, H. T., Chua, G., O'Rourke, K., Detsky, A. S. (1998). Conflict of interest in the debate over calcium-channel antagonists. *The New England Journal of Medicine, 338*, 101-106. Retrieved June 20th, 2003 from http://content.nejm.org/cgi/content/full/338/2/101.

Steneck, N. H. (2000). Assessing the integrity of publicly funded research. In *Proceedings of the First ORI Research Conference on Research Integrity.* Office of Research Integrity (pp. 1-16). Retrieved August 14th, 2006 from http://www-personal.umich.edu/~nsteneck/publications/Steneck_N_02.pdf.

Swaan, P. W. (2010). Publication ethics--a guide for submitting manuscripts to Pharmaceutical Research. *Pharmaceutical research, 27(9),* 1757-1758.

Swazey, J.P., Anderson, M.S., & Lewis, K.S. (1993). Ethical problems in academic research. *American Scientist, 81,* 542-553.

Tarnow, E., (1999). The Authorship List in Science: Junior Physicists' Perceptions of Who Appears and Why. *Science and Engineering Ethics, 5,* 73-88, retrieved August 14th, 2006 from http://onlineethics.org/essays/author/authorship.html.

Taylor, D. (2002). The appropriate use of references in a scientific paper. *Emergency Medicine, 14,* 177-170.

The PLoS Medicine Editors (2009). Ghostwriting: The Dirty Little Secret of Medical Publishing That Just Got Bigger. *PLoS Medicine, 6(9),* http://journals.plos.org/plosmedicine/article?id=10.1371/journal.pmed.1000156.

Tramer, M. R., Reynolds, D. J., Moore, R. A., & McQuay, H. J. (1997). Impact of covert duplicate publication on meta-analysis: a case study. *British Medical Journal, 315(7109),* 635–640.

U.S. Copyright Office (September 30, 1996). *Copyright law of the United States.* Library of Congress, Washington, D. C.: U.S. Government Printing Office, Circular 92.

71

U.S. Public Health Service. (August 8, 1989). Responsibility of PHS awardee and applicant institutions for dealing with and reporting possible misconduct in science. *54 Federal Register* 151; 42 CRF Part 50, 32446-51.

Vasconcelos, S., Leta, J., Costa, L., Pinto, A., & Sorenson, M. (2009). Discussing plagiarism in Latin America. *EMBO Reports, 4,* 677–682

Vasconcelos, S. M. and Roig, M. (2015 in press). Prior publication and redundancy in contemporary science: Are authors and editors at the crossroads? *Science and Engineering Ethics.*

von Elm, E., Poglia, G., Walder, B., & Tramer, M. R. (2004). Different patterns of duplicate publication: an analysis of articles used in systematic reviews. *Journal of the American Medical Association, 291(8),* 974–980.

Wager, E., Fiack, S., Graf, C., Robinson, A., & Rowlands, I. (2009). Science journal editors' views on publication ethics: results of an international survey. *Journal of Medical Ethics, 35*(6), 348–353.

Walker, A. L. (2008). Preventing unintentional plagiarism: A method for strengthening paraphrasing skills. *Journal of Instructional Psychology. 35*(4), 387-395.

Watson, J. B. and Rayner, R. (1920). Conditioned emotional reactions. *Journal of Experimental Psychology, 3,* 1-14. Retrieved on August 14th, 2006 from http://psychclassics.yorku.ca/Watson/emotion.htm.

Wheeler, A. G. (1989). The pressure to publish promotes disreputable science. *The Scientist, 3* (14): 11. Retrieved March 6, 2003 from http://www.the-scientist.com/yr1989/jul/opin_890710.html.

Witherspoon, A. (1995). This Pen for Hire. *Harper's Magazine, 290,* 1741, 49-57.

Wilhite, A. W., & Fong, E. A. (2012). Coercive citation in academic publishing. *Science, 335(6068),* 542-543.

Woloshin, S. and Schwartz, L. M. (2002). Press Releases: Translating Research into News. *Journal of the American Medical Association, 287,* 2856-2858. Retrieved June 18th, 2003 from http://jama.ama-assn.org/cgi/content/full//287/21/2856.

Woolley, K. L. (2006). Goodbye Ghostwriters! How to work ethically and efficiently with professional medical writers. *Chest, 130(3),* 921-923.

World Association of Medical Editors (2005) Ghost writing initiated by commercial companies. Available: http://www.wame.org/resources/policies#ghost.

Zigmond, M. J. and Fischer, B. A. (2002). Beyond fabrication and plagiarism: The little murders of everyday science. Commentary on "Six Domains of Research Ethics". *Science and Engineering Ethics, 8,* 229-234.

7.4   'Dear "Plagiarist': A Scientist Calls Out His Double-Crosser

Adam Marcus and Ivan Oransky

Marcus, A, Oransky, I. "Dear plagiarist": A scientist calls out his double-crosser. *STAT News* (December 12, 2016).

STAT

'Dear plagiarist': A scientist calls out his double-crosser

By Adam Marcus @armarcus *and* Ivan Oransky @ivanoransky

December 12, 2016

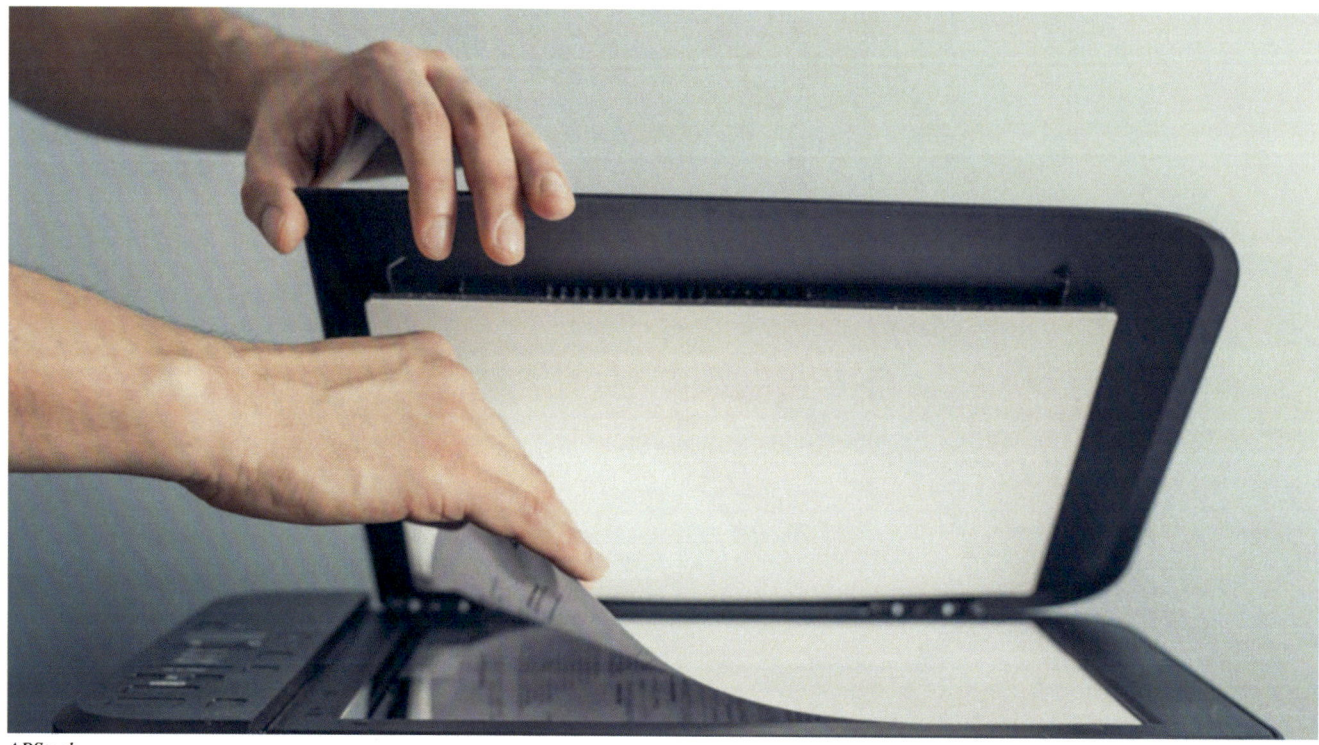

APStock

It's a researcher's worst nightmare: Pour five years, and at least 4,000 hours, of sweat and tears into a study, only to have the work stolen from you — by someone who was entrusted to confidentially review the manuscript.

But unlike many sordid tales of academia, this one is being made public. Dr. Michael Dansinger, of Tufts Medical Center, has taken to print to excoriate a group of researchers in Italy who stole his data and published it as their own.

Writing in the prestigious Annals of Internal Medicine — which unwittingly facilitated the episode by farming the paper out for review and then rejecting it — Dansinger calls out the scientists[1] who published their nearly identical version in the somewhat less prestigious EXCLI Journal.

"As you must certainly know, stealing is wrong ..." he writes. "Physicians and patients depend on the integrity of the [peer review] process. Such cases of theft, scientific fraud, and plagiarism cannot be tolerated because they are harmful and unethical."

Related Story: [2]
Do scientific fraudsters deserve a second chance? [2]

The offending individuals are with the Center of Obesity and Eating Disorders at Stella Maris Mediterraneum Foundation in Potenza, a hilly town in the ankle of Italy. Dansinger was tipped off to their duplication while searching the internet for papers bearing his name.

In September the copycat paper was retracted, and corresponding author of the paper Carmine Finelli wrote that he and his coauthors acknowledged the "unauthorized reproduction of confidential content of another manuscript." "We deeply regret these circumstances and apologize to the scientific community," the retraction letter read. Finelli told Retraction Watch that he "had the responsibility for the plagiarism."

The bogus article claims, among other things, to include data from "160 consecutive subjects referred to our out-patient Metabolic Unit in South Italy." That, in short, is a lie. In fact, those patients were from the United States — which is, of course, far from South Italy geographically, and, more importantly, medically.

As Dr. Christine Laine, editor in chief of the Annals, writes[3], fabricating a group of patients is a "particularly egregious act that could have resulted in clinicians (unknowingly) basing decisions about patient care on fraudulent data." Laine tells STAT she left out the name of the responsible author because "readers can easily identify who the guilty party" was.

Perhaps. But given the long list of coauthors, failing to name the shamed here opens a door to unnecessary ambiguity, risking tarring underlings[4] in Finelli's lab with crimes in which they may have had no role. (Though, since all authors should attest to their role in a paper, every coauthor was at least partly complicit in this fraud.)

Related Story: [4]
For young scientists, a supervisor's fraud can derail a career [4]

Dansinger says his goal in writing the letter was not to humiliate the thief, whom he identifies as Carmine Finelli, the first author of the offending article. "My aim is to raise awareness in the scientific/academic community and general public that it is possible for peer reviewers to steal an entire manuscript and publish it as their own in an unsuspecting academic journal," Dansinger told STAT. "I'm not looking to 'tattle' on the perpetrator — doing so starts to look like revenge rather than achieving the more important objectives, and may even draw attention away from those objectives."

Dansinger is far from the only scientist to be ripped off by unscrupulous reviewers[5], a particularly "heinous intellectual theft," as the Annals puts it. Indeed, we've heard this story before from others. And, whether plagiarists are reviewers or readers, their victims share a sense of shock and disgust at discovering the con[6].

A more subtle, but in many ways more insidious, kind of theft, likely happens even more often. Many researchers can tell stories of being beaten to publication by competitors whom they are fairly sure reviewed their work and delayed it long enough to make sure their own study was published first.

But perhaps the most telling part of the letter is how, from the victim's perspective, it's not just the words that plagiarists take from them, but the associated years of work that the project represents. "When you published our work as your own," Dansinger writes, "you were falsely claiming credit for all of this work and for the expertise gained by doing it."

Dansinger says he is still working to get a paper out of the study, which would be some consolation. But if this open letter of his manages to deter a few cases of misconduct, it could be the most significant publication of his career.

About the Authors

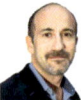

Adam Marcus[7]
Columnist, The Watchdogs
Adam covers scientific publishing and retractions.
adam.marcus@statnews.com[8]
@armarcus[9]

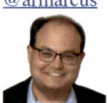

Ivan Oransky[10]
Columnist, The Watchdogs
Ivan covers scientific publishing and retractions.
ivan.oransky@statnews.com[11]
@ivanoransky[12]

Tags

Links

1. http://annals.org/aim/article/doi/10.7326/M16-2551
2. https://www.statnews.com/2016/06/24/science-fraud-second-chance/
3. http://annals.org/aim/article/doi/10.7326/M16-2550
4. https://www.statnews.com/2016/11/25/postdocs-grad-students-fraud/
5. http://retractionwatch.com/2013/01/08/university-of-waterloo-suspends-researcher-who-published-plagiarized-paper-in-his-own-journal/
6. http://retractionwatch.com/2012/03/12/how-does-it-feel-to-have-your-scientific-paper-plagiarized-and-what-can-you-do-about-it/
7. https://www.statnews.com/staff/adam-marcus/
8. https://www.statnews.com/2016/12/12/plagiarist-study-science/mailto:adam.marcus@statnews.com

9. https://twitter.com/armarcus
10. https://www.statnews.com/staff/ivan-oransky/
11. https://www.statnews.com/2016/12/12/plagiarist-study-science/mailto:ivan.oransky@statnews.com
12. https://twitter.com/ivanoransky
13. https://www.statnews.com/tag/research/

7.5   Defining the Role of Authors and Contributors

International Committee of Medical Journal Editors

International Committee of Medical Journal Editors. Defining the role of authors and contributors. http://www. icmje.org/recommendations/browse/roles-and-responsibili- ties/defining-the-role-of-authors-and-contributors.html. For official, most recent version of ICMEJ recommendations, see: www.icmje.org

Reprinted with permission from The International Committee of Medical Journal Editors.

| Enter search terms | SEARCH |

Recommendations   **Conflicts of Interest**   Journals
Following the ICMJE Recommendations   **About ICMJE**   **News & Editorials**

Recommendations

Home > Recommendations > Browse > Roles & Responsibilities > Defining the Role of Authors and Contributors

Defining the Role of Authors and Contributors

Browse

   About the Recommendations

   Roles & Responsibilities

      🔖 Defining the Role of Authors and Contributors

      Author Responsibilities —Conflicts of Interest

      Responsibilities in the Submission and Peer-Review Process

      Journal Owners and Editorial Freedom

      Protection of Research Participants

   Publishing & Editorial Issues

   Manuscript Preparation

Translations

Archives

Subscribe to Changes

PAGE CONTENTS

1. Why Authorship Matters
2. Who Is an Author?
3. Non-Author Contributors

1. Why Authorship Matters

Authorship confers credit and has important academic, social, and financial implications. Authorship also implies responsibility and accountability for published work. The following recommendations are intended to ensure that contributors who have made substantive intellectual contributions to a paper are given credit as authors, but also that contributors credited as authors understand their role in taking responsibility and being accountable for what is published.

Because authorship does not communicate what contributions qualified an individual to be an author, some journals now request and publish information about the contributions of each person named as having participated in a submitted study, at least for original research. Editors are strongly encouraged to develop and implement a contributorship policy. Such policies remove much of the ambiguity surrounding contributions, but leave unresolved the question of the quantity and quality of contribution that qualify an individual for authorship. The ICMJE has thus developed criteria for authorship that can be used by all journals, including those that distinguish authors from other contributors.

2. Who Is an Author?

The ICMJE recommends that authorship be based on the following 4 criteria:

✉ **KEEP UP-TO-DATE**

Request to receive an E-mail when the Recommendations are updated.

Subscribe to Changes

- Substantial contributions to the conception or design of the work; or the acquisition, analysis, or interpretation of data for the work; AND

- Drafting the work or revising it critically for important intellectual content; AND

- Final approval of the version to be published; AND

- Agreement to be accountable for all aspects of the work in ensuring that questions related to the accuracy or integrity of any part of the work are appropriately investigated and resolved.

In addition to being accountable for the parts of the work he or she has done, an author should be able to identify which co-authors are responsible for specific other parts of the work. In addition, authors should have confidence in the integrity of the contributions of their co-authors.

All those designated as authors should meet all four criteria for authorship, and all who meet the four criteria should be identified as authors. Those who do not meet all four criteria should be acknowledged—see Section II.A.3 below. These authorship criteria are intended to reserve the status of authorship for those who deserve credit and can take responsibility for the work. The criteria are not intended for use as a means to disqualify colleagues from authorship who otherwise meet authorship criteria by denying them the opportunity to meet criterion #s 2 or 3. Therefore, all individuals who meet the first criterion should have the opportunity to participate in the review, drafting, and final approval of the manuscript.

The individuals who conduct the work are responsible for identifying who meets these criteria and ideally should do so when planning the work, making modifications as appropriate as the work progresses. It is the collective responsibility of the authors, not the journal to which the work is submitted, to determine that all people named as authors meet all four criteria; it is not the role of journal editors to determine who qualifies or does not qualify for authorship or to arbitrate authorship conflicts. If agreement cannot be reached about who qualifies for authorship, the institution(s) where the work was performed, not the journal editor, should be asked to investigate. If authors request removal or addition of an author after manuscript submission or publication, journal editors should seek an explanation and signed statement of agreement for the requested change from all listed authors and from the author to be removed or added.

The corresponding author is the one individual who takes primary responsibility for communication with the journal during the manuscript submission, peer review, and publication process, and typically ensures that all the journal's administrative requirements, such as providing details of authorship, ethics committee approval, clinical trial registration documentation, and gathering conflict of interest forms and statements, are properly completed, although these duties may be delegated to one or more coauthors. The corresponding author should be available throughout the submission and peer review process to respond to editorial queries in a timely way, and should be available after publication to respond to critiques of the work and cooperate with any requests from the journal for data or additional information should questions about the paper arise after publication. Although the corresponding author has primary responsibility for correspondence with the journal, the ICMJE recommends that editors send copies of all correspondence to all listed authors.

When a large multi-author group has conducted the work, the group ideally should decide who will be an author before the work is started and confirm who is an author before submitting the manuscript for publication. All members of the group named as authors should meet all four criteria for authorship, including approval of the final manuscript, and they should be able to take public responsibility for the work and should have full confidence in the accuracy and integrity of the work of other group authors. They will also be expected as individuals to complete conflict-of-interest disclosure forms.

Some large multi-author groups designate authorship by a group name, with or without the names of individuals. When submitting a manuscript authored by a group, the corresponding author should specify the group name if one exists, and clearly identify the group members who can take credit and responsibility for the work as authors. The byline of the article identifies who is directly responsible for the manuscript, and MEDLINE lists as authors whichever names appear on the byline. If the byline includes a group name, MEDLINE will list the names of individual group members who are authors or who are collaborators, sometimes called non-author contributors, if there is a note associated with the byline clearly stating that the individual names are elsewhere in the paper and whether those names are authors or collaborators.

3. Non-Author Contributors

Contributors who meet fewer than all 4 of the above criteria for authorship should not be listed as authors, but they should be acknowledged. Examples of activities that alone (without other contributions) do not qualify a contributor for authorship are acquisition of funding; general supervision of a research group or general administrative support; and writing assistance, technical editing, language editing, and proofreading. Those whose contributions do not justify authorship may be acknowledged individually or together as a group under a single heading (e.g. "Clinical Investigators" or "Participating Investigators"), and their contributions should be specified (e.g., "served as scientific advisors," "critically reviewed the study proposal," "collected data," "provided and cared for study patients", "participated in writing or technical editing of the manuscript").

Because acknowledgment may imply endorsement by acknowledged individuals of a study's data and conclusions, editors are advised to require that the corresponding author obtain written permission to be acknowledged from all acknowledged individuals.

NEXT: Author Responsibilities—Conflicts of Interest

References

Amos KA. The ethics of scholarly publishing: exploring differences in plagiarism and duplicate publication across nations. J Med Libr Assoc. 2014;102(2):87–91.

Higgins JR, Lin F-C, Evans JP. Plagiarism in submitted manuscripts: incidence, characteristics and optimization of screening—case study in a major specialty medical journal. Res Integr Peer Rev. 2016;1(13):1–8.

Pecorari D, Petric B. Plagiarism in second-language writing. Lang Teach. 2014;47(3):269–302.

Shafer SL. Plagiarism is ubiquitous. Anesth Analg. 2016;122(6):1776–80.

Additional Suggested Reading

Garner H. The case of the stolen words. Sci Am 2014 310(3):64–67. *(Describes early development of Deja-Vu.)*

Shafer SL. Plagiarism is ubiquitous. Anesth Analg 2016; 122(6):1776–1780. (*Judgments about plagiarism made by journal editors cannot be rote but must be thought through.*)

Peer Review

Arthur L. Caplan and Barbara K. Redman

Many date editorial peer review to the 1752 Royal Society of London's use of a "Committee on Papers" to oversee the review of text for publication in the journal *Philosophical Transactions*. Initially, peer review was created to help editors decide what to publish. In the twentieth century it evolved into a system in which qualified peers not only judge publication merit but also evaluate the quality of scientific work including grant applications, conference proposals, books, and academic personnel actions. Today, it is the major tool in scientific self-regulation. It is often undertaken double 'blinded' so that reviewers do not know the names of those they review and vice versa. Peer reviewers names for undertaking specific tasks are often expected to be confidential.

Reviews can be open, single-blind (reviewer knows author but not vice versa), or double-blind (neither knows the other). Post-publication review is now common, although the mechanisms by which it accomplished are fragmented. PubMed Commons (https://www.ncbi.nlm.nih.gov/pubmed-commons), in which comments are attached to an article's PubMed record, is one such mechanism for post peer-review commentary. So are journals that utilize the format of target articles with extensive commentaries.

Complaints about peer review include erroneous rejection of important findings, unreliability in the detection of errors and fraud, intellectual plagiarism by reviewers, purposeful delay and undisclosed conflict of interest when reviewers and authors compete for the same funds or publications. Poor agreement among reviewers is seen as both a weakness and as a strength in bringing diverse perspectives to bear. Several kinds of reviewer bias have been noted: confirmation bias in which current beliefs are affirmed rather than challenged, publication bias for positive rather than negative outcomes or replications, bias against certain kinds of methodology (qualitative studies), and embargoing clinically important findings until all peer review is completed. (Manchikanti et al. 2015).

Two studies of peer review are helpful. A review of papers submitted to *Annals of Internal Medicine, British Medical Journal*, and *Lancet* concluded that peer review added value by filtering out submissions of poor quality but had problems dealing with exceptional or unconventional papers published later in other journals (Siler et al. 2015). A study in the social sciences found reviewers made considerable useful contributions to manuscript revision, particularly of interpretations of findings (Strang and Siler 2015).

Peer review is a prime duty of being part of a scientific community and enforcing norms of research integrity. Peer review fraud has been uncovered and dealt with. In 2015, Springer retracted 64 articles from ten different journals in which an individual invented fake email addresses and reviewed his own manuscripts (Haug 2015). Peer review will continue to be a major form of quality control in science but reviewers must disclose conflicts of interest and describe any limitations in their ability to undertake peer review to those making requests.

Advice: Expect that peer review will be imperfect but know that you can always learn from reviewers' comments. Address them directly and explicitly when you revise a manuscript or grant application for resubmission.

Sometimes reviewer comments mean that your manuscript or application is a mismatch with a journal or funding source so you should find other alternatives. Mentors should spend time explaining how to do peer review, and if they do not, mentees should ask before undertaking peer review work.

A. L. Caplan · B. K. Redman (✉)
New York University Langone Medical Center,
New York, NY, USA
e-mail: Arthur.Caplan@nyumc.org

8.1 Let's Make Peer Review Scientific

Drummond Rennie

Rennie, D. Let's make peer review scientific. *Nature* 535, 31–33 (2016). © 2016 Macmillan Publishers Limited. All rights reserved. An imprint of SpringerNature.

Illustration reproduced courtesy of David Parkins.

uncertainty is needed, as is standard practice in other fields — even bathroom scales come with uncertainties printed on them. A mark should signify that the sensor meets a minimum quality standard

If such a stamp of approval sounds bureaucratic, think of how the data might be used. People with asthma might use their local sensor data to make personal decisions on medication; an air-pollution sensor is not meant as a medical device, but its real-world application could make it function like one. Privately owned sensor data could trigger legal actions in areas that apparently exceed local air-quality standards. The economic and socially disruptive costs of closing roads or banning cars based on live sensor data would be huge.

NEXT STEPS

The academic air-pollution community must do the hard yards in the lab and field on calibration and testing. It must also find ways to overcome some measurement challenges. Researchers should take the lead on evaluating sensor performance, creating better devices and designing research applications that are suited to the quantified capabilities of sensors.

More creativity is needed in experimental design. If the long-term performance of sensors is a problem, as is likely, then we need

to design shorter-term experiments that can be performed reliably. For example, a fine-scale but qualitative measure of pollution might help to simulate the turbulent flows of pollution in street canyons or tree canopies over a few days. There might be experiments in which a fast-responding bulk sensor — one that measures the sum of many organic compounds, for example — might be able to track rapid temporal changes that add context to a slower but more quantitative instrument, such as a gas chromatograph or diffusion tube. Statistical and machine-learning methods might be developed to enable better extraction of signals from a mix of pollutants[8].

"Manufacturers and regulators need to define how and where sensors can be used."

However, academics should not become gatekeepers or validation bodies. This is a job for manufacturers and regulators, who need to define how and where sensors can and cannot be used effectively.

Governments must provide advice now to potential 'professional users', such as in cities and regional environmental agencies. For sensors that might be used for public policy, health studies or any type of infrastructure control, independent testing and verification is essential, as is already being done through

long-standing environment-agency committees and national air-pollution schemes. Even sensors that are designed for entertainment or awareness-raising need appropriate labelling to define their capabilities.

Well designed sensor experiments, that acknowledge the limitations of the technologies as well as the strengths, have the potential to simultaneously advance basic science, monitor air pollution — and bring the public along. ■

Alastair Lewis *is a science director at the National Centre for Atmospheric Science in Leeds, UK, and professor of atmospheric chemistry at the University of York, UK.*
Peter Edwards *is a research fellow in the Wolfson Atmospheric Chemistry Laboratories at the University of York, UK.*
e-mails: ally.lewis@ncas.ac.uk;
pete.edwards@york.ac.uk

1. Lim, S. S. *et al. Lancet* **380,** 2224–2260 (2012).
2. Kumar, P. *et al. Environ. Int.* **75,** 199–205 (2015).
3. Piedrahita, R. *et al. Atmos. Meas. Tech.* **7,** 3325–3336 (2014).
4. Nieuwenhuijsen, M. J. *et al. Environ. Sci. Technol.* **49,** 2977–2982 (2015).
5. Mead, M. I. *et al. Atmos. Environ.* **70,** 186–203 (2013).
6. Kamionka, M., Breuil, P. & Pijolat, C. *Sens. Actuators B Chem.* **118,** 323–327 (2006).
7. Lewis, A. C. *et al. Faraday Discuss.* http://dx.doi.org/10.1039/C5FD00201J (2015).
8. De Vito, S., Piga, M., Martinotto, L. & Di Francia, G. *Sens. Actuators B Chem.* **143,** 182–191 (2009).

Make peer review scientific

Thirty years on from the first congress on peer review, **Drummond Rennie** reflects on the improvements brought about by research into the process — and calls for more.

Peer review is touted as a demonstration of the self-critical nature of science. But it is a human system. Everybody involved brings prejudices, misunderstandings and gaps in knowledge, so no one should be surprised that peer review is often biased and inefficient. It is occasionally corrupt, sometimes a charade, an open temptation to plagiarists. Even with the best of intentions, how and whether peer review identifies high-quality science is unknown. It is, in short, unscientific.

A long time ago, scientists moved from alchemy to chemistry, from astrology to astronomy. But our reverence for peer review still often borders on mysticism. For the past three decades, I have advocated for research to improve peer review and thus the quality of the scientific literature. Here are some reflections on that winding, rocky path, and some thoughts about the road ahead.

I trained as a physician, studying the pathophysiology of exposure to high altitudes. In 1977, I became deputy editor of *The New England Journal of Medicine* (*NEJM*), working with what I assumed was a smoothly oiled peer-review system. I found myself driving an enormous machine whose operation was sometimes interrupted by startling hiccups. The first big one occurred a year after I arrived. An author who had submitted a paper to our journal accused one of our reviewers, who worked at a competing lab, of plagiarizing parts of her paper. She sent us a manuscript that her lab chief had been sent to assess for another journal, one that I could see had been typed on the same typewriter that the reviewer had used to write his review. I was told to sort it out.

This was more than a decade before a formal definition of research misconduct and systems for its investigation were established. Several careers fell apart. That

of the actual plagiarist, and also that of his chief, our reviewer, who was the senior co-author of the manuscript that contained the plagiarism. Tragically, our innocent submitting author also gave up research when her accusations were rebuffed, and she was bullied and demeaned for her persistence and integrity.

This slow-motion catastrophe angered me. How common was such incompetence, confusion and corruption? Did peer review root it out — or just lob it down the road? A few years later, revelations of fabricated data in scores of papers by US cardiologist John Darsee, in *NEJM* and other journals, showed that peer review was usually helpless in detecting gross fraud. More recently, the cases of Dutch psychologist Diederik Stapel and US-based cancer researcher Anil Potti underline how easily false data continue to get through the system. Even if peer review could not detect outright

COMMENT

SELECTING GOOD SCIENCE
Milestones in modern peer review and reporting.

1978–79 Revelations of scientific fraud at Yale and Harvard universities publicizes the issue.

1978–92 The Oxford Database of Perinatal Trials is set up by Iain Chalmers. He later establishes the Cochrane Collaboration and its systematic analyses.

1986 Studies demonstrate publication bias in clinical trials; it is caused by the failure of trial authors to submit results for publication.

1989 Regulations defining scientific misconduct and a procedure to address allegations are codified into US law. Peer review is revealed to be ineffective against misconduct.

1989 The first Peer Review Congress held in Chicago, Illinois. It includes a trial of blinding reviewers to authors' identities.

1993 The Cochrane Collaboration, founded to review published reports relevant to health, reveals inherent biases.

1996 The CONSORT statement on reporting clinical trials is released, with a checklist to assist authors and reviewers.

1999 The *British Medical Journal* adopts open peer review on the basis of evidence from randomized trials of the practice.

2000–PRESENT Online-only journals rise in prominence along with new models of peer review.

2004 Clinical-trial pre-registration is made a condition of publication.

2006 The EQUATOR Network is founded to assemble reporting guidelines.

2010 'Beall's list' warns against 'predatory' journals with questionable peer review.

2014–PRESENT Groups (including ORCID, CASRAI, F1000 working group) are founded to support and credit reviewers.

2017 Eighth Peer Review Congress to be held in Chicago.

fabrications, could it sniff out error in honest scientific work, I wondered? There had to be a way to find out.

QUESTIONS ASKED

In 1985, an influential commentary[1] asserted that "the arbiters of rigor, quality, and innovation in scientific reports" did not "apply to their own work the standards they use in judging the work of others". Ouch! Peer review had to be studied, it said, and the most urgent need was leadership within the scientific community.

I had been working at *The Journal of the American Medical Association* (*JAMA*) since 1983. The chief editor was interested in holding a conference on peer review; I jumped at the chance. I insisted that all presentations describe research — and then worried whether we would get a single abstract.

The inaugural Peer Review Congress was held in a distinctly shabby hotel in Chicago, Illinois, in 1989. It was engaging and contentious: presenters studied the demography of reviewers at various journals, how often individuals conducted reviews, blinding, statistical reporting and much more. I was thrilled to see actual data.

A distinguished editor in the audience took another view, excoriating presentation after presentation. Finally, Iain Chalmers (who later co-founded the Cochrane Collaboration) stood and addressed him: "We have listened to your incessant criticisms of everyone who has gone to the trouble of obtaining data. What we have not heard from you is one single piece of evidence for your opinions." There was loud applause, and the future of these congresses was assured. They have taken place every four years since — in much better hotels.

Thanks to such research, we now know a great deal about the mechanics of peer review — the time taken to appraise papers, rates of disagreement between reviewers, the cost at certain journals, even the occurrence of misconduct during review.

Research has brought clear improvement to the biased reporting of clinical trials. Randomized clinical trials cost millions of dollars, are rarely repeated, and greatly influence what treatments patients receive. My colleagues and I showed that most trial results in submitted manuscripts favoured the treatment tested, and this was reflected in the results that were published[2]. Other work revealed that more than 90% of the bias was due to authors failing to submit manuscripts that are unfavourable to the treatment, and that commercial sponsorship drove decisions not to submit[3]. Although any single trial might have been conducted well, the system was skewed. Publication bias made drugs look better than they were.

This line of investigation provided evidence that convinced journals to require

that clinical trials be 'pre-registered' at inception. Compliance is still patchy, but journal editors now routinely check that trials were announced publicly (typically at ClincialTrials.gov) before results were collected. We can now expect that when drugs are found to cause serious harm during the trials, the existence of those trials will no longer be hidden from the world.

Meta-research has revealed other sources of distortion. For instance, when trial reports fail to account for control patients or do not fully describe methods for randomization and blinding, they are also more likely to report exaggerated effects.

Such observations led to new standards for reporting clinical trials. An early version of the guidelines was tested in *JAMA* and produced a report that our readers found unreadable[4]. The next version of the guidelines, published in 1996 and called CONSORT (Consolidated Standards of Reporting Trials, of which I am a co-organizer), was much better accepted. These proved a highly successful model for reporting, say, epidemiologic studies, or reports of assessing clinical tests[5]. A collection of more than 300 reporting guidelines have been gathered into the EQUATOR Network (www.equator-network.org), and their use is spreading widely among biomedical researchers, journals and reviewers.

Meta-research on clinical trials has been further advanced by the Cochrane Collaboration, which systematically collects studies across disease types to weigh up the evidence. Cochrane has developed 'risk of bias' assessments to help its reviewers to evaluate possible weaknesses in trial reports.

OPEN REVIEW

Blinding of reviews is another fertile area of study. In 1998, my colleagues and I conducted a five-journal trial[6] of double-blind peer review (neither author nor reviewer knows the identity of the other). We found no difference in the quality of reviews. What's more, attempts to mask authors' identities were often ineffective and imposed a considerable bureaucratic burden. We concluded that the only potential benefit to a (largely unsuccessful) policy of masking is the appearance, not the reality, of fairness. Since then, online technologies for blinding have increased, as have numbers of scientists (and thus the difficulty of guessing who authors may be). It will be interesting to see how similar studies work out now, and whether double-blind reviewing affects acceptance rates for women and under-represented minorities.

More than a decade ago, the *British Medical Journal* (*BMJ*) ran trials in which the identities of both author and reviewer were disclosed to each other during review, and, if the paper was published, the reviewers' names were made public. The *BMJ* did not suffer a loss of manuscripts or reviewers, and

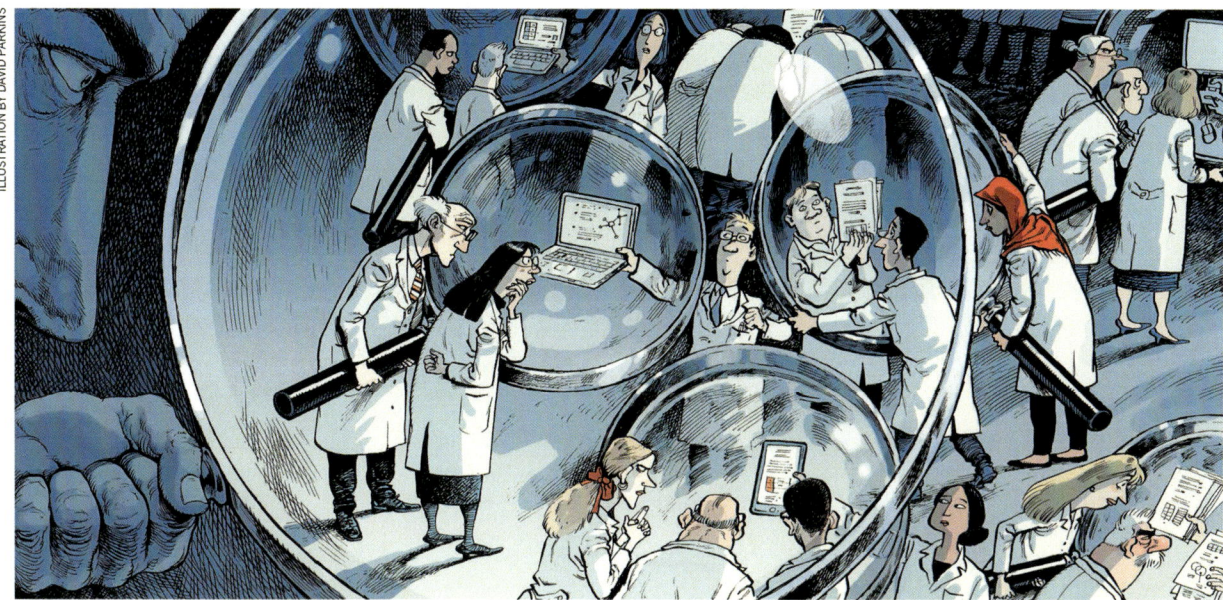

now makes such disclosures compulsory. Its experience suggests that how questions are posed is crucial. If a survey asks: "Would you like to sign your review?", most will decline. But if an editor says: "Our journal requires signed reviews. Will you review?", the *BMJ*'s experience is that very few will refuse[7]. I believe that this brand of open review is the most ethical variety, and its practicability is established. In the present system, authors frequently misidentify reviewers with complete confidence, so blame falls on innocent bystanders.

THE FUTURE

The past 15 years have seen an exciting surge of experimentation with new models of peer review — open, blinded, pre- and post-publication, portable and so on[8]. Some of these systems were tried and abandoned decades ago, before the Internet eased testing and logistics.

We need rigorous studies to tell us the pros and cons of these approaches today. Until then any advertised advantages of new arrangements are unsupported assertions. A 2015 survey[9] of more than 1,000 manuscripts was encouraging about the ability of review to identify important papers, but still found lapses.

After all, online technologies don't give reviewers more time or stamina. A common claim of new journals, whether legitimate or 'predatory' (those that charge fees to publish, but that do not offer standard publishing services), is rapid review and publication. This is a powerful pull for authors, but the detailed attention and mature reflection required for a constructive review takes time.

So what now? In my field, and perhaps in many others: follow the triallists. First,

develop evidence-based lists of items to be included in reporting (mission-sort-of-accomplished for many clinical journals). Journals must accept and promote these guidelines and ensure that reviewers hold authors to them; perhaps they should facilitate training in peer review, which has been shown to improve performance. Finally, manuscript editors and copy editors must uphold the standards. For example, we now routinely reject trial reports that cannot prove registration before inception. This change is large for all involved — authors, reviewers and journal staff — and it is taking years.

And we must continue to study what we have done. Assessment of review is more likely now than ever before. The two-year-old Meta-Research Innovation Center (METRICS) Institute at Stanford University in California, which is devoted to researching and improving the process of science,

"We need rigorous studies to tell us the pros and cons of these approaches."

shows that the field is maturing and gaining respect. So does last year's launch of the journal *Research Integrity and Peer Review*, a home for research on the topic.

In 1986, we were lucky with our timing. The peer-review congresses came just as others were trying to see what could be learned from the literature to arrive at the best treatments for patients, developing methods for systematic review, and nailing down the biases that pervade clinical research (see 'Selecting good science'). These people did the work.

To announce that first Peer Review Congress, I wrote: "There are scarcely any bars

to eventual publication. There seems to be no study too fragmented, no hypothesis too trivial, no literature citation too biased or too egotistical, no design too warped, no methodology too bungled, no presentation of results too inaccurate, too obscure, and too contradictory, no analysis too self-serving, no argument too circular, no conclusions too trifling or too unjustified, and no grammar and syntax too offensive for a paper to end up in print"[10].

Unfortunately, that statement is still true today, and I'm not just talking about predatory journals. That said, I am confident that the Peer Review Congress scheduled for 2017 will be asking more incisive, actionable questions than ever before. ■

Drummond Rennie *is a co-organizer of CONSORT, a former member of the Commission on Research Integrity for the US Public Health Service, and former president of the World Association of Medical Editors.*
e-mail: drummond.rennie@ucsf.edu

1. Bailar, J. C. & Patterson, K. *N. Engl. J. Med.* **312**, 654–657 (1985).
2. Olson, C. M. *et al. J. Am. Med. Assoc.* **287**, 2825–2828 (2002).
3. Dickersin, K. & Rennie, D. *J. Am. Med. Assoc.* **290**, 516–523 (2003).
4. Rennie, D. *J. Am. Med. Assoc.* **273**, 1054–1055 (1995).
5. Begg, C. *et al. J. Am. Med. Assoc.* **276**, 637–639 (1996).
6. Justice, A. C. *et al. J. Am. Med. Assoc.* **280**, 240–242 (1998).
7. Groves, T. *Br. Med. J.* **341,** c6424 (2010).
8. Paglione, L. D. & Lawrence, R. N. *Learn. Publ.* **28**, 309–316 (2015).
9. Siler, K., Lee, K. & Bero, L. *Proc. Natl Acad. Sci. USA* **112**, 360–365 (2015).
10. Rennie, D. *J. Am. Med. Assoc.* **256**, 2391–2392 (1986).

ILLUSTRATION BY DAVID PARKINS

8.2   A Stronger Post-Publication Culture Is Needed for Better Science

Hilda Bastian

    Bastian H (2014) A Stronger Post-Publication Culture Is Needed for Better Science. PLoS Med 11(12): e1001772. doi:https://doi.org/10.1371/journal.pmed.1001772

OPEN ⦾ ACCESS Freely available online

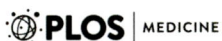

Editorial

A Stronger Post-Publication Culture Is Needed for Better Science

Hilda Bastian*

Scientist and Editor, National Center for Biotechnology Information, National Library of Medicine, National Institutes of Health, Bethesda, Maryland, United States of America

A research report or idea needs to clamber over more than the hurdle of publication to move science, practice, or policy forward. It's not only a matter of authors waiting for kudos and citations to roll in. If their work is not to sink into oblivion, or be acted on when it shouldn't be, publication is just the beginning. Both improving research quality [1,2] and reducing waste in science [3] require a stronger post-publication culture.

Early Enlightenment science was rooted in ongoing discussion among scientists. Scientific discourse in a small, widely scattered community was in person and via books and the "erudite letters" that were the precursor of journal articles [4]. The journal system, capturing fragments of research, enabled massive expansion and acceleration of scientific activity [4].

These days the system does not keep up well with the speed of activity and the volume of research from a vast community. Articles are, by and large, too uncorrectable and unconnected [5], and much significant intellectual effort is not captured at all. Substantive discussions in journal clubs, in email lists, in social media, and at conferences are not distilled into a concise, permanent, accessible record. Most of the unaddressed content of pre-publication peer review is also lost.

Post-publication evaluation is highly fragmented. It often appears within future articles, either embedded in the introduction and discussion sections, or in formal research syntheses. Dedicated review journals (and journal sections) select, summarize, and critique publications, usually in an "expert picks" way. There are also rigorously structured systems of post-publication evaluation inside and outside journals [6,7].

There are more immediate channels to respond to published research, such as letters and comments to the editor, commentaries, and editorials in journals, and discussion in blogs. Dedicated websites have been developed for discussing and sharing research among authors [8], and PubMed Commons (for which I am editor) enables post-publication commenting and

linkages by the PubMed authorship community and journal clubs [9].

Somewhere within this activity is the amorphous phenomenon that people call post-publication peer review. For some, post-publication peer review is simply shifting pre-publication peer review to after an article's release [10]. For others, it's any evaluation of an article that is similar to pre-publication peer review. Post-publication peer review overlaps with post-publication commenting, but does not encompass all of that activity.

Post-Publication Commenting

Many associate post-publication commentary with only the negative "yin" of criticism, correction, retraction, and failed replication. It is essential to prevent research-led error, harm, and futile studies. But there is a vital positive "yang" aspect, too, incorporating research aftercare [11]. Answers to questions may be critical for other studies, for adequate research assessment and synthesis, and for considering practice and policy implications [12]. Discussion can build, apply, connect, and update ideas and ongoing work.

For some, though, the success of post-publication commentary is concerned only with the "yin" of correction and retraction. For others, post-publication evaluation only "works" if it occurs for all articles, making pre-publication peer review redundant. From these perspectives,

post-publication evaluation would always be shortchanged, and be seen to fall short. However, success includes rescuing important work from obscurity, and building work and capacity, not just tearing it down. Updating is at least as critical as correction to improving published research.

Furthermore, the scientific evidence base for effects of routine pre-publication peer review on article quality remains weak [13]. Pre-publication peer review can also worsen the quality of research, as when peer reviewers demand unplanned analyses of clinical trials [14]. With an oversaturation of publication in many areas, assessing it all only exacerbates the waste. Post-publication review faces the same problems.

Cultural Challenges to Post-Publication Activity

Many are wary or worse about post-publication culture. For some, any un-peer-reviewed response to peer-reviewed work is impertinent, and the Internet's removal of constraints to adding both substantive and trivial post-publication commentary to the public space is hard to accept. The Internet has also increased the quantity of incivility out in public view (Figure 1).

Disputes between scientists have always been common, and it has always been the case that "in the bitter social conflict that ensues, the standards governing behavior

Citation: Bastian H (2014) A Stronger Post-Publication Culture Is Needed for Better Science. PLoS Med 11(12): e1001772. doi:10.1371/journal.pmed.1001772

Published December 30, 2014

Funding: HB has received funding from the Intramural Research Program of the National Center for Biotechnology Information at the National Library of Medicine, National Institutes of Health. The funders had no role in study design, data collection and analysis, decision to publish, or preparation of the manuscript.

Competing Interests: HB is a member of the Editorial Board of *PLOS Medicine*, and lead editor for PubMed Commons, a forum for scientific discourse.

* Email: hilda.bastian@nih.gov

Provenance: Commissioned; not externally peer reviewed

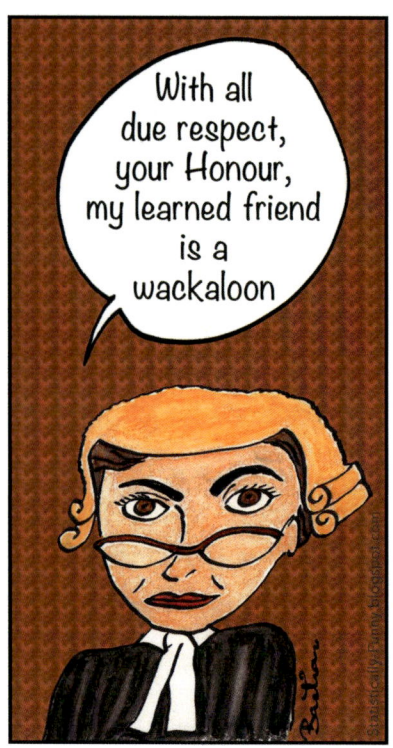

Figure 1. The melding of Internet culture and traditional communication. (Wackaloon: Internet slang for a kook; believed to derive from wacky and loon [33].) doi:10.1371/journal.pmed.1001772.g001

deteriorate" [15]. According to sociologist Robert Merton, the example of Edmond Halley calling another astronomer a "lazy and malicious thief" in the 17th century was, and remains, more commonplace than aberrant [15]. He saw these conflicts as arising from the same "deep devotion to the advancement of knowledge" that fuels the passion for engaging in intellectual labor. We need to study and improve the way we communicate and cope with our errors and criticisms of our work.

The fear of repercussions for junior scientists in particular is high. This fear lies at the heart of the contentious issue of anonymous post-publication commenting.

Some argue, though, that the risks for young scientists of openly commenting on others' work do not necessarily outweigh the advantages of visibility and recognition [16].

Even if the cost is reticence about participating, I believe the balance tips towards the requirement for transparency. Readers need to be able to judge whether writers are commenting outside their areas of expertise. Concerned readers need to have a chance of recognizing writers who have conflicts of interest, or be able to investigate whether or not potential conflicts exist.

However, addressing the obstacle to scientific progress posed by social dominance and aggression is a critical cultural issue, and not only—or even necessarily predominantly—for young researchers. Stereotype threat (anticipating discrimination) and other social issues may deter women scientists and other groups from commenting, too. Social influences can make women less talkative and less assertive than men in mixed gender groups [17], especially where "participants' concerns for self-presentation are heightened" [18].

Women scientists seem to be underrepresented in science activities that make their reflections public. In some fields and countries at least, women may still publish less [19–21], present less at conferences [22,23], and blog less [24,25]. A small body of research since the 1990s has identified some disturbingly low rates of participation by women as peer reviewers [26–28], though double-blind peer review might increase women's participation [29].

During the first year of PubMed Commons, less than 20% of those commenting were women. Research on gender bias in research and editorial peer review has been somewhat reassuring [26,27,30]. But the subject of this research has been the effect on publication fairness. The effect of under-participation on the development of confidence with the core

science career skill of formulating valuable and effective critique was not considered.

I don't think that anonymity is a good solution. We need to consider skill development in critiquing research [13,31]. That may also be valuable for those who are not scientific peers, but have contributions to make [32]. Developing a much more encouraging communication climate about errors and weaknesses of scientific communication is critical. This situation reminds me of the imperative identified decades ago to create a safety and quality culture in hospitals. A mature culture of responsiveness to complaints and problem identification is as much a prerequisite for research quality improvement as it was in health care.

Rewards for substantive intellectual effort post-publication and for the aftercare of research publications and sharing of data would help. Formal recognition is also necessary to undo the perverse incentive for authors to keep important insights and additional data until a subsequent publication. Such delays can last for months, if not years.

Passive consumption of scientific papers, and the withholding of adequate information by authors, cannot advance science. Thinking and talking about our responses to research reports is still science's vibrant and compelling intellectual core. Capturing that post-publication intellectual effort more rigorously is essential for better science.

Acknowledgments

The views expressed are personal, and do not necessarily reflect those of the National Institutes of Health. My views and knowledge on post-publication evaluation have benefited greatly from ongoing discussions with David Lipman and Melissa Vaught.

Author Contributions

Wrote the first draft of the manuscript: HB. Wrote the paper: HB. ICMJE criteria for authorship read and met: HB. Agree with manuscript results and conclusions: HB.

References

1. Collins FS, Tabak LA (2014) Policy: NIH plans to enhance reproducibility. Nature 505: 612–613. Available: http://www.nature.com/news/policy-nih-plans-to-enhance-reproducibility-1.14586. Accessed 30 October 2014.

2. Ioannidis JP (2014) How to make more published research true. PLoS Med 11: e1001747. Available: http://www.plosmedicine.org/article/info%3Adoi%2F10.1371%2Fjournal.pmed.1001747. Accessed 30 October 2014.

3. Glasziou P, Altman DG, Bossuyt P, Boutron I, Clarke M, et al. (2014) Reducing waste from incomplete or unusable reports of biomedical research. Lancet 383: 267–276. Available: http://

www.thelancet.com/journals/lancet/article/PIIS0140-6736(13)62228-X/fulltext. Accessed 30 October 2014.

4. Kronick DA (1984) Literature of the life sciences: the historical background. Bull NY Acad Med 60: 857–875. Available: http://www.ncbi.nlm.nih.gov/pmc/articles/PMC1911798/. Accessed 30 October 2014.

5. The PLOS Medicine Editors 2013) Getting closer to a fully correctable and connected research literature. PLoS Med 10: e1001408. Available: http://www.plosmedicine.org/article/info%3Adoi%2F10.1371%2Fjournal.pmed.1001408. Accessed 30 October 2014.

6. Haynes RB, Cotoi C, Holland J, Walters L, Wilczynski N, et al. (2006) Second-order peer review of the medical literature for practitioners. JAMA 295: 1801–1808. Available: http://jama.jamanetwork.com/article.aspx?articleid=202708. Accessed 30 October 2014.

7. NHS Centre for Reviews and Dissemination (2002) The Database of Abstracts of Reviews of Effects (DARE). Eff Matters 6: 1–4. Available: http://www.york.ac.uk/inst/crd/EM/em62.pdf. Accessed 30 October 2014.

8. Van Noorden R (2014 Mar 14) The new dilemma of online peer review: too many places to post? Nature News Blog. Available: http://blogs.

nature.com/news/2014/03/the-new-dilemma-of-online-peer-review-too-many-places-to-post.html. Accessed 30 October 2014.

9. National Center for Biotechnology Information (2014) PubMed Commons. Available: http://www.ncbi.nlm.nih.gov/pubmedcommons/. Accessed 30 October 2014.

10. Hunter J (2012) Post-publication peer review: opening up scientific conversation. Front Comput Neurosci 6: 63. Available: http://journal.frontiersin.org/Journal/10.3389/fncom.2012.00063/full. Accessed 30 October 2014.

11. Rennie D (1998) Freedom and responsibility in medical publication: setting the balance right. JAMA 280: 300–302. Available: http://jama.jamanetwork.com/article.aspx?articleid=187765. Accessed 30 October 2014.

12. Hoffmann TC, Glasziou PP, Boutron I, Milne R, Perera R, et al. (2014) Better reporting of interventions: template for intervention description and replication (TIDieR) checklist and guide. BMJ 348: g1687. Available: http://www.bmj.com/content/348/bmj.g1687.long. Accessed 30 October 2014.

13. Jefferson T, Rudin M, Brodney Folse S, Davidoff F (2007) Editorial peer review for improving the quality of reports of biomedical studies. Cochrane Database Syst Rev 2007: MR000016.

14. Hopewell S, Collins GS, Boutron I, Yu LM, Cook J, et al. (2014) Impact of peer review on reports of randomized trials published in open peer review journals: retrospective before and after study. BMJ 349: g4145. Available: http://www.bmj.com/content/349/bmj.g4145.long. Accessed 30 October 2014.

15. Merton RK (1963) The ambivalence of scientists. Bull Johns Hopkins Hosp 112: 77–97.

16. Goetz A (2014) Reexamining reviewer anonymity—more costs than benefits. Open Science Collaboration. Available: http://osc.centerforopenscience.org/2014/10/22/reexamining-reviewer-anonymity/. Accessed 30 October 2014.

17. Leaper C, Robnett RD (2011) Women are more likely than men to use tentative language, aren't they? A meta-analysis testing for gender differences and moderators. Psychol Women Q 35: 129–142.

18. Leaper C, Ayres MM (2007) A meta-analytic review of gender variations in adults' language use: talkativeness, affiliative speech, and assertive speech. Pers Soc Psychol Rev 11: 328.

19. Jagsi R, Guancial EA, Worobey CC, Henault LE, Chang Y, et al. (2006) The "gender gap" in authorship of academic medical literature—a 35-year perspective. N Engl J Med 355: 281–287. Available: http://www.nejm.org/doi/full/10.1056/NEJMsa053910. Accessed 30 October 2014.

20. Kelly CD, Jennions MD (2006) The h index and career assessment by numbers. Trends Ecol Evol 21: 167–170.

21. Larivière V, Ni C, Gingras Y, Cronin B, Sugimoto CR (2013) Bibliometrics: global gender disparities in science. Nature 504: 211–213. Available: http://www.nature.com/news/bibliometrics-global-gender-disparities-in-science-1.14321. Accessed 30 October 2014.

22. Isbell LA, Young TP, Harcourt AH (2012) Stag parties linger: continued gender bias in a female-rich scientific discipline. PLoS ONE 7: e49682. Available: http://www.plosone.org/article/info%3Adoi%2F10.1371%2Fjournal.pone.0049682. Accessed 30 October 2014.

23. Jones TM, Fanson KV, Lanfear R, Symonds MR, Higgie M (2014) Gender differences in conference presentations: a consequence of self-selection? PeerJ 2: e627. Available: https://peerj.com/articles/627/. Accessed 30 October 2014.

24. Shema H, Bar-Ilan J, Thelwall M (2012) Research blogs and the discussion of scholarly information. PLoS ONE 7: e35869. Available: http://www.plosone.org/article/info%3Adoi%2F10.1371%2Fjournal.pone.0035869. Accessed 30 October 2014.

25. Maynard A (2014 Mar 24) Gender balance in science blog networks: how has the male/female science blogger ration changed over the past three and a half years? Medium. Available: https://medium.com/2020-science-comms/gender-balance-in-science-blog-networks-71a1efb79958. Accessed 30 October 2014.

26. Gilbert JR, Williams ES, Lundberg GD (1994) Is there gender bias in JAMA's peer review process? JAMA 272: 139–142.

27. Zuber MA (2001) [Underrepresentation of women among peer reviewers and textbook authors in medicine in Germany.] Med Klin (Munich) 96: 173–180.

28. Mutz R, Bornmann L, Daniel HD (2012) Does gender matter in grant peer review? Z Psychol 220: 121–129. Available: http://www.ncbi.nlm.nih.gov/pmc/articles/PMC3414231/. Accessed 30 October 2014.

29. Budden AE, Tregenza T, Aarssen LW, Koricheva J, Leimu R (2008) Double-blind review favours increased representation of female authors. Trends Ecol Evol 23: 4–6.

30. Grod ON, Budden AE, Tregenza, Koricheva J, Leimu R, et al. (2008) Systematic variation in reviewer practice according to country and gender in the field of ecology and evolution. PLoS ONE 3: e3202. Available: http://www.plosone.org/article/info%3Adoi%2F10.1371%2Fjournal.pone.0003202. Accessed 30 October 2014.

31. Galipeau J, Moher D, Skidmore B, Campbell C, Hendry P, et al. (2013) Systematic review of the effectiveness of training programs in writing for scholarly publication, journal editing, and manuscript peer review (protocol). Syst Rev 2: 41. Available: http://www.systematicreviewsjournal.com/content/2/1/41. Accessed 30 October 2014.

32. Bastian H (2003) Non-peer review: consumer involvement in research review. In Godlee F, Jefferson T, editors. Peer review in health sciences, 2nd edition. London: BMJ Books. pp. 248–262.

33. Wiktionary (2014) Wackaloon. Available: https://en.wiktionary.org/w/index.php?title=wackaloon&oldid=21379171. Accessed 4 November 2014.

8.3 Reviewing Post-Publication Peer Review

Paul Knoepfler

Knoepfler, P. Reviewing post-publication peer review. *Trends in Genetics* 31(3), 221–223 (2015). © 2015 Elsevier Ltd. All rights reserved.

Reprinted with permission from Elsevier.

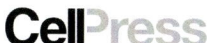

Scientific Life

Reviewing post-publication peer review

Paul Knoepfler[1,2,3]

[1] Department of Cell Biology and Human Anatomy, University of California Davis School of Medicine, 4303 Tupper Hall, Davis, CA 95616, USA
[2] Genome Center, University of California Davis School of Medicine, 451 Health Sciences Drive, Davis, CA 95616, USA
[3] Institute of Pediatric Regenerative Medicine, Shriners Hospital For Children Northern California, 2425 Stockton Boulevard, Sacramento, CA 95817, USA

Post-publication peer review (PPPR) is transforming how the life sciences community evaluates published manuscripts and data. Unsurprisingly, however, PPPR is experiencing growing pains, and some elements of the process distinct from standard pre-publication review remain controversial. I discuss the rapid evolution of PPPR, its impact, and the challenges associated with it.

The rise of PPPR in the life sciences

PPPR is having a rapidly increasing impact on science. Rigorous post-publication assessment of papers is crucial for the filtering and potential integration of meritorious data into the scientific collective. It is also faster than traditional forms of evaluation. Despite this, adoption of PPPR has been relatively slow in the life sciences. As early as 2007 Todd Gibson suggested that post-publication review could be helpful [1], but it did not really catch on until recently. It now shows every sign of continuing to have a major influence on the life sciences.

This rapid growth in PPPR has been made possible by several key factors. First, although cultural acceptance within the life science community of PPPR had consistently been rather minimal for decades, it has grown substantially in the past few years, largely due to the broader, perhaps generational shift towards the Internet culture. Second, PPPR is also gaining traction because of the wider availability of popular web platforms where the review can readily take place, such as Faculty of 1000 (F1000), ResearchGate, and PubPeer, as well as blogs (Table 1). The US National Institutes of Health (NIH) is even getting into the act. PubMed Commons now allows and even encourages comments on any article in the database. Sometimes PPPR even happens in real time on social media platforms such as Twitter. Websites that are wholly or in part dedicated to PPPR are popular and influential, as evidenced by their relatively high ranking on the web, which is often similar to or higher than that of journal websites (Table 1).

Together, these factors have shifted laboratory journal club type discussions of new papers out of the confines of conference rooms into the public domain online where commentary can be rapidly disseminated and discussions with any interested individual can be facilitated. Although a quantitative assessment of the influence of this invigorated

post-publication review in the life sciences is currently difficult [2], direct observations 'in the field' of the phenomenon suggest a strongly growing influence. For example, numerous article retractions and corrections have been catalyzed by PPPR, attracting the attention of journal editors, and some authors are directly responding to criticisms in the same online platforms in the public domain.

Fast and furious?

In the stem cell field there has been significant debate over so-called 'ground state pluripotency' of human cells and the role of the factor MBD3 (methyl-CpG-binding domain protein 3) in cellular reprogramming to make induced pluripotent stem cells (IPSC). Surprisingly, much of that debate has played out on PubPeer (dubbed the 'stem cell shoot out' https://pubpeer.com/topics/1/2B2B490DD36C55707411830 470926D), as well as on bioRxiv, a preprint server for biology, where PPPR is occurring as well. The two main scientists involved in this debate, Jose Silva and Jacob Hanna, are engaged in an almost real-time, public PPPR and scientific interaction (http://biorxiv.org/content/early/2015/01/16/ 013904) that seems unprecedented in biology. Hanna has even publicly addressed specific criticisms of his papers and as a result submitted corrections to journals (https:// pubpeer.com/publications/C278F3DE939616C4ADBD B9C15DB268#fb21519) only weeks or months after the issues were first raised via PPPR, demonstrating the extraordinary speed at which this process can catalyze concrete outcomes.

Another illustrative recent example of problematic issues in science being resolved strikingly fast largely via PPPR also comes from the stem cell arena in the form of the stimulus-triggered acquisition of pluripotency (STAP) cell case. In late January 2014, two papers on so-called STAP cells were published in *Nature* reporting a seemingly too good to be true method of cellular reprogramming [3,4]. On PubPeer and other sites, including my own blog, the STAP story quickly started to unravel, ultimately leading to the retraction of those papers and correction of the scientific record with an unprecedented rapidity of only a few months (Table 1) [5,6]. If the STAP cell papers had been published 5 or 10 years ago, I believe it would have taken several years for the record to be corrected. In the meantime valuable resources would have been squandered on STAP and trainee careers redirected to work on STAP could have been in serious jeopardy. Fortunately that did not happen, and I believe that PPPR deserves much of the credit.

Corresponding author: Knoepfler, P. (knoepfler@ucdavis.edu).

0168-9525/

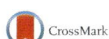

Table 1. Ranking and influence of PPPR sites and blogs

	Started	MozRank[a]	Link	Notes
F1000	2002	5.958	http://www.f1000.com	Early adopter, focused on positive reviews
Tree of Life Blog	2005	5.407	http://phylogenomics.blogspot.com/	Jonathan Eisen blog, some PPPR
RRResearch	2006	5.01	http://rrresearch.fieldofscience.com/	Rosie Redfield blog, debunked arsenic life
ResearchGate	2008	6.387	http://www.researchgate.net/	Community focused, non-anonymous
Wiring the Brain	2009	5.008	http://www.wiringthebrain.com/	Kevin Mitchell brain research-focused blog
Knoepfler Blog	2010	5.261	http://www.ipscell.com	Author's blog
PubPeer	2012	4.601	http://www.pubpeer.com	Largely anonymous post-publication review site
PubMed Commons	2013	6.718	http://www.ncbi.nlm.nih.gov/pubmedcommons/	NIH moderated venue for post-publication comments
bioRxiv	2014	5.102	http://biorxiv.org/	Pre-print server that includes PPPR
Trends in Genetics	–	4.52	http://www.cell.com/trends/genetics/home	Example reference site for MozRank

[a]The MozRank tool is an indicator of online authority and popularity in which higher numbers reflect relatively higher predicted impact. MozRank data shown are from February 2015.

Certainly, problematic life science and a corrective role for PPPR are not limited to the stem cell field. Another valuable, earlier example is the 'arsenic life' story. Scientist Felisa Wolfe-Simon at the US National Aeronautics and Space Administration (NASA) led a team reporting that they had found a microorganism that could live on arsenic instead of phosphorous. The work was eventually published in *Science* in 2011 [7]. Both in PPPR on her blog (Table 1) and in traditional publication format [8], Rosie Redfield debunked the arsenic life story in a rapid manner that limited the negative fallout from the flawed science. Even so, it is notable that the original arsenic life paper in *Science* has to date not been retracted or even corrected.

Although a clear majority of respondents to a poll I carried out on attitudes regarding PPPR was generally positive about it, a minority expressed concern over a 'gotcha' mentality (http://www.ipscell.com/2015/01/thumbs-up-for-post-pub-review-in-poll-dissenters-fault-gotcha-mentality/). Indeed, the vast majority of PPPR is negative and sometimes intensely so. In part this inclination may not be surprising given that many view it as a corrective mechanism for dealing with hyped science and inadequacies of standard peer review, particularly for high-profile papers that are perceived to have been given a 'soft' review. A potential example is the first paper on successful human therapeutic cloning, which was published in *Cell* after only a 4 day review process; it contained numerous image duplications rapidly identified on PubPeer (http://news.sciencemag.org/people-events/2013/05/cell-investigating-breakthrough-stem-cell-paper) [9].

Challenges for PPPR

A difficult issue frequently raised regarding PPPR that enables the 'gotcha' mentality that surfaces at times is the fact that the reviewers who participate are often anonymous. Although anonymity protects reviewers during both pre- and post-publication peer review from potential retaliation from authors, there is also a possible cost associated with anonymity. Some anonymous participants in PPPR feel emboldened to cross the line to engage in non-constructive criticism. In some cases PPPR comments have seemed targeted at specific individuals, and negative comments about researchers have even been sent to

institutions – with negative repercussions leading to litigation against PubPeer (http://news.sciencemag.org/scientific-community/2014/10/researcher-files-lawsuit-over-anonymous-pubpeer-comments). It would be beneficial if more post-publication reviews noted the strengths of papers, and this does occur at times on blogs and on sites such as F1000, but realistically PPPR is likely to continue to be negative more often than not. The scientific community needs to consider how this inclination could limit the positive impact of PPPR and brainstorm ways to balance this culture.

These types of issues likely take place in pre-publication review as well, but in principle the fact that editors know the identity of the reviewers is a partial deterrent. In PPPR that safety net is at best incomplete, and often entirely inoperative, because commenter identities can be masked with pseudonyms and blocked IP addresses. Anonymity also can be a roadblock to fruitful give-and-take discussions between different scientists that largely depend on knowing with whom you are engaged. So-called 'sockpuppetry', where commenters are not merely pseudonymous but sometimes actively take on false identities, or even the identities of real people, has also emerged at times in anonymous PPPR and has had a negative impact. Notably, there has recently been some constructive dialogue and brainstorming about ways to manage the potential downsides to anonymity, including better moderation, comment filtering, a set of standards, and a proposed PPPR editorial board (https://pubpeer.com/publications/F2A7891E2259B6AAD71E7F5BDA1849).

An additional concern about PPPR centers around the role that unpublished data could play. Commenters might be reluctant to publicly back-up challenges to published data with unpublished data of their own for fear of being scooped, by others or by themselves. For example, it remains unclear if a journal might consider the posting of such data online to be 'prior publication'. This very real concern limits the extent of data-based give-and-take during PPPR.

The power of a new paradigm in peer review

Skeptics or outright opponents of PPPR point out that science is already self-correcting, and that scientists can comment on each other's articles via what are supposed to be relatively rapid journal-based mechanisms such as

Scientific Life

Trends in Genetics May 2015, Vol. 31, No. 5

letters or similar formats. However, the reality is that such mechanisms are sometimes slow, and face their own challenges. For example, journals might be reluctant [10] to publish such responses if they challenge research that the journal has published, which might in some cases even lead to retractions, because no journal is likely to want to see increased retraction numbers. In the STAP case, a response article rebutting the original findings was submitted to *Nature* by Kenneth Lee, but the journal rejected it without clearly articulating why; it was only later published elsewhere [11]. Although there could have been many valid reasons why *Nature* rejected the Lee piece, this example is indicative of the complex interplay between multiple stakeholders that can in some cases tend to slow down this type of journal-centered post-publication communication, a limitation that is largely avoided in the dynamic interactions that post-publication review so nicely facilitates.

Rapid PPPR is here to stay, and, if anything, it is only likely to grow in influence and speed. A case has been made that, despite the hurdles remaining, PPPR will improve the quality of research and reduce waste in science [12]. I agree with that sentiment. Ultimately the goal is to make science more efficient, accurate, and reproducible. However, that does not mean that the evolution of PPPR will be painless or simple. Instead it is likely to be a fascinating rollercoaster ride with many twists awaiting us along the way. Hang on.

References
1 Gibson, T.A. (2007) Post-publication review could aid skills and quality. *Nature* 448, 408
2 Eyre-Walker, A. and Stoletzki, N. (2013) The assessment of science: the relative merits of post-publication review, the impact factor, and the number of citations. *PLoS Biol.* 11, e1001675
3 Obokata, H. *et al.* (2014) Bidirectional developmental potential in reprogrammed cells with acquired pluripotency. *Nature* 505, 676–680
4 Obokata, H. *et al.* (2014) Stimulus-triggered fate conversion of somatic cells into pluripotency. *Nature* 505, 641–647
5 Obokata, H. *et al.* (2014) Retraction: bidirectional developmental potential in reprogrammed cells with acquired pluripotency. *Nature* 511, 112
6 Obokata, H. *et al.* (2014) Retraction: stimulus-triggered fate conversion of somatic cells into pluripotency. *Nature* 511, 112
7 Wolfe-Simon, F. *et al.* (2011) A bacterium that can grow by using arsenic instead of phosphorus. *Science* 332, 1163–1166
8 Reaves, M.L. *et al.* (2012) Absence of detectable arsenate in DNA from arsenate-grown GFAJ-1 cells. *Science* 337, 470–473
9 Tachibana, M. *et al.* (2013) Human embryonic stem cells derived by somatic cell nuclear transfer. *Cell* 153, 1228–1238
10 Macbeth, F.R. (2010) Post-publication review. A tale of woe. *BMJ* 341, c5147
11 Tang, M.K. *et al.* (2014) Transient acid treatment cannot induce neonatal somatic cells to become pluripotent stem cells. *F1000Research* 3, 102
12 Bastian, H. (2014) A stronger post-publication culture is needed for better science. *PLoS Med.* 11, e1001772

References

Haug CJ. Peer-review fraud – hacking the scientific publication process. N Engl J Med. 2015;373(25):2393–5.

Manchikanti M, Kaye AD, Boswell M, Hirsch JA. Medical journal peer review: process and bias. Pain Physician. 2015;18:E1–14.

Siler K, Lee K, Bero L. Measuring the effectiveness of scientific gatekeeping. Proc Natl Acad Sci. 2015;112(2):360–5.

Strang D, Siler K. Revising as reframing: original submissions versus published papers in administrative science quarterly, 2005 to 2009. Sociol Theory. 2015;33(1):71–96.

Walker R, da Silva PR. Emerging trends in peer review – a survey. Front Neurosci. 2015;9(109):1–18. (*New channels of pre- and post-publication review are described.*)

Knoepfler P. Reviewing post-publication peer review. Trends Genet. 2015;31(5):221–3. (*Post-publication review, largely stimulated by the Internet, is thriving.*)

Vercellini P, Buggio L, Vigano P, Somigliana E. Peer review in medical journals: beyond quality of reports towards transparency and public scrutiny of the process. Eur J Intern Med. 2016;31:15–9. (*A number of measures could be instituted to improve peer review, including instituting more transparency.*)

Additional Suggested Reading

Ferreira C, et al. The evolution of peer review as a basis for scientific publication: directional selection towards a robust discipline? Biol Rev. 2016;91(3):597–610. (*Evolution of peer review as a method of quality control reflects a cultural lag.*)

Research Misconduct

Arthur L. Caplan and Barbara K. Redman

As defined by US federal regulations for Public Health Service (PHS) agencies (NIH, CDC, etc.), research misconduct means:

…fabrication, falsification, or plagiarism in proposing, performing, or reviewing research, or in reporting research results.

(a) Fabrication is making up data or results and recording or reporting them,
(b) Falsification is manipulating research materials, equipment, or processes or changing or omitting data or results such that the research is not accurately represented in the research record.
(c) Plagiarism is the appropriation of another person's ideas, processes, results, or words without giving appropriate credit.
(d) Research misconduct does not include honest error or differences of opinion.
42 CFR 93.103

A finding of research misconduct made under this part requires that—

(a) There be a significant departure from accepted practices of the relevant research community; and
(b) The misconduct be committed intentionally, knowingly, or recklessly; and
(c) The allegations be proven by a preponderance of the evidence.
42 CFR 93.104

Institutions receiving PHS research funds are responsible for developing policies and responding to allegations of research misconduct. These policies are administered by the US Office of Research Integrity (ORI). Similar policies govern funding by the National Science Foundation, although the processes used by the NSF are somewhat different.

Research misconduct policy has been developed in the wake of scandalous cases from all over the world in addition to falsification and fabrication, violations of subjects' protection, financial mismanagement and conflicts of interest. While the amount of research misconduct is unknown, pooled data from several surveys suggest that 2% of biomedical scientists admit to having fabricated or falsified at least once (Fanelli 2009), a level consistent with other fields such as economics (Necker 2014).

Research misconduct policies (or lack of them) vary widely across countries. For example, in the United Kingdom there are currently no statutory frameworks that regulate research integrity or sanction research misconduct except for those embedded in the regulation of the medical profession (Jacob 2016). The province of Quebec has issued guidelines for managing misconduct. Recently, Japan has established policies including monetary penalties to institutions (Asai et al. 2016). The majority of countries lack guidelines and a national organization to respond to allegations of research misconduct (Rasanen and Moore 2016).

Efforts to avoid and detect research misconduct are ongoing. Statistical anomalies in reported data can be suggestive of data fabrication/falsification. Currently, one of the most common forms of laboratory misconduct is image manipulation that does not match the original data (Shuchman 2016). Requiring shared, open, original data that can be subjected to replication by independent scientists may detect falsification, fabrication, and plagiarism (FFP). Protection of good faith complainants, also known as whistleblowers, from retaliation may encourage them to come forward and identify misconduct.

A. L. Caplan · B. K. Redman (✉)
New York University Langone Medical Center,
New York, NY, USA
e-mail: Arthur.Caplan@nyumc.org

© Springer International Publishing AG, part of Springer Nature 2018
A. L. Caplan, B. K. Redman (eds.), *Getting to Good*, https://doi.org/10.1007/978-3-319-51358-4_9

Advice: If you see what your think is FFP, document the evidence and then speak with a trusted source to verify your concerns. Be clear that changing data points, leaving data out, altering images - even if common in your field - may be considered FFP. Know if the professional society in your field has issued statements on research misconduct. Be aware of which institutional officials at your place of work are responsible for responding to concerns about research misconduct.

9.1   Shattuck Lecture: Misconduct in Medical Research

John D. Dingell

Dingell, J. Shattuck Lecture – Misconduct in Medical Research. *New England Journal of Medicine* 328(22), 1610–1615 (1993). Copyright © 1993 Massachusetts Medical Society. All rights reserved.

1610   THE NEW ENGLAND JOURNAL OF MEDICINE   June 3, 1993

SPECIAL ARTICLE

SHATTUCK LECTURE — MISCONDUCT IN MEDICAL RESEARCH

The Honorable John D. Dingell

ONE of the distinguishing characteristics of American society, noted long ago by Alexis de Tocqueville, has been optimism and a belief, bordering on faith, in progress. That characteristic is evident in our popular culture and in our politics. We recall — nostalgically — the 1939 New York World's Fair, the General Motors Parade of Progress, the can-do spirit of the New Frontier, and the hopes of the Great Society.

Our sometimes misplaced sense of optimism is at its core an expression of confidence in science and the scientific method. We believe that honest intellectual inquiry can lead us to theories or laws that, after testing and prodding, will yield truths that will light our path to the future.

For good reason, the public, through its elected representatives, has been willing to devote more and more resources to science and research. Despite the best efforts of the Reagan administration, public spending for research — and I grant that much of it was for defense — continued to rise in real and relative terms.

The foundation of public support for science, or for any public endeavor, is trust — in this case, trust that scientists and research institutions are engaged in the dispassionate search for truth. We are willing to spend great sums in the service of a higher value. And no value is believed to be more dear to a scientist than the truth.

Our support for science reflects our fascination with it. We avidly devour the news of the latest discoveries. Full sections of *The New York Times* and other newspapers are devoted to scientific coverage. The recent revelations about the big-bang theory of the cosmos led the network news broadcasts. When *60 Minutes* airs a story on a study detailing the health benefits of drinking red wine, shelves are emptied of wine and advertising campaigns are launched. Sitting in traffic listening to the radio, you are likely to hear a news story on the latest cholesterol study published in the *New England Journal of Medicine*.

Increasingly, in the modern era, cutting-edge scientific discoveries move rapidly from the laboratory to the legislature and the regulatory agencies. Scientists, hospitals, and institutes convene press conferences to publicize their findings and satisfy a public both eager for scientific advance and troubled by every new report of a threat to health and the environment. Scientific findings largely determine the agendas of govern-ment agencies with thousands of employees — the Environmental Protection Agency, the Food and Drug Administration, and the Occupational Safety and Health Administration, to name but a few.

In this climate, the publication of a paper claiming that a food additive causes cancer or that a building material retards the mental development of infants can trigger a massive public outcry and demands for government action. Americans are not a patient people. The public is rarely content to wait 5, 10, or 15 years for further research and study.

The consequences can be serious. A report that an additive causes cancer may drive a manufacturer out of business, throwing hundreds or thousands out of work. A report about the toxicity of paint or insulation can cause homeowners to spend thousands on testing kits (some of them fraudulent) and on the removal and replacement of the offending material. Housing units may even be closed, leaving low-income people homeless. School districts will strip carpet, paint, or insulation from buildings, leaving themselves unable to afford new textbooks.

Some of these regulatory actions will ultimately prove unwarranted; that is an inherent and understandable risk of relying on cutting-edge research. But there is a difference between honest error and various forms of misconduct, such as plagiarism and fraud. Blatant forms of misconduct attracted the interest of the Subcommittee on Oversight and Investigations of the U.S. House of Representatives, and the subcommittee's interest has in turn caused the scientific community to pay attention to the issue of misconduct.

What, exactly, is misconduct? Legitimate questions have been raised about precisely how misconduct should be defined, but the subcommittee has never sought to explore the outer reaches of this concept. We leave those efforts to others. Rather, we have looked only at clear-cut cases involving fabrication, falsification, or plagiarism. We follow these cases carefully to see how the system deals with them, how speedily complaints are addressed, and how fairly and accurately issues are resolved. Although many cases are referred to our subcommittee, once preliminary investigation establishes that only differences of opinion or mistakes arising from honest error are at stake, we leave the matter to the scientific community. The subcommittee does not assess the substance of scientific theories themselves, concentrating instead on such factual matters as whether data really exist and whether allegations have been seriously and properly handled.

Subcommittee investigators have pursued cases in which published papers claimed to present data that,

Presented as the 102nd Shattuck Lecture to the Annual Meeting of the Massachusetts Medical Society in Boston on May 9, 1992.

Congressman Dingell (D-Mich.) is chairman of the Subcommittee on Oversight and Investigations of the U.S. House of Representatives.

in fact, never existed or described the results of experiments that, in reality, had never been performed. They have pursued cases in which researchers abused the peer-review process to obtain advance copies of papers and appropriated their insights or accomplishments. They have followed cases in which evidence of misconduct was covered up or whitewashed by institutions apparently more interested in the appearance of integrity than in the reality of it.

Unfortunately, the nature and the purpose of the subcommittee's inquiries have been misrepresented, particularly by persons who have everything to lose from the truth. Some have said that we are putting science itself on trial. That is false. Others have said that we seek to punish people for honest errors. That is false. It has been suggested that we do not understand that mistakes are inevitable in scientific inquiry. False again.

Science is the search for truth at the boundaries of what is known about the natural world. It is a difficult and perplexing task, one in which we make progress by finding and correcting errors. In the uncharted waters of discovery, mistakes are bound to happen. To condemn scientific error would be tantamount to stopping scientific progress.

There is a corollary to the inevitability of errors, however, and it is that when errors are recognized, scientists have a duty to make them known. A "no fault" process of recognizing and correcting error is essential to progress. But in some of the cases examined by the subcommittee, this proposition was turned on its head: it was said that since errors are inevitable, there is no need to acknowledge or correct them.

For a time, the Subcommittee on Oversight and Investigations was excoriated as a band of philistines incapable of understanding science and as a troop of inquisitors engaged in a senseless witch hunt. Indeed, some of the more intemperate accounts portrayed the very concept of scientific independence as under siege by the subcommittee's efforts to uncover the truth.

As a result of this campaign, at times orchestrated for profit by public-relations firms, the subcommittee was deluged with well-meaning but misinformed letters urging us to leave scientists and universities alone. (Many advised that we go after corrupt defense contractors, a suggestion more amusing to us than to General Dynamics, Northrop, or TRW, all of which were the subjects of extensive subcommittee investigations. In fact, those are among the investigations for which we are best known.) Despite this barrage of criticism, the subcommittee has persisted, because what is at stake is too important to abandon.

Why are the inquiries by our subcommittee so important? I have already mentioned the policy implications, but there is another, equally important reason. We have an obligation to the American taxpayer. As chairman of an oversight subcommittee with responsibility for the National Institutes of Health (NIH), I have a duty to see that taxpayer dollars appropriated for scientific research are actually used for research.

Currently, taxpayers spend about $9 billion per year on the NIH. Most biomedical research performed in this country is federally funded.

Every time a researcher takes taxpayer money and publishes fabricated, falsified, or plagiarized findings, the taxpayer has in effect been swindled. Furthermore, given our budget deficit, there is never enough money to go around. Each dollar wasted on a dishonest researcher is a dollar that might have gone to another, more worthy candidate who might have made a real contribution. In short, there is an opportunity cost for each grant that is abused.

Moreover, the nature of scientists and the scientific method is to build on the interesting results obtained by others. Every paper published with fabricated or falsified data will spur other scientists using still other federal grants to try to replicate or extend the results, wasting even more money and time.

How widespread, then, is the problem of scientific misconduct? The only honest answer is that we do not know. One indicator is a study conducted by a small research group called the Acadia Institute.[1,2] This study found that approximately 40 percent of the deans of the nation's major graduate schools knew of confirmed cases of scientific misconduct occurring in their own institutions within the previous five years.

Another indicator is the recent survey sponsored by the American Association for the Advancement of Science.[3] It found that 27 percent of a group of scientists surveyed said that they had personally encountered, during the previous 10 years, research that they suspected was falsified, fabricated, or plagiarized. Those 27 percent reported, on average, witnessing at least two such incidents. Furthermore, close to half of the respondents said that the incidence of fraud was on the rise, whereas only 2 percent thought it was declining. More than half characterized university investigations of misconduct as lax. Although I would not characterize these findings as scientific, it is difficult to call them inconsequential.

Equally notable, however, were the scientists' responses when asked what they had done about the misconduct they had recognized. The vast majority had done little or nothing. The few who took action generally confined themselves to discussing the incident privately with a few people. Only 2 percent brought the matter to the attention of the public. Ironically, although large numbers had seen misconduct, although virtually none who had seen it had acted, and although the majority viewed university investigations as ineffectual, nearly all claimed that scientists should monitor themselves and that outsiders should not become involved.

The subcommittee also found disturbing attitudes when we contacted some 20 leading scientists to solicit their views on misconduct. In private interviews, almost all these scientists cited examples of misconduct they had witnessed, whistle-blowers they had seen harassed, or other matters engendering concern. Yet none were willing to testify, write open letters, or even have their names used public-ly, for fear of retaliation.

Whether misconduct is widespread or not, let us examine the argument of those who say that miscon-duct need be taken seriously only if it is widespread. The suggestion that a single bank robbery need not be investigated unless and until it can be proved that that particular form of bank robbery is rampant would be correctly regarded as ludicrous. Believe it or not, I have found that the vast majority of members of Con-gress are honest. But does that mean that a particular member of Congress should not be investigated if there are allegations of wrongdoing? Of course not. Very simply, every professional — lawyer, journalist, mechanical engineer, member of Congress — has a clear ethical obligation to handle each and every alle-gation of misconduct fairly. My concern is that in the field of science, that has until recently not happened.

I am sorry to say that the case studies pursued by the subcommittee have provided still more evidence of the disturbing reality. My descriptions here are of ne-cessity quite condensed, but I urge all interested par-ties to obtain the subcommittee's hearing reports, which run approximately 1000 pages, for more detail.

One of the first cases to capture the subcommittee's attention was that of Dr. John Darsee of Harvard Medical School.[4,5] Dr. Darsee's federally supported research in cardiology and his long list of publications marked him as a rising star until it was discovered almost by chance that he had committed an act of fraud. Two investigations were conducted at the medi-cal school — the first by Dr. Darsee's immediate su-pervisor and department chairman, and the second by a committee of faculty members from Harvard and elsewhere that the dean had appointed. Both reported no misconduct in Darsee's published research. A third committee, appointed by the NIH, discovered a mas-sive fraud: the data for a number of Dr. Darsee's pub-lished experiments did not exist. This was particularly awkward for Harvard, which had maintained up to that point that its investigators had reviewed the data fully — the same data that later turned out not to exist.

Another major case involved Dr. Stephen E. Breun-ing, a professor at the University of Pittsburgh who had risen to national prominence as an expert on drug treatment for the mentally retarded.[5-7] Dr. Breuning's research purportedly showed that the condition of se-verely retarded children improved markedly when they were taken off certain tranquilizers. From 1979 to 1983, Dr. Breuning reportedly published a third of all the articles in his field. Some states changed their treatment protocols in response to his purported findings.

In 1983, however, in a letter to the National Insti-tute of Mental Health, Dr. Breuning's mentor, Dr. Robert Sprague, raised serious questions about the integrity of Dr. Breuning's research. The University of Pittsburgh investigated and reported to the govern-ment that it found no problem. The National Institute of Mental Health sat on the matter for years, and the whistle-blower, Dr. Sprague, suffered apparent repri-sals. During this three-year period, Dr. Breuning trav-eled the country propagating his theories further to an unknowing public. It turned out that, among other things, Dr. Breuning's data had in large part never existed and that subjects had not been tested. Dr. Sprague's allegations were eventually substantiated in almost every detail. Dr. Breuning eventually pled guilty to two felonies and served time in a halfway house. Yet even after Dr. Breuning was publicly un-masked, several scientific journals actually fought the efforts of coauthors to retract articles on which he had worked.

In a more recent case involving faculty members from Tufts University and the Massachusetts Insti-tute of Technology (MIT), a scientist named Dr. Margot O'Toole was vilified and effectively driven from her profession after she revealed that a paper in *Cell* coauthored by, among others, her supervisor, Dr. Thereza Imanishi-Kari, and Nobel laureate Dr. David Baltimore relied in large part on data that were falsified.[8-11] Senior scientists at both MIT and Tufts University contended that Dr. O'Toole's allegations were unfounded and reported that the paper was vir-tually error-free. These senior scientists informed Dr. O'Toole that the article could not be corrected be-cause any correction would damage Dr. Imanishi-Kari's career[5] and because the scientific literature was so full of error anyway that one more error would not matter. Dr. Baltimore himself said, in a letter to Dr. Herman Eisen, that he did not favor the retrac-tion of the paper because of possible adverse con-sequences for another scientist who had been listed as an author, even though he, Dr. Baltimore, admitted that the paper was grossly defective and that he would never fully trust Dr. Imanishi-Kari's work again. Even after forensic analysis by the Secret Service had established that the data Dr. Imanishi-Kari did have were largely a recent fabrication, she and her coauthors continued to portray themselves as innocent victims.

At the end of a lengthy investigation by the Of-fice of Scientific Integrity, Dr. Baltimore retracted the *Cell* article. He later resigned from the presidency of Rockefeller University. Still later, he announced his intention to retract the retraction. Dr. Imanishi-Kari came under prolonged investigation by a grand jury.[12-14]

In another case, involving the Cleveland Clinic, a researcher, Dr. Rameshwar K. Sharma, was ultimate-ly found to have falsified his grant application, but was initially exonerated by the clinic's own investi-gation on the strange theory that all he had done was engage in "anticipatory writing."[15] In anticipato-ry writing, a researcher claims to have already per-formed certain experiments and obtained certain data, and then justifies the false claims on the grounds that he or she "anticipated" being able to achieve the results at some point in the future.

It later emerged that the Cleveland Clinic's ready exoneration of the anticipatory writer had been based on a two- or three-hour inquiry in which no data were reviewed and no witnesses were interviewed. The person who handled this investigative effort, Dr. Bernadine Healy, now directs the NIH. Among her early actions in that post were efforts to undermine the Office of Scientific Integrity and compromise its independence — efforts that included inappropriate verbal attacks on a critical draft report and on the office itself, a demand that a second important draft report be rewritten, an unjustified attempt to initiate an investigation of one of the office's chief investigators, and an instruction that the office reverse its decision to remove a scientific-panel member who had failed to inform the office of a possibly serious conflict of interest.

Finally, there is the matter of Dr. Robert Gallo, the NIH's world-famous AIDS researcher. Because the subcommittee has not yet completed its investigation, I cannot tell you what our conclusion will be. I can say, however, that one of the things that puzzles and troubles us is Dr. Gallo's entanglement in a large number of unusual circumstances that he claims are misunderstandings and coincidences.

After Dr. Zaki Salahuddin, one of his longtime laboratory scientists, was convicted of a felony in connection with his activities at Dr. Gallo's laboratory, Dr. Gallo explained that he had been unaware of Dr. Salahuddin's activities. In short order, Dr. Prem Sarin, Dr. Gallo's deputy laboratory chief, was indicted for activities unrelated to those of Dr. Salahuddin but also stemming from work at the laboratory.[16,17] Dr. Gallo explained that he knew nothing of his deputy laboratory chief's misconduct and that these two separate criminal cases involving his laboratory scientists were unfortunate coincidences.

Then we learned that two subjects described in an article in the *Lancet* coauthored by Dr. Gallo and French researcher Dr. Daniel Zagury had died, but that Dr. Gallo had failed to report these deaths to the NIH as was required by grant regulations and had erroneously reported in the *Lancet* that he had observed no adverse reactions in the human subjects.[18,19] Dr. Gallo again had an explanation. He explained that the statement in the *Lancet* was an inadvertent error and that his failure to comply with NIH procedure was a result of unfamiliarity with the regulations — this despite some 20 years of employment at the NIH.

More recently, in the controversy over the AIDS blood test, Dr. Gallo is under investigation because of, among other things, allegations that statements he made in the patent application and thereafter in the patent dispute were deliberately misleading. Dr. Gallo first stated that the virus he used was definitely different from that used by the competing French team. When genetic sequencing proved that the viruses were identical, he suggested that the French must have taken his virus. When that claim was challenged, Dr. Gallo explained that there must have been an inadvertent contamination in his laboratory. Meanwhile, there were also questions about the cell line in which Dr. Gallo grew his viruses. Initially, Dr. Gallo seemed to suggest that the cell line was his own development. It eventually emerged that the cell line belonged to Dr. Adi Gazdar, a researcher at another NIH institute. Dr. Gallo explained that this was a misunderstanding and that he had never intended to deprive Dr. Gazdar of credit, but merely renamed the cell line for convenience.

This is a deeply troubling case. An eminent scientist who heads one of the most important laboratories in the world is embroiled, directly or indirectly, in many different serious situations, which Dr. Gallo himself invariably characterizes as inadvertent errors, miscommunications, and unfortunate coincidences. And the NIH's now defunct Office of Scientific Integrity found Dr. Gallo innocent of fraud or serious misconduct, a finding about which I had serious questions. We understand that the NIH itself receives millions of dollars each year in royalties from the blood test, but that should be no impediment to its assessing the charges against Dr. Gallo objectively.

Although the cases the subcommittee has examined differ considerably in their particulars, common threads run through them. First, in most cases, the dishonest scientist engaged in misconduct for years. Those in a position to know ignored the warning signs or turned a blind eye. Second, in nearly every case, the whistle-blower was treated badly, often far worse than the offender, for having put truth ahead of personal convenience or career advantage. Third, in virtually every case we examined, the internal procedures that are supposed to allow universities and other research institutions to police themselves failed. At best, internal investigations appeared careless and inept; at worst, they appeared to be conducted in bad faith. Fourth, the offices within the NIH that are responsible for monitoring issues of scientific integrity showed a marked disinclination to perform their job, a reluctance to pursue scientific-misconduct cases aggressively, a dilatoriness in developing evidence, and an overall lack of dedication to the goal of confronting scientific misconduct. Fifth, many prominent scientific-misconduct cases are accompanied by a barrage of erroneous and misleading reports in the media in which the long-suffering whistle-blower is labeled as vindictive and irresponsible, those investigating the allegations are lambasted as ignorant troublemakers, and blatant acts of dishonesty — such as the wholesale theft of another researcher's article or the fabrication of data — are trivialized as minor mistakes, misrepresented as differences of interpretation, or dismissed as mere communication problems.

What, then, can be done about misconduct in sci-

1614   THE NEW ENGLAND JOURNAL OF MEDICINE   June 3, 1993

ence? Every case of misconduct is difficult for those accused, for those making the allegations, for the institutions involved, for the funding agencies, and for the profession. To their credit, a great many scientists and professionals have begun addressing the issue. They realize that public esteem for science and scientists can only be harmed when ego and career are valued more highly than the accuracy of the scientific literature and the welfare of the public. The reality of scientific misconduct is painful for everyone who loves science and respects those who devote their lives to it — myself included. But if the reality is unpleasant, the solution is to change it.

Some have proposed that the problem be attacked with ethics courses for junior scientists. But no ethics seminar can counteract the example set by leading scientists who engage in misconduct or who excuse it in others. Dr. Margot O'Toole can tell you that it is often idealistic young scientists who pay the heaviest price for honorably seeking to protect the integrity of science.

Some have claimed that more "due process" is needed. Due process is certainly appropriate and desirable. But the problem is not so much the amount of process as its quality. It is difficult for a group of professors to investigate impartially someone who is a colleague and, in many instances, a personal friend. It is asking a great deal to hope that an institution will assiduously pursue charges that, if substantiated, may cause it embarrassment, bad publicity, and the loss of funds. In many instances, it is unrealistic to expect the NIH to investigate aggressively the possibility that it erred in its selection of grant recipients.

Who, then, should resolve allegations of misconduct? And what procedures should be followed? These questions are being debated intensely today, and I have no ready answer. Scientists and their institutions are better equipped than others to do this job, and I would greatly prefer to see the scientific community handle the problem. The worst place to resolve these questions is in a congressional hearing. Congressional hearings are rather blunt instruments, poorly suited to making fine distinctions of fact. They are a forum of last resort, whose function is to shine light on severe problems not being addressed. The subcommittee would not have needed to pursue any of the cases I have described here had the institutions and people involved pursued them properly from the start. I would go even further: there is absolutely no good reason why a congressional subcommittee should be doing a job that scientists can and should do themselves.

Encouraging science to police itself is far preferable to the alternatives. I have heard the phrase "science police" bandied about, and that is a ghastly idea. But with every Darsee or Breuning whose case is covered up or mishandled, pressure builds for such extreme measures. Scientists are allowed to monitor themselves on the theory that they are honorable and devoted to truth. They are granted considerable leeway

on the theory that their work is of transcendent value and serves the public good. Only so many times can prominent scientists refuse to correct an article on the grounds that a correction may hurt a wrongdoer's career or is not worth the trouble because the journals are riddled with error anyway, before the public begins to wonder why it should fund literature that scientists themselves treat with disrespect. Scientists need to understand that the best way, perhaps the only way, to avoid the threat of "science police" is for scientists themselves to show that they have the ability and the will to police themselves. It is a matter of morality, but also of self-interest.

I hope that the roots of my interest in this issue are understood, and not just the policy or budgetary roots. In 1943 my father, then a member of Congress from Michigan, cosponsored a pioneering bill on national health insurance, and throughout his career he was one of Congress's strongest supporters of federally funded research and of the NIH. My brother is a research scientist, and my wife devotes much time to efforts on behalf of medical research.

One of the most upsetting and wrongheaded criticisms of the subcommittee's work on scientific misconduct is the charge that it would cause young idealists to pursue careers elsewhere. In all too many of the cases with which we are familiar, young, idealistic scientists challenged the system and blew the whistle. We do not need courses in ethics to teach young scientists to be idealistic. We need institutions that will say to them, Don't be afraid to ask hard questions. Don't ever lose that idealism. After all, I remember what it was like to be a young, idealistic member of Congress.

I began this discussion by talking about our innate American sense of optimism. After years of fighting uphill battles, after accumulating layers of scar tissue, I may no longer believe in the perfectibility of human institutions or societies, but I do believe in their improvement. One of the most valuable tools we have toward that end is science.

ADDENDUM

Since I gave the Shattuck Lecture last year, judgments have been handed down in three of the cases I cited. In the case of Dr. Imanishi-Kari, in July 1992 the U.S. attorney in Baltimore formally declined to prosecute her. In statements to the press as well as in correspondence with the subcommittee and the Secret Service, U.S. Attorney Robert Bennett stressed that the declination was based on the difficulty of presenting the complex scientific facts to a lay jury, which would have to understand them fully to find guilt beyond a reasonable doubt in a criminal trial. Bennett emphasized that the declination was not an exoneration of David Baltimore or Thereza Imanishi-Kari, nor did it reflect doubt on the part of the prosecutor's office that the data had been falsified.

In the case of the Cleveland Clinic, the Office of Research Integrity of the Department of Health and

Human Services ruled late last year not only that the scientist, Dr. Sharma, had committed scientific misconduct, but also that the initial inquiry "lacked competence, thoroughness, and objectivity" and "was hurried and superficial."

After a six-day trial, a jury convicted Dr. Prem Sarin on July 8, 1992, on three counts of embezzlement and false statements to the NIH.

Finally, in the case of Dr. Robert Gallo, the Office of Research Integrity found last December that Dr. Gallo had intentionally misled the scientific community by claiming that he had not grown the lymphadenopathy-associated virus obtained from French investigators in a permanent cell line.

With respect to Dr. Gallo's service as a referee on a manuscript submitted to a journal by scientists from the Institut Pasteur, the Office of Research Integrity found that "Dr. Gallo's actions reflect Dr. Gallo's propensity to misrepresent and mislead in favor of his own research findings or hypotheses." The office also faulted Dr. Gallo's laboratory supervision, asserting that it "reflects irresponsible laboratory management that has permanently impaired the ability to trace the important steps taken" in Dr. Gallo's early AIDS research. The Office of Research Integrity noted that the importance for science and the public health of the work relating to AIDS "imposed an obligation in reporting the methodologies and results of this groundbreaking research" — an obligation, the office said, that Dr. Gallo "failed to meet."

I am indebted to Reid P.F. Stuntz, Peter D.H. Stockton, Bruce F. Chafin, Dennis Fitzgibbons, and Janina A. Jaruzelski for their assistance as congressional staff members in the subcommittee's investigations and the preparation of this lecture, and to Dr. Margot O'Toole, Dr. Ned Feder, Mr. Walter Stewart, Dr. Suzanne Hadley, and other subcommittee witnesses courageous enough to speak the truth, for their invaluable contributions to the subcommittee's work.

REFERENCES

1. Swazey JP, Louis KS, Anderson MS. University policies and ethical issues in research and graduate education: highlights of the CGS deans' survey. CGS Communicator 1989;22(3):1-3, 7-8.
2. Panel on Scientific Responsibility and the Conduct of Research. Responsible science: ensuring the integrity of the research process. Washington, D.C.: National Academy of Sciences, 1992:91-3.
3. Hamilton DP. In the trenches, doubts about scientific integrity. Science 1992;255:1636.
4. The brilliant John Darsee. In: Kohn A. False prophets: fraud and error in science and medicine. Oxford, England: Blackwell, 1986:84-8.
5. United States House of Representatives Subcommittee on Oversight and Investigations of the Committee on Energy and Commerce. Fraud in NIH grant programs. Washington, D.C.: Government Printing Office, 1989. (Serial no. 100-189.)
6. Willcox BL. Fraud in scientific research: the prosecutor's approach. Accountability 1992;2:139-51.
7. National Institute of Mental Health. Final report: investigation of alleged scientific misconduct on MH32206 and MH37449. 1987. Washington, D.C.: Office of Research Integrity, Department of Health and Human Services, 1987.
8. United States House of Representatives Subcommittee on Oversight and Investigations of the Committee on Energy and Commerce. Scientific fraud. Washington, D.C.: Government Printing Office, 1989. (Serial no. 101-64.)
9. *Idem.* Scientific fraud. Washington, D.C.: Government Printing Office, 1989. (Serial no. 101-187.)
10. Hilts PJ. Crucial research data in report biologist signed are held fake: Nobelist to ask retraction on paper he defended. New York Times. March 21, 1991:A1, B10.
11. Gosselin PG. U.S. finds fraud in research at MIT: report also assails Nobel laureate. Boston Globe. May 21, 1991:1, 25.
12. Hilts PJ. Researcher accused of fraud in her data will not be indicted: the prosecutor calls the case too complex to take to court. New York Times. July 14, 1992:C3.
13. Gladwell M. Prosecutors halt scientific fraud probe: researcher Baltimore claims vindication, plans to "unretract" paper. Washington Post. July 14, 1992:A3.
14. Wheeler DL. U.S. attorney will not seek indictment of researcher accused in "Baltimore case." Chron Higher Educ 1992;36(46):A7.
15. United States House of Representatives Subcommittee on Oversight and Investigations of the Committee on Energy and Commerce. Scientific fraud. Washington, D.C.: Government Printing Office, 1992. (Serial no. 102-75.)
16. Valentine PW. Ex-NIH official convicted. Washington Post. July 9, 1992:A12.
17. Crewdson J. Ex-Gallo aide guilty of pocketing $25,000. Chicago Tribune. July 8, 1992:4.
18. Picard O, Giral P, Defer MC, et al. AIDS vaccine therapy: phase I trial. Lancet 1990;336:179.
19. Crewdson J. U.S. agency faulted in AIDS vaccine study. Chicago Tribune. July 16, 1991:6.

9.2   Ethical Modernization: Research Misconduct and Research Ethics Reforms in Korea following the Hwang Affair

Jongyoung Kim and Kibeom Park

Kim, J, Park, K. Ethical modernization: Research misconduct and research ethics reforms in Korea following the Hwang affair. *Science and Engineering Ethics* 19, 355–380 (2013). © Springer Science+Business Media B.V. 2012. A SpringerNature imprint.

Sci Eng Ethics (2013) 19:355–380
DOI 10.1007/s11948-011-9341-8

ORIGINAL PAPER

Ethical Modernization: Research Misconduct and Research Ethics Reforms in Korea Following the Hwang Affair

Jongyoung Kim · Kibeom Park

Received: 15 October 2009 / Accepted: 23 February 2011 / Published online: 5 January 2012
© Springer Science+Business Media B.V. 2012

Abstract   The Hwang affair, a dramatic and far reaching instance of scientific fraud, shocked the world. This collective national failure prompted various organizations in Korea, including universities, regulatory agencies, and research associations, to engage in self-criticism and research ethics reforms. This paper aims, first, to document and review research misconduct perpetrated by Hwang and members of his research team, with particular attention to the agencies that failed to regulate and then supervise Hwang's research. The paper then examines the research ethics reforms introduced in the wake of this international scandal. After reviewing American and European research governance structures and policies, policy makers developed a mixed model mindful of its Korean context. The third part of the paper examines how research ethics reform is proactive (a response to shocking scientific misconduct and ensuing external criticism from the press and society) as well as reactive (identification of and adherence to national or international ethics standards). The last part deals with Korean society's response to the Hwang affair, which had the effect of a moral atomic bomb and has led to broad ethical reform in Korean society. We conceptualize this change as ethical modernization, through which the Korean public corrects the failures of a growth-oriented economic model for social progress, and attempts to create a more trustworthy and ethical society.

J. Kim (✉)
Department of Sociology, Kyung Hee University, 1 Hoegi-Dong,
Dongdaemun-Gu, Seoul 130-701, Republic of Korea
e-mail: jykim24@khu.ac.kr; kim24uiuc@hanmail.net

K. Park
Science and Technology Policy Institute, Specialty Construction Center,
26th floor, 375-70 Shindaebang-Dong, Dongjak-Gu, Seoul 156-714, Republic of Korea
e-mail: soli@stepi.re.kr

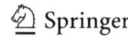 Springer

A. L. Caplan and B. K. Redman

Keywords   Hwang affair · Ethical modernization · Research ethics ·
Scientific misconduct · Regulation · Stem cell research

The Hwang affair, one of the biggest frauds in the history of science, needs to be scrutinized in order to prevent similar debacles. As various books and articles on the affair were published (Han 2006; Kang et al. 2006; Kakuk 2009), this vexing and perplexing case has elevated consciousness of research ethics around the world. In particular, the scientific community and regulatory agencies in Korea experienced a collective guilt, leading to self-criticism and research ethics reforms. Korea's full institutionalization of research ethics was initiated by this shocking scientific misconduct rather than by a self-correcting mechanism operating within the scientific community. Historical research on scientific misconduct and the institutionalization of research ethics provides similar incidents. For example, the role of German scientists and physicians in the brutal murder of people during World War II, and the subsequent Nuremberg trials, led researchers to take actions against scientific misconduct (Cornwell 2003; Ehrenfreund 2007). The Tuskegee affair was also triggered by press revelations of inhuman behavior at a time when some members of the scientific community believed that the search for medical and biological knowledge could justify the research team's treatment of research subjects (Reverby 2000; Jones 1993). These incidents led to implementation of a code of ethics, proper laws, and research ethics in the twentieth century. From an historical perspective, then, the Hwang affair is the most recent example of a pattern in which the self-correction mechanism of the scientific community failed to regulate scientific misconduct, and external criticism mounted to push science to reform its research ethics and its institutionalization.

Facts regarding the fraudulent research published by Hwang and colleagues in *Science* have been well documented by others (J. Kim 2006, 2009; H. S. Kim 2006; Gottweis and Triendle 2006). But they lack some details of the kinds of misconduct that occurred in Hwang's team because many key Korean documents and informants were not available to scholars outside of Korea (Prosecutors' Office 2006; Seoul National University Investigation Committee 2006a, b). Therefore, it is worthwhile to examine in detail the misconduct of Hwang and members of his research team, and the institutional failure to oversee and direct the research. Furthermore, it is necessary to examine how the Hwang affair has led to research ethics reform and broad ethical changes in Korea to understand a society's response to an ethical debacle. Therefore, compared to previous literature on the Hwang scandal, what is new in this paper is, first, examination of details of the misconduct reported by the prosecutor's office and Seoul National University, as well as our in-depth interviews with two whistle-blowers. Second, no prior publication has addressed the issue of research reform in Korea subsequent to the affair. The Korean academic and scientific communities have attempted to implement research ethics programs in several ways. From these efforts, we can learn something about how research ethics evolve in a society and about how participants in science and academia respond to an ethical debacle. Third, we will examine how the Hwang

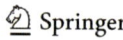 Springer

affair has led Korean society to reorganize its modernization project toward what we call ethical modernization. Discourses on the failure of Korean modernity and the need for a more ethical and fair society have penetrated a number of social realms, including academia, government, business, culture, religion, and even entertainment. Very rarely does scientific misconduct lead to questions about the entire modernization project of a society, and our analysis sheds light on how egregious scientific misconduct, interpreted as a national failure, has led to the reformation of that society's modernization project.

This paper consists of five parts. First, it details scientific misconduct by Hwang's team. Recent investigations in Korea have revealed how thoroughly Hwang's team violated research ethics. Second, we discuss the institutional failure of science governance. The roles of three responsible parties—the Korean government, media, and the scientific community—will be examined. Third, we examine the boom in research ethic discourse in Korea after the Hwang affair. This discourse has produced various types of suggestions and action to implement real policy changes. Fourth, we scrutinize policy changes in research ethics that have been implemented in three sectors: government regulatory agencies, university and research institutions, and academic and research associations. Finally, we discuss how the Hwang affair questions the dominant model of Korean modernization and how it has led to what we call "ethical modernization." Beyond academia and scientific fields, unethical misconduct in the areas of business, politics, and culture was revealed, and in response the media and general public set higher moral standards. At the same time, faith in economy-centered progress and resultism was subjected to close scrutiny. As a form of reflexive modernization, Korean society has undertaken ethical modernization to reform various institutions' programs as well as members' beliefs and attitudes.

For this study, we rely on four types of materials. First, previous literature on the Hwang affair provides diverse interpretations and perspectives helping us to understand the complex relationships among various actors in the affair. Second, the Korean prosecutor officer's report (Prosecutors' Office 2006) and Seoul National University's two reports (Seoul National University Investigation Committee 2006a, b) on Hwang's scientific misconduct are valuable resources identifying specific instances of scientific misconduct. Third, we conducted in-depth interviews, each lasting for about 2 h, with seven people who were directly involved in the Hwang affair.[1] Particularly important are the revelations of two "whistle-blowers" who worked in Hwang's laboratory and gave us detailed information about how Hwang's lab operated and how Hwang's working style and his lab culture contributed to the scientific misconduct. Last but not least, our study depends on research on research ethics published in Korea after the affair. We also conducted

---

[1] We interviewed two whistle-blowers (former researchers in Hwang's lab), Hak-Soo Han (Producer of PD Notebook who debunked the Hwang's scientific misconducts in a national television program in Korea), Byung-Soo Kim (activist who protected two whistle-blowers and helped Producer Han to battle against Hwang's ally), Jae-Kak Han (policy maker who ardently opposed Hwang's research before the affair), Yang-Koo Kang (journalist who also revealed Hwang's research misconducts during the affair) and Mr. M (activist who organized anti-Hwang protesters). All interviews are recorded and transcribed in verbatim.

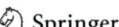 Springer

various types of research on this subject, including survey research, ethnography, and policy reports. Finally, we synthesize information from these multiple sources and perspectives to analyze Hwang's scientific misconduct and the ensuing diverse reactions from Korean society.

"Devil's Means with Angel's End": Scientific Misconduct by Hwang's Team

Woo-Suk Hwang attracted world-wide renown after publishing papers in 2004 and 2005 on cloning human stem cell lines in *Science* magazine (Hwang et al. 2004, 2005). Hwang, who became at the height of his popularity the most famous and influential person in Korea, established connections with the president of South Korea, politicians, CEOs, and leading scientists (Kang et al. 2006; J. Kim 2006). The Korean government, pronouncing him "the Supreme Scientist," gave him millions of dollars in funding. The Korean media were frantic, praising his diligence, humility, and perseverance; they depicted him as a national hero, and Hwang enjoyed rock-star status in Korea (Park et al. 2009). The scientific community, especially in the field of biotechnology [BT], used Hwang's research to gain research funding and social legitimacy. Laypeople influenced by strong feelings of national pride and hopes for a promising future inspired by stem cell research were proud of him because his accomplishment brought global recognition of Korea's scientific excellence (J. Kim 2009).

Meanwhile, after Hwang's 2005 publication in *Science*, his former senior researcher, who was the second author of the 2004 *Science* paper, quit his position, and then contacted "PD Notebook," a long-running and famous investigational program sponsored by the Munhwa Broadcasting Corporation (MBC) that has publicized various social problems as well as cases of corruption and injustice (Han 2006). From October of 2005 to May of 2006, the Hwang network and "PD Notebook" battled in several dramatic rounds over accusations of unethical acquisitions of eggs, data fabrication, mismanagement of lab members, and conflicts of interest, thus begetting tremendous shocks and controversies. Eventually, Hwang and his scientific-political alliance collapsed. As the Hwang affair unfolded, Seoul National University [SNU] investigated allegations of Hwang's possible scientific misconduct and confirmed that no cloned human stem cell lines existed. Subsequently, the prosecutors' office examined the entire body of Hwang's work and announced that it had found detailed misconduct, indicting him in May of 2006. This section is mainly based on the two reports published by SNU (Seoul National University Investigation Committee 2006a, b) and the prosecutor's office (Prosecutors' Office 2006). It also makes use of two whistle-blowers' in-depth interviews to analyze the culture of scientific behavior in the Hwang affair.

SNU's report focused on the fabrication and falsification of Hwang's 2004 and 2005 *Science* papers and 2005 *Nature* paper. The investigational committee, which was formed on December 15, 2005, conducted its investigation for 26 days. It investigated a total of 58 people, and announced the results on January 10, 2006, revealing that both *Science* papers were fabricated. But it also found that the Hwang team's first *Nature* paper, regarding the cloned dog, SNUPPY, was genuine (Seoul

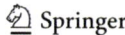 Springer

National University Investigation Committee 2006a, p. 46). After this report, Hwang resigned his position in SNU and made a public apology. The prosecutor's report is more intensive and extensive than that of SNU. On January 11, 2006, a special investigational team was formed within the prosecutor's office; it comprised 63 people altogether, including attorneys, police detectives, and supporting personnel (Prosecutors' Office 2006, p. 2). This investigation lasted for 120 days, much longer than SNU's 4 weeks of investigation. Because all Koreans were scrutinizing the results and the affair referred to highly scientific matters, the prosecutor's investigators were very cautious in coming to a conclusion. They subpoenaed and examined all but one of the co-authors who were responsible for the 2004 and 2005 *Science* papers. They also brought in hundreds of people who were involved in Hwang's research, as well as independent stem cell scientists who helped prosecutors understand and interpret Hwang's research. Altogether, they investigated 930 people, devoting extraordinary energy and time to Hwang himself. Finally, the investigational team announced its findings on May 12, 2006, indicting Hwang and five collaborators.

According to the two reports, Hwang's team violated many different principles of research ethics; its transgressions included data fabrication, gift authorship, unethical procedures on human subjects, mismanagement of funds, and exploitation of students and researchers. In short, the report revealed total and complete violation of research ethics. Here, we will summarize five types of research misconduct enacted by Hwang's team.

First, the two *Science* papers by Hwang's team were fabricated. The 2004 *Science* paper is somewhat controversial because scientists have debated whether the alleged first human embryonic stem cell line (so-called NT-1) is created by SCNT (denucleation of human egg and insertion of a nucleus from an ordinary somatic cell into the egg) or by parthenogenesis (development of an embryo without fertilization). SNU's supplementary report, published on May 1, 2006, focused on this problem and confirmed that the cell line is made by parthenogenesis. But another scientist who supported Hwang declared that Hwang had told him that the cell line was created using the SCNT method. Regardless of the truth of this declaration, four types of tests and their subsequent data were fabricated (Prosecutors' Office 2006, pp. 51–60): DNA fingerprinting, the teratoma experiment, the immunohistochemistry experiment, and genetic imprinting by PT-PCR (reverse transcriptase-polymerase chain reaction). These experiments are usually utilized to prove whether the cloned gene is a real one, but Hwang's team fabricated these tests primarily because they had failed to organize egg donors' identifications. The Hwang team did actually succeed in obtaining the stem cell line (NT-1), but they did not know the egg donor (Prosecutors' Office 2006, pp. 48–49). This very basic mistake caused chain reactions as Hwang's team ardently sought to create the first human embryonic stem cell line in the history of science. Hwang, who strongly believed in the existence of NT-1, ordered his researchers to fabricate data, and his researchers were also actively involved in building sham results (Prosecutors' Office 2006, pp. 52–57).

The data fabrication in Hwang's 2005 *Science* paper is preposterous in retrospect, because the 11 cloned stem cell lines were all sham, as were all of the experimental

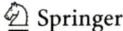 Springer

processes. Originally, in 2005, Hwang's team reported in *Science* that his team created 11 human embryonic stem cell lines with patients' nuclei. This implied that his team had raised efficiency and success rates, and the cloning process had been stabilized. But the whistle-blower who did not participate in this series of testing has speculated that the creation of 11 stem cell lines was impossible, based on his very close knowledge of the experiment (Prosecutors' Office 2006, pp. 115–116). With good reason, he suspected that Hwang's 2005 paper was a fake, and asked PD Notebook to investigate. This was the most important trigger in the revelation of Hwang's misconduct. As was revealed in the SNU's and prosecutor office's reports, Sun-Jong Kim, a senior researcher in Hwang's lab, and Dr. Hwang himself were actively engaged in fabricating experiments and data (Prosecutors' Office 2006, pp. 62–75). At that time, they also grew nine stem cell lines, but failed to gain cloning cells for various complicated reasons. Hwang "wanted to believe" that his team succeeded in creating 11 stem cell lines, and ordered his researchers to fabricate data and experiments. But, in fact, Sun-Jong Kim had made 2 stem cell lines, not by SCNT but by IVF, and fabricated the 9 other stem cell lines by manipulating pictures. Furthermore, the Hwang team fabricated DNA fingerprinting, the teratoma experiment, embryoid bodies, isotype matches, and karyotyping. According to the report, Sun-Jong Kim deceived Hwang about his success in creating two stem cell lines due to tremendous pressure from Hwang. Hwang stated that he wanted to win the stem cell competition with foreign scientists, and did not want to waste time.

Second, the two *Science* papers reveal many authorship problems. Of these, the most serious was the fact that Hwang assigned co-authorship of the 2004 *Science* paper to Ky-yong Park, advisor to the President of Korea for Science and Technology. Park was a leading figure who used her position to give Hwang's team policy favors and funding. For example, she was deeply involved in creating the "Supreme Scientist Program" with its multi-million dollar funding prize, which intended to select Dr Hwang as the first awardee. Consequently, Hwang was indeed named the "Supreme Scientist," but the program was abolished after the affair. The prosecutor's report added that two other people were also inappropriately named as co-authors of the 2004 *Science* paper (Prosecutors' Office 2006, pp. 60–61). Further, at least two people were included as co-authors of the 2005 *Science* paper, although they did not contribute to the research. The report also raised question about Schatten's role as corresponding author, since all he did for the 2005 paper was to respond to reviewers' comments and edit its English.[2]

Third, the Hwang affair also raised serious questions regarding its unethical process of dealing with human subjects. Korea's National Bioethics committee reported that Hwang's team used a total of 2,221 eggs from 121 women (National Bioethics Committee 2006, p. 9). These women were not told that their eggs would be used for Hwang's research, and many of them received no information about potential serious side effects of the ova extraction process. In other words, the egg

---

[2] Korea's prosecutor office attempted to investigate Schatten in a face-to-face setting, as they did with all Korean witnesses and suspects. But because Schatten resides in Pittsburgh in the US, the office did not have legal authority to bring him to Korea. Instead, the prosecutor sent him a questionnaire on his role in Hwang's research, and Schatten denied his involvement in Hwang's fraud.

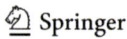

extraction team did not procure relevant "informed consent" from egg donors (National Bioethics Committee 2006, p. 20). In addition, 96 women were paid for their contributions, which suggests that Hwang's team took advantage of financially desperate women (Prosecutors' Office 2006, p. 112). Another disturbing part of this story, first identified by *Nature*, is that two women researchers in Hwang's lab also contributed their eggs because Hwang forced them to do so.

Fourth, Hwang's team mismanaged its research funds in several ways. The Korean government funding agencies decided to give a total of 40 million dollars to Hwang's lab from 2001 to 2005. Of this amount, the Hwang team had already spent 16 million dollars. The team also received 6 million dollars from supporting networks, most of which came from major Korean corporations. The problem is that Hwang diverted the research funds to his private bank accounts and 63 borrowed-name bank accounts, mixing his own money with research funds. Although Hwang insisted that he used his own bank account for his lab, prosecutors found that the account was used to pay for his wife's car, personal gifts, and donations to politicians (Prosecutors' Office 2006, p. 107). In addition, Hwang laundered the research funds through false-name bank accounts, which is illegal in Korea. Two junior professors, Hwang's right-hand men, also misused research funding in various ways.

Fifth, Hwang exploited his students and researchers. As we already mentioned, Hwang pushed female researchers to donate their eggs. He also usurped researcher's labor costs from the research fund. Usually, researchers were expected to wake up early and arrive at the lab by 6: 30 AM. Hwang's famous phrase—"Monday, Tuesday, Wednesday, Thursday, Friday, Friday, and Friday"—meant that his team was expected not to take days off. But when Hwang talked about these working conditions, as he did several times in the mass media, he depicted them as a sign of his researchers' diligence, and the media raised no questions. A subsequent in-depth interview with a whistle-blower revealed that the reality was quite different, however: Hwang's students hated Hwang intensely because of their working conditions. Many people wanted to escape Hwang's lab, and Hwang's three senior researchers joined Schatten at the University of Pittsburgh after making fraudulent stem cell lines.

After Hwang's research misconduct was revealed, he was fired from Seoul National University in April 2006 and indicted by the prosecutor's office in May 2006. Also indicted were Hwang's five collaborators, mainly due to their violation of the Bioethics and Safety Act and mismanagement of funds. Because of many people's involvement in the Hwang affair and the complicated nature of stem cell research, the first trial had 42 hearings, lasting almost 3 and one-half years. On October 16, 2009, the verdict stated that Dr. Hwang was guilty of embezzlement of research funds and violation of the Bioethics and Safety Act, punishing him with a suspended prison sentence (Segye Daily 2009). The ruling also clearly indicated that Dr. Hwang and his research collaborators had fabricated data published in *Science* and deceived the scientific community and general public (Hankyoreh 2009). Hwang appealed the ruling, but the appealing court also reached the same conclusion on December, 2010 (Hankuk Daily 2010).

We have summarized the major instances of the scientific misconduct of Hwang's team in order to ask how such a shocking, even crazy, development could

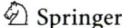

have transpired in Korea's most prestigious university. The whistle-blower describes Hwang's misconduct as "the devil's means with an angel's end." Hwang insisted that stem cell research would cure human disease, and he publicly hoped that a famous but disabled singer would stand up in the near future. Many disabled patients supported Hwang because of the great potential of stem cell research, and the Korean people saw the "angel's end" in Hwang's promise. In actual laboratory situations, however, the "devil's means" fabricated data, gave authorship to the powerful, violated ethical codes regarding human subjects, mismanaged funds, and exploited students and researchers. But this "devil's means" was linked with institutional failure to govern science appropriately.

The Institutional Failure of Science Governance: Government, Media, & Scientific Community

It seems obvious that the Hwang "affair" is not just a scientific fraud but a more institutional collapse that developed into a social crisis (Gottweis et al. 2009; Hong 2008). No scientific event received more social attention and controversy than the Hwang affair in Korea. Hwang's popularity peaked before October 2005; before that, major Korean social institutions had strongly supported Dr. Hwang without posing questions or criticism. In this section, we describe the three institutions most responsible in the Hwang affair: the Korean government, the media, and the scientific community.

Hwang was strongly supported by the Korean president, Moo-Hyun Roh (2003–2008), and his science and technology advisor, Ky-Yong Park (J. Kim 2006; S. Lee 2006). As we have mentioned, Park contrived to set up funding and regulatory policies favoring Hwang. President Roh visited Hwang's laboratory in person and promised to support him; Roh commented during this visit that he felt a sort of magic when he saw Hwang's stem cell technology (L. Kim 2008, p. 402). Later, when Dr. Hwang opened the World Stem Cell Hub in Korea, President Roh pledged that his government would manage ethical problems so as not to inhibit Dr. Hwang's research. Regardless of their party affiliations, many leading Korean politicians and presidential candidates supported Hwang. Hwang and his team members even received the Order of Science and Technology Merit from the president. With the President's backing, the National Bioethics Committee (NBC) was presided over by Hwang's lawyer, Sam-Sung Yang (Gottweis and Triendle 2006, p, 143). When the Bioethics and Biosafety Act, a new law on stem cell technology, was promulgated in 2005, the NBC and the Ministry of Health and Welfare gave an exclusive right to research on human stem cell lines to Hwang's team. When the Hwang scandal broke, the Korean president and government first defended Hwang, but as the evidence of scientific misconducts mounted they fell silent; to this day, the Korean government has never made a public apology regarding the Hwang affair.

In the same way, the Korean media contributed to the Hwang affair by producing enormous publicity as they extolled the dreams and promise inspired by stem cell research (Ban 2006; Chun 2006; H. W. Kim 2006; Haran and Kitzinger 2009).

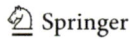

Various national television specials were devoted to Hwang and stem cell research. Without giving sufficient caution, such broadcasts depicted a rosy future in which illness and disease would be conquered by the stem cell revolution. Simultaneously, the media described Hwang as a diligent and sincere person who rose from a humble rural background to the top of the science world. His too-good-to-be-true character in the media drew enormous popular support from Korean people. His two papers appearing in *Science* magazine gave Hwang additional legitimacy and authority, and the Korean press raised no questions about his research. Meanwhile, Hwang's expressions of nationalism received applause from the media, thus disseminating feelings of nationalist pride through the popular imagination (Chekar and Kitzinger 2007). Hwang stated that his breakthrough had planted a Korean national flag on the summit of biotechnology in the US, and added that his stem cell line was "made in Korea" (Donga Science 2004). Korea's conservative and progressive media alike were captivated by his nationalist rhetoric, and described his every activity in a constant stream of articles and broadcasts. During the battle between Hwang and "PD Notebook," Korean media outlets such as *YTN*, *Chosun Daily*, and *Donga Daily* attacked "PD Notebook" for various reasons. For example, *YTN* accused "PD Notebook" of unethical journalism when a producer threatened Hwang's senior researcher in order to get important information about scientific misconduct (Han 2006, pp. 425–432). Rather than referring to social justice or the need to establish the scientific validity of Hwang's research, influential Korean newspapers appealed to Korean nationalism, arguing that other foreign scientists, especially in Japan and the US, would take over stem cell research if Koreans continued to attack Hwang (J. Kim 2006, p. 99). Furthermore, the Korean press revealed one whistleblowers' identity, and depicted him as a traitor rather than a person intent on telling the truth.

In addition, the scientific community—both within Korea and outside its borders—shares responsibility for the Hwang affair. Inside Korea, scientists forged a complete complicity with Hwang (Kang et al. 2006; S. Lee 2006; T. H. Kim 2008). Because Hwang's research promoted funding and popular support for science, many Korean scientists chose to remain silent about Hwang's research ethics. Scientists who were involved in the IRB examination of Hwang's research did not seriously investigate the Hwang's team's research process and its treatment of human subjects (Gottweis and Triendle 2006, p. 143). Instead, they indulged Hwang, and bioethicists even gave Hwang a measure of legitimacy when they failed to raise serious questions about his research. Even after Hwang's ethical problems regarding egg donation were revealed, the scientific community remained silent. During the battle between Hwang and "PD Notebook," the dominant factions in the scientific community were reluctant to raise their voices. Instead, it was the young and obscure scientists who were actively engaged in discovering the scientific misconduct that eventually brought Hwang down (Chong and Normile 2006).

For its part, the scientific community outside Korea was also guilty of neglect (Resnik et al. 2006): *Science* magazine mishandled peer review of Hwang's paper, and Schatten, Hwang's American partner, played a significant role in getting Hwang's paper accepted by the journal. Furthermore, *Science* magazine deliberately used Hwang's research to push the Bush government to change its policy opposing funding of stem-cell research (Han 2006). However, in the process of the Hwang affair, the

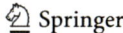

journal delivered details on how it proceeded and how stakeholders responded (Chong 2006; Wohn 2006). After the affair, it dealt not only with the trials of Hwang's team and Korean society's responses, but also with policy issues regarding scientific misconduct (Wohn and Normile 2006; Cho et al. 2006). In particular, Donald Kennedy, the editor-in-chief of *Science*, formed a committee to examine the review process on Hwang's papers. The committee reported that *Science* magazine followed the normal review process, but Hwang's intentional and deliberate fraud produced an unfortunate outcome (Brauman 2006). However, it also recommended a more cautious review procedure that includes audits of submitted manuscripts, formal risk-assessment, and enhanced data request. The committee report recognizes that because publication in a leading journal is motivated by self-interest, trust within the scientific community can be broken. More specifically, the review process should take extra caution concerning highly visible and influential research like stem cell research. The editor promised that the journal would set up a more rigorous and cautious review process to prevent scientific frauds like Hwang's (Kennedy 2006).

In sum, the Hwang affair occurred in the midst of total institutional failures of science governance. The Korean president and the Ministry of Science and Technology, the Korean media, and the scientific community all contributed to the worst scandal in the history of modern science. The coupling of one scientist's blind pursuit of fame and interest with the institutional collapse of science governance engendered a serious danger to science, the public, government, and the press.

Discourses on Research Ethics in Korea After the Hwang Affair

Scientific misconduct in the Hwang affair caused enormous shocks and aftermaths in Korean society. In those processes, Korean lay people and academics alike experienced other shocks. The Korean mass media alleged that several candidates for positions such as university chancellors, government ministers, and cabinet members were guilty of various sorts of misconduct, including duplicate publications, gift or honorary authorship, and mismanagement of funds (Editorial 2008). In fact, some cabinet members and chancellors resigned their positions. Doubts and suspicions regarding notable scientists and scholars were widespread, especially when some were appointed to high positions. In addition, the Korean press found that tens of professors had fabricated their doctoral degrees (Kim and Lee 2007). In one such notable case, which drew enormous attention, Jungah Shin, who was hired as an assistant professor by Dongguk University in Seoul in 2005, was found to have submitted forged documents indicating that she had received a Ph.D. from Yale University (Economy Daily 2007). More strikingly, a high-ranking senior director for the Korean president had supported her through his connection with Dongguk University's top officials. Shin was eventually arrested, facing several charges. Suddenly, Korean media also found that other very famous figures, including actors, actresses, and social notables, had forged their university degrees (Economy Today 2007). Corruption and dishonesty in the academy led to several rounds of public turmoil as famous social figures were found guilty of scientific misconduct or of forging degrees.

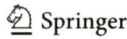

The Korean academy and scientific communities scrambled to understand the research ethics situation, and focused on how to repair misconduct and enhance research ethics in general (Ministry of Science and Education 2007; Ministry of Education, Science, and Technology 2008; Song 2007). Problems of research ethics had never drawn any serious attentions in the academy in South Korea, but suddenly it seemed that everyone in academia was talking about research ethics and misconduct regardless of disciplinary backgrounds. The discourses on research ethics that flourished in Korea after the Hwang affair can be assigned to four categories: (1) definition of scientific misconduct and responsible research practices, (2) the actual conditions and situations of research ethics in Korea, (3) the institutionalization of research ethics, and (4) education for research ethics. Some of those discourses were directly linked to research ethics policies and reforms.

First, scholars sought to define research ethics and misconduct. These discourses of definition diverged in two directions. On the one hand, they attempted to find broad definitions and boundaries. Many countries, including the US and European countries, have experience in implementing research ethics, and Korean scholars wanted to learn from them. The American definition of research misconduct focuses on FFP (fabrication, falsification, and plagiarism). Meanwhile, the general European definition, broader and more diverse, includes authorship problems, mismanagement of data, and misuse of funds. Korean scholars generally agreed that while the US definition is too narrow, the European definition is too broad and ambiguous to apply to Korean situations. Because the US definition focuses only on the writing process, many argued that it cannot regulate the other serious instances of research misconduct that occurred in the Hwang affair (Park 2006). As we will show later, when the Korean government implemented government orders regarding research ethics, it combined US and European definitions. On the other hand, commentators on research ethics focused on defining specific types of research misconduct, such as duplicate publishing and authorship problems as well as fabrication, falsification, and plagiarism (I. Lee 2007, 2009; Choi and Shin 2007). Duplicate publication received much attention because many Korean scientists and scholars have been unaware of this problem. In the April of 2010, on the Korean Broadcasting System (KBS), a national broadcast revealed that one-fourth of professors in the college of social science and the college of humanities at Seoul National University had duplicate publications during their publication career, for various reasons (Korean Broadcasting System 2010). For instance, simultaneous publication in Korean and English without quotation, practiced by some professors in the past, also can be defined as duplicate publication. Debates on specific types of research misconduct continue to this day in Korea.

Second, researchers examined actual cases and situations of research ethics and misconduct in South Korea. Along with the now-infamous Hwang affair, other less-legendary examples of research misconduct were studied and classified. For example, the Science and Technology Policy Institute in Korea (Park 2008, pp. 22–23) examined 364 research institutes, including universities, to determine frequency and kinds of research misconduct perpetrated between 2007 and the first half of 2008. According to this study, 39 cases were identified as examples of research misconduct, including duplicate publication (19), plagiarism (15),

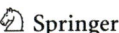

fabrication (5), authorship problem (5), and other research misconduct (6—cases can violate multiple rules). An overview of actual case studies concluded that the number of violations was not more serious than expected. This report also detailed how scientific misconducts occurred. After reviewing the case studies, many researchers agreed that Korea lacks the institutional supports and programs needed to foster research ethics. Before the Hwang affair, there were no research ethics institutions in Korea like the ORI (Office of Research Integrity) of the US that are empowered to investigate and adjudicate research misconduct. In addition, programs for educating about research ethics were almost non-existent before the Hwang affair. Furthermore, journals and academic associations did not implement codes of ethics, and few academic associations had set up guidelines for research ethics and ethical misconduct. This diagnosis led to the third type of discourse—the institutionalization of research ethics.

Scholars agreed that the Korean system lacks institutions that regulate and guide research ethics. They studied various countries' approaches to institutionalization, and discussed the ORI and European systems. Northern European countries' regulation systems, in particular, drew the attention of Korean scholars. They found that governments in the US and Northern European countries are more engaged in the research ethics, but those in most Western European countries, with some variation, do not have explicit involvement in research ethics regulation. Instead, funding organizations and research organizations guide and regulate research ethics and misconducts. Korean researchers compared the strength and weaknesses of several systems. While Pro-US scholars urged the government to be directly involved in creating and maintaining a central regulation system like the ORI of the US, others supported the Western European style (Park 2006). Despite this difference of opinion, Korean researchers agreed that the Korean system needs to institutionalize research ethics by making appropriate laws and creating the equivalents of an IRB, ORI, and ombudsperson program.

The fourth category of discourse, education on research ethics, received much attention. Many criticized the Korean system for its lack of educational programs teaching the nature of scientific misconduct and how researchers and scientists can promote good, responsible research practices. For example, students in universities had no concrete guides showing them how to avoid plagiarism, and many committed this type of misconduct because of their ignorance (W. Son 2007, p. 146). The discourse of education on research ethics displayed three types of interests: the current status of research education in Korea, the implementation of research ethics in a formal curriculum, and the problem of situating ethics education within disciplinary backgrounds. Many sought to determine how many research ethics programs existed in Korea: they found that many universities provided very few courses on the topic, reflecting the institutions' lack of genuine interest in research ethics. As a consequence, critics suggested that universities should implement research ethics education in their curricula (Oh 2008). Some argued that every student should be required to take such a course, while others proposed that only students in science and engineering programs should take it (K. Son 2007). Some scholars maintained that stand-alone courses that focus only on research ethics should be provided, while many believed that a number of basic courses in

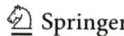 Springer

science and engineering should include some coverage of research ethics (Han et al. 2009, p. 37). In addition, many have pointed out that each discipline maintains a different type of research ethics. For instance, people in the social sciences and the humanities were more interested in plagiarism and duplicate publication, whereas researchers in biology were more concerned about the ethics related to using human and animal subjects (Kang et al. 2007; Shin 2008).

Within this buzz of research ethics discourse, Korean researchers considered every aspect of scientific ethics and misconduct. At no prior time was this discussion as intense as it has been in the past 6 years. Naturally, many urged institutional reforms of research ethics. Academics, the media, and government officials all agreed on this point, but they needed to negotiate the kinds of concrete programs, regulations, and institutions needed within a specifically Korean context and culture.

Research Ethics Reforms in Korea After the Hwang Affair

Due to the enormous criticism from all directions (academic members, the media, social critics, and even laypeople), institutions responsible for science governance and regulation were pressed to respond immediately after the Hwang affair. At the national level, the government was asked to set up regulations. At the local level, universities and academic associations were pushed to establish certain institutional devices to guide research ethics and educate their members on the subject. In this section, we will summarize responses to the call for research ethics reforms from three institutions—the Korean government, universities, and academic organizations.

The Korean government received intense criticism because of its connection with Hwang, even though the government turned its back on Hwang as the evidence of his scientific misconduct mounted (Kakuk 2009 ; Gottweis and Triendle 2006; J. Kim 2006). In response, the government convened leading professionals on research ethics, government policy makers, and academics to determine what government should do, but several problems arose (Park 2006). First, neither the government nor any research institution in Korea had comprehensively defined scientific misconduct. Second, the role of the government and its relationship with research institutions in research ethics have been debated because Korean scientists and academics wanted to protect academic freedom as well as keep government regulation of research to a minimum. Third, the question of what kinds of institutions, programs, and procedures are necessary proved to be a source of dissent among the three different groups represented at the meeting. The government's main regulation was articulated in official order number 236 by the Ministry of Science and Technology, "Guides for Securing Research Ethics," which was released on February 8, 2007 (Ministry of Science and Technology 2007). Universities and research institutes funded by the Korean government are required to follow this order in principle, but strict adherence to every detailed prescription is not mandated. The order consisted of three parts: a definition of research misconduct, the research institution's role in research misconduct and ethics, and a verification process and criteria for response to suspected research misconduct.

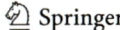 Springer

When they discussed the definition of scientific misconducts, the members of the committee agreed that the US definition of FFP is too narrow to apply in Korean contexts because the Hwang affair and other incidents revealed a wide variety of violations of scientific norms (Park 2006). For instance, authorship problems (gift authorship, honorary authorship), mentor–mentee problems, mismanagement of funds, and mistreatment of human subjects are the most common violations of research ethics. Also, mistreatment of whistleblowers became an important issue in the Hwang affair, as a result of which two whistleblowers lost their jobs, had their identities revealed, and were treated as traitors to their organization (D. Kim 2007). Meanwhile, the European definitions, such as the German version, are too broad to apply. The committee members reached agreement as they combined the US and the European models. As a result, the order defines scientific misconduct as follows: (1) fabrication, (2) falsification, (3) plagiarism, (4) inappropriate authorship, (5) activities that interfere with a research ethics committee's examination of research misconducts, or activities that harm a whistleblower, and (6) activities that go beyond generally acceptable norms in scientific community (Ministry of Science and Technology 2007, p. 1). These definitions are a "guide" for research institutions, and the sixth category provides flexibility as each organization builds its own definitions.

The government order also required universities and research institutes to create a committee that would verify or examine alleged scientific misconducts in their own institutions. The need to set up a central regulatory agency on scientific misconduct, like the ORI of the US, has been debated, but policy-makers concluded that this kind of government regulation might threaten academic freedom (O. Kim 2007; Park 2006). As an alternative, each research organization was required to set up an investigative committee to examine allegations of scientific misconduct (Ministry of Science and Technology 2007, pp. 1–2). Therefore, each university and research institute has its own "Research Integrity Committee," without having any centralized regulation agency in government sector like the ORI of the US.[3] The order also mandates that research organizations should provide appropriate educational programs for research ethics, protect whistleblowers, and secure the rights of researchers accused of misconduct.

The order also suggested guidelines for a verification process and criteria for investigation (Ministry of Science and Technology 2007, pp. 4–7). It proposes that investigation can be applicable only to misconduct occurring within the preceding 5 years. The burden of proof is on the investigative committee in the research organization. The investigation process is composed of three steps: preliminary inquiry, main investigation, and adjudication. The preliminary inquiry should start within 30 days after scientific misconduct is reported. If the alleged researcher admits his/her misconduct, it is not necessary to move into the next step of investigation. If s/he denies it and further investigation is needed, the main

---

[3] We cannot define the Korean system as a hybrid of US and European models, because Europe has various models of research ethics. It is safer to say that Korean policy makers and research ethics professionals pulled good models of various types of research ethics governance and combined them to fit the Korean context.

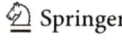 Springer

investigation is initiated. The main investigation should be completed within 6 months.

Because there were no official procedures and regulations on scientific misconduct before the Hwang affair, individual institutions did not know how to deal with it, but the government guidelines provided examples showing how each research institution should set up its research integrity committee and a program to examine scientific misconduct. A survey conducted by the Science and Technology Policy Institute revealed that more than 80% of researchers agreed that this government order is appropriate and its recommendations are satisfactory (Park 2009). They also agreed that of the several government actions regarding research ethics, this official order is the most important and necessary because it provided the definition of scientific misconduct and the process that each institution should follow (Park 2009, p. 36).

The government also established the Division of Research Integrity Team to regulate universities and research organizations (Park 2008, p. 11). This team does not have the right to investigate research misconduct, but functions to collect all types of information on research misconduct and coordinate policy choices and different opinions from the government, university, and academic organizations. In addition, responsible government agencies in the Ministry of Science and Technology and the Ministry of Human Resources and Developments produced books and bulletins to disseminate good research practices (Ministry of Science and Education 2007; Ministry of Education, Science, and Technology 2008). These agencies also made a concerted effort to educate middle- and high- school students on academic ethics (Yoo 2007). In addition, these agencies organized international symposiums on research ethics, through which directors of research ethics regulation agencies from foreign counties shared their experiences and policies with Korean policy makers. They also formed several types of research ethics forums to educate researchers in Korea. Other regulations to support the office order followed. An official order (22 June 2009) strongly recommended that researchers should write their research processes, not only to present any research misconduct, but also to promote responsibility (Ministry of Science, Technology, and Education 2009). Another government order (22 July 2009) requires that any government-funded research program must follow appropriate research procedures so as not to violate research ethics (Ministry of Government Legislation 2009). As for stem cell research, the Bioethics and Biosafety Act was revised (5 June 2008) (Korean National Assembly 2008). Previously, this law allowed only Hwang's team to conduct SCNT experiments in stem cell research with human eggs, but all clauses written to favor Hwang's research program were stripped from its language. In response to the problematic treatment of human subjects in Hwang's lab, the revision also strengthened the egg donor's legal rights to information regarding health consequences, and enhanced punishment for the illegal trafficking of human eggs and sperm.

Major Korean universities immediately followed the government official order. Although the order is not a law, major universities have been forced to abide by it in order to obtain research funds. While the order also gave flexible conditions to universities, universities that receive more than 10 million dollars per year are

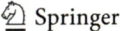 Springer

expected to create and maintain research integrity committees. Consequently, 27 universities established such a committee within 3 months after the order, and another 47 universities did so by September 30, 2007 (Hong 2007, pp. 21–22). The most recent study found that 75.7% of 4-year colleges in Korea had created a research integrity committee by September of 2008 (I. Lee 2008, p. 150). This finding suggests that the institutionalization of research ethics is quite successful, especially in view of the situation before the Hwang affair, when no such committee existed in Korea. The government order also gave universities latitude to set up their own procedures determining the composition and procedures of the committee, although it made some recommendations. All of the research integrity committees now present in Korean universities were established after the Hwang affair. The establishment of such committees in each university has sent strong signals to university members and enhanced university members' consciousness of research ethics.

Universities have also created educational programs to promote research ethics. A recent study revealed that 56.8% of 4-year colleges in Korea have educational programs on research ethics (W. Son 2007, p. 155). Some universities require undergraduate and graduate to take research ethics courses at the early stages of their programs. A comprehensive study found that large research universities have newly installed those kinds of programs. Generally speaking, there are two types of courses in the educational program (Han et al. 2009). The first type of course deals with research ethics directly, so that students learn various ethical situations and solutions. The second type of course deals with the broad relationship between science and society, or between engineering and society. In this process, students learn how society and their research activities are linked, and the range of their social responsibilities. Furthermore, in daily experimental situations and writing processes, advisors or mentors emphasize research ethics to students.

Academic and scientific associations have also reformed their policies on research ethics after the Hwang affair. The biggest movement came from an effort combining the largest and most influential organizations and most highly honored associations in Korea. On April 20, 2007, the Korean Federation of Science and Technology Society (540,766 members), the Korean Academy of Science and Technology, the National Academy Engineering of Korea, and the Korean branch of UNESCO declared the Code of Ethics for Scientists and Engineers (Science Times 2007). They clearly expressed that this declaration was motivated by the Hwang affair. This code broadly articulated scientists' and engineers' social responsibilities, and promoted good research practices. This declaration raised scientists' consciousness on research ethics.

Most of the journals and academic associations lacking a policy on research ethics before the Hwang affair have now instituted codes of ethics, research integrity committees, and educational programs. Journals linked with academic associations that already have those policies have revised and enhanced their codes of ethics. A recent study found that 85.4% of academic associations in Korea now have a code of ethics, and 63.3% have established their own research integrity committee (I. Lee 2008, p. 123). However, only 21.9% of these associations have implemented educational programs on research ethics (I. Lee 2008, p. 45).

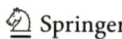

Meanwhile, many academic organizations have promoted good publication practices, noting that most instances of scientific misconduct occur in the process of writing and publication. For example, the Korean Association of Medical Journal Editors published and disseminated "Good Publication Guidelines for Medical Journals" to its members (January 31, 2008) (Korean Association of Medical Journal Editors 2008). Furthermore, some academic associations have convened special forums to promote research ethics and educate their members. For instance, in October of 2008, the Korean Chemical Society held a special symposium on research ethics to educate its members and emphasize the importance of research ethics (The Korean Chemical Society 2008). Virtually all academic associations in Korea have discussed and implemented new ethical codes and procedures.

Government agencies, universities, and academic members have also worked together to promote research ethics, and organized a number of domestic and international symposiums and conferences to discuss institutionalization of research ethics. Following is a list of the major symposiums and conferences held in Korea after the Hwang affair.

- International Symposium for Securing Research Ethics (June 14, 2007)
- Research Ethics Forum: Directions and Themes for Good Research Practice (October 23–31, 2007)
- Good Research Practice Forum: Education and Activities for Good Research Practice toward a Strong Research Nation (June 26, 2008)
- Good Research Practice 4th Forum: Challenges and Practices for Ensuring Research Ethics and toward a Developed Nation in Research Ethics (December 3, 2008)
- 2008 Workshop for Research Ethics Professionals (December 11–12, 2008)
- Research Ethics and the Value of Community (February 5, 2009)
- Good Research Can Be Guided by Research Ethics Education (December 2, 2009)
- 2010 Research Ethics Forum: Problems and Prospects for Establishing Research Ethics (July 30, 2010)
- Educational Program for the Research Ethics Professional as Professor (December 13–15, 2010)

In these meetings, all types of issues and problems were raised and discussed. Government officials also participated in the meetings in order to find solutions to problems of scientific misconduct in Korean academia, and foreign professionals were invited to describe their experiences and policies. As the meetings' titles indicate, the problem of research ethics has been connected with a "national" project. Because the Hwang affair was regarded as the failure of Korea, and not just the scientific misconduct of one scientist, Korean researchers and policy makers have strived to improve research ethics reform at the national level rather than just promoting individual scientists and academic organizations.

Though the efforts by responsible agencies are encouraging, the reforms have confronted several problems as they are applied to actual situations. Because each organization has its own definition of scientific misconduct, and its own investigative procedures despite the government guideline, determinations of

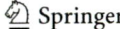 Springer

misconduct and the levels of punishment vary from one institution to the next (Park 2008). Also, because the committee members of research integrity had no procedural experience, and limited professional knowledge of research ethics (there was no such committee in Korean universities and academic organizations before the Hwang affair), the committee members were confused when they treated actual cases (Park 2008, pp. 101–103). Furthermore, top university officials and academic members still tend to conceal any alleged scientific misconduct for fear of tarnishing the university's or academic organization's reputation (Park 2008, pp. 104–105). As a result, the research integrity committee tends to devote less energy to investigation, and instead tries to minimize the alleged cases. For example, the press raised serious questions about the committee's activities and judgment. Because of the media pressure, some universities tightened their policies and imposed serious punishment on researchers who violated research ethics. The actual case study found that the self-correction process in academic organizations has limitations and that more comprehensive government actions will be needed. The current institutionalization of research ethics in Korea remains open to revisions and criticisms. Because of its short history, it will evolve to adjust to several confrontations and dissents. We cannot predict how it unfolds in the future, but it will receive continuous attention from the government, universities, and academic organizations. But the ethical reformation has gone beyond the academic and research world in Korea.

Ethical Modernization: The Failure of Korean Modernity and Its Reformulation

What is unique in the Hwang affair compared to other cases is that it made the Korean society question the whole modernization project the country has pursued. Korea has successfully achieved economic development within a relatively short time, but the country also experienced dictatorship, environmental deterioration, labor oppression, and moral hazards (Lie 2000). As the democratic system gradually has been implemented since 1987, many suppressed social spheres such as labor, gender, and the environment have become central issues, challenging economic modernity and developmentalism (Oh 1999). Thanks to social movements and political struggles in various sectors, the Korean society has addressed the problems of undemocratic cultures and various types of inequalities (Choi 2005). Even so, an economy-first policy and mentality has still dominated the country and people, and as a result violations of laws and ethics committed by prominent organizations and individuals have met with soft punishments, for a variety of reasons. For instance, the owners of Korean conglomerates (Chabol) broke a variety of laws, ranging from unlawful bequeathals to offspring and funding for politicians to illegal acquisition of real estate and environmental damages caused by industrial development (Ji 2006). Response to these violations has usually amounted to a slap on the wrist because Chabol has contributed to the Korean economy at large. Similar logics have applied to the Korean elites' misconduct in various realms. But the Hwang affair seriously questioned propensities for an economy-first policy, success without morality, and

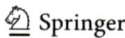

result-oriented centrism (J. Kim 2006; Gottweis and Kim 2010). In other words, the Hwang affair questioned the entire modernization project that Koreans have pursued.

The impact of the Hwang affair went beyond the meaning of scientific fraud because it seriously questioned the Korean society's pursuit of development and progress. Dr. Hwang had strongly linked his research to the Korean economy's progress as well as to the symbolic success of the Korean nation (S. Lee 2006). He specifically predicted that the Korean economy would benefit from stem cell technology (J. Kim 2006). The media then spread hopes and expectations that the technology would beget billions of dollars in profit (Chun 2006). Ordinary people regarded Dr. Hwang as a patriot who epitomized the superiority of Korean science as well as the future of the nation (J. Kim 2009). After revelation of the fraud, the whole nation confronted a moral crisis which debunked the collective complicity and led many to question the values of growth and development.

The Hwang affair involved various important institutions such as the Korean government, leading political elites, the economic sector, the media, and ordinary people. The Korean government has been criticized for its failure in biotech governance. But more importantly, its moral leadership was broken because when the fraud unfolded it still supported the fraudulent scientist. The media also received serious attacks because it disseminated nationalistic sentiment and unreasonable expectations, instead of critically examining Dr. Hwang's research (Han 2006; Ban 2006). Politicians were shameless, in that many of them chose to support Hwang since they still believed in the economic promise of stem cell research (Kang et al. 2006; S. Lee 2006). Hwang supporters, who were ordinary Korean citizens, formed a social movement to save the fraudulent scientist (J. Kim 2009). These moral failures produced a moral discourse that sought to reformulate the Korean nation as well as Koreans' ethics. We conceptualize this reform movement as ethical modernization, through which Koreans seriously question economy-centered growth and instead promote "social changes" for a more ethical and fair society.

The move for ethical reforms in Korean society after the Hwang affair, which started in the academic field, spread to economic, governmental, and public sectors, and then to the cultural and entertainment sector. Response to Hwang's fraud rippled from the academic field, which as the epicenter of the moral blast has been thoroughly scrutinized, leading to institutional ethical reforms in universities, research organizations, scientific associations, and journals (Park 2006; I. Lee 2008). The Hwang fraud produced a "culture of distrust" in which nobody can be fully trusted before being fully investigated and proven in public. Authorities involved in the Hwang affair ethically mishandled the research process, and as a consequence trust of authorities collapsed. For instance, because Hwang was a professor at Seoul National University, the most prestigious academic institution in Korea, the university lost credibility and authority. The institutional review board in Seoul National University did not work properly, and many collaborators in the same university were also involved in the fraud (Prosecutors' Office 2006; Seoul National University Investigation Committee 2006a). *Science* magazine also lost its authority and credibility in the eyes of the Korean public. Furthermore, it used

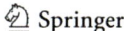 Springer

Hwang's paper politically to promote stem cell research in the US and to pressure the US federal government (Han 2006; Kang et al. 2006).

Higher ethical standards also started to be applied to broad social realms. Prior to the Hwang affair, misconduct in the economic sector often received soft punishment, and complicity among politicians, capitalists, journalists, judges, and the general public led to remarkably generous responses to economic and financial misconduct. But this quiet complicity was shattered after the Hwang affair as the public and media harshly attacked unethical management in the economic sector (Y. Kim 2010; Hankyoreh 2008). In consequence, businessmen and capitalists launched an "ethical management movement" through which they vowed not only to manage their companies ethically, but also to pursue public services for a better society beyond their interests (Hankuk Daily 2009). The discourse on "corporate social responsibility" gained popularity in the media and academia alike, and some CEOs who had pursued ethical management and contributed to social welfare rose to celebrity status (Han 2008; Hankuk Daily 2007). Owners' and CEOs' unethical behaviors in daily life also received serious scrutiny from media and ordinary people's online moral politics. For instance, Sueng-yon Kim, an owner of a Korean conglomerate, mobilized a gang to punish a group of men who hurt his son in a karaoke bar (Donga Daily 2007). The media and ordinary citizens attacked his unethical behavior, and eventually he was imprisoned. Another owner of a Korean chabol, who battered a worker with a baseball bat, was also arrested (Kyunghang Daily 2010). Those instances would hardly be visible before the Hwang affair because ethical standards and expectations for powerful corporations and owners were very low.

The political sector also received close scrutiny from the media and the general public. As doubts about ministers' and politicians' misconduct were publicly revealed, many of them resigned their positions (Donga Daily 2006; Hankuk Daily 2010). If they came from academia, their previous academic activities were questioned. Before the Hwang affair, this kind of scrutiny was unknown in Korea: not only were publication problems not taken seriously, but other types of illegal misconduct, such as embezzlement, speculative investment in real estate, and illegal inheritance, had prevailed in politicians' and top government officials' careers. Moral standards to evaluate politicians and top officials have been strengthened, and public and media investigations have become harsher. In this process, their unlawful behaviors and misconduct in public life created more distrust in Korean society. Finally, the current Korean president declared that Koreans should advance toward the "Fair Society" in which citizens should behave ethically to promote mutual trust and public goods (Kyunghang Daily 2010).

The cultural, spiritual, and entertainment sectors that influence ordinary people's attitudes and perceptions also experienced a moral crisis after revelations that many artists, actors, singers, religious leaders, and writers had faked their university degrees or stolen others' ideas on various occasions. In Korean society, where degrees function as a caste system, one's university diploma is highly sensitive because people tend to judge one's ability in terms of one's alma mater. Several dozen professors and researchers in the academic field were the subjects of serious investigations, and the investigations then moved from the academic to the cultural

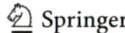 Springer

sector. As reporters and journalists started to examine high-profile figures, they found that notable actors and entertainers had also fabricated their diplomas and deceived the Korean public (Hankuk Daily 2007; Donga Daily 2007; Kwangju Daily 2007). A dozen such deceptions were publicly revealed, and most of those who were culpable apologized for their misconducts. For the first time, the media rigorously pursued cultural figures' alleged unethical past conduct. In addition, some singers and writers confronted plagiarism issues that produced heated controversies, which also led to public apologies (Hankuk Daily 2010). Even some famous religious leaders came under attack because they faked their degrees or professional accomplishments to enhance their public image (Seoul Daily 2007). In addition, citizens used the Internet to detect and unmask such misrepresentations. In this surveillance culture, everybody has become a watchdog who constantly keeps a vigilant and doubtful eye on others' unethical misconduct or illegal activities.

It is safe to say that after the Hwang affair the Korean public became more aware of, and more sensitive to, questions of ethics and morality; more than that, it functioned as a moral atomic bomb shattering a culture of unethical behavior in Korean society. It led to ethical modernization, through which the growth-centered modernization project would have to be reformulated to allow for creation of a more ethical and trustworthy society. We conceptualize ethical modernization as a form of reflexive modernity in which the previous economy- and industry-centered social projects are reformulated to become more ethical and fairer. Scholars have underscored that modernity is not a homogeneous whole, but instead has heterogeneous dimensions in which different societal realms have changed with different speeds, logics, and elements (Eisenstadt 2000; Kaya 2004; Gaonkar 1999). In this respect, Beck and Giddens have argued that modernization itself has been reformulated reflexively to correct its failures and thus reenergize the utopian agendas that modernization pursues (Beck et al. 1994; Beck 1992). From these perspectives on modernity, we can fairly conclude that the meaning of modernity has become multiplied and reformulated, depending on interpretation, differences in social background, and political contexts. The Hwang affair played a significant role in rethinking Korea's pathway of unethical success. The affair involved professors in the most renowned university, politicians, top corporations, and even the Korean president. It has shown the prevailing problems of Korean modernity, such as success without morality, a result-first culture, exploitation of the weak by the strong, and illegitimate connection. Korean society has felt an enduring shock, and reformers in many sectors have implemented ethical codes and regulations in hopes of changing a culture of mistrust. Turns to a more ethical and fairer society have gained momentum in Korean society, and Koreans have learned a significant lesson from a spectacular scientific fraud. In short, the unexpected consequence of the Hwang affair has been the call for ethical modernization in Korean society and beyond.

Summary

First, this paper detailed the instances of scientific misconduct perpetrated by Hwang's team, and connected them with the failure of science governance. Second,

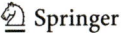 Springer

it analyzed the kinds of discourses on research ethics that arose and how regulatory agencies and academic organizations institutionalized research ethics. Third, this paper investigated how Korean society reformulated their pathway to modernity and attempted to build a more ethical and fairer society beyond the realm of research. Korean society, as well as the Korean scientific community, had never experienced the moral and social crisis caused by one of the biggest frauds in the history of science. This shock led to heated discussion of research ethics, and beyond science governance, Koreans have recognized the importance of ethics in the making of their own society.

The characteristics of the Hwang affair and its effects on the institutionalization of research ethics can be summarized as follows. The scientific misconduct in the Hwang affair surpassed imagination. It violated many different principles of research ethics. Neither the scientific community, nor the press, nor the government, nor the lay people of Korea had experienced a crisis in scientific ethics prior to the Hwang scandal, which led to social and moral crisis. Responsible institutions and the scientific community were forced to respond to preclude similar fraud in the future. Their findings revealed that the fraud resulted in large part from the absence of scientific governance. The Korean press and people also came to realize that scientific misconduct is not confined to rare cases, and that other notable people had also violated certain types of research ethics. The critique and request for reforms gained momentum and legitimacy. In particular, critiques issuing from outside the scientific community pushed it to supervise and self-correct its scientific activities. Because institutions for research ethics did not exist in Korea, reformers and policy-makers searched US and European models. In the actual implementation process, they drew on many models and policies, modifying each to suit Korean contexts and cultures. But the institutionalization of these reforms is not a magic bullet, and the ambiguity of regulations and of definitions of research ethics has led to confusion, requests for clarifications, and further revision. Despite these limitations, the reform and institutionalization of research ethics in Korea has achieved a certain level of success. A substantial majority of academic organizations have implemented a code of ethics, a research integrity committee, and educational programs on research ethics. This Korean case might shed light on how certain types of research ethics reforms and institutionalization arise, and how a shocking instance of scientific misconduct informs the normative structure of scientific activity and regulation.

But beyond academia, the Hwang affair forced the Korean public to investigate other social realms, where it also found various types of unethical misconduct. Notables, businessmen, and journalists, as well as scientists and scholars, had to apologize for their misconduct or resign from their positions. As a result of these moral crises, Korean society seriously questioned its modernization project. The previous model for modernization had been based upon an economy-first policy, a result-based centrism, and desire for success at whatever cost. But because of the Hwang affair, forgotten values such as morality, fairness, trust, and balance suddenly came to the forefront. A moral discourse claiming that Korean development should be reformulated to include ethical principles gained legitimacy. Attempts to reformulate Korean modernization in various sectors have subsequently taken place. Those reforms intend to correct the previous failures of Korean

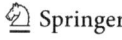

modernity, and to redirect it toward a new modernization—ethical modernization. Therefore, this study shows how the overall system failure in Korean led to the Hwang affair, and in turn how the Hwang affair propelled ethical modernization in society beyond merely correcting the governance of science.

Acknowledgments   We would like to thank reviewers for their valuable comments and criticisms. We are also grateful to Gardner Rogers who edited this paper. This research was funded by Science and Technology Policy Institute in Korea.

References

Ban, H. (2006). The Hwang affair and television news. In: Y. Won & K. Chun (Eds.), *The fall of myth, ghost of national interest: Woo Suk Hwang, PD notebook, and Korean journalism* (pp. 151–210). Seoul: Hanarae. (in Korean).

Beck, U. (1992). *Risk society: Toward a new modernity*. London: Sage Publications.

Beck, U., Giddens, A., & Lash, S. (1994). *Reflexive modernization*. Stanford, CA: Stanford University Press.

Brauman, J. (2006). *Science*'s response to the committee report on Hwang et al., *Science* 2004 and 2005. Supporting online material for "Responding to fraud." doi:10.1126/science.1137840.

Chekar, C., & Kitzinger, J. (2007). Science, patriotism, and discourses of nation and culture: reflections on the South Korean stem cell breakthroughs and scandals. *New Genetics and Society, 26*, 289–307.

Cho, M., McGee, G., & Magnus, D. (2006). Lessons of the stem cell scandal. *Science, 311*, 614–615.

Choi, J. (2005). *Democracy after democratization*. Seoul: Humanitas. (in Korean).

Choi, H., & Shin, J. (2007). Research misconduct and research norms. *Philosophy of Science, 10*, 103–126. (in Korean).

Chong, S. (2006). Investigations document still more problems for stem cell researchers. *Science, 311*, 754–755.

Chong, S., & Normile, D. (2006). How young Korean researchers helped unearth a scandal. *Science, 311*, 22–23.

Chun, K. (2006). Failures to protect public interest and democratic journalism's responsibility: The limitations of Korean journalism in the Hwang affair. In: S. Kim, K. Choi & S. Hong (Eds.), *The Hwang affair and Korean society* (pp. 151–180). Seoul: Nanam Publications. (in Korean).

Cornwell, J. (2003). *Hitler's scientists: Science, war and the devil's pact*. New York: Viking.

Donga Daily. (2006). *Byongjun Kim, the Minister of education and human resource development, resigned*. August 3, 2006.

Donga Daily. (2007). *Sungyon Kim, the CEO of Hanhwa Group, is arrested and jailed*. May 12, 2007 (in Korean).

Donga Daily. (2007). *Soojong Choi, a top actor, also faked his university degree*. August 22, 2007 (in Korean).

Donga Science. (2004). *Hwang Woo Suk says "We have placed a Korean flag at the summit of global bioengineering research."* February 19, 2004 (in Korean). http://news.dongascience.com/HTML/News/2004/02/19/20040219200000000001.

Economy Daily. (2007). *Jungah Shin's degrees are all fabricated*. July 12, 2007. (in Korean) http://news.mk.co.kr/outside/view.php?year=2007&no=366214.

Economy Today. (2007). *Twister of diploma fabrication reveals ugliness at the bottom*. December 22, 2007. (in Korean). http://www.eto.co.kr/?Code=20071222112152310&ts=124949.

Editorial. (2008). *Fabrication and plagiarism of papers cannot reach world-class universities*. March 2, 2008. Donga Daily. (in Korean) http://news.donga.com/fbin/output?n=200803020119.

Ehrenfreund, N. (2007). *The Nuremberg legacy: How the Nazi war crimes trials changed the course of history*. New York: Palgrave Macmillan.

Eisenstadt, S. N. (2000). Multiple modernities. *Daedalus, 129*, 1–29.

Gaonkar, D. (1999). On alternative modernities. *Public Culture, 11*(1), 1–18.

Gottweis, H., & Kim, B. (2010). Explaining Hwang-Gate: South Korean identity politics between bionationalism and globalization. *Science, Technology and Human Values, 35*(4), 501–524.

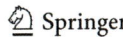 Springer

Gottweis, H., Salter, B., & Waldby, C. (2009). *The global politics of human embryonic stem cell science.* New York: Palgrave Macmillan.

Gottweis, H., & Triendle, R. (2006). South Korean policy failure and the Hwang debacle. *Nature Biotechnology, 24*, 141–143.

Han, H. (2006). *Folks, how can I tell you this news?: A journalist's investigation of the Hwang affair.* Seoul: Sahoepyungron. (in Korean).

Han, C. (2008). Corporate social responsibility: Today's assignment. *Studies on Corporate Law, 22*(1), 149–175. (in Korean).

Han, K., Hur, J., & Lee, C. (2009). Engineering ethics education: Issue and strategy. *Studies in Engineering Ethics, 12*, 31–41. (in Korean).

Hankuk Daily. (2007). *Missionary for ethical management: Kookhyun Moon, the CEO of Yuhan-Kimberly.* March 12, 2007. (in Korean).

Hankuk Daily. (2007). *Mihee Jang, a famous actress, faked her degree.* August 18, 2007. (in Korean).

Hankuk Daily. (2009). *In the era of CEO ordeal, ethical management rises.* September 26, 2009. (in Korean).

Hankuk Daily. (2010). *The appealing court also ruled to give Hwang a suspended prison sentence.* December 17, 2010. (in Korean).

Hankuk Daily. (2010). *Serial resignations of candidates for prime minister and ministers: Lie is lethal to politicians and cabinet members.* August 30, 2010. (in Korean).

Hankuk Daily. (2010). *Songwriter was guilty and jailed due to the plagiarism of Hyori Lee's song.* October 25, 2010. (in Korean).

Hankyoreh. (2008). *Socially responsible corporations that practice ethical and transparent business are rising.* June 21, 2008. (in Korean).

Hankyoreh. (2009). *The court ruled that Woo Suk Hwang fabricated papers: Hwang got a suspended prison sentence.* October 27, 2009. (in Korean).

Haran, J., & Kitzinger, J. (2009). Modest witnessing and managing the boundaries between science and media: A case study of breakthrough and scandal. *Public Understanding of Science, 18*(6), 634–652.

Hong, S. (2007). *Research on the program of establishing research ethics in the scientific and engineering community.* Seoul: Ministry of Science and Technology. (in Korean).

Hong, S. (2008). The Hwang scandal that "shook the world of science". *East Asian Science, Technology and Society, 2*(1), 1–7.

Hwang, W. S., et al. (2004). Evidence of a pluripotent human embryonic stem cell line derived from a cloned blastocyst. *Science, 303*, 1669–1674.

Hwang, W. S., et al. (2005). Patient-specific embryonic stem cells derived from human SCNT blastocysts. *Science, 308*, 1777–1783.

Ji, D. (2006). *Korean conglomerates.* Seoul: Samgakhyung Biz. (in Korean).

Jones, J. (1993). *Bad blood: The Tuskegee syphilis experiment* (2nd ed.). New York: Free Press.

Kakuk, P. (2009). The legacy of the Hwang case: Research Misconduct in biosciences. *Science and Engineering Ethics, 15*(4), 545–562.

Kang, Y., Kim, B., & Han, J. (2006). *Silence and frenzy: Seven years of documents on the Hwang affair.* Seoul: Humanitas. (in Korean).

Kang, E., Yi, S., & Cho, E. (2007). Current status of research ethics education for life scientists and its curriculum. *Journal of ELSI Studies, 5*, 35–55. (in Korean).

Kaya, I. (2004). Modernity, openness, interpretation: A perspective on multiple modernities. *Social Science Information, 43*(1), 35–57.

Kennedy, D. (2006). Editorial: Responding to fraud. *Science, 314*, 1353.

Kim, H. S. (2006). The cause of the Hwang affair and its social implications. *Economy and Society, 71*, 237–255. (in Korean).

Kim, J. (2006). Science as multiple social phenomena and Hwang Woo Suk as a techno-scientific alliance. *History Review, 74*, 82–114. (in Korean).

Kim, J. (2009). Public feeling for science: The Hwang affair and Hwang supporters. *Public Understanding of Science, 18*(6), 670–686.

Kim, H. W. (2006). *Mass media's strategy for covering uncertainty: Research on journalists covering Dr. Hwang's scandal.* Master's thesis. Sogang University. Seoul. Korea. (in Korean).

Kim, O. (2007). *Establishing and promoting research ethics: Cases of foreign universities.* Seoul: Ministry of Education and Human Resources Development. (in Korean).

Kim, D. (2007). A study on the researcher's whistle-blowing from an ethical perspective. *Ethics Studies, 66*, 27–49. (in Korean).

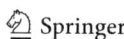

Kim, T. H. (2008). How could a scientist become a national celebrity: Nationalism and Hwang Woo-Suk scandal. *East Asian Science, Technology, and Society, 2*, 27–45.

Kim, L. (2008). Explaining the Hwang scandal: National scientific culture and its global relevance. *Science as Culture, 17*, 397–415.

Kim, Y. (2010). *Thinking about Samsung conglomerate.* Seoul: Sahoipyungron. (in Korean).

Kim, S., & Lee, W. (2007). Why and how are people seduced to fabricate their diplomas?: Various cases on diploma fabrication. *Joongang Monthly, 382*, 129–133. (in Korean).

Korean Association of Medical Journal Editors. (2008). *Good publication practice guidelines for medical journals.* Seoul: Aramedit. (in Korean).

Korean Broadcasting System. (2010). *Scholar and paper: Asking the way of study at Seoul National University.* Broadcasted on April 20, 2010. (in Korean).

Korean National Assembly. (2008). *Law number 9100: The bioethics and biosafety act.* June 5, 2008. (in Korean). http://www.law.go.kr/LSW/LsInfoP.do?lsiSeq=87356.

Kwangju Daily. (2007). *Younghun Ju, a famous songwriter, faked his degree and his explanation was also revealed as a lie.* August 22, 2007 (in Korean).

Kyunghang Daily. (2010). *Chabol's fist beyond the law.* December 14, 2010. (in Korean).

Kyunghang Daily. (2010). *President Lee's theory of the fair society.* September 7, 2010. (in Korean).

Lee, S. (2006a). *Hwang Soo Suk's nation.* Seoul: Bada Publishers. (in Korean).

Lee, I. (2007). The understanding of citation and plagiarism for establishment of the research ethics. *Ethics Research, 66*, 1–25. (in Korean).

Lee, I. (2008). *A survey on research ethics activities in Korea.* Seoul: Ministry of Education, Science, and Technology. (in Korean).

Lee, I. (2009). Problems of redundant publication and the establishment of ways of research. *Korean Discourses on Philosophy, 26*, 305–323. (in Korean).

Lie, J. (2000). *Han unbound: The political economy of South Korea.* Stanford, CA: Stanford University Press.

Ministry of Education, Science, and Technology. (2008). *Establishing and promoting research ethics: At national and transnational level.* Seoul: Ministry of Education, Science, and Technology. (in Korean).

Ministry of Government Legislation. (2009). Presidential decree number 21634: Regulations for management of government-funded research projects. July 22, 2009. (in Korean). http://www.law.go.kr/LSW/LsBdyPrint.do.

Ministry of Science and Education. (2007). *Practical research ethics.* Kyunggi, Korea: Ministry of Science and Education. (in Korean).

Ministry of Science and Technology. (2007). Government order number 236: Guides for securing research ethics. February 8, 2007. http://kautm.net/kautm02/data/view.asp?bname=pds&no=445.

Ministry of Science, Technology, and Education. (2009). *Government order number 128: Guides for writing research notes in government-funded research projects.* June 22, 2009. (in Korean). http://www.law.go.kr/LSW/jsp/ls05/AdmRulPrint.jsp?id=print.

National Bioethics Committee. (2006). *Report on ethical problems in Professor Hwang Woo-Suk's research.* February 1, 2006. (in Korean).

Oh, J. (1999). *Korean politics: The quest for democratization and economic development.* Ithaca, NY: Cornell University Press.

Oh, S. (2008). Thesis on general education plan for research ethics. *Korean Language Literature 67*, 515–536. (in Korean).

Park, K. (2006). *Government policy and guideline on research misconduct and integrity.* Seoul: Science and Technology Policy Institute. (in Korean).

Park, K. (2008). *Settlement of actual issues in implementing the system securing research integrity through case studies.* Seoul: Science and Technology Policy Institute. (in Korean).

Park, K. (2009). *A survey on Korean researchers' perceptions of research ethics.* Seoul: Science and Technology Policy Institute. (in Korean).

Park, J., Jeon, H., & Logan, R. (2009). The Korean press and Hwang's fraud. *Public Understanding of Science, 18*(6), 653–669.

Prosecutors' Office. (2006). *Criminal investigation report on the fabrication of stem cell research.* May 12, 2006. (in Korean).

Resnik, D., Shamoo, A., & Krimsky, S. (2006) Fraudulent human embryonic stem cell research in South Korea: Lessons learned. *Accountability in Research, 13*, 101–109.

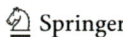

Reverby, S. (2000). *Tuskegee's truth: Rethinking Tuskegee syphilis study*. Chapel Hill: The University of North Carolina Press.

Science Times. (2007). *Declaration for the code of ethics for scientists and engineers*. (in Korean). http://www.sciencetimes.co.kr/article.do?atidx=0000019590.

Segye Daily. (2009). *The court ruled that Hwang is guilty*. October 27, 2009. (in Korean).

Seoul Daily. (2007). *Famous Buddhist monk, Jikwan, suspected of faking his degree*. September 13, 2007. (in Korean).

Seoul National University Investigation Committee. (2006a). *Final report on Professor Woo Suk Hwang's research allegations*. January 10, 2006. (in Korean).

Seoul National University Investigation Committee. (2006b). *Supporting material on former Professor Woo Suk Hwang's research misconduct*. May 1, 2006. (in Korean).

Shin. K. (2008). *Research ethics in social science research. Conference for Korean Association of Social Work*. (in Korean).

Son, W. (2007a). Analysis of current research ethics education in Korean universities. *Philosophical Thought, 24*, 143–183. (in Korean).

Son, K. (2007b). The study on the case-based approach in the research ethics education program. *Ethics Research, 64*, 53–80. (in Korean).

Song, S. (2007). Discussion of science ethics in a Korean context. *Journal of ELSI Studies, 5*, 1–18. (in Korean).

The Korean Chemical Society. (2008). *Research ethics symposium*. October 17, 2008. Jeju International Convention Center. Jeju, Korea.

Wohn, Y. (2006). Seoul National University dismisses Hwang. *Science, 311*, 1695.

Wohn, Y., & Normile, D. (2006). Prosecutors allege elaborate deception and missing fund. *Science, 312*, 980–981.

Yoo, H. (2007). *Making a research ethics educational program for elementary, middle, and high school students*. Seoul: Korea Research Foundation. (in Korean).

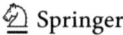

9.3   Research Misconduct and Data Fraud in Clinical Trials: Prevalence and Causal Factors

Stephen L. George

George S. Research misconduct and data fraud in clinical trials: prevalence and causal factors. International Journal of Clinical Oncology 2016; 21:15–21. © Japan Society of Clinical Oncology 2015.

Table 2 and Table 3 were reprints without modification of Figure 2 in Fanelli D (2009) How many scientists fabricate and falsifyresearch? A systematic review and meta-analysis of survey data. PLoS One 4(5):e5738. doi:https://doi.org/10.1371/journal.pone.0005738. **Copyright:** © 2009 Fanelli.

Int J Clin Oncol (2016) 21:15–21
DOI 10.1007/s10147-015-0887-3

CrossMark

REVIEW ARTICLE

Research misconduct and data fraud in clinical trials: prevalence and causal factors

Stephen L. George[1]

Received: 28 July 2015 / Accepted: 1 August 2015 / Published online: 20 August 2015
© Japan Society of Clinical Oncology 2015

Abstract The disclosure of cases of research misconduct in clinical trials, conventionally defined as fabrication, falsification or plagiarism, has been a disturbingly common phenomenon in recent years. Such cases can potentially harm patients enrolled on the trials in question or patients treated based on the results of those trials and can seriously undermine the scientific and public trust in the validity of clinical trial results. Here, I review what is known about the prevalence of research misconduct in general and the contributing or causal factors leading to the misconduct. The evidence on prevalence is unreliable and fraught with definitional problems and with study design issues. Nevertheless, the evidence taken as a whole seems to suggest that cases of the most serious types of misconduct, fabrication and falsification (i.e., data fraud), are relatively rare but that other types of questionable research practices are quite common. There have been many individual, institutional and scientific factors proposed for misconduct but, as is the case with estimates of prevalence, reliable empirical evidence on the strength and relative importance of these factors is lacking. However, it seems clear that the view of misconduct as being simply the result of aberrant or self-delusional personalities likely underestimates the effect of other important factors and inhibits the development of effective prevention strategies.

Keywords Research misconduct · Fraud · Clinical trials

✉ Stephen L. George
   stephen.george@duke.edu

[1] Department of Biostatistics and Bioinformatics, Duke
     University School of Medicine, 2424 Erwin Road, Suite
     1102, Room 11082, Durham, NC 27705, USA

Introduction

Cases of data fraud in clinical trials, defined as the fabrication or falsification of data, are uncovered on a regular basis [1, 2]. Some prominent recent examples are summarized in Table 1.

These cases include Roger Poisson, who falsified eligibility data for patients entered on multi-center breast cancer trials sponsored by the National Surgical Adjuvant Breast and Bowel Project (NSABP) [3, 4]; Werner Bezwoda, who reported strikingly positive findings from a single-institution trial using high-dose chemotherapy stem cell rescue in patients with high-risk breast cancer but the data on which the results were based could not be verified in an independent audit [5, 6]; Robert Fiddes, who was a lead investigator for a large number of clinical trials sponsored by pharmaceutical companies but was discovered to have committed a wide range of fraud and misconduct in these trials over many years [7, 8]; Harry Snyder and Renee Peugeot, a husband and wife team who falsified data on a clinical trial of a topical agent for the treatment of psoriasis and cutaneous T-cell lymphoma [9, 10]; Yoshitaka Fujii, an anesthesiologist who fabricated data on a large number of clinical trials of agents used to control postoperative nausea and vomiting in humans and animals [11–16]; Anil Potti, who developed predictive models for therapeutic agents in cancer that were used in subsequent clinical trials but the details underlying the development of those models could not be independently validated [17]; and Hiroaki Matsubara, who resigned his university position in the wake of allegations of data fabrication and falsification in clinical trials of valsartan [18, 19].

Since clinical trials are a special type of research study, such cases are part of the general problem of research misconduct, with the added risk of potentially serious consequences

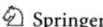 Springer

16   Int J Clin Oncol (2016) 21:15–21

Table 1 Some prominent cases of data fraud in clinical trials

Name	Allegations/findings	Outcome	Key references
Roger Poisson	Falsification of eligibility data on multi-center breast cancer trials	Barred from research funding (8 years)	Fisher and Redmond [3], Weir and Murray [4]
Werner Bezwoda	Fabrication and falsification of data on single institution breast cancer trials	Dismissed from position	Horton [5], Weiss et al. [6]
Robert Fiddes	Fabrication and falsification of data and entering ineligible patients on multi-center industry-supported clinical trials	Prison sentence (15 months)	Eichenwald and Kolata [7], Swaminathan and Avery [8]
Harry Snyder Renee Peugeot	Falsification of data on single-institution clinical trials for a biotech firm	Prison sentences (3 years; 2.5 years), financial restitution	Birch and Cohen [9], Grant [10]
Yoshiaka Fujii	Fabrication of data on clinical trials in post-operative nausea and vomiting	Dismissed from position, 183 papers retracted	Kranke et al. [14], Carlisle [11]
Anil Potti	Falsification of genomics data used in predictive modelling for cancer clinical trials	Resigned position, 11 papers retracted	Baggerly and Coombes [17]
Hiroaki Matsubara	Fabrication and falsification of data on clinical trials of antihypertensive agent valsartan	Resigned position, 9 papers retracted	Husten [19], Oransky [18]

for patients treated on trials or treated based on the results of those trials. Here, I discuss the definitions of misconduct, ranging from the narrow definition of 'fabrication, falsification or plagiarism' to wider definitions which include other questionable research practices; evaluate the available evidence on the prevalence or incidence of misconduct; and discuss potential contributing or causal factors leading to misconduct and the implications for preventive measures.

Definitions of research misconduct and data fraud

A single universally accepted definition of research misconduct does not exist among the various professional societies, scientific journals, government agencies and regulatory bodies concerned with the issue. However, fabrication, falsification and plagiarism are so egregious that all definitions implicitly or explicitly include these practices. The US Public Health Service defines research misconduct specifically limited to these practices [20]:

> "Research misconduct means fabrication, falsification, or plagiarism in proposing, performing, or reviewing research, or in reporting research results.
>
> (a) Fabrication is making up data or results and recording or reporting them.
> (b) Falsification is manipulating research materials, equipment, or processes, or changing or omitting data or results such that the research is not accurately represented in the research record.
> (c) Plagiarism is the appropriation of another person's ideas, processes, results, or words without giving appropriate credit.

> (d) Research misconduct does not include honest error or differences of opinion."

The National Institutes of Health [21], National Science Foundation [22], American Psychological Association [23] and others use identical or nearly identical definitions. This is a very narrow definition, covering only the most serious unethical behaviors. For clinical investigators, the US Food and Drug Administration use a much broader definition of investigator misconduct, targeting practices that might create a safety risk for patients, including:

> "Failure to report serious or life-threatening adverse events; serious protocol violations, such as enrolling subjects who do not meet the entrance criteria because they have conditions that put them at increased risk from the investigational drug, or failing to carry out critical safety evaluations; repeated or deliberate failure to obtain adequate informed consent, including falsification of consent forms or repeated or deliberate failure to disclose serious risks of the investigational drug in the informed consent process; falsification of study safety data; failure to obtain IRB review and approval for significant protocol changes; failure to adequately supervise the clinical trial such that human subjects are or would be exposed to an unreasonable and significant risk of illness or injury" [24].

There are also other organizations that take a broader perspective, including the Council of Scientific Editors, who in a white paper on integrity in scientific publications [25], defined research misconduct as

> "Behaviour by a researcher, intentional or not, that falls short of good ethical and scientific standard."

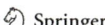

Similarly, Universities UK defines research misconduct to include "behaviour or actions that fall short of the standards of ethics, research and scholarship are required to ensure that the integrity of research is upheld" [26]. These definitions are both broader and vaguer than the PHS definition, leaving open the question of the definition of 'good ethical and scientific standard' or 'research and scholarship standards' and what exactly constitutes falling short of those standards.

There has been much discussion in the literature on questionable research practices other than fabrication, falsification or plagiarism that may nevertheless result in unreliable results and other serious problems [27–34]. Some of these practices relevant to clinical trials are listed in Table 2.

In Table 2, these questionable practices are grouped into several categories—Design and analysis, such as the use of improper design or analysis techniques, misrepresentation of the methodology used, or selective reporting; publication and authorship, such as failure to publish or gift authorship; patient safety, such as failure to follow protocol safety requirements or failure to obtain proper informed consent;

Table 2 Questionable research practices in clinical trials other than fabrication, falsification and plagiarism

Design, conduct and analysis
  Improper design or analysis
  Selective reporting
  Over-interpretation of results
  Data dredging (P-hacking)
  Study weaknesses not described
  Misrepresentation of design, statistical methodology or data
  Subgroup and post hoc analysis not identified as such
  Improper analysis of missing data
  Ignoring outliers
  Sloppiness or incompetence
Publication and authorship
  Failure to publish
  Agreement not to publish
  Gift authorship
  Redundant publications
Patient safety
  Failure to follow protocol safety requirements
  Failure to obtain proper informed consent
  Failure to obtain appropriate prior approval for research
  Failure to report adverse events
Other
  Misuse of funds
  Conflicts of interest
  Refusal to share data

and other practices, such as misuse of funds, conflicts of interest, or refusal to share data.

One view of data fraud in clinical trials is that it represents the extreme end of a spectrum of sources of data errors in clinical trials, ranging from the inevitable honest errors at one end of the spectrum to data fraud at the other end, with misunderstandings, incompetence and sloppiness in between. This spectrum is illustrated graphically in Fig. 1 where there is a clear dividing line between data fraud and other sources of error defined by intent. Other sources of data errors are regrettable but data fraud involves a deliberate intent to deceive or 'intent to cheat', a qualitatively different source of data errors.

It is arguable that in aggregate more damage is caused by the less serious forms of questionable research practices and from sloppiness or incompetence than from data fraud—largely because these other sources of data errors are more common.

Prevalence

There are fundamental difficulties in trying to estimate the prevalence of research misconduct in science in general and clinical trials in particular. First, there are definitional problems. Does 'misconduct' include only fabrication, falsification and plagiarism as in the PHS definition or should it include some of the other types of questionable research practices listed in Table 2?

Second, there are difficulties in the assessment of prevalence when applied to research misconduct. In epidemiology, prevalence is defined as the proportion of people in a defined population with a given condition at a specific time (point prevalence), or that have (or had) the condition during a specified time period (period prevalence), or that have ever had the condition at any time (lifetime prevalence). For assessing the prevalence of research misconduct there needs to be clarity in the type of prevalence being assessed as well as a clear statement of the population being studied, the defined population. Is it everyone engaged in research, or just primary investigators, or some other defined group of individuals? Even if the population can be defined in principle, how are the numbers of people in the population estimated? And how can we take a reasonable random sample, or some other reasonably representative sample,

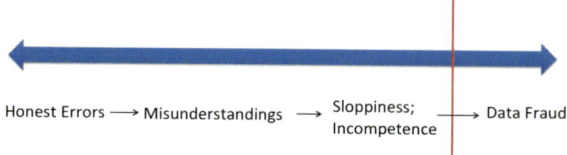

Honest Errors ⟶ Misunderstandings ⟶ Sloppiness; Incompetence ⟶ Data Fraud

Fig. 1 Spectrum of sources of data errors in clinical trials

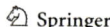
  Springer

18   Int J Clin Oncol (2016) 21:15–21

from the population in order to construct an estimate of prevalence?

Lastly, there is an ascertainment problem. Accurate responses to questions about misconduct may be difficult to obtain. This is a well-known problem when attempting to elicit responses from individuals for questions about behavior that is embarrassing, illegal or that is otherwise liable to result in evasive answers.

Because of these difficulties, the true prevalence of research misconduct in general or in clinical trials in particular is unknown, perhaps even unknowable. Nevertheless, there have been many attempts to address the issue. These efforts may be classified into studies providing indirect estimates of prevalence through assessing the detected cases [35–37] and surveys providing direct evidence by asking questions in some supposedly representative sample of subjects about knowledge of misconduct by others [28, 38–42] or about the respondent's own behavior [29, 40, 43, 44]. The detected cases alone are obviously less than the actual number of cases and thus lead to an unreliable and biased underestimate of prevalence. Such indirect evidence on prevalence has resulted in speculations that range from the 'tip of the iceberg' metaphor, often favored by science journalists, at one extreme to the conclusion that fraud is extremely rare at the other extreme ('99.9999 % of all reports are accurate and truthful' [45]).

The evidence from sample surveys has the advantage of producing a direct estimate of prevalence, despite the caveats noted earlier. However, these surveys differ greatly in study designs, sample sizes, questions asked, and other features, resulting in inconsistent outcomes. In addition, as noted above, the surveys ask questions about topics for which respondents might be expected not to be truthful. Although there is a 50-year history of using randomized response designs in this setting to minimize this problem [46, 47], only one survey of misconduct actually used this type of design to address the issue [48].

In order to make some sense of the published survey results, Fanelli [49] conducted a meta-analysis of 21 surveys published in 1987–2008, restricting attention to those surveys asking direct questions about the misconduct of researchers or about the misconduct of their colleagues. Only studies addressing fabrication, falsification or other questionable research practices that could produce biased or misleading results in the analysis were included (e.g., plagiarism was not included). In addition, only studies that clearly separated fabrication/falsification from other questionable practices were included.

Figure 2 gives a Forest plot of the results from the meta-analysis of self-reported fabrication or falsification. Figure 3 gives similar results for personal knowledge of fabrication or falsification by others (i.e., of the respondent's colleagues).

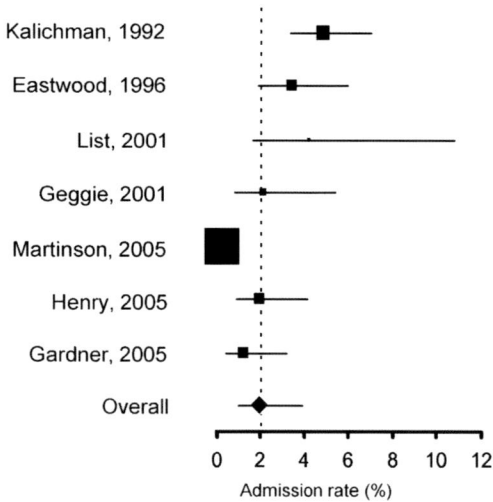

Fig. 2 Forest plot of admission rates of data fabrication, falsification and alteration in self reports. Area of *squares* represents sample size, *horizontal lines* are 95 % confidence interval, *diamond* and *vertical dotted line* show the pooled weighted estimate. This figure is a reproduction without modification of Fig. 2 in Fanelli [49]

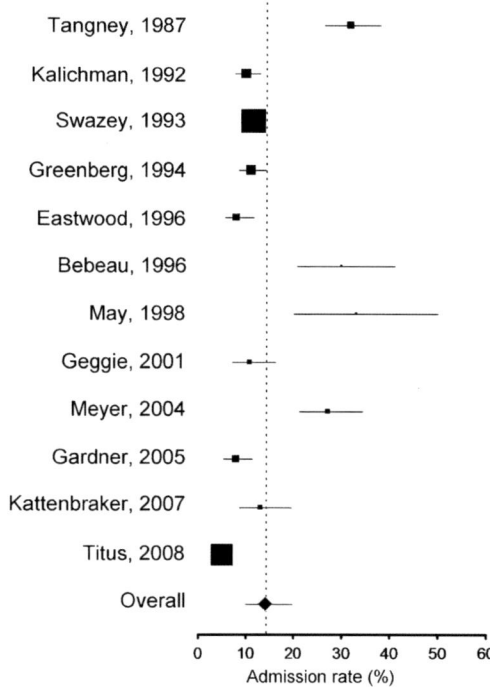

Fig. 3 Forest plot of admission rates of data fabrication, falsification and alteration in non-self reports. Area of *squares* represents sample size, *horizontal lines* are 95 % confidence interval, *diamond* and *vertical dotted line* show the pooled weighted estimate. This figure is a reproduction without modification of Fig. 2 in Fanelli [49]

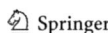 Springer

The pooled weighted estimate of the self-reported admission rate, rounded to one decimal, was 2.0 % (95 % CI 0.9–4.5) and the pooled weighted estimate of those who reported fabrication or falsification by others was 14.1 % (95 % CI 9.9–19.7). Significant heterogeneity among the surveys was observed. It is likely that the self-reported admission rates are biased (low) for the reasons noted above.

Other questionable research practices are likely to be much more prevalent than fabrication, falsification or plagiarism. For example, in a large survey of US scientists funded by the National Institutes of Health, Martinson et al. [29] reported that 15.5 % of the respondents admitted to 'changing the design, methodology or results of a study in response to pressure from a funding source' and 33 % admitted to at least one of the 'top 10' questionable practices.

Causal factors and prevention

"Why does research misconduct happen? The answer that researchers love is 'pressure to publish', but my preferred answer is 'Why wouldn't it happen?' All human activity is associated with misconduct. Indeed, misconduct may be easier for scientists because the system operates on trust. Plus scientists may have been victims of their own rhetoric: they have fooled themselves that science is a wholly objective enterprise unsullied by the usual human subjectivity and imperfections. It is not. It is a human activity."
R. Smith [50]

Unfortunately, in common with estimates of prevalence, reliable data concerning the possible causes of misconduct do not exist [30]. We are left largely with expert opinions and speculation. The lack of data is problematic for formulation of effective prevention strategies; however, in most cases of research misconduct it is reasonable to assume that the motivation for the perpetrator lies at least partly in the potential for personal gain. In some cases there may be financial advantages, either direct personal financial gain or indirect financial gain for research funding. In other cases seeking promotion or tenure or scientific prestige may be primary motivating factors. Finally, there is always the possibility of some type of psychiatric condition or illness behind the misconduct. In any specific case, even when the perpetrator has admitted to the misconduct and offered some explanations for it, the testimony itself may be unreliable and the true motivating factors may remain unclear. Generalizations from individual cases are unreliable at best.

Despite the lack of reliable empirical evidence, there is a considerable literature addressing the contributing factors

in misconduct, with three broad general narratives about three primary contributing factors—individual traits, institutional issues, and structural problems in science itself [28, 51, 52].

Individual traits include characteristics of the individual researcher that may lead to misconduct, including the inability to handle the 'publish or perish' and other competitive pressures, personal ambition, the desire for personal recognition or the wish for direct or indirect financial gain [53]. Some ascribe the presence of research misconduct or fraud primarily to 'bad apples' since, as in all human endeavor, there are individuals who violate established norms of behavior. Some of these individuals may have self-delusional, even self-destructive, tendencies.

Institutional issues include the 'publish or perish' pressures inherent in the promotion and tenure requirements, inadequacies of training and mentoring, lack of detailed oversight of research, competition for federal support and other issues [54, 55]. Structural issues in the way modern science is conducted may also contribute to the problem [51].

In discussing the causes of research misconduct and their implication for potentially effective prevention methods, information from the broader context of other illegal, immoral, inappropriate or unethical behavior in society may be useful. Adams and Pimple [56] address this directly. Reduction of criminal/deviant behavior has proven resistant to strategies based on rational decision analysis and to setting appropriate norms and values, however laudable these may be. This approach can be called the 'individualist' approach, based on the 'bad actor' or 'bad apple' assumption. A new approach from recent theories in criminology, 'opportunity theory', starts with the assumption that the population of potential offenders is essentially everyone (see Ariely [57] for support of this assumption). If this is so, then we need to create physical settings or situations that reduce the opportunity for misconduct and encourage appropriate behavior, especially via effective supervision and internal controls. As Adams and Pimple state: "It is sometimes far easier and more effective to control or change situations than it is to control or change individuals" [56].

In the case of clinical trials, especially multi-center clinical trials, institutional issues and structural issues in science in general are likely to be less important than individual factors. In addition, with a few exceptions such as the Fiddes case and the Snyder–Peugeot case noted in the introduction, direct financial gain does not appear to be a major motivating factor. One intriguing suggestion is that physician-scientists simply may be less rigorous than other scientists in their approach to clinical trials:

"It is our sense, primarily experiential and impressionistic in nature, that honesty in research work as

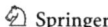

20

Int J Clin Oncol (2016) 21:15–21

a fundamental rule is valued more strongly among scientists than among physicians... Physicians tend to evaluate research in terms of harm or benefit to patients rather than in terms of adherence to the rigorous norms of scientific investigation" [58].

Years after this speculation was published, some support for this view was inadvertently supplied by Poisson in his explanation of why he falsified eligibility data on NSABP trials:

"I believed I understood the reasons behind the study rules, and I felt that the rules were meant to be understood as guidelines and not necessarily followed blindly. My sole concern at all times was the health of my patients. I firmly believed that a patient who was able to enter into an NSABP trial received the best therapy and follow-up treatment... Maintaining the proper balance between good clinical care and rigid research methods is not an easy task" [59].

In addition to the usual suggestions for preventing misconduct implied by consideration of the various factors involved (training in the ethics of research, improved mentoring, increased supervision, etc.), none of which have been proven to be effective, statistical procedures may also play a role. In particular, central statistical monitoring, an effective tool for detecting data fraud in clinical trials as part of a general data quality assurance program, may also function as a deterrent to committing such fraud in the first place for trials in which such monitoring is known to be in place [1, 60, 61]. Such procedures should be applied more commonly in multi-center clinical trials.

Summary

Despite the large and growing literature on the prevalence, causes and prevention of research misconduct in science in general and in clinical trials in particular, reliable empirical evidence to support the discussion remains in short supply. This situation exists in part because of the difficulties in definitions and in part because of the difficulties in designing and conducting studies in this area. However, the available evidence taken as a whole suggests that the most serious forms of misconduct, fabrication and falsification, are relatively rare, albeit perhaps higher than assumed by most scientists, whereas other questionable research practices are quite common. In addition, most discussions of the causal factors in misconduct are not based on reliable empirical evidence. Thus, prevention measures which are based on assumptions about causal factors are also liable to be misguided. More rigorous studies of the prevalence, causal factors and potential prevention strategies for research misconduct are needed.

Compliance with ethical standards

Conflict of interest The author declares that he has no conflict of interest.

References

1. George SL, Buyse M (2015) Data fraud in clinical trials. Clin Investig (Lond.) 15(2):161–173
2. George SL (1997) Perspectives on scientific misconduct and fraud in clinical trials. Chance 10(4):3–5
3. Fisher B, Redmond CK (1994) Fraud in breast-cancer trials. N Engl J Med 330(20):1458–1460
4. Weir C, Murray G (2011) Fraud in clinical trials. Significance 8(4):164–168. doi:10.1111/j.1740-9713.2011.00521.x
5. Horton R (2000) After Bezwoda. Lancet 355(9208):942–943. doi:10.1016/s0140-6736(00)90006-0
6. Weiss RB, Rifkin RM, Stewart FM et al (2000) High-dose chemotherapy for high-risk primary breast cancer: an on-site review of the Bezwoda study. Lancet 355(9208):999–1003
7. Eichenwald K, Kolata G (1999) A doctor's drug studies turn into fraud. The New York times on the Web, A1–A16
8. Swaminathan V, Avery M (2012) FDA enforcement of criminal liability for clinical investigator fraud. Hastings Sci Tech Law J 4:325–356
9. Birch DM, Cohen G (2001) How a cancer trial ended in betrayal. http://www.baltimoresun.com/bal-te.research24jun24-story.html#page=1. Accessed 12 Jan 2015
10. Grant B (2009) Biotech's baddies. Scientist 23(4):48
11. Carlisle J (2012) The analysis of 168 randomised controlled trials to test data integrity. Anaesthesia 67(5):521–537
12. Fujii Y (2000) Reply to "Reported data on granisetron and postoperative nausea and vomiting by Fujii et al. are incredibly nice!" [letter]. Anesth Analg 90(4):1004
13. Fujii Y (2012) Reply to "The analysis of 168 randomised controlled trials to test data integrity" [letter]. Anaesthesia 67(6):669–670
14. Kranke P, Apfel CC, Roewer N (2000) Reported data on granisetron and postoperative nausea and vomiting by Fujii et al. are incredibly nice! [letter]. Anesth Analg 90(4):1004
15. Miller D (2012) Retraction of articles written by Dr. Yoshitaka Fujii. Can J Anesth/J Can Anesth 59(12):1081–1088. doi:10.1007/s12630-012-9802-9
16. Normile D (2012) A new record for retractions? http://news.sciencemag.org/education/2012/04/newrecord-retractions. Accessed 13 Aug 2015
17. Baggerly KA, Coombes KR (2009) Deriving chemosensitivity from cell lines: Forensic bioinformatics and reproducible research in high-throughput biology. Ann Appl Stat 3:1309–1334
18. Oransky I (2014) Novartis Diovan scandal claims two more papers. http://retractionwatch.com/2014/04/02/novartis-diovan-scandal-claims-two-more-papers/. Accessed 4 May 2015
19. Husten L (2013) Diovan data was fabricated, say Japanese Health Minister and university officials. http://www.forbes.com/sites/larryhusten/2013/07/12/diovan-data-was-fabricated-say-japanese-health-minister-and-university-officials/. Accessed 3 July 2015
20. Federal Register (2005) Public health service policies on research misconduct final rule (42 CFR part 93.103). http://www.ecfr.gov/cgi-bin/text-idx?SID=0b07ed68cf889962cae6c2b45d89150b&node=pt42.1.93&rgn=div5. Accessed 4 July 2015
21. National Institutes of Health (2015) Research integrity. http://grants.nih.gov/grants/research_integrity/research_misconduct.htm. Accessed 4 July 2015

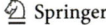 Springer

Int J Clin Oncol (2016) 21:15–21   21

22. Federal Register (2002) National science foundation policies on research misconduct (45 CFR part 689) http://www.nsf.gov/oig/regulations/. Accessed 4 July 2015

23. American Psychological Association (2015) Research misconduct. https://apa.org/research/responsible/misconduct/index.aspx. Accessed 4 July 2015

24. U.S. Food and Drug Administration (2004) Guidance for industry: the use of clinical holds following clinical investigator misconduct. http://www.fda.gov/downloads/regulatoryinformation/guidances/ucm126997.pdf. Accessed 25 July 2015

25. Scott-Lichter D, Editorial Policy Committee, Council of Scientific Editors (2006) CSE's white paper on promoting integrity in scientific journal publications. CSE, Reston

26. Universities UK (2012) The concordat to support research integrity http://www.universitiesuk.ac.uk/highereducation/Pages/Theconcordattosupportresearchintegrity.aspx#.VZgN03J3EdU. Accessed 4 July 2015

27. Breen KJ (2003) Misconduct in medical research: whose responsibility? Intern Med J 33(4):186–191

28. Habermann B, Broome M, Pryor ER et al (2010) Research coordinators' experiences with scientific misconduct and research integrity. Nurs Res 59(1):51–57

29. Martinson BC, Anderson MS, De Vries R (2005) Scientists behaving badly. Nature 435(7043):737–738. doi:10.1038/435737a

30. Weed DL (1998) Preventing scientific misconduct. Am J Public Health 88(1):125–129

31. Wilmshurst P (1997) The code of silence. Lancet 349(9051):567–569

32. Sarwar U, Nicolaou M (2012) Fraud and deceit in medical research. J Res Med Sci 17(11):1077–1081

33. Steneck NH (2006) Fostering integrity in research: definitions, current knowledge, and future directions. Sci Eng Ethics 12(1):53–74

34. Claxton LD (2005) Scientific authorship: part 1. A window into scientific fraud? Mutat Res 589(1):17–30

35. Hone J (1993) Combating fraud and misconduct in medical research. Scrip Mag 14(March):14–15

36. Reynolds SM (2004) ORI findings of scientific misconduct in clinical trials and publicly funded research, 1992–2002. Clin Trials 1(6):509–516. doi:10.1191/1740774504cn048oa

37. Weiss RB, Vogelzang NJ, Peterson BA et al (1993) A successful system of scientific data audits for clinical trials. A report from the Cancer and Leukemia Group B. J Am Med Assoc 270(4):459–464

38. Hamilton D (1992) In the trenches, doubts about scientific integrity. Science 255(5052):1636. doi:10.1126/science.11642983

39. Ranstam J, Buyse M, George SL et al (2000) Fraud in medical research: an international survey of biostatisticians. Control Clin Trials 21(5):415–427. doi:10.1016/s0197-2456(00)00069-6

40. Kalichman MW, Friedman PJ (1992) A pilot study of biomedical trainees' perceptions concerning research ethics. Acad Med 67(11):769–775

41. Swazey JP, Anderson MS, Lewis KS (1993) Ethical problems in academic research. Am Sci 81:542–553

42. Titus SL, Wells JA, Rhoades LJ (2008) Repairing research integrity. Nature 453(7198):980–982

43. John LK, Loewenstein G, Prelec D (2012) Measuring the prevalence of questionable research practices with incentives for truth telling. Psychol Sci 23(5):524–532. doi:10.1177/0956797611430953

44. Martinson BC, Crain AL, Anderson MS et al (2009) Institutions' expectations for researchers' self-funding, federal grant holding, and private industry involvement: manifold drivers of self-interest and researcher behavior. Acad Med 84(11):1491–1499

45. Koshland DE (1987) Fraud in science. Science 235:141–142

46. Blair G, Imai K, Zhou Y-Y (2015) Design and analysis of the randomized response technique (in press). J Am Stat Assoc

47. Warner SL (1965) Randomized response: a survey technique for eliminating evasive answer bias. J Am Stat Assoc 60(309):63–69

48. List JA, Bailey CD, Euzent PJ et al (2001) Academic economists behaving badly? A survey on three areas of unethical behavior. Econ Inq 39(1):162–170

49. Fanelli D (2009) How many scientists fabricate and falsify research? A systematic review and meta-analysis of survey data. PLoS One 4(5):e5738. doi:10.1371/journal.pone.0005738

50. Smith R (2006) Research misconduct: the poisoning of the well. J R Soc Med 99(5):232–237. doi:10.1258/jrsm.99.5.232

51. Sovacool BK (2008) Exploring scientific misconduct: isolated individuals, impure institutions, or an inevitable idiom of modern science? Bioeth Inq 5(4):271–282. doi:10.1007/s11673-008-9113-6

52. Davis MS, Riske-Morris M, Diaz SR (2007) Causal factors implicated in research misconduct: evidence from ORI case files. Sci Eng Ethics 13(4):395–414. doi:10.1007/s11948-007-9045-2

53. Chubin DE (1985) Misconduct in research: an issue of science policy and practice. Minerva 23(2):175–202. doi:10.1007/bf01099941

54. De Vries R, Anderson MS, Martinson BC (2006) Normal misbehavior: scientists talk about the ethics of research. J Empir Res Hum Res Eth 1(1):43–50

55. Gaddis B, Helton-Fauth W, Scott G et al (2003) Development of two measures of climate for scientific organizations. Account Res 10(4):253–288

56. Adams D, Pimple KD (2005) Research misconduct and crime lessons from criminal science on preventing misconduct and promoting integrity. Account Res 12(3):225–240

57. Ariely D (2012) The honest truth about dishonesty. Harper Collins Publishers, New York

58. Swazey JP, Scher SR (1982) Whistleblowing in biomedical research. Government Printing Office, Washington

59. Poisson R (1994) Fraud in breast-cancer trials [letter]. N Engl J Med 330(20):1460

60. Buyse M, George SL, Evans S et al (1999) The role of biostatistics in the prevention, detection and treatment of fraud in clinical trials. Stat Med 18(24):3435–3451

61. Knatterud GL, Rockhold FW, George SL et al (1998) Guidelines for quality assurance in multicenter trials: a position paper. Control Clin Trials 19(5):477–493. doi:10.1016/s0197-2456(98)00033-6

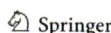

9.4   Repairing Research Integrity

Sandra L. Titus, James A. Wells, and Lawrence J. Rhoades

Titus S, Wells J, Rhoades L. Repairing research integrity. Nature 2008;190 June 453(7198):980–982. © 2008 Macmillan Publishers Limited. All rights reserved. Reprint of SpringerNature.

nature

Vol 453|19 June 2008

COMMENTARY

Repairing research integrity

A survey suggests that many research misconduct incidents in the United States go unreported to the Office of Research Integrity. **Sandra L. Titus**, **James A. Wells** and **Lawrence J. Rhoades** say it's time to change that.

Misconduct jeopardizes the good name of any institution. Inevitably, the way in which research misconduct is policed and corrected reflects the integrity of the whole enterprise of science. The US National Academy of Sciences has asserted that scientists share an 'obligation to act' when suspected research misconduct is observed[1]. But it has been unclear how well scientists are meeting that obligation. In the United States, the Office of Research Integrity (ORI) evaluates all the investigation records submitted by institutions and plays an oversight role in determining whether there has been misconduct at institutions that receive support from the Department of Health and Human Services (DHHS). The reported number of investigations submitted to ORI has remained low: on average 24 institutional investigation reports per year[2].

ORI focuses resources, not only on evaluating institutional reports of research misconduct but also on preventing misconduct and promoting research integrity through deterrence and education. To evaluate these initiatives, we investigated whether the low number of misconduct cases reported to ORI is an accurate reflection of misconduct incidence, or the tip of a much larger iceberg. The latter seems to be the case.

The 2,212 researchers we surveyed observed 201 instances of likely misconduct over a three-year period. That's 3 incidents per 100 researchers per year. A conservative extrapolation from our findings to all DHHS-funded researchers predicts that more than 2,300 observations of potential misconduct are made every year. Not all are being reported to universities and few of these are being reported to the ORI.

No regulatory office can hope to catch all research misconduct and we think that the primary deterrent must be at the institutional level. Institutions must establish the culture that promotes safeguards for whistleblowers and establishes zero tolerance both for those who commit misconduct and for those who turn a blind eye to it.

Defining misconduct

A first step in developing that culture is taking stock of misconduct's frequency. Several investigators have addressed research misconduct incidence with limited results because of methodological problems, such as applying

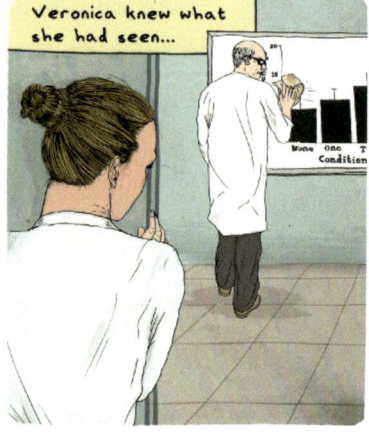

inconsistent definitions of misconduct or not accounting for duplicate reports of the same incident[3-5]. So, we used the US federal definition of research misconduct[6] — fabrication, falsification or plagiarism in proposing, performing or reviewing research, or in reporting research results — and verified whether reports accurately fitted that definition. The possibility of duplicate reports was virtually eliminated by selecting only one National Institutes of Health (NIH)-funded researcher in a given department to respond. We asked about events only from

> "Institutions must establish safeguards for whistleblowers."

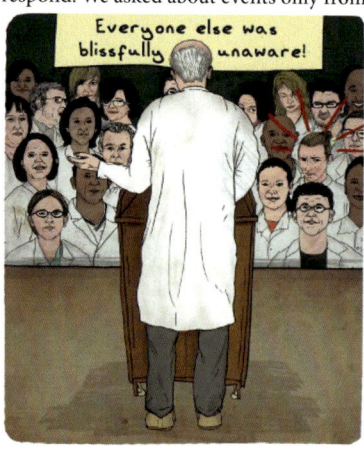

the past three academic years to avoid inclusion of distant events and to have a consistent time parameter. We used frequent and varied reminders to secure a high response rate to the survey. Previous research has treated survey reports of misconduct as if the observer could make the determination that they had observed misconduct. Instead, we consider the observations to be 'possible research misconduct' and not all such observations will result in a finding of misconduct. In all we asked 4,298 scientists holding NIH extramural research funds at 605 institutions to respond to the survey so that our findings would be representative of a broad spectrum of research fields as well as varied sizes of institutions.

What scientists saw

In 2006, we asked participants to indicate the number of times they had observed suspected research misconduct in their own department in the past three academic years (2002–05). 2,212 scientists provided complete responses to questions concerning research misconduct (51% response rate). Of these, 192 scientists (8.7%) indicated that they had observed or had direct evidence of researchers in their own department committing one or more incidents of suspected research misconduct over the past three academic years. The 192 scientists described a total of 265 incidents.

Scientists were asked to indicate how they became aware of the possible misconduct and were told to report observations and not hearsay (see table, page 982). Suspected misconduct was observed at all scientific ranks including postdocs, students, and tenured faculty members. The following are examples of how scientists described such incidents. We used these descriptions to validate whether the observation met the federal definition of research misconduct.

> "A post doc changed the numbers in assays in order to 'improve' the data."

> "A colleague duplicated results between three different papers but differently labelled data in each paper."

> "A co-investigator on a large, interdisciplinary grant application reported that a postdoctoral fellow in his laboratory falsified data submitted as preliminary data in the grant. As principal investigator of the grant, I submitted

NATURE|Vol 453|19 June 2008

supplementary data to correct the application."

"A colleague used Photoshop to eliminate background bands on a western blot to make the data look more specific than they were."

Two people independently coded and evaluated the 265 descriptions to determine whether each met the federal definition of research misconduct. In all, 64 reports (24% of the total) did not meet the threshold of the federal definition — which left 201 observations of potential misconduct made by 164 scientists (7.4%). These 201 misconduct observations included fabrication or falsification (60%) and plagiarism only (36%).

According to our respondents, 58% of the observed incidents had been reported to officials at their institutions. In 24% of incidents it was the survey respondent who reported it and in 33% of the incidents it was someone other than the respondent. Responses indicated that 37% of incidents were not reported by anyone and for 5% of the cases respondents did not know.

Study limitations

Several limitations may have affected the study results. As the sample only includes one observer per department, the number of suspected research-misconduct incidents found in this study is likely to be a very conservative estimate. Because the sample only represented scientists holding research awards given to established researchers, we lack the views of postdoctoral fellows, graduate students, clinical-trial coordinators and lab technicians who might report a different quantity and type of suspected research misconduct. The study is also probably more representative of the biomedical, behavioural and life sciences than it is of the physical and social sciences, reflecting the mission of the NIH.

Although the scientists we sampled were receiving research support from the NIH, we know nothing about the funding of those they suspected to be committing misconduct. This means that the findings do not exclusively apply to NIH investigators. And because of the possibility of human error from respondents, our method of measurement may have failed to elicit all instances of suspected research misconduct or may have included erroneous instances. Some observations, for example, may have occurred outside the time period specified because of 'telescoping' — including salient events that occurred before the period of interest. Still, the questionnaire was careful to specify the period of interest as the past three academic years.

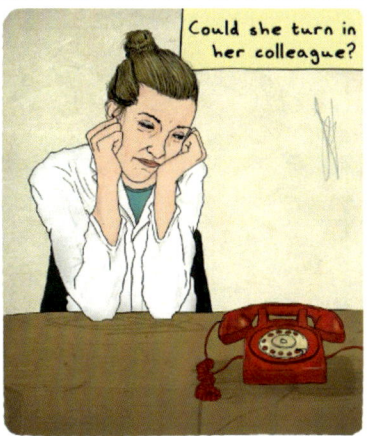

Could she turn in her colleague?

Extrapolating the survey results — even conservatively — projects an alarming picture of under-reporting. NIH extramural research grants in 2007 supported an estimated 155,000 people, which includes principal investigators and other research personnel[7]. In our survey, 201 cases were observed over three years by 2,212 respondents, essentially 3 cases per 100 people per year. Most conservatively, we assumed that non-responders (roughly half of our sample) did not witness any misconduct. Thus, applying 1.5 cases in 100 scientists to 155,000 researchers suggests that there could be, minimally, 2,325 possible research misconduct observations in a year. If 58% of these cases were reported to institutional officials as in our survey, approximately 1,350 would have been reported whereas almost 1,000 could be assumed to go unreported to any official.

> " Extrapolating the survey results projects an alarming picture of under-reporting ."

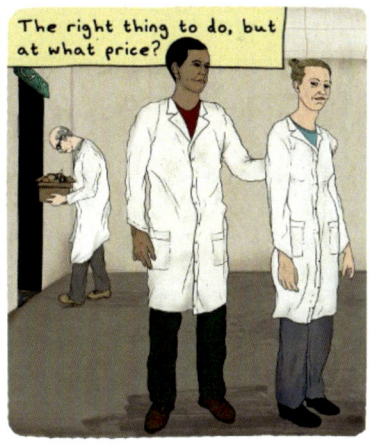

The right thing to do, but at what price?

These numbers indicate a sizeable disconnect between what universities are seeing and the 24 investigations evaluated by the ORI annually. Could all the predicted cases be found to lack evidence? Could all the cases be concluded at the inquiry stage? Could the cases be primarily occurring in research that is not funded by the Public Health Service and hence not reportable to the ORI? Can duplicate observations of misconduct account for this disparity?

We doubt that affirmative answers to these questions could sufficiently explain the discrepancy. We recognize that this estimate is not perfect. First we are applying our findings from a defined context to a much larger context and one that also includes the staff of the investigator. Another weakness of the prediction is the fact that scientists in our study would have been narrowly reporting observations restricted to their own experience. A single observer in a department cannot be expected to have been exposed to all instances of misconduct. Thus, our estimate may be off by an order of magnitude in either direction.

On an individual level, many reasons for under-reporting are easy to understand because they involve motivations we might all have experienced. For example, one does not want to accuse falsely. One may also fear that reporting would take time away from research, or have concerns and fears about possible retaliation. One may assume someone else will or should report it. Or one may have sympathy towards a researcher, and might think "it's not too bad", it can be sorted out without a career-damaging investigation. Reporting also necessitates confidence that the issue will be examined carefully and thoroughly.

Keeping it quiet

The leaders of institutions may also have concerns about handling research misconduct. Because public image is important to institutions, some may try to minimize reporting and keep unfavourable information from reaching the ORI and the press. An institution may choose to ignore conducting an investigation and instead they may simply dismiss an accused person or even a whistleblower in the hope that the problem will go away without needing further examination. Additionally, institutional leaders may wish to ignore or minimize allegations of possible research misconduct to protect the revenue that the researcher generates; some may avoid investigations because they are costly in terms of time and money. Administrators may not recognize the significance of evaluating research misconduct and of course they may be poorly equipped to conduct an investigation in an appropriate manner.

Fundamentally all explanations seem to

OPINION

NATURE|Vol 453|19 June 2008

share a common denominator — the failure to foster a culture of integrity. An analysis commissioned by the ORI found in 2000 that only 29% of institutional misconduct polices explicitly obligate members to report scientific misconduct[8]. Individuals and institutions, not the federal government, are the guardians of research integrity. Therefore, we urge action and recommend six strategies to champion integrity.

Adopt zero tolerance

To create a zero-tolerance culture, we think that it is essential that an institution specifies and implements the requirements that all suspected misconduct must be reported, and all allegations must be thoroughly and fairly investigated. Social responsibility to the academic community and to the public who fund the research will be strengthened when it is apparent that an institution has a real commitment to integrity.

Protect whistleblowers

Careful attention must be paid to the creation and dissemination of measures to protect whistleblowers. Responders to our survey said that reporting would be most likely to improve if institutions and the federal government increased the whistleblower protection. Indeed, more than two-thirds of whistleblowers, in a Research Triangle Institute study, experienced at least one negative outcome as a direct result of their actions[9]. Plus, 43% reported that institutions encouraged them to drop the allegation.

Clarify how to report

Researchers in our study also emphasized what would promote reporting: establishing a reporting system that clearly identifies the individuals to whom allegations should be brought, and establishing clear policies, procedures and guidelines related to misconduct and responsible conduct.

Train the mentors

If we want to build a stronger culture of integrity, then the current generation of researchers has to be educated to pay more attention to how they work with their junior team members. Social science has a long history of describing how group standards affect individual behaviour. Mentors specifically need to become more aware of their roles in establishing and maintaining research rules and minimizing opportunities to commit research misconduct[10]. Only 34% of scientists in a study with 2,206 laboratory directors strongly agreed that their mentor had prepared them to be a good mentor to others[11]. An institutional

SUSPECTED MISCONDUCT: 201 CASES OBSERVED BY 164 SCIENTISTS

	Number of cases
Type of misconduct	
Fabrication or falsification	120 (59.7%)
Plagiarism only	73 (36.3%)
Unknown	8 (4.0%)
Rank of those suspected*	
Professor or senior scientist	44 (21.9%)
Associate professor or scientist	28 (13.9%)
Assistant professor or scientist	34 (16.9%)
Postdoctoral fellow	50 (24.9%)
Graduate student	29 (14.4%)
Other (includes 1 unknown)	24 (11.9%)
How it was discovered	
Directly observed	23 (11.4%)
Observed products	53 (26.4%)
Told first, then observed	60 (29.9%)
Other direct evidence	30 (14.9%)
Other	30 (14.9%)
Don't recall	1 (0.5%)
No answer	4 (2.0%)
Was it reported?	
Yes, reported by responder	49 (24.4%)
Yes, reported by someone else	67 (33.3%)
No, not reported	75 (37.3%)
Don't know	5 (2.5%)
No answer	5 (2.5%)

* Eight cases identified more than one person involved in incident.

investment in building better mentors is an important vehicle to promoting research integrity.

Use alternative mechanisms

Institutions must start to use other means to protect the integrity of their studies. The Institute of Medicine recommends that "Universities should not rely upon formal complaints of scientific misconduct as the sole source of monitoring the integrity and quality of the research conducted under their auspices. They need continuing

mechanisms to review and evaluate the research and training environment of their institution."[12] Auditing research records would be one such means. Mechanisms of review are needed to reduce deficient record keeping, improper protection of human or animal subjects or the utilization of questionable research behaviour[13].

Model ethical behaviour

People imitate the behaviour of powerful role models. Institutions successfully stop cheating, for example, when they have leaders who communicate what is acceptable behaviour, encourage faculty members and staff to follow the policies, develop fair and appropriate procedures for handling misconduct cases, focus on ways to develop and promote ethical behaviour, and provide clear deterrents that are communicated[14].

Nearly one generation after the effort to reduce misconduct in science began, the responses by NIH scientists suggests that falsified and fabricated research records, publications, dissertations and grant applications are much more prevalent than has been suspected to date. Our study calls into question the effectiveness of self-regulation. We hope it will lead individuals and institutions to evaluate their commitment to research integrity. ■

Sandra L. Titus is director of intramural research, Office of Research Integrity, 1101 Wootton Parkway, Suite 750, Rockville, Maryland 20852, USA. James A. Wells is director of the Office of Research Policy, University of Wisconsin-Madison, 205 Bascom Hall, 500 Lincoln Drive, Madison, Wisconsin 53706, USA. Lawrence J. Rhoades is the retired former director of the Division of Education and Integrity, Office of Research Integrity, 1101 Wootton Parkway, Suite 750, Rockville, Maryland 20852, USA.

1. www.nap.edu/html/obas/
2. http://ori.dhhs.gov/research/intra/documents/ Investigations1994-2003-2.pdf
3. Swazey, J., Anderson, M. & Lewis, K. Am. Sci. **81,** 542-553 (1993).
4. St James-Roberts, I. New Sci. **72,** 466-469 (1976).
5. Rankin, M. & Esteves, M. D. Nurs. Res. **46,** 270-276 (1997).
6. Department of Health and Human Services Public Health Service Policies on Research Misconduct 42 CFR 93 (2005).
7. Lederhendler, I. National Institutes of Health, personal communication.
8. http://ori.dhhs.gov/documents/institutional_policies.pdf
9. http://ori.hhs.gov/documents/consequences.pdf
10. Adams, D. & Pimple, K. D. Account. Res. **12,** 225-240 (2005).
11. http://ori.dhhs.gov/documents/research/intergity_ measures_final_report_11_07_03.pdf
12. Institute of Medicine The Responsible Conduct of Research in Health Sciences (National Academies Press, Washington DC, 1989).
13. Martinson, B., Anderson, M. & DeVries, R. Nature **435,** 737-738 (2005).
14. McCabe, D. L., Trevino, L. K. & Butterfield, K. D. Ethics Behav. **11,** 219-232 (2001).

A more detailed report discussing this study can be found at http://tinyurl.com/3keo6h.

See Editorial, page 957.

References

Asai A, Okita T, Enzo A. Conflicting messages concerning current strategies against research misconduct in Japan: a call for ethical spontaneity. J Med Ethics. 2016;42(8):524–7.

Fanelli D. How many scientists fabricate and falsify research? A systematic review and meta-analysis of survey data. PLoS One. 2009;4(5):e5738.

Jacob M. On the scope and typology of research misconduct: The gaze of the General Medical Council, 1990–2015. Med Law Rev. 2016;24(4):497–517.

Necker S. Scientific misbehavior in economics. Res Policy. 2014;43:1747–59.

Rasanen L, Moore E. Critical evaluation of the guidelines of the Finnish Advisory Board on Research Integrity and of their application. Res Integr Peer Rev. 2016;1:15.

Shuchman M. False images top form of scientific misconduct. Can Med Assoc J. 2016;188(9):645.

Additional Suggested Reading

Asai A, Okita T, Enzo A. Conflicting messages concerning current strategies against research misconduct in Japan: a call for ethical spontaneity. J Med Ethics. 2016;42(8):524–7. (*Describes Japan's effort to deal with research misconduct.*)

Ahmed B, Ahmad A, Herekar A, Uqaili U, Effendi J, Alvi S, Herekar A, Steiner T. Fraud in a population-based study of headache: prevention, detection and correction. J Headache Pain. 2014;15:37. (*Provides an example of one field dealing with RM.*)

O'Leary P. Policing research misconduct. Albany Law J Sci Technol. 2015;25(1):39–93. (*Explores options for controlling research misconduct, well beyond current policy.*)

Whistleblowing

Arthur L. Caplan and Barbara K. Redman

Whistleblowers (also called complainants) are persons with access to information about wrongdoing. As such they are indispensable to self-regulation in science. While allegations can be filed in any regulatory area (research misconduct, human or animal subjects protection, conflict of interest), most attention has been paid to their role in identifying research misconduct (FFP) since other methods of detection such as routine nonfinancial audits, are not required. Federal regulations and many state laws require institutions to: publish policies about how to receive whistleblower/complainant allegations, investigate them including determining whether they are made in good faith and to protect the complainant.

In research misconduct, allegations of FFP are in the US received by research integrity officers (RIOs), who are named by their institutions. A recent study showed that even experienced RIOs frequently do not inform potential complainants about four essential elements necessary for them to make an informed decision about whether to file a complaint. Those elements are: the allegation review process, the availability of anonymity and confidentiality, institutional responsibilities to complainants, and potential adverse consequences to reporting an allegation (Bonito et al. 2012).

Whistleblowers are often caught in a conflict in loyalty between their institution or organization and to society. Many do not report their concerns, frequently because they fear being seen as disloyal or untrustworthy. Sometimes they keep their concerns to themselves because they do not believe any change will be made. In deciding to report they consider seriousness of the issue and magnitude of the consequences as well as potential for personal harm from retaliation (Culiberg and Mihelic 2016).

While little research on whistleblowing in biomedical and social science research is available, case studies show that allegations have been lodged by statisticians concerned that reported findings do not match with the data (Gewin 2012), by clinical trial coordinators, colleagues, research technicians, students, and others. The whistleblower in the case of Woo Suk Hwang, the cloning expert in South Korea who committed fraud, kept his silence for eight years. When he eventually reported his allegations to the media, he had to go into hiding to deal with threatening levels of retaliation (Cyranoski 2014).

Two decades ago, the Commission on Research Integrity addressed the issue of appropriate whistleblower policy (Commission on Research Integrity 1995). Their proposal was met by a firestorm of criticism and never adopted as formal regulation (Redman 2016). While the evidence is far from complete, it would appear that self-regulation in this area is insufficiently effective. Advancing research integrity requires strengthened protection of good-faith whistleblowers and identification and deterrence of bad-faith whistleblowers – those whose intent is only revenge or to protect a commercial interest or slow a competitor's program of research. Developments such as data transparency and sharing will likely expose data fabrication/falsification in ways that can support whistleblowing.

Advice: Check out processes and people in your organization that deal with whistleblowing complaints. Some institutions have an anonymous call-in line, but expect that if you wish to lodge a complaint, your identity will possibly be known through inference or deduction. That said, whistleblowing is a noble and central aspect of maintaining ethical integrity in science and medicine.

A. L. Caplan · B. K. Redman (✉)
New York University Langone Medical Center,
New York, NY, USA
e-mail: Arthur.Caplan@nyumc.org

10.1   Integrity and Misconduct in Research

Commission on Research Integrity

Report of the Commission on Research Integrity. Integrity and Misconduct in Research; US Department of Health and Human Services (1995).

Responsible Whistleblowing

Introduction

The scientific endeavor requires creating and maintaining an environment in which good-faith questions about the integrity of scientific information or methods can be raised without penalty, and in which such issues are reviewed objectively and impartially. The scientific community's response to questions about the validity of research should be consonant with these goals and processes. Neither the scientific community nor the public can afford to let secrecy in misconduct cases shield scientists from accountability.

Whistleblowers in research--those who raise questions that lead to concerns about the integrity of research--have at times found themselves penalized and retaliated against by the individuals they question, by their colleagues, and by their institutions, rather than being recognized for their effort. The Commission heard testimony and reviewed documentation confirming that good-faith whistleblowers are not always as protected as they should be.

Whistleblowers provided extensive testimony to the Commission alleging destructive and painful retaliation they had experienced in response to their allegations of research misconduct. The public record demonstrates that good-faith whistleblowers, some publicly vindicated, have experienced harm or ruin to their professional careers through threats, censorship, physical isolation, retaliatory investigations, accusations of racial bias or of the very misconduct they challenged, academic expulsion, denial of access to their data and laboratories, and even threatened deportation or physical injury.[38] [39] [40] [41] The research community must squarely address this issue.[42]

Members of the scientific community with knowledge of research misconduct have an ethical responsibility to come forward. But few are likely to fulfill this responsibility in the absence of a system that provides a fair review of concerns and effective protection from retaliation.

---

[38] U.S. Merit Systems Protection Board (1981): Whistleblowing and the Federal Employee: Blowing the Whistle on Fraud, Waste, and Mismanagement--Who Does It and What Happens? Washington, D.C.: U.S. Government Printing Office.

[39] U.S. Merit Systems Protection Board (1984): Blowing the Whistle in the Federal Government: A Comparative Analysis of 1980 and 1983 Survey Findings. Washington, D.C.: U.S. Government Printing Office.

[40] U.S. Merit Systems Protection Board (1993): Whistleblowing in the Federal Government: An Update. Washington, D.C.: U.S. Government Printing Office.

[41] Lubalin, J.S., Ardini, M.E., and Matheson, J.L. "Consequences of Whistleblowing for the Whistle Misconduct in Science Cases: Final Report." Unpublished. Submitted to ORI by Research Triangle Inst: No. 282-92-0045, October 2, 1995.

[42] This concern was shared by the NAS panel; see NAS report Recommendation #11, pp 15-16.

To strengthen whistleblower protection, the Commission has taken several steps:

a. It has developed a Whistleblower's Bill of Rights (see Section 2 below), which is intended to encourage institutions to treat good-faith whistleblowers fairly, shield them from retaliation, and articulate the responsibilities of any individual who accuses another of research misconduct.

b. During the Commission's tenure, the Office of Research Integrity, in consultation with the Commission, developed institutional guidelines to protect whistleblowers against retaliation. The draft guidelines proposed by ORI (Appendix E) support the principles articulated in the Whistleblower's Bill of Rights, below. The final regulation that is required by law should ensure these principles.

c. In its proposed definition of research misconduct and other forms of professional misconduct, the Commission has stated clearly that obstruction of investigations of research misconduct is a major concern of the Federal Government--a step that provides an explicit foundation for the protection of whistleblowers. The Commission also recommends strengthening the capacity of ORI/DHHS to respond to instances of alleged retaliation against whistleblowers and institutional complicity in or indifference to such retaliation.

An issue repeatedly raised by whistleblowers who risked retaliation is the absence of an independent, credible forum free from inherent institutional conflicts of interest, providing them with a right to develop the record and seek corrective action on their concerns. During its deliberations, the Commission considered the potential roles of an independent advocate or ombudsperson for whistleblowers at the institutional level. Members failed to agree, however, that individuals with such a narrow focus of concern would improve matters sufficiently, either for whistleblowers or for scientific research in general, to warrant recommendation. The Commission nonetheless endorses the broad role of ombudspersons as a source of improved communication, useful information, and reduced interpersonal strife.

The Commission believes that the best protection for whistleblowers and witnesses lies not in federal regulation, but in an institutional culture that is committed to integrity in research. To establish such a culture, committed institutional leadership is an essential component. Institutional commitment expedites good-faith resolution of disputes over alleged research misconduct and helps to prevent prolonged adversarial proceedings.

Each institution must accept responsibility for adopting a structure and procedures that protect the rights summarized below. This responsibility includes implementing the Commission's recommended assurance on research integrity education.[43]

Recommendation:

The Commission recommends that the Secretary develop regulations guaranteeing the standards expressed in the following statement of principles:

---

[43] See Recommendations #3 and 4, Section F.

Responsible Whistleblowing: A Whistleblower's Bill of Rights

a. *Communication:* Whistleblowers are free to disclose lawfully whatever information supports a reasonable belief of research misconduct as it is defined by PHS policy. An individual or institution that retaliates against any person making protected disclosures engages in prohibited obstruction of investigations of research misconduct as defined by the Commission on Research Integrity. Whistleblowers must respect the confidentiality of sensitive information and give legitimate institutional structures an opportunity to function. Should a whistleblower elect to make a lawful disclosure that violates institutional rules of confidentiality, the institution may thereafter legitimately limit the whistleblower's access to further information about the case.

b. *Protection from retaliation:*[44] Institutions have a duty not to tolerate or engage in retaliation against good-faith whistleblowers. This duty includes providing appropriate and timely relief to ameliorate the consequences of actual or threatened reprisals, and holding accountable those who retaliate. Whistleblowers and other witnesses to possible research misconduct have a responsibility to raise their concerns honorably and with foundation.

c. *Fair procedures:* Institutions have a duty to provide fair and objective procedures for examining and resolving complaints, disputes, and allegations of research misconduct. In cases of alleged retaliation that are not resolved through institutional intervention, whistleblowers should have an opportunity to defend themselves in a proceeding where they can present witnesses and confront those they charge with retaliation against them, except when they violate rules of confidentiality.

   Whistleblowers have a responsibility to participate honorably in such procedures by respecting the serious consequences for those they accuse of misconduct, and by using the same standards to correct their own errors that they apply to others.

d. *Procedures free from partiality:* Institutions have a duty to follow procedures that are not tainted by partiality arising from personal or institutional conflict of interest or other sources of bias. Whistleblowers have a responsibility to act within legitimate institutional channels when raising concerns about the integrity of research. They have the right to raise objections concerning the possible partiality of those selected to review their concerns without incurring retaliation.

---

[44] The Commission on Research Integrity supports the Institute of Medicine recommendation universities should "provide mediation and counseling services for faculty, staff, and students who concerns about professionally questionable training or research practices." Institute of Medicine (1 Responsible Conduct of Research in the Health Sciences. Washington, D.C.: National Academy Press, p. 4.

e.   *Information*: Institutions have a duty to elicit and evaluate fully and objectively information about concerns raised by whistleblowers. Whistleblowers may have unique knowledge needed to evaluate thoroughly responses from those whose actions are questioned. Consequently, a competent investigation may involve giving whistleblowers one or more opportunities to comment on the accuracy and completeness of information relevant to their concerns, except when they violate rules of confidentiality.

f.   *Timely processes*: Institutions have a duty to handle cases involving alleged research misconduct as expeditiously as is possible without compromising responsible resolutions. When cases drag on for years, the issue becomes the dispute rather than its resolution. Whistleblowers have a responsibility to facilitate expeditious resolution of cases by good-faith participation in misconduct procedures.

g.   *Vindication*: At the conclusion of proceedings, institutions have a responsibility to credit promptly--in public and/or in private as appropriate--those whose allegations are substantiated.

Every right carries with it a corresponding responsibility. In this context, the Whistleblower Bill of Rights carries the obligation to avoid false statements and unlawful behavior.

Administrative Processes and Investigations in Research Misconduct

Structures and Procedures of Research Institutions[45]

An environment that protects and nurtures research integrity is one in which questions can be freely raised. All individuals actually or potentially involved in maintaining scientific integrity need the security of knowing that open-mindedness and fair procedures are ensured. Rigorous adherence to fair procedures must occur from the very first exploration by an individual who questions the behavior of another, to the final disposition of formal inquiries and hearings.

Institutions must guard against all factors that may undermine impartiality and fairness in such proceedings, including those that place narrow views of institutional self-interest above all others. When conduct is questioned in research institutions, even the earliest and least formal phases of proceedings are vulnerable to mishandling, and power inequalities can contribute to unfair treatment of both whistleblowers (who may be of junior status) and the accused. Testimony to the Commission underscored the potential dangers of partiality in the

---

[45] This section draws on concepts developed by C.K. Gunsalus and others within and outside (Commission.

institutional handling of misconduct allegations from the inception to the completion of investigations.

Mediation by an ombudsperson or mediator from inside or outside the institution should be possible if agreeable to all parties. When academic institutions offer mediation or conciliation, it should be provided by an individual who is independent of the dispute. (See Whistleblower's Bill of Rights, section (d).)

Whatever processes individual institutions develop or adopt, they must achieve a fair balance of impartiality and advocacy in all proceedings. Guidelines for adequate process are required to ensure that allegations are addressed through procedures that are impartial, fair, fact-based, accessible, and open.

The Commission examined diverse model assurances and guidelines developed by institutions, professional organizations, and the Federal Government, and considered suggestions for their implementation.[46][47][48][49] No single specific set of guidelines can ensure satisfactory procedures in all settings because institutions vary considerably in style, size, and structure. Nonetheless, existing policies and guidelines offer important principles and procedures that must be borne in mind. Based on these, the Commission believes institutional procedures must be:

> *Accessible from multiple entry points,* such as through the mentor, lab supervisor, department head or other scientific colleagues, and the research integrity officer or ombudsperson. The existence of multiple entry points requires consistent mechanisms for assessing allegations, as well as adequate communications among these components.

> *Overseen by individuals or by committees whose members are free from bias and conflict of interest.* At every stage of the process, institutions must demonstrate that none of those assessing the allegations have substantial personal or professional involvement with the facts at issue or the individual(s) whose conduct is in question. In whatever manner institutional committee membership is determined, those making the determination must not be directly involved with the unit in which the allegation is made. At least one person who is not from the

---

[46] Gunsalus CK. (1993): Institutional structure to ensure research integrity. Academic Medicine (Supplement 3).

[47] Framework for Institutional Policies and Procedures to Deal with Fraud in Research. Washington, D.C.: Association of American Universities, National Association of State Unive Land-Grant Colleges, Council of Graduate Schools, Nov. 4, 1988; reissued Nov. 10, 1989; developed by an ir working group.

[48] AAMC Ad Hoc Committee on Misconduct and Conflict of Interest in Research: Beyond the "Framework": Institutional Considerations in Managing Allegations of Misconduct in Research. Washington, D.C.: Association of American Medical Colleges, Sept. 1992.

[49] Office of Research Integrity advisory document: "Model Policy and Procedures for Respon‹ Allegations of Scientific Misconduct," April 1995.

institution in which the allegation arose should be included in the investigation phase. It is also good practice to include one or more experts in the scientific field, also from outside the institution. The rosters of professionals that the Commission has suggested be developed by professional societies could provide one useful source of such "outside" professional expertise. Whenever possible, the whistleblower and the accused should have equal input in assembling the committee.

Based on independent investigation. The factual basis for allegations of misconduct must be established without regard to the personality and motivations of whistleblowers or the reputations of those whose behavior they question. The only relevant issue is the facts.

Overseen by bodies that are separated in their investigatory and adjudicatory functions.
It is well established that justice is not usually served by having a single individual or group function as investigator, prosecutor, judge, and jury. The checks and balances provided by separating investigatory and adjudicatory functions are essential to fair process.[50]

Balanced in advocacy.
Testimony to the institutional committee from both sides of the dispute must be reasonably balanced. Institutions must recognize and adjust for differences in power and resources among participants.

Capable of preventing retaliation against participants.
To protect the integrity of the investigative process, the accuser and the accused should receive protection from being silenced, or punished, whether by retaliation or by damage to reputation or resources. Methods for achieving this protection include notifying all faculty members of acceptable and unacceptable procedures; making available an independent ombudsperson; and appointing a senior advisor to both accuser and accused.

Open.
While confidentiality is necessary to protect reputations from inappropriate damage, excessive secrecy undermines justice. Proceedings, or at a minimum their results, should be open whenever possible. Anyone whose conduct is questioned should have an opportunity to respond.

---

[50] This principle applies equally to federal proceedings.

Processing Whistleblower Retaliation Complaints

Responsible Official

1. Covered institutions shall designate a "responsible official" to establish and implement the institution's whistleblower policies according to 42 C.F.R. § 50.103(d)(13) and these Guidelines. The responsible official also serves as a liaison between the institution and ORI for transmitting such information as ORI may require.

2. The responsible official shall be free of any real or apparent conflicts of interest in any particular case.

3. If involvement of the responsible official in a particular case creates a real or apparent conflict of interest with the institution's obligation to protect good faith whistleblowers, and the conflict cannot be satisfactorily resolved for that case, the administrative head shall appoint a substitute responsible official who has no conflict of interest.

Notice of Institutional Policy

The institution shall provide to all its members notice of its whistleblower policies and these Guidelines with Appendices (Whistleblower's Bill of Rights and Attachment to this guideline). The notice shall include the requirement set forth below regarding a whistleblower's deadline for filing a retaliation complaint. The institution's policies and these Guidelines shall be either disseminated or be publicized and made readily available to all institutional members.

Filing Complaints

1. A whistleblower who wishes to receive the procedural protections described by these Guidelines shall file his or her retaliation complaint with the responsible official at the appropriate institution within 180 days[1] from the date the whistleblower became aware or should have become aware of the alleged adverse action. Covered institutions shall review and resolve all whistleblower retaliation complaints and should do so within 180 days after receipt of the complaint. If the whistleblower fails to receive an institutional response to the complaint in accordance with these Guidelines within ten (10) working days,[2] the whistleblower may file the retaliation complaint directly with ORI at the following address:

Office of Research Integrity
Division of Policy and Education
5515 Security Lane, Suite 700
Rockville, MD 20852

Telephone: (301) 443-5300
Fax: (301) 594-0042

ORI will forward such complaints to the institution's responsible official for appropriate action.

2. In addition to prospective complaints, institutions may apply these Guidelines to complaints of retaliation made prior to the effective date of the institution's adoption of these Guidelines.

3. The retaliation complaint must include a description of the whistleblower's scientific misconduct allegation and the asserted adverse action, or threat thereof, against the whistleblower, by the institution or its members in response to the allegation. If the retaliation complaint is incomplete, the responsible official shall describe to the whistleblower

---

[1] The institution may establish a longer period of time.

[2] The institution may establish a shorter period of time.

what additional information is needed in order to meet the minimum requirements of a complaint under this Part.

Responding to Complaints

1. Upon receipt of a whistleblower retaliation complaint, the responsible official shall notify the whistleblower of receipt within ten (10) working days[3] after receipt. The notice shall also inform the whistleblower of which process under Section V of the Guidelines the institution proposes to follow in resolving the retaliation complaint and the necessary actions by the whistleblower required under that process. The notice shall also notify the whistleblower of his/her choice of responses listed below.

2. The whistleblower may raise any concerns about the proposed process and the institution may modify the process in response the whistleblower's concerns.

3. The whistleblower has five working days from the date of the initial notification in Part 1 above to

   a. accept the proposed process, although the whistleblower may also submit documentation for the official record about any concerns he/she may have about the proposed process; or

   b. not accept the proposed process and may seek other remedies.

4. If the whistleblower does not accept the proposed process, the institution may, but is not required to, propose the alternative option under Section V of the Guidelines.

5. The institution shall notify ORI of any whistleblower retaliation complaint it receives within ten (10) working days[4] after receipt of the complaint.

Interim Protections

1. At any time before the merits of a whistleblower retaliation complaint have been fully resolved, the whistleblower may submit a written request to the responsible official to take interim actions to protect the whistleblower against an existing adverse action or credible threat of an adverse action by the institution or member.

2. Based on the available evidence, the responsible official shall make a determination of whether to provide interim protections and shall advise the whistleblower of its decision in writing. Documentation underlying the decision whether to provide interim protections shall become part of the record of the complaint. When the whistleblower retaliation complaint is fully resolved, any temporary measure taken to protect the whistleblower shall be discontinued or replaced with permanent remedies.

---

[3] The institution may establish a shorter period of time consistent with footnote 2.

[4] The institution may establish a shorter period of time.

Resolving Complaints

1. For each whistleblower retaliation complaint received, a covered institution shall adhere to one of the two alternative processes for resolving the whistleblower retaliation complaint, or settle the complaint, as described below.

2. Whichever process is elected shall be implemented in a timely fashion. The process should be completed within 180 days of the date the complaint is filed, unless the whistleblower agrees to an extension of time. The institution shall promptly report the final outcome of either process or any settlement to ORI.

3. If the whistleblower declines the institution's proposed process according to these Guidelines, he/she may pursue any other legal rights available to the whistleblower for resolution of the retaliation complaint. However, ORI will deem the institution to have met its obligation under 42 C.F.R. § 50.103(d)(13) and will not pursue the whistleblower complaint further.

Option A: Institutional Investigation

1. If the institution elects Option A, the institution shall conduct an investigation of the whistleblower retaliation complaint according to these Guidelines and implement appropriate administrative remedies consistent with the investigation's finding and institutional decision thereon.

2. An investigation of whistleblower retaliation shall be timely, objective, thorough, and competent. The investigation should be conducted by a panel of at least three (3) individuals appointed by the responsible official. The members of the investigation panel, who may be from outside the institution, shall have no personal or professional relationship or other conflict of interest with the whistleblower or the alleged individual retaliator(s), and shall be qualified to conduct a thorough and competent investigation.

3. The investigation shall include the collection and examination of all relevant evidence, including interviews with the whistleblower, the alleged retaliator(s), and any other individual who can provide relevant and material information regarding the claimed retaliation.

4. The institution shall fully cooperate with the investigation and use all available administrative means to secure testimony, documents, and other materials relevant to the investigation.

5. The confidentiality of all participants in the investigation shall be maintained to the maximum extent possible throughout the investigation.

6. The Panel members shall evaluate objectively and respond accordingly to any concerns raised by the whistleblower, including the identity of the deciding official, responsible official and specific panel members prior to resolution of the complaint.

7. The conclusions of the investigation shall be documented in a written report and made available to the parties. The report should include findings of fact, a list of witnesses interviewed, an analysis of the evidence, and a detailed description of the investigative process.

8. The deciding official shall make a final institutional determination as to whether retaliation occurred. This decision shall be based on the report, the record of the investigation, and a preponderance of evidence standard.

9. If there is a determination that retaliation has occurred, the deciding official shall determine what remedies are appropriate to satisfy the institution's regulatory obligation to protect whistleblowers. The deciding official shall, in consultation with the whistleblower, take measures to protect and/or restore the whistleblower's position and reputation, including making any public or private statements, as appropriate. In addition the deciding official may impose any protections against further retaliation by establishing a system to monitor or discipline the retaliator.

10. The institution shall promptly notify ORI of its conclusions and remedies, if any, and forward the underlying investigation report to ORI.

11. The ORI will review the institutional report to determine whether the institution has substantially followed the process described herein. If the institution has substantially conformed to the process, ORI will not review the merits of the institutional determination under Paragraph 8.

12. Institutional compliance with Section V does not bar the whistleblower from challenging the process or the objectivity, thoroughness, competence, or results of the process, under State law, institutional procedure, policy or agreement, or as otherwise provided by law.

Option B: Arbitration

1. If the institution elects Option B, the institution shall offer the whistleblower the opportunity to submit the retaliation dispute to binding arbitration. The parties shall sign a written agreement that the retaliation dispute will be decided by final and binding arbitration, identifying by whom the arbitration will be conducted.

2. The arbitration agreement shall specify that the institution and the whistleblower abrogate all other rights under Federal, State and local law, and other institutional policies or employment agreements pertinent to the resolution of the whistleblower retaliation complaint, other than enforcement of the arbitration award. However, the parties may enter into any legally enforceable settlement agreement before a final arbitration award is made. A sample arbitration agreement is attached.

3. Any retaliation complaint submitted to arbitration shall be arbitrated according to the rules and procedures of the presiding arbitrator and designated arbitration association.

4. An arbitration under these Guidelines shall be conducted by an arbitrator who has no personal or professional relationship or conflict of interest with the whistleblower, the

institution, the alleged retaliator(s), or any person who is the subject of the underlying scientific misconduct allegation. The institution and the whistleblower shall agree on the choice of arbitrator. The arbitration should be facilitated by the American Arbitration Association or any other recognized non-profit arbitration association.

5. The institution and the whistleblower shall share equally the administrative costs of the arbitration. Each party is responsible for the cost of presenting its own case.

6. The arbitration agreement shall specify that the arbitrator shall require the institution to compensate the whistleblower for part or all of his or her arbitration costs, including attorney fees, if the arbitrator finds that the institution, or its members, retaliated against the whistleblower.

7. The arbitration agreement shall also specify that the arbitrator shall require the whistleblower to compensate the institution for part or all of any filing fees and arbitrator's costs if the arbitrator finds that the whistleblower's allegation of scientific misconduct was not made in good faith. If an institution seeks compensation on this basis, it shall make a preliminary motion to dismiss the retaliation complaint prior to commencement of a hearing. The arbitrator shall, if possible, make a threshold decision on the question of good faith based on written submissions prior to commencement of a hearing on the merits of the retaliation dispute. The institution has the burden of proving by a preponderance of the evidence that the allegation of scientific misconduct was not made in good faith.

8. The arbitration agreement shall specify a preponderance of the evidence standard in determining whether retaliation occurred or any other standard mutually agreed to by the parties.

9. The arbitration agreement shall state that the arbitrator's award is final and binding on all parties, and enforceable as provided by law.

10. If the arbitrator finds that the institution, or its members, retaliated against the whistleblower, the arbitrator may order any relief necessary to make the whistleblower whole for the direct or indirect consequences of retaliation, including protection against further retaliation through imposing a system to monitor or discipline the retaliator. The institution shall abide by the arbitrator's final award and shall implement any additional administrative actions it determines is necessary to correct the retaliation.

11. The institution shall promptly forward a copy of the final arbitration award to ORI.

Settlement

In lieu of the two options described above, an institution and whistleblower may, at any time after the retaliation complaint is made, enter into any binding settlement agreement which finally resolves the retaliation complaint. If both parties agree, the responsible official shall facilitate such settlements. If such an agreement is reached, the institution and the whistleblower shall sign a statement indicating that the retaliation complaint has been resolved.

The institution shall within 30 days send a copy of the signed statement to ORI. ORI does not require a copy of the actual terms of the settlement. The settlement may not restrict the whistleblower from cooperating with any investigation of an allegation protected by 42 C.F.R. Part 50, Subpart A. ORI shall consider a settlement meeting these requirements as fulfilling the institution's regulatory obligation under 42 C.F.R. § 50.103(d)(13).

Institutional Compliance

At any time ORI may review a covered institution's compliance with 42 C.F.R. § 50.103(d)(13) and these Guidelines to the extent that the institution relies on these Guidelines for regulatory compliance. Covered institutions and their members shall cooperate with any such review and provide ORI access to all relevant records. If a covered institution's procedures and implementation thereof substantially conforms to Sections IV and V above, it shall be deemed to have met its whistleblower protection obligation under 42 C.F.R. § 50.103(d)(13).

ATTACHMENT

Sample Arbitration Agreement to Resolve Whistleblower Retaliation Complaint

1. <u>Name of whistleblower</u> ("Complainant") and <u>institution</u> agree that Complainant's whistleblower retaliation complaint against <u>institution and/or members</u> will be submitted to an arbitration proceeding for final resolution of that complaint. Specifically, the parties agree to abide by all of the provisions of this Agreement. Moreover, the parties agree to abrogate all other rights under Federal, State, or local law, and other institutional policies or employment agreements pertinent to the resolution of the whistleblower retaliation complaint, other than enforcement of the arbitration award. This Agreement may not be modified in any manner absent the consent of both parties.

2. Complainant and <u>institution</u> agree that the arbitration shall be conducted by <u>name of arbitrator</u> according to the rules of <u>arbitration association.</u> The parties agree that <u>arbitrator</u> has no professional or personal relationship or conflict of interest with any of the parties.

3. <u>Institution</u> and Complainant agree to share equally the administrative costs of the arbitration proceeding subject to modification by the arbitrator as part of his/her final award. Each party shall be responsible for the costs of presenting its own case subject to modification by the arbitrator as part of his/her final award. The arbitrator shall modify the allocation of costs in favor of the whistleblower including the award of attorney's fees if the arbitrator finds that <u>institution and/or members</u> retaliated against the whistleblower.

The arbitrator shall modify the allocation of costs and dismiss the retaliation dispute in favor of <u>institution</u> if the arbitrator finds that Complainant's allegation of scientific misconduct was not made in good faith. The institution, however, shall be compensated only if it has timely made a preliminary motion to dismiss the retaliation claim on the basis that the allegation of scientific misconduct was not made in good faith, and proves its contention by a preponderance of the evidence.

4. The arbitrator's award shall be limited to Complainant's whistleblower retaliation claim. By submitting this dispute to arbitration under this Agreement, the parties agree that the retaliation claim will be fully settled under this Agreement, shall be dropped from all pending suits, and shall not be part of any future suits in any court of law other than suits to enforce the arbitration award.

5. The arbitrator shall apply a preponderance of the evidence standard in determining whether retaliation occurred [or any other standard mutually agreed to by the parties].

6. Upon completion of the parties' presentations, the arbitrator shall render an award which is final and binding upon both parties. The arbitrator shall grant any remedy or relief that the arbitrator deems just and equitable and is consistent with 42 C.F.R. § 50.103(d)(13) and

Sections IV and V of the ORI Guidelines. The arbitrator's award is not appealable before any court of law and may be enforced by the prevailing party in court or otherwise.

_____ _____

(whistleblower)   Date

_____ _____

(institution)   Date

10.2 Whistle-Blower Breaks His Silence

David Cyranoski

Cyranoski, D. Whistle-blower breaks his silence. *Nature* 505, 593–594 (2014). © 2014 Macmillan Publishers Limited. All rights reserved. An imprint of SpringerNature.

NEWS IN FOCUS

MEDICINE Stress proves to be a simple recipe for turning body cells into stem cells **p.596**

BUSINESS Synthetic biologists seek the sweet smell of success **p.598**

POLITICS Ukraine's scientists square up to the government over European links **p.599**

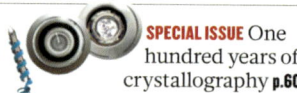

SPECIAL ISSUE One hundred years of crystallography **p.601**

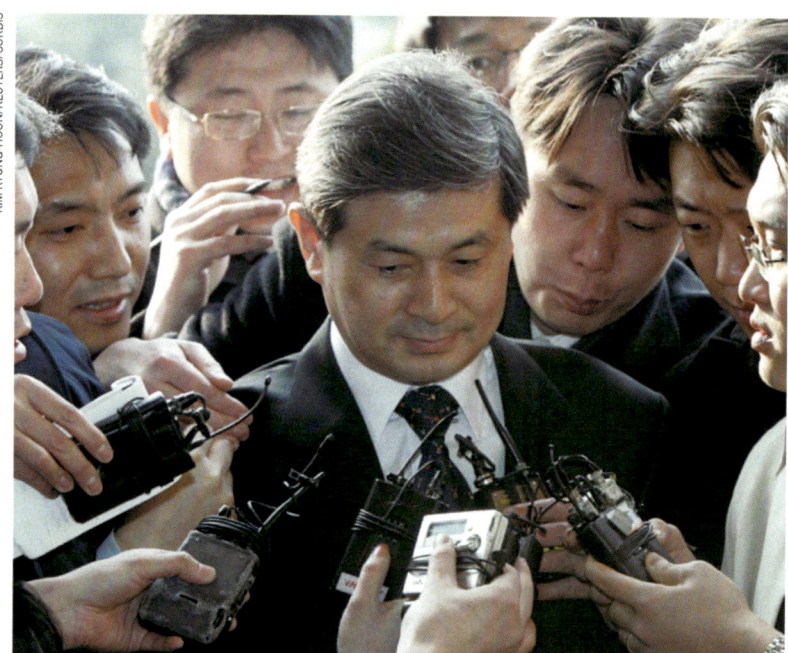

Woo Suk Hwang's human-cloning research was deemed fraudulent by Seoul National University in 2006.

MISCONDUCT

Whistle–blower breaks his silence

South Korean researcher reveals the fallout he faced from his tip-offs about former cloning fraudster Woo Suk Hwang.

BY DAVID CYRANOSKI

The whistle-blower who played a key part in exposing the fraud of South Korean cloning specialist Woo Suk Hwang has spoken for the first time about his role in the scandal — and the suffering he endured as a result.

Young-Joon Ryu, who was a key figure in Hwang's laboratory for several years, kept his silence for eight years. But in a blog post in December 2013 and a subsequent interview with *Nature,* he revealed that he was responsible for initiating the investigation that uncovered one of the biggest frauds in science. He has since received both support and abuse, highlighting just how divided South Korean society still is over the legacy of its fallen hero.

"The nature of the Hwang scandal is the abuse of other people's sacrifice and other people's lives for personal success," Ryu, now in the pathology department at Kangwon National University in Chuncheon, told *Nature.*

Hwang claimed in 2004 to have cloned a human embryo and produced stem cells from it, potentially opening the way for new disease treatments. In 2006, he admitted fabricating his findings, but despite being convicted of fraud, has since made a controversial comeback (see *Nature* **505,** 468–471; 2014).

Ryu joined Hwang's laboratory at Seoul National University in 2002, and that year led the team that attempted to create cloned human embryos and stem-cell lines from them. He wrote the first manuscript of an article on the work, which was published with great fanfare in February 2004 (W. S. Hwang *et al. Science* **303,** 1669–1674; 2004).

While Hwang basked in its glory, Ryu started to have misgivings about Hwang's tendency to seek publicity. He also felt that human cloning had little potential for clinical applications. In April 2004, he left the laboratory and soon began work at the Korea Cancer Centre Hospital.

When Hwang's group published a dazzling follow-up the next year that suggested that the previous proof-of-principle was almost ready for the clinic (W. S. Hwang *et al. Science* **308,** 1777–1783; 2005), Ryu was suspicious. He knew that important lab members had left, yet the team had pumped out 11 embryonic stem-cell lines in a short time. "I knew how difficult it was," he says. "It wasn't logical."

He then heard that Hwang was preparing a clinical trial for a 10-year-old with a spinal-cord injury, whom Hwang had promised to make walk again. Ryu had known the boy and worried that a trial could hurt him. "I was furious," he says. "I wanted to stop all of that."

Lacking evidence and worried that his identity might be revealed, Ryu baulked at approaching the university or police. Instead, on 1 June 2005, he e-mailed television network Munhwa Broadcasting Corporation (MBC) to recommend an investigation.

MBC producers were initially intimidated by Hwang's star status, but decided to work with Ryu to develop their case. A first programme on the subject, about ethical violations in the way that Hwang recruited egg donors, aired on 22 November 2005, and forced a confession from him. A storm of support for Hwang ensued. A second programme, concerning the fraudulent research, was postponed ▶

▶ after sponsors withdrew support for the TV network and producers faced legal and physical threats. But suspicion was mounting. Posts on the website of the Biological Research Information Center (BRIC), in which volunteers noted errors in the papers, helped to force Seoul National University to open an investigation. By the time the second show aired, on 15 December, Hwang's fate was sealed.

Ryu's identity was leaked after MBC's first programme, and his worst fears about the militancy of Hwang's supporters were borne out. Ryu says that they hacked his blog and sent threatening e-mails to him, his employer and his wife, another former researcher in Hwang's laboratory. On 6 December 2005, Ryu resigned from his hospital job under pressure.

Ryu, his wife and their 8-month-old daughter went into hiding for the next six months. "We cried a lot," says Ryu. It was 2007 before the ostracized Ryu could find paid employment, as a pathology resident at Korea University in Seoul.

On 23 December 2013, Ryu posted a note on the BRIC site to thank those who supported him

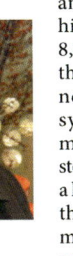

DAVID CYRANOSKI/NATURE

"The nature of the Hwang scandal is the abuse of other people's sacrifice."
Young-Joon Ryu

and signed off with his real name. Some 8,000 people viewed the post, which garnered a few dozen sympathetic comments. But then the story was picked up by a local newspaper and the tone changed. Of more than 1,000 comments on the popular Daum news-aggregator website, 90% have been negative. Online commenters have said that by "revealing a petty truth", Ryu caused South Korea to "fall behind in the stem-cell business". Another accuses him of "satisfying his arrogance" while "seriously injuring the nation" as the "entire project was stolen by other nations".

Ryu says that he has no regrets about what he did. The scandal did not ruin his faith in science either. He completed a PhD in bioethics and safe research in 2011 and is now pursuing a doctoral degree in animal reproductive biology at Seoul National University.

The episode shows how whistle-blowing still carries risks, especially for junior researchers, says Bernd Pulverer, head of scientific publications at the European Molecular Biology Organization in Heidelberg, Germany. "The Hwang case was a wake-up call for many journals to police [fraud] more seriously," he says. But he adds that "little has formally changed regarding the protection and encouragement of constructive whistle-blowing". ■

Additional reporting by Soo Bin Park.

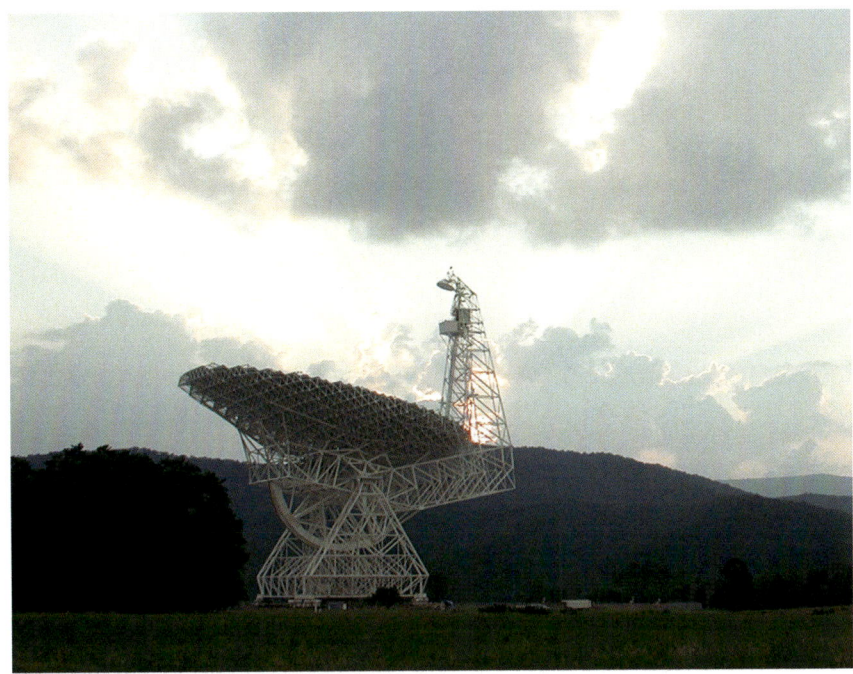

West Virginia's Green Bank Telescope needs partners to pay half of its US$8-million operating costs.

ASTRONOMY

US struggles to offload telescopes

West Virginia radio observatory seeks money from partners to fend off closure by the National Science Foundation.

BY ALEXANDRA WITZE

Astronomer D. J. Pisano got to spread some good news last month. He and his colleagues at West Virginia University in Morgantown announced a US$500,000 grant from the National Science Foundation (NSF). The money will allow his team to build an antenna-like detector to speed up sky surveys at the Green Bank Telescope (GBT), the nearby 110-metre-wide radio dish that is the largest steerable radio telescope in the world.

There is just one problem. Even as the NSF funding goes towards improving the telescope, the agency is trying to get rid of it.

Following an independent 'portfolio review' in 2012 (see *Nature* **488**, 440; 2012), the NSF is exploring closing the GBT and nine other telescopes it operates (see 'Closing time'). The alternative is to find partners to share the cost. West Virginia University has already shelled out $1 million to buy time on the GBT to bolster its growing astronomy faculty — a first hint of what a future for these jettisoned telescopes might look like.

Still, such partnerships are frustratingly hard to achieve. Last month, the NSF reported that, thanks to the slow pace of discussions and the complex environmental reviews required to shut national facilities, it is not close to making any permanent decisions. That leaves the future of the telescopes in limbo — and puts the careers of astronomers such as Pisano on edge. "We were obviously upset by it, we were somewhat confused," he says.

For the NSF, there is some urgency to replace the old with the new. By offloading the old telescopes, the agency could free up about 10% of its $233-million astronomy budget. That would allow more money for research grants. More importantly, it would regain money for future telescopes, such as the Large Synoptic Survey Telescope, which astronomers are slated to begin building in Chile this year (see *Nature* **505**, 461–462; 2014). "Our job is to foster frontier science," says James Ulvestad, who heads the NSF's astronomy division. "Within a constrained budget there is nothing you can do that isn't going to hurt somebody."

10.3   No One Likes a Snitch

Barbara Redman and Arthur Caplan

Redman, B, Caplan, A. No one likes a snitch. *Science and Engineering Ethics* 21(4), 813–819 (2015). © Springer Science+Business Media Dordrecht 2014. An imprint of SpringerNature.

Sci Eng Ethics (2015) 21:813–819
DOI 10.1007/s11948-014-9570-8

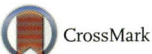

COMMENTARY

No One Likes a Snitch

Barbara Redman · Arthur Caplan

Received: 29 January 2014 / Accepted: 10 June 2014 / Published online: 17 June 2014
© Springer Science+Business Media Dordrecht 2014

Abstract   Whistleblowers remain essential as complainants in allegations of research misconduct. Frequently internal to the research team, they are poorly protected from acts of retribution, which may deter the reporting of misconduct. In order to perform their important role, whistleblowers must be treated fairly. Draft regulations for whistleblower protection were published for public comment almost a decade ago but never issued (Dahlberg 2013). In the face of the growing challenge of research fraud, we suggest vigorous steps, to include: organizational responsibility to certify the accuracy of research including audit, required whistleblower action in the face of imminent or grave harm to subjects, strengthened legal protections against retaliation including prompt enactment of Federal whistleblower protections and consideration of criminalizing the most egregious cases of research misconduct.

Keywords   Research misconduct · Whistleblowers · Research ethics · Fair

Introduction

Most considerations of ethics in research focus appropriately on the protection of subjects. But there are others within the three regulated domains of research ethics (subjects protection, research misconduct and conflict of interest) who, if subjects

B. Redman (✉)
Division of Medical Ethics, NYU Langone Medical Center, New York, NY, USA
e-mail: bkredman@comcast.net

A. Caplan
Drs. William F and Virginia Connolly Mitty Chair, Division of Medical Ethics,
NYU Langone Medical Center, New York, NY, USA
e-mail: Arthur.caplan@nyumc.org

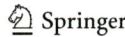

are to be protected, merit protection as well—whistleblowers. It is rare that an institution or the US Office of Research Integrity (ORI) identifies possible research misconduct on its own. The regulation of research misconduct, defined as falsification, fabrication and plagiarism (FFP)(42 CFR part 93 2005) requires a complainant—a whistleblower (WB) for the detection of these actions. Anonymous complaints in fact often preclude ORI from obtaining adequate information (Pascal 2006).

Some have interpreted the growth of anonymous online allegations as a sign that whistleblowers are not being adequately protected in academic environments (Yong et al. 2013). ORI confirms an increase of allegations of this sort, received directly or by institutions. ORI relies on local institutional investigation of allegations. If ORI deems the allegations specific and credible and the charge falls under their funding jurisdiction, ORI refers the allegation to the institution where the violation is alleged to have occurred for assessment and further formal review if warranted (Dahlberg 2013).

Aside from anonymous complaints, there is overwhelming dependence on identifiable WBs to bring forth complaints of research misconduct. Those who do are often placed at high risk in terms of retribution. Although protected by ORI and frequently by institutional policy and state laws, nearly a quarter of whistleblowers report job loss and loss of research support. In ORI cases 43 % reported pressure to drop the allegation (Research Triangle Institute 1995).

The only available study shows that more than two-thirds of identifiable WBs reported experiencing at least one negative outcome including on their physical (28 %) and mental (52 %) health. Seventy-five percent felt stigmatized. Despite these consequences and even though many are in vulnerable junior positions, nearly 80 % of WB said they would or would probably blow the whistle again (Research Triangle Institute 1995).

ORI has not compiled data on whistleblowers in recent years because it lacks resources for internal review, and because its attorney's interpretation of routine use exceptions to the Privacy Act precludes allowing its records to be used for research purposes (Dahlberg 2013). This ongoing lack of data puts WBs, and therefore, human subjects at risk.

A series of more recent studies summarized by Kornfeld (2012), document that fear of retaliation causes many students and faculty to refrain from reporting suspected research misconduct. One researcher is quoted as indicating that consistently, almost no one reports misconduct to the proper authorities (Gewith 2006). And a survey of NIH extramurally funded researchers found significant under-reporting of incidents thought to be research misconduct concluding that better WB protection is needed to improve reporting (Titus et al. 2008). Dahlberg (2013) reports that ORI has taken an average of about a dozen compliance actions per year concerning institutions failing to adequately investigate allegations of misconduct.

A recent study of WBs in nonprofits showed that they had a stronger than usual sense of loyalty to these organizations, believed they were asked to be complicit in bad conduct if they didn't speak up. Many hoped their actions would return the organization to its values and public purposes. In very few cases did the WB

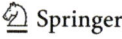 Springer

anticipate or prepare for the level of retaliation they incurred which included job loss and damage to their personal reputation. In the end, the majority did not feel their disclosures led to any significant organizational change. Yet, ninety percent said they would engage in whistleblowing again (Rothschild 2013).

Those internal to a research group alleging research misconduct may share motivations found in a non-profit setting. However, others may be motivated by malice, for example, to stop a competitor's program of research. And still others are part of a movement to detect errors in others' studies, in order to improve the replicability of research.

In the absence of a comprehensive national WB protection law, the False Claims Act (FCA) has been used by WBs involved in research misconduct cases. Well known cases often feature those who have been successful. Walter DeNino, the WB in the case of Eric Poehlman, the first academic in the United States to be jailed for falsifying data in a grant application, was described as "self assured" (Interlandi 2006). He used the False Claims Act and eventually received a relator's fee of $21,600 (Dahlberg 2006).

DeNino's success appears to be the exception. Kohn (2011) warns that without competent legal counsel, WBs are likely to lose FCA actions. Attorney fees often exceed the amount of damages awarded to the complainant WB. The absence of a national law and difficulties in using the FCA leave WB without adequate protection.

Kohn (2011; p7) notes a study of the corporate world showing evidence that WBs uncover more fraud (43 %) than do auditors (19 %). This illustrates their essential role. Sadly, this crucial social role does not square with the level of protection currently provided.

This editorial suggests weaknesses in current regulations and supports adoption and evaluation of more rigorous policies to hold institutions accountable, further buttress protections for WBs and possible criminalization of the most egregious cases of misconduct.

Are We Doing Right by WBs?

The stated purpose of current research misconduct regulations is "…to protect the health and safety of the public, promote the integrity of PHS supported research and conserve public funding…" (42 CFR 93.101 2005). These goals emphasize an aggregate greater good and while they do not preclude concern about WBs, the procedures they depend upon have apparently not been effective in protecting them. A more expanded set of goals for research misconduct policy might include: (A) protect scientific capital (knowledge, scientists, research teams, institutions, norms of science, (B) support fair competition in scientific research, and (C) contain harms to end users (Redman 2009). This set of goals suggests more emphasis on protection of members of the scientific community who must be willing to act as WBs to maintain the integrity of research and the welfare of human subjects. There is little empirical evidence as to whether any of these goals is being met.

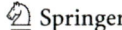 Springer

In 2000, a section on WB protection was developed and published for public comment but never issued in final form. Its revision and reissuance, almost a decade later, would require significant revision (Dahlberg 2013). The ANPRM contains a number of differences from current regulations including authorization of remedies for the WB (reinstatement, back pay, rehabilitation of reputation.) and sanctions toward institutions found to have been engaged in WB retaliation. These include probation status for the institution, recovery of PHS funds misspent in connection with retaliatory action, termination of current and future funding, and public notice of the determination (Handling 2000). In 1996 the Commission on Research Integrity's recommendation of a whistleblower's bill of rights drew sharp criticism from the scientific community (Wadman 1996).

There is acknowledgement that research misconduct is under-reported in part because WBs are reluctant to come forward. At the same time, there is concern that some are experiencing the use of allegations by WBs wielded as political or economic weapons to discredit or slow a competitor's program of research or to extract revenge on a rival. While institutional Research Integrity Officers report an increase in frivolous or malicious allegations, few if any data exist regarding how often accusations are in error or malicious (Wright 2013; Goldenring 2010). An allegation is not in good faith "if made with knowing and reckless disregard for information that would negate the allegation or testimony" (42 CFR Part 93). The existing regulation is silent on how such allegations should be handled (Dahlberg 2013). Future regulations concerning whistleblowers and their protection should define grounds on which allegations could be considered to be in bad faith, with sanctions.

Table 1 outlines benefits and risks of the current WB system, one potentially damaging to WBs. It suggests that risks outweigh benefits to all relevant stakeholders, and are sufficiently significant to require testing of additional regulatory approaches. Suppression of the reporting of evidence of FFP by not protecting WB, not controlling malicious WB and not using other methods of discovery such as regular audits can diminish the quality and integrity of scientific research. It can also obscure an accurate estimate of the amount of FFP, damage from it and how to prevent it.

This analysis leaves key concerns about the roles WBs must play, about how this allocation of roles contributes to ineffective research misconduct policy, and about how risks can be better controlled. First, organizations will apparently always need corrective action from those willing to point out their faults. Some suggest that an increase in WB activity would serve as a deterrent, by increased and earlier exposure and thereby minimize flawed data in the scientific record (Kornfeld 2012).

Second, in the face of overwhelming competition and commercial incentives in science, WBs are one of several mechanisms (including open access data) necessary to keep science centered on its collective objectives (Dal-Re and Caplan 2014). While it is reasonable to expect that required posting of new data will increase the number of WBs external to the research team, internal WB will still be important and need stronger protection. Third, spreading the burden to institutions which must certify that scientific work done under their auspices is free of research misconduct should create a fairer system.

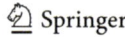 Springer

Table 1 Benefits and risks of whistleblowers as complainants in research misconduct

	Benefits of current system	Risks of current system
Whistleblower	Hope to correct a wrong	Ruins careers and lives (75 % stigmatized, 25 % lose jobs, <10 % cases reported to ORI result in finding of RM)
	Potential notoriety and sense of ethical superiority	Can be used to stop competitor's program of research
Institution	Believed to support loyalty to the institution as steward of research funds	Impact unknown
Science	Appears that RM is under control	Appears that RM is under control
		Potentially suppresses quality control and transparency of the scientific endeavor
Society	Supports trust in science and its institutions	Many potential WB unwilling to take risks so RM underreported; effects on WB unfair and could eventually be corrosive of trust in science

RM research misconduct, *WB* whistleblower

So what ought to be done? First, organizations should have a responsibility to certify as part of their General Assurance to the NIH, other Federal funders and regulatory agencies such as ORI, that they maintain protections for WBs and strive to create an environment of utmost integrity for all. Current research misconduct regulations (42 CFR 93.304) require institutions to protect the confidentiality of complainants and to take "all reasonable and practical efforts to protect and restore the position and reputation of any complainant…and to counter potential or actual retaliation against these complainants…" Available evidence does not support their effectiveness. Certification should require an organizational official to present specific evidence showing what "reasonable and practical efforts" have been taken.

Second, some form of random auditing should be required to detect and correct instances of FFP. Currently it is not expected practice for institutions to monitor non-financial aspects of research projects (Richman Richman and Richman 2012). Some believe that a real threat of an audit would be a more significant deterrent than is the remote chance that a WB will act. It will be important to establish the audit pattern that will optimize the detection of research misconduct for the associated costs.

Third, regulations could be changed to require or obligate WBs to act when they have direct knowledge of an imminent grave harm to animals or humans. Even in the absence of recent data, it is reasonable to assume that incentives to WBs operating in the current system are not optimal for protecting subjects. Under an "imminent grave harm" regulation, any harm to a subject reported or found through subject complaint or IRB review would lead to an investigation of who knew or should have known.

Fourth, to protect WBs in this requirement, the Federal legal protections for WBs ought to be strengthened. These should include creating a penalty should a WB experience a negative job action within a specified time period post reporting a concern. The many ways employers can avoid claims of retaliation are well

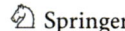 Springer

known—layoffs due to lack of work, poor performance evaluations, shifts to 'makework' jobs, offers to quit and drop the case so one will be able to find new work—and proof of causation is subtle (Kohn 2011). Federal regulations have languished far too long given the key role that WBs play.

Fifth, criminalizing those who commit the most egregious cases of research misconduct and prosecuting them would surely deter research misconduct (Sovacool 2005; Redman and Caplan 2005) and demonstrate that if confirmed WBs' charges have serious consequences for wrongdoers. It has been argued that scientific fraud is no different from financial fraud, which is criminalized, as each involves the misuse of resources. Both misuse taxpayer money and have been prosecuted in both state and federal courts including under charges of making false statements. Scientific fraud can also cause harm through use of ineffective and dangerous treatments (Smith 2005).

These are admittedly tough and vigorous steps to try and encourage and protect whistleblowing while also utilizing other strategies to try and secure research integrity. The growing challenges of misconduct and fraud justify a serious exploration of each of the merits of toughening whistleblower protection and instituting additional measures to detect and discourage fraud and misconduct.

References

Code of Federal Regulations 42 CFR Part 93 2005.

Dahlberg, J. (2013) Email correspondence to the author 12/19/13.

Dahlberg, J., & Mahler, C. (2006). The Poehlman case: Running away from the truth. *Science and Engineering Ethics, 12,* 157–173.

Dal-Re, R., & Caplan, A. (2014). Time to ensure that clinical trial appropriate results are actually published. *European Journal of Clinical Pharmacology.* doi:10.1007/s00228-013-1635-0.

Gewith, V. (2006). Uncovering misconduct. *Nature, 485,* 1137–1139.

Goldenring, J. (2010). Innocence and due diligence: Managing unfounded allegations of scientific misconduct. *Academic Medicine, 85,* 527–530.

Handling Misconduct NPRM-Regulation, 65 Fed Reg 70830 and Fed Reg 82972, (Nov 28, 2000). May be obtained on ORI's web site.

Interlandi, J. (2006). An unwelcome discovery. *New York Times,* October 22, 2006.

Kohn, S. M. (2011). *The whistleblowers handbook.* Guilford, CT: Lyons Press.

Kornfeld, D. S. (2012). Research misconduct: The search for a remedy. *Academic Medicine, 87,* 877–882.

Pascal, C. B. (2006). Complainant issues in research misconduct: The Office of Research Integrity experience. *Experimental Biology in Medicine, 231,* 1264–1270.

Redman, B. K. (2009). Research misconduct and fraud. In V. Ravitsky, A. Fiester, & A. L. Caplan (Eds.), *Penn center guide to bioethics* (pp. 213–222). New York: Springer.

Redman, B. K., & Caplan, A. L. (2005). Off with their heads: The need to criminalize some forms of scientific misconduct. *Journal of Law, Medicine and Ethics, 33*(2), 345–348.

Research Triangle Institute. (October 30, 1995). *Consequences of whistleblowing for the whistleblower in misconduct in science cases.* ORI Website.

Richman, V., & Richman, A. (2012). A tale of two perspectives: regulation versus self-regulation, a financial reporting approach (from Sarbanes-Oxley) for research ethics. *Science and Engineering Ethics, 18,* 241–246.

Rothschild, J. (2013). Rising in defense of nonprofit organizations' social purposes: How do whistle-blowers fare when they expose corruption in nonprofits? *Nonprofit and Voluntary Sector Quarterly, 42,* 1–13.

Smith, R. (2005). Should scientific fraud be a criminal offense? *British Medical Journal, 331,* 288.

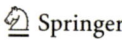

Sovacool, B. (2005). Using criminalization and due process to reduce scientific misconduct. *American Journal of Bioethics, 5*(5), W1–W7.

Titus, S., Wells, J., & Rhoades, L. (2008). Repairing research integrity. *Nature, 453*, 980–982.

Wadman, M. (1996). Hostile reception to US misconduct report. *Nature, 301*, 639.

Wright, D. E. (2013). Guest editorial. *Accountability in Research, 20*, 287–290.

Yong, E., Ledford, H., & Van Noorden, R. (2013). Three ways to blow the whistle. *Nature, 502*, 454–457.

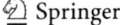 Springer

References

Bonito A, Titus S, Greene A, Amoozegar J, Eicheldinger C, Wright D. Preparing whistleblowers for reporting research misconduct. Account Res. 2012;19:308–28.

Culiberg B, Mihelic K. The evolution of whistleblowing studies: a critical review and research agenda. J Bus Ethics. 2016; on-line 20 June.

Cyranoski D. Whistle-blower breaks his silence. Nature. 2014;505:593–4.

Gewin V. Uncovering misconduct. Nature. 2012;485:137–9.

Redman B. Commentary: legacy of the commission on research integrity. Sci Eng Ethics. 2016; on-line January 13.

Report of the Commission on Research Integrity: Integrity and Misconduct in Research. 1995. US Department of Health and Human Services.

Additional Suggested Reading

Gewin V. Uncovering misconduct. Nature. 2012;485:137–139. (*Statisticians from another university had to persist for some time to gain attention to findings that did not match an investigator's data.*)

Yong E, Ledford H, Van Noorden R. 3 ways to blow the whistle. Nature. 2013;503:454–457. (*Some whistleblowers obtain evidence by statistical analysis, others by prolonged efforts to persuade authorities and others by anonymous allegations.*)

Conflict of Interest

Arthur L. Caplan and Barbara K. Redman

Conflict of interest (COI) describes a situation in which the impartiality of research may be compromised by the researcher standing to profit in some way from conclusions drawn in the research. This can be a conflict among roles as when a researcher takes on too many outside consulting duties and neglects mentoring students, or misses classroom teaching, or a conflict of trust when the ability to make money from offering a particular interpretation of findings distorts trust in the analysis or conclusions reached. COI can occur at individual, institutional, or industry level or in a particular case, at several of these levels at once. Conflicts can arise from financial, ideological, political, religious beliefs, or personal relationships. Transparency through the disclosure of financial COIs has been the main management technique for handling COI. But it is suboptimal because it provides no way to know for sure whether competing interests have compromised the research (Dunn et al. 2016). There is no detailed federal policy in the USA on identifying or managing institutional conflicts of interest. A survey by Resnik (2016) found that only 38% of top grant getting institutions had such policies.

Cases in this chapter and in the suggested supplementary readings provide examples of COI and how they might be handled. Historical evidence of an NIH institute being captured by the sugar industry while setting its research priorities yielded unfortunate results for controlling disease. Tactics were similar to those used by tobacco, lead, and other industries – using funding to divert the research agenda to protect their products (Kearns et al. 2015). In the case of the death of Jesse Gelsinger in a gene therapy trial at the University of Pennsylvania, both individual and institutional conflicts of interest involving patents for vector technology were present. The principal investigator of that trial in various subsequent writings identified lessons learned, which included more rigorous restrictions to separate the investigator and physician caretaker roles and limitation of trial involvement by an investigator with a stake in a company whose value could be affected by the outcome of the trial (Wilson 2009). Elliott (2016) describes a complex web of conflicts by a university in its oversight role in the protection of human subjects. Review of this situation by an independent external group provided insights into best practices for minimizing conflicts including a greater role for those not affiliated with the institution on review committees.

Potential COIs can be found in many areas of research production, dissemination and oversight. Campbell et al. (2015) found industry COI on the part of 30% of IRB members and noted that 25% of conflicted members voted on a protocol on which they were conflicted, which is an ethical violation—they should have recused themselves. At the same time, since discussion of the commercial purpose of a study and researcher compensation are not part of IRB review, members cannot discuss how interests of the researcher may conflict with interests of the research subject (participant). Meta-analyses (MA) of antidepressant trials found 30% of authors to be employees of the drug manufacturer with a total of 79% of authors having industry links. Those with employee authors were much less likely than were other studies to have negative statements about the drug.

COIs do not automatically invalidate scientific work but rather raise a question about whether a scientist or institution

A. L. Caplan · B. K. Redman (✉)
New York University Langone Medical Center,
New York, NY, USA
e-mail: Arthur.Caplan@nyumc.org

has been careful in their role and impartial. Some COIs could be seen as inherent in certain structures (IRB action on proposals that bring money to the university that appoints IRB members) but may be counterbalanced with benefits from this arrangement such as local knowledge of the trustworthiness of investigators.

Advice: Know how to identify potential COIs, how to evaluate evidence when they are present. Seek to minimize COI by not undertaking outside work that greatly interferes with your primary duties and never accepting support that is contingent on reaching a particular conclusion in your work. If you are evaluating your own work prior to publishing or that of others, do not be the only one to do so if you have COI. Always disclose any concerns you have about possible COI to editors, regulatory bodies, and colleagues.

11.1 Sugar Industry Influence on the Scientific Agenda of the National Institute of Dental Research's 1971 National Caries Program: A Historical Analysis of Internal Documents

Cristin E. Kearns, Stanton A. Glantz, and Laura A. Schmidt

Kearns, C, Glantz, S, Schmidt, L. Sugar industry influence on the scientific agenda of the National Institute of Dental Research's 1971 National Caries Program: A historical analysis of internal documents. *PLoS Medicine* 12(3), e1001798 (2015). Copyright: © 2015 Kearns et al.

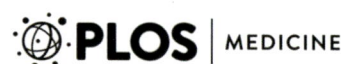

RESEARCH ARTICLE

Sugar Industry Influence on the Scientific Agenda of the National Institute of Dental Research's 1971 National Caries Program: A Historical Analysis of Internal Documents

Cristin E. Kearns[1,2,3], **Stanton A. Glantz**[1,2,4,5]*, **Laura A. Schmidt**[1,2,6,7]

1 Philip R. Lee Institute for Health Policy Studies, University of California San Francisco, San Francisco, California, United States of America, 2 Department of Medicine, University of California San Francisco, San Francisco, California, United States of America, 3 Department of Orofacial Sciences, University of California San Francisco, San Francisco, California, United States of America, 4 Center for Tobacco Control Research and Education, University of California San Francisco, San Francisco, California, United States of America, 5 Helen Diller Family Comprehensive Cancer Center, University of California San Francisco, San Francisco, California, United States of America, 6 Clinical and Translational Science Institute, University of California San Francisco, San Francisco, California, United States of America, 7 Department of Anthropology, History and Social Medicine, University of California San Francisco, San Francisco, California, United States of America

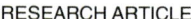

* glantz@medicine.ucsf.edu

G OPEN ACCESS

Citation: Kearns CE, Glantz SA, Schmidt LA (2015) Sugar Industry Influence on the Scientific Agenda of the National Institute of Dental Research's 1971 National Caries Program: A Historical Analysis of Internal Documents. PLoS Med 12(3): e1001798. doi:10.1371/journal.pmed.1001798

Academic Editor: Simon Capewell, University of Liverpool, UNITED KINGDOM

Received: October 30, 2014

Accepted: January 29, 2015

Published: March 10, 2015

Funding: This work was supported by the UCSF Philip R. Lee Institute for Health Policy Studies, a donation by the Hellmann Family Fund to the UCSF Center for Tobacco Control Research and Education, the UCSF School of Dentistry Department of Orofacial Sciences and Global Oral Health Program, National Institute of Dental and Craniofacial Research

Abstract

Background

In 1966, the National Institute of Dental Research (NIDR) began planning a targeted research program to identify interventions for widespread application to eradicate dental caries (tooth decay) within a decade. In 1971, the NIDR launched the National Caries Program (NCP). The objective of this paper is to explore the sugar industry's interaction with the NIDR to alter the research priorities of the NIDR NCP.

Methods and Findings

We used internal cane and beet sugar industry documents from 1959 to 1971 to analyze industry actions related to setting research priorities for the NCP. The sugar industry could not deny the role of sucrose in dental caries given the scientific evidence. They therefore adopted a strategy to deflect attention to public health interventions that would reduce the harms of sugar consumption rather than restricting intake. Industry tactics included the following: funding research in collaboration with allied food industries on enzymes to break up dental plaque and a vaccine against tooth decay with questionable potential for widespread application, cultivation of relationships with the NIDR leadership, consulting of members on an NIDR expert panel, and submission of a report to the NIDR that became the foundation of the first request for proposals issued for the NCP. Seventy-eight percent of the sugar industry submission was incorporated into the NIDR's call for research applications. Research that could have been harmful to sugar industry interests was omitted from priorities

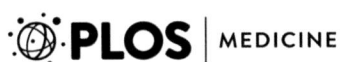

grant DE-007306 and National Cancer Institute Grant
CA-087472. The funders had no role in study design,
data collection and analysis, decision to publish, or
preparation of the manuscript.

Competing Interests: The authors have declared
that no competing interests exist.

Abbreviations: FAO, Food and Agriculture
Organization; FDA, Food and Drug Administration;
ISRF, International Sugar Research Foundation; NCI,
National Cancer Institute; NCP, National Caries
Program; NIDR, National Institute of Dental
Research; NIDCR, National Institute of Dental and
Craniofacial Research; NIH, National Institutes of
Health; RFC, request for contracts; SA, the Sugar
Association; SRF, Sugar Research Foundation;
TIRC, Tobacco Industry Research Committee; TWG,
Tobacco Working Group; WHO, World Health
Organization; WSRO, World Sugar Research
Organisation.

identified at the launch of the NCP. Limitations are that this analysis relies on one source of sugar industry documents and that we could not interview key actors.

Conclusions

The NCP was a missed opportunity to develop a scientific understanding of how to restrict sugar consumption to prevent tooth decay. A key factor was the alignment of research agendas between the NIDR and the sugar industry. This historical example illustrates how industry protects itself from potentially damaging research, which can inform policy makers today. Industry opposition to current policy proposals—including a World Health Organization guideline on sugars proposed in 2014 and changes to the nutrition facts panel on packaged food in the US proposed in 2014 by the US Food and Drug Administration—should be carefully scrutinized to ensure that industry interests do not supersede public health goals.

Introduction

Despite overwhelming consensus on the causal role of sugars in tooth decay [1] and recommendations by expert committees [2–4], quantitative targets restricting the intake of sugars to control dental caries have not been widely implemented [5]. In 2003, a joint committee of the World Health Organization (WHO) and the Food and Agriculture Organization (FAO) recommended limiting "free" or added sugars, defined as "monosaccharides and disaccharides added to foods by the manufacturer, cook or consumer, and sugars naturally present in honey, syrups, fruit juices and fruit concentrates" to 10% of total calories [3]. The World Sugar Research Organisation (WSRO), a trade organization representing more than 30 international members with economic interests in the cane and beet sugar industry, including the Sugar Association (SA) in the US and Coca-Cola [6], successfully blocked the 2003 WHO/FAO joint committee recommendation from becoming WHO policy [7]. The WHO/FAO joint committee quantitative recommendation to limit free sugars [3] was replaced with the nonspecific recommendation to "limit the intake of free sugars" [8]. In 2014, based largely on the global burden of dental disease, the WHO Nutrition Guidance Expert Advisory Group issued draft guidelines with strong quantitative recommendations to limit daily consumption of free sugars to 10% of total calories, with a further suggestion to limit free sugars to less than 5% of total calories [4]. As with the 2003 WHO recommendation, WSRO and its members have submitted comments in opposition to the 2014 WHO draft recommendation [9,10] and have signaled willingness to contest the 2014 recommendations with equal force as in 2003 [11,12]. WSRO argued that dental public health interventions should focus on reducing the harm of sugar consumption with methods such as the "regular use of fluoride toothpaste" rather than restricting sugar intake [9,13].

Publications about food industry influence on public health policy are growing [14–21], but analyses of food industry documents are rare [22]. Historical analyses of internal tobacco industry documents have proven key to informing policy and litigation successes in tobacco control [23–27]. There are similar historical internal documents related to WSRO that could inform public health efforts by illuminating sugar industry activities designed to undermine or subvert policies to restrict sugar consumption [28].

We analyzed previously unexplored sugar industry documents to trace industry interactions with the US National Institute of Dental Research (NIDR, which changed its name to the

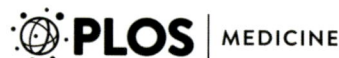
National Institute of Dental and Craniofacial Research [NIDCR] in 1998) between 1966 and 1971, a critical period for dental caries control policy when the NIDR planned the launch of the National Caries Program (NCP) with the goal of eradicating dental caries within one decade [29]. Reflecting the research priorities of the sugar industry, the 1971 NCP research priorities ignored strategies to limit sugar consumption and focused instead on fluoride delivery, reducing the virulence of oral bacteria, and modifying food products with additives to counter sugar's harmful effects [30]. Ultimately, the NCP, which drove the US dental caries research agenda for more than a decade, failed to significantly reduce the burden of dental caries [31], a preventable disease that remains the leading chronic disease in children and adolescents in the US [32].

Methods

Data Sources

Sugar industry documents.   This study drew substantially on previously unexplored WSRO-related internal documents from between 1959 and 1971 [33]. WSRO was formed from a number of related sugar industry trade organizations including the Sugar Research Foundation (SRF) and the International Sugar Research Foundation (ISRF) (Fig. 1) [6,34–36]. The first author located these documents in 2010 in an inventory of the papers of Roger Adams housed in the University of Illinois Archives through a Google search using the terms "International Sugar Research Foundation" and "archives" [33]. Roger Adams, Emeritus Professor of Organic Chemistry, served on the SRF and then ISRF Scientific Advisory Board [37] from 1959 until his death in 1971 [38,39]. Adams's files contain correspondence with sugar industry executives, meeting minutes, and other relevant reports. After reviewing the inventory

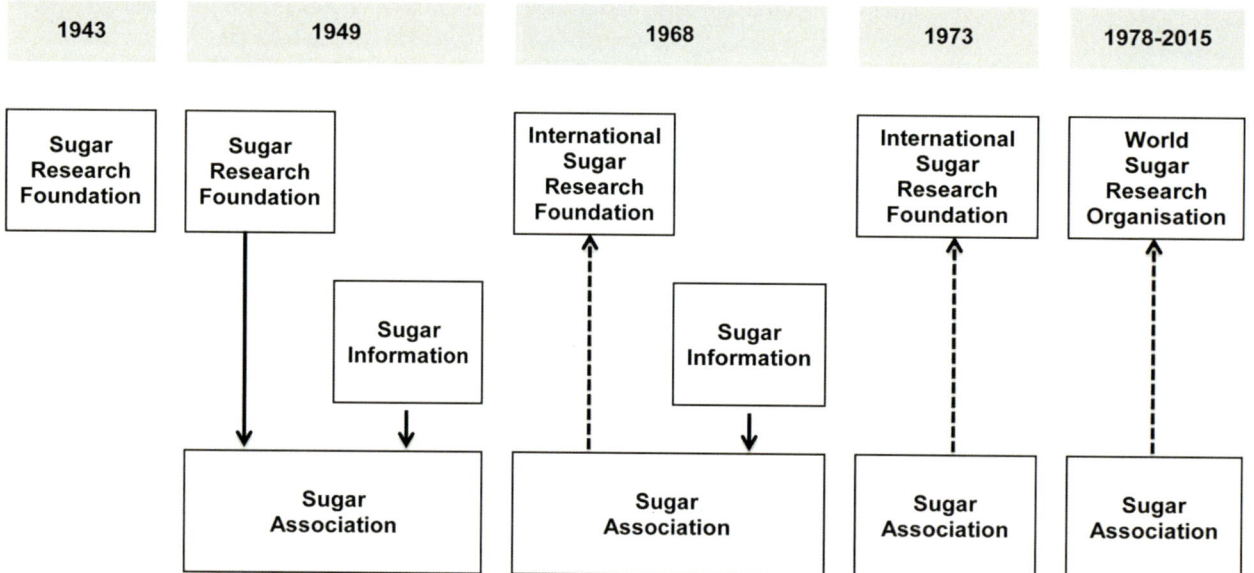

Fig 1. Two sugar industry organizations operating as of 2015, the World Sugar Research Organisation and the Sugar Association, evolved out of the Sugar Research Foundation. In 1943, SRF was founded in New York, New York. In 1949, SA was created to oversee the research activities of SRF (the research arm) and the newly created Sugar Information (the public relations arm). In 1968, SRF dissociated from SA and was reorganized as ISRF. SA joined ISRF as a member (shown as a dotted line). In 1973, SA discontinued Sugar Information because there was no longer a meaningful separation of duties between SA and Sugar Information. In 1978, ISRF was reorganized to become WSRO, and SA joined WSRO as a member.

doi:10.1371/journal.pmed.1001798.g001

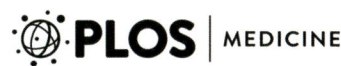

of the Roger Adams papers and consulting with University of Illinois archivists, the first author identified 319 documents (1,551 pages) related to SRF/ISRF. Additional material authored by SRF, ISRF, and WSRO was located through a WorldCat search, including annual reports, symposium proceedings, and reviews of research. Documents were carefully reviewed for relevance to dental caries research and policy.

National Institute of Dental Research documents.   We located sources related to the NIDR NCP through searches of PubMed and WorldCat, and by contacting NIDCR directly. Materials included NCP primary publications [40–45] and two historical reviews commissioned by the NIDR: a description of the first decade of the NCP by its project officer, William E. Rogers [29], and a history of the NIDR by historian Ruth Roy Harris [31].

Findings were assembled chronologically into a narrative case study. Part of the analysis called for systematically comparing two key reports for similarities: (1) *Dental Caries Research—1969* [46], a document submitted by ISRF to the NIDR, and (2) the NIDR's 1971 *Opportunities for Participation in the National Caries Program* [30], which defined the research priorities at the launch of the NCP. Both documents were entered into Microsoft Word using a monospaced font at 12 characters per inch (average of 12 words per line). After line numbering both documents, we compared the documents, classifying each line of the 1971 NIDR document and the 1969 ISRF document as different, paraphrased, or verbatim. "Paraphrased" was defined as some identical words with the same overall meaning.

Results

Emergence of the National Caries Program, 1966–1967

Table 1 provides a timeline of events during the planning and launch of the NCP.

In June 1966, President Lyndon Johnson initiated a major reappraisal of National Institutes of Health (NIH) research agendas, requesting that directors of NIH institutes submit their programs' "priorities and objectives in the national attack on disease and disability" [29]. The NIDR Director Seymour Kreshover's report to President Johnson in November 1966 stated that "an accelerated program of research during the next decade could reasonably provide the means for virtual eradication of dental caries" [31].

The threat of the NIDR's dental research program to the sugar industry began to crystallize in July 1967, after the president praised Kreshover's report [31]. While it had long been known that bacteria caused tooth decay [54], Kreshover based his plans on the work of NIDR scientists Robert Fitzgerald and Paul Keyes, who had singled out the bacterial strain *Streptococcus mutans* as a major culprit in the production of acids that caused dental caries [55,56]. Research suggested that sucrose was more hazardous than other types of sugars because it caused *S. mutans* to form dextrans, sticky molecules that caused the bacteria to tenaciously adhere to one another in the plaque and on the tooth's surface [57]. The NIDR's increased interest in *S. mutans* brought renewed scrutiny to sucrose consumption and dental caries risk.

In October 1967, the NIDR's National Dental Advisory Council identified three main areas of emphasis to inform research priorities to eradicate caries: reducing the virulence of bacteria once exposed to sugars, fluoride delivery, and, of most concern to the sugar industry, dietary modification [31]. A particular threat was research conducted by NIDR scientist Robert Stephan, initiated in the 1940s, on the "cariogenic" (decay-causing) potential of foods [58–60]. According to Stephan, as of 1966:

There have been a great many observations, discussions, and controversies published in the literature concerning the role of different foods and particularly sweets in the etiology [of

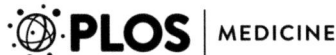
Table 1. Timeline of events of sugar industry influence on the scientific agenda of the National Institute of Dental Research's 1971 National Caries Program.

Key Dates	NIDR	SRF and ISRF
1959		Roger Adams becomes member of SRF Scientific Advisory Board [37]
June 1966	NIDR Director Seymour Kreshover initiates planning for what would become NCP [29,31]	
1967		SRF funds Project 269 to develop dextranase enzyme and vaccine [47]
June 1968	Announcement of Caries Task Force [31]	Philip Ross (with ties to the US National Institutes of Health) elected ISRF president [48,49], coordinates meetings with the NIDR prior to NCP launch [50]
June 1969		Symposium on the Status of Research in Sucrochemistry, Diet and Heart Disease, Obesity, Dental Caries, and Clinical Nutrition held; Prof. G. Neil Jenkins speaks on "Sugar and Dental Caries" [51]
Sept. 1969		Symposium held: Seeking New Approaches to Old Problems; the NIDR's Richard Greulich speaks on "The Future of Caries Control" [52]
Oct. 1969	Caries Task Force Steering Committee meeting on research priorities; planning for Role of Human Foodstuffs in Caries Workshop Conference [29]	ISRF convenes Panel Meeting of the Dental Caries Task Force—members of the NIDR Caries Task Force Steering Committee participate [53]
Late 1969		Submission of ISRF report *Dental Caries Research—1969* to the NIDR Caries Task Force [46]
Jan. 1970	NIDR Laboratory of Microbiology chief Henry Scherp submits *A National Caries Program of the National Institute of Dental Research: Ten-Year Program of Research and Development*; Nixon selects NCP as special health initiative to be funded in fiscal year 1971 [41]	
Feb. 1970	President Nixon endorses NCP [31]	Celebratory *International Sugar Research Foundation Special Report: Dental Caries* mailed to Roger Adams [50]
March 1970	Caries Task Force holds Role of Human Foodstuffs in Caries Workshop Conference [42]	
March 1971	NCP becomes operational [29]; Omnibus request for contracts, *Opportunities for Participation in the National Caries Program*, released [30]	

doi:10.1371/journal.pmed.1001798.t001

dental caries]. However. . .there seems to be little controlled experimental proof to show which foods are cariogenic and which noncariogenic in humans. [61]

Stephan had initiated work to develop an animal model that could "evaluate cariogenicity and anticariogenicity of different foods and beverages that people like and commonly consume" [61]. Based on existing research at the time, foods containing sucrose were in danger of being placed at the top of the list of harmful cariogenic products [62].

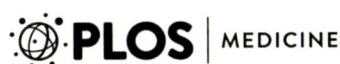

Industry Deflection of Attention Away from Limiting Sugar Intake

Industry position on caries control.   At least as early as 1950, SRF knew its product damaged teeth and appreciated that both the scientific evidence and the dental community favored restricting sugar intake as a key way to control caries [63]. The 1950 SRF annual report stated:

> The ultimate aim of the Foundation in dental research has been to discover effective means of controlling tooth decay *by methods other than restricting carbohydrate intake.* This program has both laboratory and clinical aspects.

> *There is evidence tending to show that carbohydrates, including sugar, and perhaps other food types, are implicated in tooth decay.* There is also evidence, though less convincing, that soluble sugars may play a bigger role than starches. Besides the relatively clear evidence there are many conjectures, traditions and myths that confuse the picture.

> *Until recently the great majority of the dental profession had adopted the view that practical control of tooth decay could be achieved only by restriction of carbohydrates, particularly sugar in the diet.* Scientific logic, nevertheless, points to many other promising possibilities and many of these are supported by preliminary laboratory observations. [63] (emphasis added)

The 1950 SRF annual report also shows that industry research was selected as part of a strategy to deflect attention away from sugar restriction as a means to control caries [63].

Funding research to divert attention from limiting sugar intake.   Consistent with a deflection strategy, between 1967 and 1970, SRF funded Project 269 to bolster research on interventions not requiring sugar restriction to control dental caries [47]. Project 269, led by Professor Bertram Cohen at the Royal College of Surgeons of England, sought to render *S. mutans* less destructive to teeth after sugar was consumed using enzymes called dextranases to break the sticky dextrans in dental plaque formed after sugar was consumed [47]. Project 269 also attempted to develop a vaccine against tooth decay that would allow people to continue to consume sugar [47]. The NIDR had investigated both methods in the 1960s [31] and found that although dextranases added to the food and water of rodents had shown some promise of being effective, more research was necessary before human applications could be developed [64], and a vaccine against *S. mutans* tested in hamsters failed to prevent tooth decay [65]. By 1962, NIDR scientists were suggesting that measures other than a vaccine would be needed to control dental caries [31].

SRF allocated US$12,000 (US$85,455 in 2014 dollars) to Project 269 between 1967 and 1970 [47]. Project 269 was primarily funded by the chocolate and confectionary industries and had an annual budget of US$120,000 (US$854,558 in 2014 dollars) [47]. A confidential report mailed to Roger Adams summarizing Project 269 indicated that SRF considered dental caries "one of the major troublesome factors in the nonacceptance of sucrose" [47]. SRF leaders hoped that their support for this new project would prove a "significant way of solving the problem" [47].

Funding from SRF and the chocolate and confectionary industry allowed Cohen to create a new laboratory to use monkeys for the development of dextranases and a tooth decay vaccine for human application [47]. SRF hoped that the work on dextranases and a vaccine could be handed over to drug companies to develop commercial quantities [47]. A 1968 *Montreal Gazette* article, "These Monkeys May Save Your Teeth," reported that one practical application for dextranase under consideration was "to mix it with raw sugar and use it as a powder on

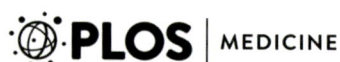
desserts and cakes and in soft drinks" [66]. Cohen was described as having "little sympathy for those who would ban sweet things," and was quoted as saying "Why should people be denied pleasure? It would obviously be far better to eliminate the harmful effects" [66]. While at the time there was less attention paid to scientific conflicts of interest than in 2015, the article mentioned that a grant from the Nuffield Foundation funded the building of the research unit that housed the monkeys, but not that the sugar or chocolate and confectionary industries were also supporting Cohen's work [66].

Setting Research Priorities for the National Caries Program, 1968–1969

At a June 1968 press conference, NIDR Director Kreshover announced the creation of the Caries Task Force chaired by NIDR Laboratory of Microbiology chief Henry Scherp to develop the NCP [31]. A subcommittee, the Caries Task Force Steering Committee, was assigned the essential task of identifying research priorities [29]. Task force members were largely drawn from federal agencies and academia (Table 2). Professor Basil Bibby, with a strong background in developing models that could evaluate the cariogenicity of foods, would be assigned a leading role in evaluating research supporting dietary interventions to eliminate tooth decay [29].

In 1968, SRF reorganized as ISRF to carry on SRF's research mission at the global level [48]. Existing SRF research projects, including Project 269, continued to be supported by ISRF [67]. ISRF was also interested in engaging federal research agencies. On July 1, 1968, Dr. Philip Ross became ISRF president [48]. Ross had ties to the NIH, having served as chief of the NIDR/NIH Research Grants Section from 1963 to 1965, then as assistant head of the NIH Special International Programs Section until 1967 [49]. Moreover, that summer, ISRF moved its headquarters from New York to Bethesda, Maryland, near the NIH [68].

Industry reviews dental caries literature. As the NIDR Caries Task Force Steering Committee began meeting to discuss research priorities in 1969, ISRF scheduled a series of meetings

Table 2. Comparison of membership of the NIDR Caries Task Force Steering Committee and ISRF Panel Meeting of Dental Caries Task Force.

Name	Affiliation	NIDR Caries Task Force Steering Committee, 1969 [31]	ISRF Panel Meeting of Dental Caries Task Force, October 20, 1969 [53]
Basil G. Bibby	Director, Eastman Dental Center	X	X
George W. Burnett	Professor of Microbiology, School of Dentistry, Medical College of Georgia	X	X
James P. Carlos	Chief, Biometry Section, NIDR		X
Charles J. Donnelly	Chief, Dental Caries and Hard Tissues Program, Extramural Programs, NIDR	X	X
Robert J. Fitzgerald	Laboratory of Microbiology, NIDR	X	
John C. Greene	Deputy Director, Division of Dental Health, Bureau of Health Professions, Education of Manpower Training, NIH	X	X
Robert S. Harris	Professor of Nutritional Biochemistry, Massachusetts Institute of Technology	X	X
John Knutson	Professor of Preventive Dentistry, School of Dentistry, University of California, Los Angeles	X	X
Bo Krasse	Professor of Cariology and Dean, Faculty of Odontology, University of Gothenburg, Sweden		X
Seymour Kreshover	Director, NIDR and Caries Task Force Steering Committee	X	X
Henry W. Scherp	Chief, Laboratory of Microbiology, NIDR, Chairman Caries Task Force	X	X

doi:10.1371/journal.pmed.1001798.t002

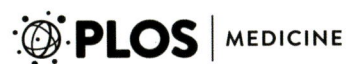

Table 3. Comparison of Research Priorities Identified by ISRF and the NIDR, 1969–1971.

Feasible Interventions to Eradicate Dental Caries	(A) Prof. G. Neil Jenkins address to ISRF, "Sugar and Dental Caries," June 1969 [51]	(B) NIDR's Richard Greulich address to ISRF, "The Future of Caries Control," September 1969 [52]	(C) NIDR Caries Task Force Steering Committee, October 1969 [29]	(D) ISRF Panel Meeting of the Dental Caries Task Force, October 1969 [71]	(E) ISRF Submission to the NIDR: *Dental Caries Research— 1969*, Late 1969 [46]	(F) NIDR Caries Task Force Role of Human Foodstuffs in Caries Workshop Conference, March 1970 [72]	(G) NIDR Request for Contracts, *Opportunities for Participation in the National Caries Program*, 1971 [30]
Dietary interventions							
Cariogenic potential of foods			Deferred to March 1970 meeting			X	
Dietary phosphates	X	X	X	X	X	X	X
Invert sugars		X	X			X	X
Dietary trace elements	X		X	X		X	X
Non-dietary interventions							
Dextranase	X	X	X	X	X	N/A	X
Low molecular weight dextrans		X	X		X	N/A	X
Antimicrobial agents			X	X	X	N/A	X
Antibiotics			X		X	N/A	X
Immunization	X		X	X	X	N/A	X
Water fluoridation	X		X	X	X	N/A	
Topical application of fluoride	X		X		X	N/A	X
Addition of fluoride to sugar, salt, flour			X	X	X	N/A	
Sealants		X	X	X	X	N/A	X
Other						N/A	
Dental epidemiology			X			N/A	
Education for motivation			X			N/A	

N/A, not applicable.

doi:10.1371/journal.pmed.1001798.t003

to select "the areas of research that [ISRF] should be attacking" [69]. Table 3 provides an overview of the research priorities discussed by the NIDR and ISRF committees at key moments leading up to the launch of the NCP. According to ISRF President Ross, ISRF meetings would consider "critical reviews of the major areas [concerning] sugar," including a range of public health topics: "dental caries, overweight and obesity, [and] atherosclerotic vascular disease" [69]. Panels of outside consultants would be convened, and the results of these activities compiled and sent to ISRF Scientific Advisory Board members by December 1969 [70].

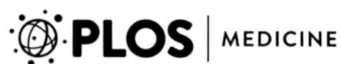
ISRF launched its critical review of dental caries by inviting Dr. G. Neil Jenkins, a professor at the University of Newcastle Dental School, to speak at an ISRF symposium in London in June 1969 [51]. Jenkins's assessment of research on interventions that reduced the harm of sugar consumption without restricting intake (Table 3, column A) was largely unfavorable [51]. Jenkins reviewed food additives, which in preliminary studies reduced the yield of bacterial acid produced after sugar consumption, and concluded that the dose of additives needed might be so high as to render the methods impractical or cause harmful side effects [51]. Perhaps unaware that ISRF was supporting research on dextranase and a tooth decay vaccine at the time under Project 269, Jenkins expressed skepticism about these lines of research:

> Several lines of evidence have tended to emphasize, and perhaps exaggerate, the importance of dextrans.…As an enzyme its instability would limit its application, and the whole basis of this idea depends on the unresolved question of the importance of dextrans. [51]

On the caries vaccine Jenkins noted, that while "a successful preliminary experiment along these lines has been reported in three monkeys," the promise of this result was limited because "it is admitted that the organisms used in the above experiment would be unsuitable for human use and it is not yet possible to incriminate any individual species [of bacteria] as the sole cause of human caries" [51]. Jenkins saw fluoridation as "the only thoroughly well-established method of reducing caries which does not require the active (and usually reluctant) participation of the patient" [51].

Industry receives a preview of the NIDR's research priorities. ISRF got a preview of the NIDR's research priorities for the NCP at the second ISRF symposium in September 1969 in Bethesda [52]. Richard Greulich, the NIDR's intramural scientific director [31], spoke on "The Future of Caries Control" one month before the NIDR Caries Task Force Steering Committee would first discuss NCP research priorities (Table 1) [52]. Greulich said that while water fluoridation (which had been accepted in the US in 1965 as a "proved highly beneficial public health measure ready for widespread implementation" [29]) had achieved some success, The NIDR knew it was not the sole answer to eradicating dental caries:

> From a public health point of view, we do not feel confident that fluoride is the only answer; and biologically speaking, it obviously is not because we have not talked to the other enterprises here. We have mentioned a host factor as represented or reflected by fluoridation. We have not talked to the microbes; we have not talked to the substrate or to nutrition. [52]

Greulich's symposium presentation downplayed the value of limiting sucrose consumption as a means to control dental caries:

> One could say, on logical grounds and good evidence, that if we could eliminate the consumption of sucrose, we could eliminate the problem—because we would be denying these pathogens their primary source of nutrient. We are realists, however, and we recognize the value of sucrose to nutrition. So *while it is theoretically possible to take this approach to demonstrate it, and it has been demonstrated certainly in animal models, it is not practical as a public health measure.* It is like saying the maximum speed of a jet plane is the speed of light. It just is not practical to try and evolve on to that point. And so in smooth surface caries, we have a more practical goal in working on the microorganism. [52] (emphasis added)

Similar to the approaches the sugar industry was promoting, Greulich identified interventions targeting bacteria as promising to the NIDR (Table 3, column B), including dextranases, for

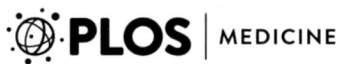

which the NIDR had been working with the pharmaceutical company Merck Sharpe & Dohme to think through the steps necessary for practical application [52]. The NIDR was also hopeful about a laboratory finding on "low molecular weight dextrans," another substance that might be delivered to keep bacteria from producing harmful acid when exposed to sugar [52].

Beyond its focus on decay-causing bacteria, Greulich told ISRF that the NIDR was investigating ways to modify sugar to reduce its harmful effects [52]. These dietary modification interventions included adding phosphates to sugar, and the possibility of replacing table sugar, in the form of sucrose, with a liquid sugar, that split the sucrose molecules into glucose and fructose, which were thought to be less harmful to teeth [47]. Just before concluding, Greulich again assured ISRF that the NIDR research was not a threat to sugar consumption: "I reiterate that the role of sucrose [in dental caries] is undeniable, yet there is very little that anyone would want to do about this other than to explore some of these possible [dietary] modifications" [52].

Industry convenes a panel that includes many members of the NIDR Caries Task Force. In October 1969, the NIDR Caries Task Force Steering Committee met to identify research priorities [29]. As Greulich predicted, the main approaches reviewed focused on interfering with bacteria and dietary modification of sugar (Table 3, column C) [29]. However, a summary of the Caries Task Force Steering Committee meeting indicates that they "also reviewed the agenda for a conference on the role of human foodstuffs in dental caries" [29]. Caries Task Force Steering Committee member Basil Bibby would participate in the conference organization [42], and would have the chance to discuss the state of research on models identifying the cariogenicity of foods with the Caries Task Force, but not until March 1970 [43].

In October 1969, the same month the Caries Task Force Steering Committee was evaluating research priorities to eradicate dental caries (Table 1) [31,71], ISRF President Ross convened his Panel Meeting of the Dental Caries Task Force to consult on ISRF's dental caries research priorities [53]. As Table 2 illustrates, the membership of ISRF's panel overlapped almost completely with the NIDR Caries Task Force Steering Committee. All members of the NIDR Caries Task Force Steering Committee sat on the ISRF expert panel, with the exception of Fitzgerald, whose research on *S. mutans* had identified sucrose as the worst offender in smooth surface cavities [31,53]. The significant overlap between the membership of the ISRF expert panel and that of the NIDR Caries Task Force Steering Committee gave ISRF direct access to the NIDR's Caries Task Force Steering Committee.

ISRF's summary of the ISRF Panel Meeting of the Dental Caries Task Force indicates that the ISRF panel "recommended that a study be made of the cariogenicity of carbohydrate-containing foodstuffs" but did not mention studying the tooth-decay-causing potential of foods in its final "major approaches to caries" [71] (Table 3, column D).

Industry submits recommendations to the NIDR. ISRF submitted the findings from its series of meetings to the NIDR Caries Task Force late in 1969 in a report titled *Dental Caries Research—1969* [46]. While recognizing the causative role of sugar in tooth decay, ISRF downplayed the feasibility of restricting consumption of sugars while promoting advances made in areas of dextranase and caries vaccine research [46]. It also summarized dental caries interventions that would reduce the harm of sugar without impacting consumption, including phosphate food additives, protective sealants, and fluoride delivery through expanded community water programs, topical application, and addition to sugar, salt, or flour [46]. The research priorities identified by the NIDR Caries Task Force Steering Committee in October 1969 (Table 3, column C) are strongly aligned with ISRF's submission (Table 3, column E), with the notable exception of developing a model to identify the cariogenicity of foods.

During fall 1969, the Nixon administration focused on biomedical research policy and showed signs of interest in supporting the NCP [31]. In January 1970, Caries Task Force

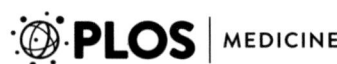

Chairman Scherp submitted the report *A National Caries Program of the National Institute of Dental Research: Ten-Year Program of Research and Development* [41] in response to a request from the Office of the Secretary of Health, Education, and Welfare for a detailed plan for developing dental caries interventions [31]. Scherp's report was based on the work of the NIDR Caries Task Force Steering Committee at its October meeting [31]. Later that month, the Assistant Secretary for Health indicated that President Nixon would endorse the program [31].

Launch of the National Dental Caries Program, 1970–1971

During his February 1970 budget message, President Nixon announced support for "substantial increases in research on cancer, heart disease, serious childhood illnesses, and dental health—where current findings promise significant advances for the future" [31]. A line item in the budget allocated US$5 million (US$30.6 million in 2014 dollars) for the NCP in fiscal year 1971 [29].

In February 1970, after President Nixon's public endorsement of the NCP but before the NIDR officially released the NCP research priorities, ISRF mailed its report *International Sugar Research Foundation Special Report: Dental Caries* [50] to its Scientific Advisory Board. The ISRF report began, "The correlation between sugar and dental decay—a practical concern of the sugar industry for many years—may become a purely academic issue within the foreseeable future," then described the work ISRF leaders had invested to influence the NCP [50]. ISRF President Ross had collaborated with the NIDR Caries Task Force Chairman Scherp and had submitted a report created by ISRF staff on dental caries research priorities directly to the NIDR Caries Task Force:

> Dental caries has been a constant worry to many consumers of sugar and sugar products. To some scientists, dental caries and sugar are considered almost "synonymous." ISRF, in its concern about this image, has supported research to uncover many of the unknowns, and has kept in close communication with other institutions which concentrate on such research. The National Institute of Dental Research, of the U.S. Public Health Service's National Institutes of Health, is the most prominent U. S. organization conducting dental caries research on a broad scale. Last year the Institute formed a Dental Caries Task Force to work "toward the goal of virtually eliminating tooth decay in the United States." Dr. Philip Ross, ISRF President, met with the Dental Caries Task Force and has worked closely with its Chairman, Dr. Henry W. Scherp. Dental Caries Research—1969, prepared several months ago by the staff of ISRF, reviewed current knowledge of the subject and was submitted to the Task Force for its consideration. [50]

The NIDR Caries Task Force held its conference on dietary research priorities one month later (Table 1) [42]. At the NIDR Role of Human Foodstuffs in Caries Workshop Conference, Caries Task Force Steering Committee member Basil Bibby presented a paper, "Methods for Comparing the Cariogenicity of Foodstuffs," which reviewed the status of research on experimental models to identify food products harmful to teeth [43]. These models were important, according to Bibby, because it was "desirable to have a relatively speedy and economical method of evaluating cariogenicity, especially of snack-type foods, so that parents can be warned against the more destructive products" [43]. Bibby's presentation summarized 12 different models to identify the cariogenicity of foods, ranging from "acid production from foods incubated in saliva" to the production of caries in rats, monkeys, and pigs [43]. During the discussion of Bibby's presentation, Caries Task Force members established that "a quick screening method was needed to provide presumptive evidence of the potential cariogenicity of accepted foods and new products that appear almost daily on the shelves of food markets," although there were differences of opinion on what the best model would be to screen for cariogenicity [44]. No one argued that the NIDR not pursue standardization of a test that would rank foods on their potential for tooth decay [44].

Comparison of ISRF and the NIDR Research Priorities

Soon after Nixon's February 1970 endorsement of the NCP, Scherp began operational planning for program implementation at the NIDR [29]. Research priorities were first published in an omnibus request for contracts (RFC) [29] titled *Opportunities for Participation in the National Caries Program* [30] in early 1971. The NIDR received 112 proposals and funded 17 contracts [29] totaling US$3 million (US$18.3 million in 2014 dollars) out of the NCP's budget of US$6 million (US$36.7 million in 2014 dollars) [31]. While the 1971 NCP RFC was the first of several RFCs [73], it established the NIDR's research priorities for years [29].

The research priorities in the 1971 NCP RFC largely reflected the research priorities identified at the October 1969 NIDR Caries Task Force Steering Committee meeting (compare columns C and G in Table 3). Despite being published nearly a year after the NIDR Caries Task Force Role of Human Foodstuffs in Caries Workshop Conference (Table 1), the 1971 NIDR RFC omitted developing a standardized model to identify the cariogenicity of foods as a research priority.

Comparison of the research priorities identified by ISRF and submitted to the NIDR in 1969 (Table 3, column E) with those published by the NIDR in its 1971 NCP RFC (column G) shows that ISRF and the NIDR research priorities were largely aligned. Indeed, a side-by-side comparison of overlapping text from the ISRF submission to the NIDR, *Dental Caries Research—1969* [46], and the 1971 NCP RFC, *Opportunities for Participation in the National Caries Program* [30], reveals that 78% of the ISRF submission to the NIDR was directly incorporated into the 1971 NCP RFC. (S1 Table provides the actual text from the ISRF submission and 1971 NCP RFC.) Of the 274 total lines in the 1971 NCP RFC describing research priorities, 110 lines, or 40%, were taken verbatim or closely paraphrased from the ISRF submission. Of these 110 lines, 34% were copied verbatim from the ISRF report, and 66% were paraphrased.

Discussion

This study analyzes a series of papers discussing previously undocumented cane and beet sugar industry activities between 1959 and 1971 regarding strategies to influence the research priorities of the NIDR's 1971 NCP. The documents show that the sugar industry knew that sugar caused dental caries as early as 1950 and did not attempt to deny the causative role of sucrose in tooth decay. Instead, through trade associations, the sugar industry adopted a strategy to deflect attention to public health interventions that would reduce the harm of sugar consumption, rather than restricting intake.

After the NIDR announced it was considering a research program to eradicate dental caries in 1966, the sugar industry used tactics designed to protect sucrose sales. In collaboration with the chocolate and confectionary industries, SRF funded research that supported the idea that enzymes and a tooth decay vaccine could be developed that could eradicate dental decay without requiring sugar restrictions. ISRF conducted reviews of the dental caries literature to identify potential interventions that might reduce the health harms of sugar consumption other than by restricting sugar intake. ISRF cultivated relationships with the NIDR leadership through meetings with the Caries Task Force chairman and through a consultation with members of the NCP steering committee charged with selecting research priorities. A sugar industry report

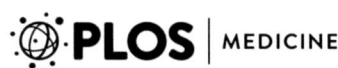

submitted to the NIDR became the basis for the research priorities published in the first NCP RFC.

While not officially recognized as participating in the NIDR Caries Task Force, the sugar industry effectively contributed to the research priorities developed for the launch of the NCP. Research priorities identified in the first NIDR NCP RFC focused on sugar harm reduction strategies, as opposed to sugar restriction, and were strongly aligned with sugar industry research priorities. The NIDR, like ISRF, took the position that sugar restriction was impractical.

The first policies related to the declaration of conflicts of interest for federal advisory committees were implemented in the early 1960s [74]. Prior to that, concern that industry interests were a threat to scientific integrity was not a majority view [75]. Significant consumer concern about corporate influence on expert committees would not surface until the 1970s, after the launch of the NCP. By contrast, in 2015, the NIH had an entire program dedicated to ethical contact within its institutes [76] because of the greater awareness of industry conflicts of interest and how they can adversely impact the scientific enterprise.

The 1970s Missed Opportunity

The majority of the research priorities promoted by the sugar industry and those selected for the 1971 NCP RFC failed to lead to widespread application [31]. By 1976, clinical studies of dextranase mouth rinses in humans had failed to duplicate the success of using dextranases to inhibit new dental caries in experimental animals [31]. The NIDR found that the pharmaceutical industry had limited interest in research, development, and distribution of antimicrobial agents, because of the high cost of regulatory approval by the Food and Drug Administration (FDA) and doubts about identifying an agent that would be successful on a large scale [31]. By 1977, NCP researchers had found that their plan to substitute sucrose with a mixture of glucose and fructose "would effect little reduction in food cariogenicity" [29]. In addition, by 1978, the NIDR had terminated clinical trials on phosphates added to foods because they were ineffective [31].

The most successful interventions selected for funding following the 1971 NCP RFP were topical fluoride and sealants [31]. While a 1980 prevalence survey found that the burden of dental disease in children had decreased by more than 30% since the last survey in 1971–1973, 64% of children still exhibited dental caries, far short of the NCP's founding goal of eradicating the disease [31].

It is not clear why the NIDR adopted the position in 1969 that reducing sugar intake as a public health measure was impractical. Proposals centered on ways to limit sucrose consumption were just around the corner. In its multi-year review of foods generally recognized as safe initiated in 1969, the FDA deemed sucrose consumption at 1976 levels as unsafe for teeth [77]. In the coming years, the FDA would consider food labels "to warn against the hazards to the teeth of consuming a particular product" and debate whether warning labels should be placed on foods based on the percentage of sugar content, or on some measure of cariogenic potential [78].

When reflecting on the NCP in 1990, Basil Bibby, a member of the Caries Task Force Steering Committee, noted that the NIDR approved only "one or two small research grants" related to food cariogenicity compared to the "hundreds of generous awards [that] were made for investigations with so-called high scientific content" [79]. He also noted that since the NIDR was the major funding source for dental research in the US, "the failure of the National Institute for Dental Research to support research on foods meant that there was no group of investigators in the United States who had enough financial support to undertake significant research on food cariogenicity" [79].

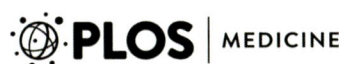

In 1977, the NIDR finally moved to develop a standardized animal model to identify the tooth-decay-causing potential of foods "with the objective of its being widely accepted in industry, and in regulatory agencies and in academic research, as a basis for distinguishing cariogenic from non-cariogenic snacks" [29]. While research on an animal model was initiated at the NIDR [29], the bulk of the research was conducted outside the NIDR, largely funded by the American Dental Association Health Foundation [80]. Based on the promise of the development of a standardized model to identify harmful foods, in 1978 the US Federal Trade Commission proposed restrictions on advertising cariogenic products to children [81]. The first US Department of Health and Human Services Healthy People objectives, issued in 1980, proposed banning cariogenic products from schools as a means to control dental caries [82]. While lobbying efforts of the food, advertising, and broadcasting industries were a major reason for the failure of the FDA, Federal Trade Commission, and Healthy People proposals, another common factor cited for these policy failures is the lack of a standardized model to identify foods harmful to teeth [78,81,83].

With industry input, consensus was finally achieved on a standard method to screen foods for cariogenicity at a conference sponsored by the Foods, Nutrition and Dental Health Program of the American Dental Association in 1985, but only to support claims that food products were safe for teeth [84]. In 1996, the FDA began allowing health claims (i.e., "does not promote tooth decay") on food products containing sugar substitutes based on a standard screening method for cariogenicity [85]. The FDA did not, however, require disclosure or labeling of harmful foods. In 1999, a group of clinicians and dental scientists updated the methodology agreed upon in 1985 with the aim of identifying which methods were "suitable as research tools but also for regulatory assessments" [86]. However, the use of these methods to identify foods harmful to teeth remained controversial [87].

With the implementation of the nutrition facts panel on packaged food products in 1993, the FDA required the declaration of total sugars [88], a requirement that remained unchanged as of January 2015. As of January 2015, the FDA was considering a proposed rule to require disclosure of added sugars on the nutrition facts panel [88], and SA was opposing it, citing "the lack of science to justify 'added sugars' labeling" [89].

Comparison to the Tobacco Industry

The sugar industry formed SRF in 1943 to fund research that supported the industry position [34], 11 years before the creation of the Tobacco Industry Research Committee (TIRC) in 1954 to play a similar role for the tobacco industry [90]. In 1954, the TIRC hired SRF's first scientific director, Robert Hockett, to serve as the TIRC's associate scientific director [91], where he was positioned to help the tobacco industry learn key science manipulation tactics from the sugar industry.

At the same time that the NIDR was planning the NCP, the National Cancer Institute (NCI) was pursuing its Smoking and Health Program [92–94]. Like NCP, which focused on sugar harm reduction strategies, the Smoking and Health Program focused on harm reduction strategies with the primary goal of developing a safe cigarette [93]. The NCI invited tobacco industry representatives to join the NCI's Tobacco Working Group (TWG), the planning committee for the effort to develop a less hazardous cigarette [93]. The NCI did so on the assumption that tobacco manufacturers were interested in promoting new, safer cigarettes and had product expertise the NCI lacked [94]. The NCI also believed industry participation was advantageous because implementation would fall to tobacco companies and, if approached in a positive way, the companies would agree to collaborate [94]. The willingness of the NIDR leaders to interact with the sugar industry during planning for the NCP may have reflected similar

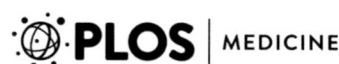
thinking, particularly because responsibility for manufacturing and incorporating additives to reduce the risk of dental caries would fall to food and pharmaceutical industries.

The tobacco industry used its involvement in the TWG to oppose funding of projects, such as smoking cessation programs, that were seen as a threat to industry interests [94]. The tobacco industry also withheld knowledge about the biological effects of cigarette smoke and human smoking behavior, which negatively impacted the NCI's efforts [94]. Indeed, industry use of the TWG to block effective tobacco control strategies was cited by federal Judge Gladys Kessler in her 2006 ruling that the major cigarette companies and their research and lobbying organizations had formed an illegal enterprise to defraud the public in violation of the Racketeer Influenced and Corrupt Organizations Act [95].

Litigation against tobacco companies has been a major factor in achieving meaningful policy change. Successful litigation could not have been achieved without industry documents research illuminating the strategies and tactics of tobacco companies. This analysis demonstrates that sugar industry documents research has the potential to define industry strategies and tactics, which may potentially prove useful in future litigation.

Limitations

While we were fortunate to discover the Roger Adams papers, we recognize that it provides a narrow window into the activities of just one sugar industry trade association, particularly because other industries had an interest in the outcome of the NCP, including the chocolate and confectionary industries, the pharmaceutical industry, and food companies interested in developing food additives and sugar substitutes. To help compensate for limited access to industry documents, we used other historical materials to cross-validate findings as they emerged throughout the analysis. Another limitation was that we could not interview key actors.

Conclusion

This historical example illustrates how industry protects itself from potentially damaging research, which can inform policy makers today. While it may be valuable in theory for the industry to contribute data about their products to the research community, industry should not have the opportunity to influence public health research priorities [94]. Regulatory science to support sensible and defensible policies to limit added sugar consumption was not pursued in the 1970s because of the alignment of the NIDR's research priorities with those of the sugar industry. Actions taken by the sugar industry to impact the NIDR's NCP research priorities, which echo those of the tobacco industry, should be a warning to the public health community. The sugar industry's current position—that public health recommendations to reduce dental caries risk should focus on sugar harm reduction as opposed to sugar restrictions—is grounded in more than 60 years of protecting industry interests. Industry opposition to current policy proposals—including a WHO guideline on sugars proposed in 2014 and changes to the nutrition facts panel proposed in 2014 by the FDA—should be carefully scrutinized to ensure that industry interests do not supersede public health goals.

Supporting Information

S1 Table. Comparison of ISRF's submission to the NIDR Caries Task Force, *Dental Caries Research—1969*, to NIDR's 1971 National Caries Program request for contracts, *Opportunities for Participation in the National Caries Program*.
(PDF)

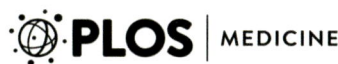

Acknowledgments

We thank Ernest Newbrun, Aubrey Sheiham, Ben Chaffee, Lauren Lempert, Rachel Barry, Lauren Dutra, Margaret Kulik, Randy Uang, and Clayton Velicer for helpful comments on the manuscript. We thank Linda Stahnke, Cara Bertram, and Willam Maher at the University of Illinois Archives for their assistance with the Roger Adams papers. We thank George Coy for his assistance locating documents related to the NCP at NIDCR.

Author Contributions

Conceived and designed the experiments: CEK SAG LAS. Performed the experiments: CEK. Analyzed the data: CEK SAG LAS. Wrote the first draft of the manuscript: CEK. Contributed to the writing of the manuscript: CEK SAG LAS. Agree with manuscript results and conclusions: CEK SAG LAS. All authors have read, and confirm that they meet, ICMJE criteria for authorship.

References

1. Sheiham A (2001) Dietary effects on dental diseases. Public Health Nutrition 4: 569–591. PMID: 11683551

2. Scientific Advisory Committee on Nutrition (2014) Draft carbohydrates and health report—scientific consultation: 26 June to 1 September 2014. http://www.gov.uk/government/uploads/system/uploads/attachment_data/file/339771/Draft_SACN_Carbohydrates_and_Health_report_consultation.pdf. Accessed 30 June 2014.

3. (2003) Joint WHO/FAO expert consultation on diet, nutrition and the prevention of chronic diseases. WHO Technical Report Series No. 916. http://whqlibdoc.who.int/trs/who_trs_916.pdf. Accessed 20 October 2014.

4. World Health Organization Nutrition Guideline Advisory Group (2014) Guideline: sugars intake for adults and children—draft guidelines on free sugars released for public consultation, 5 March 2014. Geneva: World Health Organization.

5. Food and Agriculture Organization of the United Nations (2014) Food-based dietary guidelines. http://www.fao.org/ag/humannutrition/nutritioneducation/fbdg/en/. Accessed 20 October 2014.

6. World Sugar Research Organisation (2012) About WSRO. http://www.wsro.org/AboutWSRO.aspx. Accessed 7 March 2014.

7. Norum KR (2005) World Health Organization's global strategy on diet, physical activity and health: the process behind the scenes. Food Nutr Res 49: 83–88.

8. World Health Organization (2004) Global strategy on diet, physical activity and health. http://www.who.int/dietphysicalactivity/strategy/eb11344/strategy_english_web.pdf. Accessed 19 December 2014.

9. World Sugar Research Organisation (2014) Comments from World Sugar Research Organisation on WHO draft "Guideline: Sugars Intake for Adults and Children.". http://www.wsro.org/Portals/12/Docs/public/documents/News/FINAL%20WSRO%20Comments%20on%20Draft%20WHO%20Guideline%20on%20sugars.pdf. Accessed 30 January 2015.

10. The Sugar Association (2014) Draft guidelines on free sugars released for public consultation, 5 March 2014: "Guideline: Sugars Intake for Adults and Children." http://www.sugar.org/wp-content/uploads/2014/03/Sugar-Association-Comments-Sugars-Intake-Draft-Guidelines.pdf. Accessed 22 August 2014.

11. The Sugar Association (2014) The Sugar Association voices concern regarding the World Health Organization (WHO) draft guideline development process and lack of transparency. http://www.sugar.org/sugar-association-voices-concern-regarding-world-health-organization-draft-guideline-development-process-lack-transparency/. Accessed 12 October 2014.

12. Briscoe AC, Gaine PC (2014 Aug 28) [Letter to Margaret Chan, Director General, World Health Organization.] Washington (District of Columbia): The Sugar Association. http://www.sugar.org/wp-content/uploads/2014/09/WHO-Letter-Signed-8-28-14.pdf. Accessed 10 October 2014.

13. Cottrell RC (2014) Letter to the Editor, "Effect on caries of restricting sugars intake: systematic review to inform WHO guidelines." J Dent Res 93: 530. doi: 10.1177/0022034514526408 PMID: 24595636

14. Lesser LI, Ebbeling CB, Goozner M, Wypij D, Ludwig DS (2007) Relationship between funding source and conclusion among nutrition-related scientific articles. PLoS Med 4: e5. PMID: 17214504

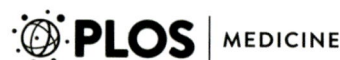

15. Brownell KD, Warner KE (2009) The perils of ignoring history: big tobacco played dirty and millions died. How similar is big food? Milbank Q 87: 259–294. doi: 10.1111/j.1468-0009.2009.00555.x PMID: 19298423

16. Taubes G, Couzens CK (2012) Big sugar's sweet little lies: how the industry kept scientists from asking, does sugar kill? Mother Jones. http://www.motherjones.com/environment/2012/10/sugar-industry-lies-campaign. Accessed 17 October 2014.

17. Moodie R, Stuckler D, Monteiro C, Sheron N, Neal B, et al. (2013) Profits and pandemics: prevention of harmful effects of tobacco, alcohol, and ultra-processed food and drink industries. Lancet 381: 670–679. doi: 10.1016/S0140-6736(12)62089-3 PMID: 23410611

18. Bes-Rastrollo M, Schulze MB, Ruiz-Canela M, Martinez-Gonzalez MA (2013) Financial conflicts of interest and reporting bias regarding the association between sugar-sweetened beverages and weight gain: a systematic review of systematic reviews. PLoS Med 10: e1001578. doi: 10.1371/journal.pmed.1001578 PMID: 24391479

19. Nestle M (2013) Food politics: how the food industry influences nutrition and health. Berkeley (California): University of California Press.

20. Brownell KD, Horgen KB (2004) Food fight: the inside story of the food industry, America's obesity crisis, and what we can do about it. Chicago: Contemporary Books.

21. Freudenberg N (2014) Lethal but legal: corporations, consumption, and protecting public health. Oxford: Oxford University Press.

22. The PLOS Medicine Editors (2012) PLOS Medicine series on big food: the food industry is ripe for scrutiny. PLoS Med 9: e1001246. doi: 10.1371/journal.pmed.1001246 PMID: 22723749

23. Todd JS, Rennie D, McAfee RE, Bristow LR, Painter JT, et al. (1995) The Brown and Williamson documents: where do we go from here? JAMA 274: 256–258. PMID: 7609236

24. Eubanks SY, Glantz SA (2013) Bad acts: the racketeering case against the tobacco industry. Washington (District of Columbia): American Public Health Association.

25. World Health Organization (2003) WHO framework convention on tobacco control. http://whqlibdoc.who.int/publications/2003/9241591013.pdf?ua=1. Accessed 20 October 2014.

26. Bero LA (2003) Implications of the tobacco industry documents for public health and policy. Annu Rev Public Health 24: 267–288. PMID: 12415145

27. California Department of Health Services Tobacco Control Section (1998) Model for change: the California experience in tobacco control. Sacramento: California Department of Health Services. http://www.cdph.ca.gov/programs/tobacco/Documents/CTCPmodelforchange1998.pdf. Accessed 2 October 2014.

28. Couzens CK (2012) How a former dentist drilled the sugar industry. Mother Jones. http://www.motherjones.com/environment/2012/10/former-dentist-sugar-industry-lies. Accessed 22 August 2014.

29. Rogers WE (1983) The National Caries Program: the first ten years, a brief history of the National Caries Program at the National Institute of Dental Research. Washington (District of Columbia): US Government Printing Office.

30. National Institute of Dental Research (1971) Opportunities for participation in the National Caries Program. http://catalog.hathitrust.org/Record/003436264. Accessed 16 May 2014.

31. Harris RR (1992) Dental science in a new age: a history of the National Institute of Dental Research. Ames (Iowa): Iowa State University Press.

32. Centers for Disease Control and Prevention Division of Oral Health (2013) Preventing dental caries with community programs. http://www.cdc.gov/oralhealth/publications/factsheets/dental_caries.htm. Accessed 23 October 2014.

33. (1889–1971) Roger Adams: an inventory of the papers of Roger Adams at the University of Illinois Archives. Record Series Number 15/5/23. Urbana (Illinois): University of Illinois Archives. http://archives.library.illinois.edu/ead/ua/1505023/1505023f.html. Accessed 10 October 2010.

34. Sugar Research Foundation (1945) Some facts about the Sugar Research Foundation, Inc. and its prize award program. New York: Sugar Research Foundation.

35. The Sugar Association (1976) The Sugar Association, Inc. Board of Directors Meeting October 14, 1976 Scottsdale, Arizona. Records of the Great Western Sugar Company. Fort Collins (Colorado); Agricultural and Natural Resources Archive, Colorado State University.

36. The Sugar Association (1978) The Sugar Association, Inc. Annual Meeting of Members May 11, 1978, Washington, D.C. Records of the Great Western Sugar Company. Fort Collins (Colorado): Agricultural and Natural Resources Archive, Colorado State University.

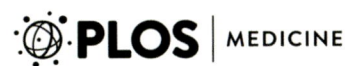

37. Adams R (1959) Letter to Ernest W. Greene, President of The Sugar Association (September 17). In: Roger Adams: an inventory of the papers of Roger Adams at the University of Illinois Archives. Record Series Number 15/5/23. Urbana (Illinois): University of Illinois Archives.

38. Ross P (1968) Letter to Roger Adams of Sugar Research Foundation Scientific Advisory Board (October 3) In: Roger Adams: an inventory of the papers of Roger Adams at the University of Illinois Archives. Record Series Number 15/5/23. Urbana (Illinois): University of Illinois Archives.

39. Adams R (1971) Letter to John L. Hickson, Vice President of International Sugar Research Foundation (February 26). In: Roger Adams: an inventory of the papers of Roger Adams at the University of Illinois Archives. Record Series Number 15/5/23. Urbana (Illinois): University of Illinois Archives.

40. National Institute of Dental Research (1970) Oral disease: target for the 70's: five-year plan of the National Institute of Dental Research for optimum development of the nation's dental research effort. http://catalog.hathitrust.org/Record/003253592. Accessed 13 May 2014.

41. National Institute of Dental Research (1970) A National Caries Program of the National Institute of Dental Research: ten-year program of research and development. Bethesda (Maryland): US Department of Health, Education, and Welfare, Public Health Service, National Institutes of Health.

42. Scherp HW (1970) Introduction: why another conference? J Dent Res 49: 1191. PMID: 5274311

43. Bibby BG (1970) Methods for comparing the cariogenicity of foodstuffs. J Dent Res 49: 1334–1336. PMID: 4991889

44. (1970) Discussion. J Dent Res 49: 1337–1338.

45. National Caries Program Evaluation Project (1980) Evaluation of the National Institute of Dental Research National Caries Program. Bethesda (Maryland): US Department of Health, Education, and Welfare, Public Health Service, National Institutes of Health.

46. International Sugar Research Foundation (1969) Dental caries research—1969. In: Roger Adams: an inventory of the papers of Roger Adams at the University of Illinois Archives. Record Series Number 15/5/23. Urbana (Illinois): University of Illinois Archives.

47. International Sugar Research Foundation (1969) The International Sugar Research Foundation quadrennial report of research for the years 1965–1969. In: Roger Adams: an inventory of the papers of Roger Adams at the University of Illinois Archives. Record Series Number 15/5/23. Urbana (Illinois): University of Illinois Archives.

48. Johnson V (1968) Letter to Scientific Advisory Board of the Sugar Research Foundation (November 19). In: Roger Adams: an inventory of the papers of Roger Adams at the University of Illinois Archives. Record Series Number 15/5/23. Urbana (Illinois): University of Illinois Archives.

49. Ross P (1968) Philip Ross, curriculum vitae. In: Roger Adams: an inventory of the papers of Roger Adams at the University of Illinois Archives. Record Series Number 15/5/23. Urbana (Illinois): University of Illinois Archives.

50. International Sugar Research Foundation (1970) International Sugar Research Foundation special report: dental caries. In: Roger Adams: an inventory of the papers of Roger Adams at the University of Illinois Archives. Record Series Number 15/5/23. Urbana (Illinois): University of Illinois Archives.

51. International Sugar Research Foundation (1969) International Sugar Research Foundation symposium on the status of research in sucrochemistry, diet and heart disease, obesity, dental caries, and clinical nutrition. In: Roger Adams: an inventory of the papers of Roger Adams at the University of Illinois Archives. Record Series Number 15/5/23. Urbana (Illinois): University of Illinois Archives.

52. International Sugar Research Foundation (1969) International Sugar Research Foundation research symposium: seeking new approaches to old problems. In: Roger Adams: an inventory of the papers of Roger Adams at the University of Illinois Archives. Record Series Number 15/5/23. Urbana (Illinois): University of Illinois Archives.

53. International Sugar Research Foundation (1969) International Sugar Research Foundation dental caries task force October 20, 1969. In: Roger Adams: an inventory of the papers of Roger Adams at the University of Illinois Archives. Record Series Number 15/5/23. Urbana (Illinois): University of Illinois Archives.

54. Miller WD (1890) The micro-organisms of the human mouth: the local and general diseases which are caused by them. Philadelphia: S. S. White Dental Manufacturing Company.

55. Fitzgerald R, Jordan H, Stanley H, Poole W, Bowler A (1960) Experimental caries and gingival pathologic changes in the gnotobiotic rat. J Dent Res 39: 923–935. PMID: 13700062

56. Fitzgerald RJ (1960) Demonstration of the etiologic role of streptococci in experimental caries in the hamster. J Am Dent Assoc 61: 9–13. PMID: 13823312

57. Fitzgerald R, Spinell D, Stoudt T (1968) Enzymatic removal of artificial plaques. Arch Oral Biol 13: 125–129. PMID: 5237550

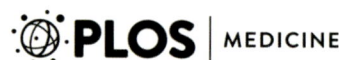

58.   Stephan R (1940) Changes in hydrogen-ion concentration on tooth surfaces and in carious lesions. J Am Dent Assoc 27: 718–723.

59.   Stephan RM (1944) Intra-oral hydrogen-ion concentrations associated with dental caries activity. J Dent Res 23: 257–266.

60.   Preston AJ, Edgar WM (2005) Developments in dental plaque pH modelling. J Dent 33: 209–222. PMID: 15725521

61.   Stephan RM (1966) Effects of different types of human foods on dental health in experimental animals. J Dent Res 45: 1551–1561. PMID: 5225331

62.   Newbrun E (1967) Sucrose, the arch criminal of dental caries. Odontol Revy 18: 373. PMID: 5234965

63.   Sugar Research Foundation (1950) Progress and prospects, scientific research in physiology, nutrition and special uses of sugar: seventh annual report, 1950. New York: Sugar Research Foundation.

64.   Fitzgerald R, Keyes PH, Stoudt TH, Spinell DM (1968) Effects of a dextranase preparation on plaque and caries in hamsters, a preliminary report. J Am Dent Assoc 76: 301.

65.   Fitzgerald R, Keyes P (1962) Attempted immunization of albino hamsters against induced dental caries [abstract]. 40th General Meeting of the International Association for Dental Research; March 1962; St. Louis, MO, US.

66.   (1968 Nov 16) These monkeys may save your teeth. Montreal Gazette. Montreal: Postmedia Network.

67.   Cheek DW (1974) Sugar Research, 1943–1972. Bethesda (Maryland): International Sugar Research Foundation.

68.   International Sugar Research Foundation (1968) The International Sugar Research Foundation, Inc. announces its move to new headquarters. In: Roger Adams: an inventory of the papers of Roger Adams at the University of Illinois Archives. Record Series Number 15/5/23. Urbana (Illinois): University of Illinois Archives.

69.   Ross P (1969) Memorandum to Executive Committee regarding Research Program (August 11). In: Roger Adams: an inventory of the papers of Roger Adams at the University of Illinois Archives. Record Series Number 15/5/23. Urbana (Illinois): University of Illinois Archives.

70.   Ross P (1969) Letter to Roger Adams, ISRF Scientific Advisory Board Member (November 14). In: Roger Adams: an inventory of the papers of Roger Adams at the University of Illinois Archives. Record Series Number 15/5/23. Urbana (Illinois): University of Illinois Archives.

71.   International Sugar Research Foundation (1969) Summary of the discussion and recommendations of the International Sugar Research Foundation panel meeting of the Dental Caries Task Force, October 20–21, 1969. In: Roger Adams: an inventory of the papers of Roger Adams at the University of Illinois Archives. Record Series Number 15/5/23. Urbana (Illinois): University of Illinois Archives.

72.   (1970) Table of contents. J Dent Res 49: 1190–1191.

73.   US Department of Health, Education, and Welfare (1972) National Caries Program: National Institute of Dental Research—status report 1972. Bethesda (Maryland): US Department of Health, Education, and Welfare, Public Health Service, National Institutes of Health.

74.   Lo B, Field MJ, Institute of Medicine, Committee on Conflict of Interest in Medical Research, Education, and Practice (2009) Conflict of interest in medical research, education, and practice. Washington (District of Columbia): National Academies Press.

75.   Parascandola M (2007) A turning point for conflicts of interest: the controversy over the National Academy of Sciences' first conflicts of interest disclosure policy. J Clin Oncol 25: 3774–3779. PMID: 17704427

76.   National Institutes of Health (2014) NIH ethics program overview. https://ethics.od.nih.gov/overview.htm. Accessed 9 February 2015.

77.   US Department of Health and Human Services (2013) Food and Drug Administration Select Committee on GRAS Substances (SCOGS) opinion: sucrose. http://www.fda.gov/Food/IngredientsPackagingLabeling/GRAS/SCOGS/ucm260083.htm. Accessed 24 March 2014.

78.   Miller SA (1981) Sugar, oral health and regulation: a strategy for prevention of oral disease. In: Hefferen JJ, Koehler MS, editors. Foods, nutrition and dental health. Park Forest South (Illinois): Pathotox Publishers. pp. 385–394.

79.   Bibby BG (1990) Food and the teeth. New York: Vantage.

80.   Hefferen JJ, Koehler MS, editors (1981) Foods, nutrition and dental health. Park Forest South (Illinois): Pathotox Publishers. 417 p.

81.   Westen T (2006) Government regulation of food marketing to children: the Federal Trade Commission and the kid-vid controversy. Loyola Los Angel Law Rev 39: 79.

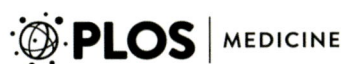

82. US Department of Health and Human Services (1980) Promoting health/preventing disease: objectives for the nation. Washington (District of Columbia): Department of Health and Human Services, Public Health Service.

83. United States Office of Disease Prevention and Health Promotion (1986) The 1990 health objectives for the nation: a midcourse review. Washington (District of Columbia): US Department of Health and Human Services, Public Health Service.

84. Hefferren J, editor (1986) Scientific consensus conference on methods for assessment of the cariogenic potential of foods: November 17–21, 1985, San Antonio, Texas: proceedings. J Dent Res 65S. 72 p.

85. US Food and Drug Administration (2014) Code of Federal Regulations Title 21, Volume 2. Part 101—food labeling. Subpart E—specific requirements for health claims. Sec. 101.80. Health claims: dietary noncariogenic carbohydrate sweeteners and dental caries. http://www.accessdata.fda.gov/scripts/cdrh/cfdocs/cfcfr/cfrsearch.cfm?fr=101.80. Accessed 20 October 2014.

86. Curzon ME, Hefferren JJ (2001) Modern methods for assessing the cariogenic and erosive potential of foods. Br Dent J 191: 41–46. PMID: 11491478

87. Zero D (2004) Sugars: the arch criminal? Caries Res 38: 277–285. PMID: 15153701

88. US Food and Drug Administration (2014) Proposed changes to the nutrition facts label. http://www.fda.gov/Food/GuidanceRegulation/GuidanceDocumentsRegulatoryInformation/LabelingNutrition/ucm385663.htm. Accessed 18 December 2014.

89. The Sugar Association (2014) The Sugar Association calls for withdrawal of 'added sugars' labeling proposal in comments filed to FDA. http://www.sugar.org/sugar-association-calls-withdrawal-added-sugars-labeling-proposal-comments-filed-fda/. Accessed 18 December 2014.

90. Glantz SA, Slade J, Bero LA, Hanauer P, Barnes DE (1996) The cigarette papers. Berkeley: University of California Press.

91. Tobacco Industry Research Committee (1954 Dec 6) Scientific associate named by tobacco research group. http://legacy.library.ucsf.edu/tid/noe6aa00. Accessed 19 December 2014.

92. Gori GB (2000) Virtually safe cigarettes: reviving an opportunity once tragically rejected. Amsterdam: IOS Press.

93. Parascandola M (2005) Science, industry, and tobacco harm reduction: a case study of tobacco industry scientists' involvement in the National Cancer Institute's Smoking and Health Program, 1964–1980. Public Health Rep 120: 338–349. PMID: 16134578

94. Parascandola M (2005) Lessons from the history of tobacco harm reduction: the National Cancer Institute's Smoking and Health Program and the "less hazardous cigarette". Nicotine Tob Res 7: 779–789. PMID: 16191749

95. US Court of Appeals for the District of Columbia Circuit (2009) United States v. Philip Morris USA Inc., 449 F. Supp. 2d 1, 157 (D.D.C. 2006), aff'd in part & vacated in part, 566 F.3d 1095 (D.C. Cir. 2009) (per curiam), cert. denied, 561 US ___, 130 S. Ct. 3501 (2010).

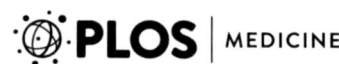
PLOS | MEDICINE

Editors' Summary

Background.

Tooth decay (dental caries) is the leading chronic disease of children and adolescents. Although largely preventable, 42% of children in the US have some decay in their baby (primary) teeth, and 59% of adolescents have cavities in their permanent teeth. Tooth decay occurs when the hard enamel covering the tooth surface is damaged by acid, which is produced by bacteria in the mouth. Plaque, a sticky substance of bacteria, food particles, and saliva, constantly forms on teeth. When you eat food—particularly sugary foods and drinks—the bacteria in plaque produce acids that attack the tooth enamel. The stickiness of the plaque keeps the acids in contact with the teeth. Plaque buildup can be prevented by regular brushing and flossing. Dentists can detect tooth decay before it causes toothache through visual examination or by taking dental X-rays, and can treat the condition by removing the decay and plugging the hole with a "dental filling." However, if the decay has damaged the nerve in the center of the tooth, root canal treatment or removal of the tooth may be necessary.

Why Was This Study Done?

Experts generally agree that sugars play a causal role in tooth decay. Consequently, in 2014, the World Health Organization (WHO) issued a draft guideline that recommended a daily limit on the consumption of "free" sugars (sugars added to food by manufacturers, cooks, or consumers). Also in 2014, the US Food and Drug Administration (FDA) proposed that the nutrition facts panels on US packaged food products should list added sugars. As with similar proposals made in the past, the World Sugar Research Organisation, a trade organization that represents companies with economic interests in sugar production, is challenging these proposals, arguing that, rather than trying to limit sugar intake, public health interventions to prevent tooth decay should focus on reducing the harms of sugar consumption. Here, the researchers explore how the sugar industry has historically sought to undermine or subvert policies to restrict sugar consumption, by examining internal industry documents related to the launch of a targeted research program to identify interventions to eradicate tooth decay—the National Caries Program (NCP)—by the US National Institute of Dental Research (NIDR) in 1971.

What Did the Researchers Do and Find?

The researchers analyzed an archive of 319 internal sugar industry documents from 1959 to 1971 (the "Roger Adams papers") and NIDR documents to explore how the sugar industry sought to influence the setting of research priorities for the NCP. Their analysis indicates that, as early as 1950, sugar industry trade organizations had accepted that sugar damaged teeth and had recognized that the dental community favored restricting sugar intake as a key way to control caries. The sugar industry therefore adopted a strategy to deflect attention towards public health interventions that would reduce the harms of sugar consumption. This strategy included tactics such as funding research into enzymes that break up dental plaque and into a vaccine against tooth decay, and cultivating relationships with the NIDR leadership. Notably, 78% of a report submitted to the NIDR by the sugar industry was directly incorporated into the NIDR's first request for research proposals for the NCP, and research that could have been harmful to sugar industry interests

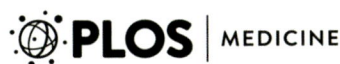

(specifically, research into methods to measure the propensity of specific foods to cause caries) was omitted from the research priorities identified at the launch of the NCP.

What Do These Findings Mean?

These findings, although limited by the researchers' reliance on a single source of industry documents and by the absence of interviews with key actors in the launch of the NCP, reveal an alignment of research agendas between the NIDR and the sugar industry in the early 1970s. The findings also suggest that the NCP was a missed opportunity to develop a scientific understanding of how to restrict sugar consumption to prevent tooth decay. Indeed, although tooth decay declined by 20% between 1971/1973 and 1980, 64% of children still developed caries a decade after the NCP was launched. Most importantly, these findings illustrate how the sugar industry has protected itself from potentially damaging research in the past; a similar approach has also been taken by the tobacco industry. These findings highlight the need to carefully scrutinize industry opposition to the proposed WHO and FDA guidelines on sugar intake and labeling, respectively, to ensure that industry interests do not interfere with current efforts to improve dental public health.

Additional Information.

Please access these websites via the online version of this summary at http://dx.doi.org/10.1371/journal.pmed.1001798.

- The US National Institute of Dental and Craniofacial Research (the successor to the NIDR) provides detailed information on tooth decay (in English and Spanish)

- The US Centers for Disease Control and Prevention also provides information on dental caries

- The UK National Health Service Choices website provides detailed information about all aspects of tooth decay; it also provides an analysis of a recent news report concerning research supporting the proposed WHO guideline for limiting sugar intake

- MedlinePlus provides links to additional information about tooth decay (in English and Spanish)

- Information about the 2014 WHO draft guideline on sugar intake and about the changes proposed to the nutrition facts label by the FDA are available (in English and Spanish)

11.2 Lessons Learned from the Gene Therapy Trial for Ornithine Transcarbamylase Deficiency

James M. Wilson

Wilson, J. Lessons learned from the gene therapy trial for ornithine transcarbamylase deficiency. *Molecular Genetics and Metabolism* 96, 151–157 (2009). © 2009 Elsevier Inc.

Reprinted with permission from Elsevier.

Molecular Genetics and Metabolism 96 (2009) 151–157

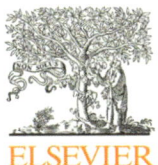

Contents lists available at ScienceDirect

Molecular Genetics and Metabolism

journal homepage: www.elsevier.com/locate/ymgme

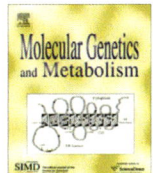

Commentary

Lessons learned from the gene therapy trial for ornithine transcarbamylase deficiency

James M. Wilson *

Department of Pathology and Laboratory Medicine, University of Pennsylvania, Suite 2000 TRL, 125 S. 31st Street, Philadelphia, PA 19104-3403, USA

ARTICLE INFO

Article history:
Received 10 October 2008
Received in revised form 23 December 2008
Accepted 24 December 2008
Available online 10 February 2009

Keywords:
Gene therapy
Ornithine transcarbamylase deficiency
Clinical trial

ABSTRACT

It has been 9 years since Mr. Jesse Gelsinger died from complications of vector administration in a liver gene therapy trial of research subjects with a deficiency of ornithine transcarbamylase (OTCD). This study was performed at the Institute for Human Gene Therapy of the University of Pennsylvania (Penn) which I directed. His tragic death provoked a series of events that had implications beyond those directly involved in the clinical trial.

The events surrounding the death of this research subject have been the topic of much coverage and commentary in the popular press. The goal of this article is to share with you my reflections on the OTCD gene therapy trial and lessons that I have learned which may be of value to others engaged in various aspects of translational medicine.

© 2009 Elsevier Inc. Open access under CC BY-NC-ND license.

The Phase I Gene Therapy Clinical Trial for OTCD

The gene encoding OTC is located on the X chromosome, meaning that males are more commonly affected with the disorder (reviewed in [1]). A complete absence of OTC function due to a severe mutation in its gene can have dramatic clinical consequences. Newborn males with a complete deficiency develop hyperammonemic coma following their first 3 days of life which, if untreated, is lethal. Even with current treatment, most survivors are left with severe cognitive deficits. Individuals who survive the newborn episode of coma can be partially treated with chronic drug therapy, although they are at risk for repeated episodes of protein-induced coma; the overall prognosis, despite excellent clinical care, is poor, and leads to the development of progressively worsening cognitive abilities and premature death in childhood. Females who carry one abnormal gene for OTC are usually without symptoms, although they can demonstrate protein intolerance especially at times of severe stress, such as following major trauma. Intermediate phenotypes are observed with males who have OTC mutations that render the enzyme partially defective.

The metabolic and clinical consequences of a deficiency of OTC can be corrected through liver transplantation, although there is significant morbidity and mortality from the procedure and the ongoing immune suppressive drugs [2]. Interestingly, the liver in patients with OTCD is generally normal except for the defect in this one gene. This suggests that an alternative approach to treating OTCD would be correction of the genetic defect or replacement with a normal version of the OTC gene in hepatocytes.

I was recruited to Penn in 1993 to establish the Institute for Human Gene Therapy. Soon after my arrival, I met with Dr. Mark Batshaw, who is a world expert in metabolic diseases with a particular interest in OTCD. Dr. Batshaw, together with his collaborators at Johns Hopkins University, developed the current pharmacologic therapy for OTCD [3]. We agreed that this disease would be an excellent initial model for testing liver-directed gene therapy and we initiated a collaboration to evaluate this possibility.

At the time of my recruitment to Penn, the field of gene therapy was still in its infancy. The first clinical trial of gene therapy for a genetic disease had been initiated, only 3 years prior to my recruitment, by Drs. Anderson and Blaese in research subjects with an inherited immune deficiency disease. Our studies would be the first to evaluate gene therapy directed to liver in humans with a genetic disease by direct administration of a vector. We were well equipped to develop the basic science and preclinical research to evaluate the feasibility of gene therapy for OTCD. The challenge, however, was to access the translational resources necessary to bring our basic research conducted in the laboratory into the clinic in the setting of first-in-human Phase I clinical trials. One approach to access these resources is through collaboration with the biopharmaceutical industry, which is more experienced than academia in issues related to translational and clinical research. This, however, was difficult to achieve in the early 1990s due to the nascent state of the field of gene therapy and the fact that OTCD was not a sufficiently large market to justify much commercial investment. Our approach, therefore, was to establish a translational capability internal to the academic program at Penn which would include production of clinical grade vector under good manufacturing practices, evaluation of the safety of the vector in animal models under good laboratory practices, design and conduct of the

* Fax: +1 215 898 6588.
E-mail address: wilsonjm@mail.med.upenn.edu

clinical trial under good clinical practices, and a quality assurance oversight group to assure compliance in all of these critical areas. This is, in fact, what we attempted to develop in the 1990s within the Institute for Human Gene Therapy. At the time the OTCD trial was put on hold in the Fall of 1999, the Institute for Human Gene Therapy was directly supporting Investigational New Drug protocols (INDs) for seven clinical trials spanning a wide range of diseases.

The key step in advancing gene therapy for OTCD was to develop a gene delivery vehicle capable of shuttling a normal version of the OTC gene into hepatocytes. This was accomplished through the use of an attenuated or disabled version of an adenovirus which had been engineered to express the normal OTC gene. Dr. Batshaw and I were able to demonstrate some level of efficacy using an adenoviral vector in a mouse model of OTCD [4,5]. Based on these preliminary data, we assembled a team of investigators to further this program and submitted a Program Project Grant to the NIH to support the work. Responsibilities were distributed amongst three scientists with complementary backgrounds in order to access the scientific and clinical experiences necessary to: (1) perform the preclinical studies, (2) to conduct the clinical trial, and (3) to manage financial and non-financial conflicts of interest of the investigators. A more thorough discussion of these conflicts of interest is provided in later sections of this commentary. I provided expertise in vectors and preclinical gene therapy and served as sponsor of the IND application to the FDA and was co-Principal Investigator on the grant. Dr. Mark Batshaw is an expert in OTCD and a practicing pediatrician. He served as Principal Investigator on the Institutional Review Board (IRB) submission to the affiliated pediatric hospital, The Children's Hospital of Philadelphia, and was the Principal Investigator on the grant to the NIH. We recruited the help of a colleague of ours, Dr. Steve Raper, who is a general surgeon and had experience in clinical gene therapy for treating liver disease using an alternative approach based on transplantation of genetically modified cells. Dr. Raper was the Principal Investigator of the protocol submitted to the IRB at the Hospital of the University of Pennsylvania where the subjects were admitted; in this capacity, he served as the physician of record for these individuals while in the hospital. He was also co-Principal Investigator on the grant.

The grant was submitted on March 23, 1994 and we soon developed promising preclinical data that led to the submission of an IND to the FDA approximately 2 years later. The preclinical data developed to support this IND application involved efficacy experiments in the mouse model of OTCD and safety assessment studies performed both in mice and in various types of non-human primates. Using the first generation of the adenoviral vector (i.e., deleted of the E1 gene), we showed a nearly complete correction of the metabolic defect in the mouse model for OTCD that lasted for several weeks to 1 month [4,5]. High doses of the first-generation vector were administered to mice and rhesus macaques in order to assess potential toxicities [6,7]. The primary toxicity we observed was related to the development of self-limited hepatitis approximately 1 week after vector administration. At the highest dose of the first-generation vector, monkeys developed a syndrome of severe liver damage and a clotting disorder that led to death or required euthanasia within several days [6]. Between the time of the initial IND submission on April 18, 1996 and when we received permission to enroll subjects on October 21, 1996, we brought forward at least two improved versions of the OTC adenoviral vector called second- and third-generation vectors. The trial proceeded with the third-generation vector which showed in mice a substantially improved toxicity profile over what was obtained with the first-generation vector [8]. In an attempt to assure safety in the clinical trial, we proposed to administer third-generation vector at a maximum dose that was 17-fold lower than the dose of first-generation vector that showed severe toxicity in macaques.

We felt that this would provide us with a 100- to 1000-fold margin of safety in terms of vector dose. Based on discussions with FDA, we designed a final study to simulate the clinical trial in which third-generation vector was administered to baboons at the starting and ending doses proposed for the clinical trial. Only minor and transient laboratory abnormalities were observed in the high dose baboon group [9].

The team engaged in an extensive set of discussions regarding the structure of the clinical trial [10]. Various aspects of the study design were quite standard such as the fact that it would be a Phase I dose escalation study using safety measures as the primary endpoints, although metabolic correction was also considered. We selected six groups of subjects, with three subjects per group, beginning with a very low dose vector, and escalating half-logs between cohorts to a maximum dose of vector as described above.

One controversial aspect of the trial related to the eligibility criteria for participation which was restricted to adults. Consideration was also given to enrolling newborns in the setting of, or immediately following, resolution of the neonatal hyperammonemic crisis. This was rejected based on concerns over informed consent which would have to be provided by a guardian and the "coercive" nature of the situation in which the guardian would need to provide this consent (i.e., at a time when the child is severely sick and at high risk of dying and/or becoming mentally retarded). The decision to proceed with adults followed extensive discussion with scientists, metabolic disease physicians, bioethicists, and representatives of the Urea Cycle Foundation. Our decision to focus on adults was fully endorsed at the time the protocol was initially reviewed by the relevant regulatory agencies and oversight committees. This decision was questioned after the trial was stopped because we had subjected volunteers with little to no disease-associated morbidity to vector-associated risks that were essentially unknown in humans. In fact, the bioethics community has debated the appropriateness of clinical trials in healthy volunteers in which participation is associated with more than minimal risk [11]. For example, the first evaluation of toxicity for many novel cancer treatments and some applications of gene therapy are performed in subjects more severely affected by their disease. In retrospect, I have questioned the wisdom of this decision, although beginning the study in younger, more severely affected individuals presents a different set of ethical dilemmas.

The first subject was dosed with vector on April 7, 1997. The clinical trial progressed through the first five cohorts without serious adverse events, although toxicity was indeed observed as described [10]. These toxicities included self-limited fever and flu-like symptoms and several transient laboratory abnormalities (e.g., transaminitis, hypophosphatemia, and thrombocytopenia). The first subject of the sixth cohort (i.e., OTC018) received the highest dose of third-generation vector which was 17-fold lower than the dose of the more immunogenic first-generation vector that caused severe toxicities in non-human primates. This 19-year-old female experienced the same toxicity seen in previous human cohorts that included fever and flu-like symptoms with some transient laboratory abnormalities. The second subject in this cohort was an 18-year-old male, Mr. Jesse Gelsinger[1] (OTC019). He received vector on September 13, 1999 and experienced a dramatically different response that ultimately led to systemic inflammation and multi-organ failure; this fulminate acute inflammatory response to vector was different from the toxicities observed in the other human research subjects and in the preclinical studies [12]. Despite attempts of the clinical team and all available consultants to support Mr. Gelsinger through this severe inflammatory episode, he died

---

[1] The name of this research subject was disclosed extensively in the popular press with the apparent consent of his family. We therefore will refer to him as Mr. Gelsinger throughout the manuscript.

J.M. Wilson/Molecular Genetics and Metabolism 96 (2009) 151–157   153

98 h after receiving vector. The trial was put on clinical hold at this time and eventually withdrawn without accruing additional research subjects. Almost 2.5 years transpired between dosing of the first and last research subjects which was due to the conservative dosing schedule in the protocol that allowed for safety assessment between subjects within a cohort and between cohorts, as well as the challenge of finding volunteers with this rare disease who were willing to participate and who fulfilled the restricted eligibility criteria.

In order to identify the mechanism(s) of this severe toxicity observed in Mr. Gelsinger, we initiated a series of studies that continue to this day. Permission to conduct an autopsy was granted from the Gelsinger family and biological samples were further analyzed suggesting vector-induced activation of innate immunity, leading to an acute release of inflammatory mediators [12]. Additional animal experiments were conducted focusing on components of the vector preparations that may activate innate immunity. Problems with the actual preparation of vector administered to Mr. Gelsinger such as contamination were ruled out. Our current hypothesis is that certain protein components of the vector capsid, which are necessary for the vector to function, inadvertently trigger antigen presenting cells to elaborate inflammatory cytokines [13,14]. Unfortunately, modifications of the vector genome will not and apparently did not circumvent these innate immune responses.

What remains unclear is why the response to vector in Mr. Gelsinger (i.e., subject 019) was so exaggerated as compared to what was observed in the other subjects, including subject 018, who received the same dose of vector. Several mechanisms are being considered, such as (1) a genetic predisposition to enhanced innate immunity or (2) immune memory to the vector and/or previous exposure to adenoviruses in the setting of natural infections that enhances the response of the host to a second exposure to the virus/vector. It is interesting that the level of pre-existing immunity to the vector as measured by neutralizing antibody was higher in Mr. Gelsinger (titer of neutralizing antibody (NAB) of 1/80) than in subject 018 (titer of NAB at limit of detection which is 1/20). Recent studies in mice and NHP, however, have not been able to demonstrate such a dramatic difference in toxicity as a function of pre-existing immunity to vector [15,16].

Consequences of the OTCD Trial

When it became clear that Mr. Gelsinger was suffering from a severe reaction to the vector, the team informed his family and notified all relevant national and local agencies including the IRBs, the Recombinant DNA Advisory Committee (RAC) of the NIH, and the FDA.

Subsequent inquiries from the press and congressional investigations about adverse events in other gene therapy trials determined that there was confusion as to the need for reporting adverse events to the RAC. Although the toxicity seen in Mr. Gelsinger was reported promptly, it appeared there was under-reporting of adverse events in many gene therapy trials, which fueled concern over the federal oversight of gene therapy.

Both Penn and the Children's National Medical Center, where Dr. Batshaw was located at the time, initiated internal investigations about the conduct of the OTCD trial. The Washington Post published a series of investigative reports alleging non-compliance in several aspects of the trial management. Parallel investigations by multiple federal regulatory agencies were initiated including the Office for Human Research Protections, the NIH, the FDA (including separate audits of the clinical trial, the safety assessment studies, and the vector manufacturing), Committees from both the United States Senate and House of Representatives, and the United States Attorney for the Eastern District of Pennsylvania.

These investigations resulted in a number of allegations of non-compliance in the formal evaluation of safety in preclinical models and in the conduct of the clinical trial. Questions were raised about non-compliance in a number of areas including: documentation of findings, timeliness and accuracy of reports to the IRB and FDA including summaries of adverse events, completeness of protocol mandated tests, adherence to eligibility criteria and stopping criteria, adequacy of training of clinical staff, delivery and content of the consent process, completeness of monitoring of subjects following vector dosing, and timely notification to FDA of animal toxicity data acquired subsequent to initiation of the study. The investigations ultimately led to a settlement with the government without admission of wrongdoing by the institutions or the individuals including Drs. Batshaw, Raper and myself.

Responding to the multiple investigations provided Drs. Raper, Batshaw and me an opportunity to review all aspects of the events that led up to the trial, as well as its conduct. It became apparent there were shortcomings in several key aspects of the trial; a number of the allegations asserted by the government indeed had merit. This level of non-compliance is inexcusable and as sponsor of the IND and Director of the Institute for Human Gene Therapy at that time, I accept full responsibility for these problems. I truly believe, however, that the team of physicians, scientists, nurses, and administrative staff that were charged with conducting the clinical trials were an extremely committed and dedicated group of individuals who did the best with what they were provided, and never intended to misrepresent or withhold information.

The events surrounding the OTCD trial occurred at a time when there was an emerging concern at a national level about the existing infrastructure to oversee clinical research. Around this time, all clinical research was temporarily shut down at several institutions, including University of Oklahoma and Duke University, due to concerns over the institution's oversight of human subject research. The Secretary of the Department of Health and Human Services at the time, Dr. Donna Shalala, in an article published in the New England Journal of Medicine, pointed out the importance of bolstering this critical infrastructure, citing the OTCD trial as an example of why this was necessary [17].

In fact, there have been substantial reforms across many institutions in the U.S. in terms of oversight of human subject research. This transformation at Penn has been dramatic. We have evolved from 1999, where we had four IRBs with a staff of five, to 2008, where we have revitalized IRBs that number eight with a current staff of 23, improved institutional SOPs, mandatory training and education, an Office of Human Research with a staff of 14, a Faculty Advisory Committee charged with monitoring and oversight, and a Clinical Research Advisory Committee. We have also received accreditation by the AAHRPP, a national non-profit agency established to accredit human research protection programs. The kind of training, support, and oversight currently provided to academic investigators involved in clinical trials at many institutions will go a long way in avoiding the kind of problems encountered in the OTCD trial. I say this not to deflect blame, but to highlight some of the positive consequences that have emerged following Mr. Gelsinger's tragic death.

The purpose of this commentary is not to respond to each of the allegations that emerged from the investigations, but rather to learn from my experience as an investigator in the OTCD gene therapy trial.

Several lessons that I have learned from this experience are presented below.

Lesson #1: The clinical protocol is a contract with the research subjects and regulatory agencies that must be strictly and literally adhered to. A major challenge was the fact that a clinical trial of this complexity using gene transfer technology not previously tested in humans had never been conducted in an academic setting, and its implementation was complicated by a variety of factors. Examples of problems with the clinical protocol and its implementation are provided below.

The protocol was designed to allow for evaluation of the consequences of gene transfer for a period of time after dosing before the next subject within a cohort could be dosed; a formal review of the cumulated data was conducted and submitted to FDA between cohorts before we were allowed to proceed to the next dose. These summary data were used to determine whether to continue dosing and, if so, whether the data would compel us to revise the protocol. An example was the observation of transient thrombocytopenia in an early cohort, which led to the inclusion of measures of disseminated intravascular coagulation (DIC) in all subsequent subjects. The ongoing evaluation and reporting of data during the trial resulted in a very active and productive dialog with FDA that included a total of 151 communications, 86 of which occurred before the trial was put on hold relating to the first 17 of 18 total research subjects. The extensive ongoing data analysis and communications with FDA contributed to the long duration of this trial which took almost 2.5 years to dose 18 volunteers.

The actual protocol became a living document with changes occurring in real time. The team attempted to capture these changes through four different protocol revisions, with up to 54 changes included in some of the revised protocols. The investigations revealed, however, that we did not adequately document and report all of the protocol modifications to the IRBs and to the FDA. This led to confusion amongst members of the team and misunderstandings between the FDA and the team.

Another problem that became evident during the investigation is that aspects of the protocols did not provide sufficient clarity regarding key issues such as eligibility criteria. This led to the allegation that Mr. Gelsinger was not eligible for participation in the trial based on several issues including a measurement of serum ammonia that was greater than the acceptable level of <70 μM. In fact, this threshold had been increased from 50 to 70 μM in an earlier revision to the protocol. In establishing this criterion, the clinical investigators did not take into account the substantial fluctuation in plasma ammonia that characterizes this disorder, nor did they specify the specific time(s) it was necessary for the serum ammonia to be below this threshold level. Multiple serum ammonia measurements were obtained prior to and immediately after dosing Mr. Gelsinger, which fluctuated around the threshold of 70 μM. The clinicians felt this kind of fluctuation was not clinically relevant and therefore enrolled Mr. Gelsinger. However, the protocol was not written to include clinical relevance of metabolic measures in assessing inclusion criteria providing credence to the FDA's concerns.

It is absolutely critical that the investigator view the protocol as a document that must be strictly adhered to. These documents need to be clearly written and any changes clearly highlighted and shared with all relevant agencies prior to incorporating the changes into the conduct of the trial.

A key question is how these problems could have occurred? The fact is that much of the study was done according to protocol in a fully compliant way. It is clear now that the Clinical and Quality Assurance (QA) groups did not have the resources necessary to assure *complete* compliance for such a dynamic and complex protocol. They were asked to cover too much territory; each clinical research nurse oversaw as many as three gene therapy protocols at any one time, while the QA group, which numbered seven staff members at its peak, was responsible for most aspects of GMP, GCP, and GLP compliance for up to seven active INDs. Support for these programs was provided primarily from grants and contracts that, individually, did not provide sufficient Clinical and QA resources to fully support specific protocols. However, it was my responsibility to secure the necessary resources to conduct each

study in a fully compliant way and we should not have proceeded if the resources were insufficient.

Lesson #2: If you think about reporting – then do so! An example of this is related to the allegation that we had not reported deaths of monkeys in a timely manner. As noted earlier, we had performed a series of studies in rhesus macaques with first-generation adenoviral vectors in which the animals did die and suffered from hemorrhagic bleeding disorders at very high doses [6]. Subsequently, in the context of a separate and unrelated liver cancer gene therapy trial, additional experiments were performed with adenoviral vectors in rhesus macaques. Animals that received first- and second-generation vectors suffered fatal consequences at the highest vector dose similar to the studies performed with first-generation vector in preparation for the OTCD IND that were reported to the RAC, IRB, and FDA. The new information from the more recent experiments related to studies with the third-generation vector of the type used in the OTCD trial administered at the dose that caused lethal toxicity with the first- and second- generation vectors; these animals did in fact survive, although they did have cutaneous manifestations of low platelets called petechiae and transient laboratory abnormalities. The OTCD team did discuss the implications of the additional primate data on the ongoing OTCD study and concluded that these additional studies did not provide additional new information beyond what was initially submitted to the RAC and FDA and did not require immediate reporting in the context of the OTCD study. The QA group recommended inclusion of the data developed for the cancer trial in a subsequent annual report to the FDA regarding the OTCD trial which at the time the trial was put on hold had not yet happened. Our conclusion regarding the new monkey data and its relevance to the ongoing OTCD trial and the plan for reporting, which was documented in team meeting minutes, was deemed by FDA to be incorrect based on the agency's review of this information first provided to them immediately after the trial was put on hold. I conclude that any preclinical or clinical data that could conceivably have an impact on an ongoing trial should be reported promptly to both the FDA and the IRB as well as potential research participants. If you think about reporting it, then do so!

My retrospective analysis of the way this issue was handled raised a potential problem with the dynamics of the research group. As described above, responsibilities for the protocol were distributed amongst three physician-scientists with complementary skills and experiences. Decisions were made in the context of "team meetings" with all constituencies present. This approach provided transparency for key decisions and invited input from all members of the group to better inform these decisions. A potential disadvantage of this approach is that it diverts responsibilities from individuals to the team, creating the sense of diminished individual accountability, which was not its intent and may have played a role in some of the decisions made during the conduct of the trial such as the one related to timing of disclosure of these additional animal studies. The fact is that this decision was ultimately mine as sponsor of the IND, irrespective of what others thought, and that I have to take sole ownership of the decision.

Lesson #3: It is very difficult to manage real or perceived financial conflicts of interest in clinical trials. One of the most troubling allegations that surfaced following the OTCD gene therapy trial was that decisions were influenced by the potential for personal financial gain, especially as it related to my affiliation with a gene therapy biotechnology company called Genovo, Inc. These allegations emerged at a time when more global concerns had been rising regarding financial conflicts of interest in other clinical trials conducted in the United States. Evaluation of this issue often attempts to differentiate real conflicts of interest due to possible financial gain from situations where there is no potential for financial gain but that there is the perception that this may occur (i.e., perception

J.M. Wilson / Molecular Genetics and Metabolism 96 (2009) 151–157   155

of conflict of interest). As I will argue below, this distinction is irrelevant when considering management strategies and consequences of conflicts of interest in clinical trials. Reference to "conflicts of interest" will encompass both real and perceived conflicts.

My analysis of this issue focuses on financial conflicts of interest of the investigator and does not address the even more complicated issue regarding financial conflicts of interest of the institution where the research is performed. The institution may benefit directly from the success of companies to which it has licensed technology and may benefit indirectly from research conducted by its faculty in terms of increased numbers of grants and donations.

My immediate response to the allegation that I had a financial conflict of interest was that it was unfounded, based on several considerations. The concept of the OTCD gene therapy program and the preparation of the grant which included the clinical trial occurred before Genovo received funding and established programs. Genovo was not the sponsor of the clinical trial, provided no direct support for the conduct of the trial, and there appeared to be little commercial interest in the disease since it was so rare.

Upon reflection, I realize my initial reaction to these allegations oversimplified what is a more complex issue and that concerns raised about the potential for financial conflicts of interest in my role as sponsor of the IND were indeed legitimate. The fact is that I was a founder in a biotechnology company focused on gene therapy while being directly involved in gene therapy clinical trials as a sponsor of the respective INDs. The juxtaposition of these two facts, independent of their connection, raised the perception of a potential financial conflict; in this kind of situation, perception can quickly become reality. Furthermore, it is virtually impossible to convincingly rule out the absence of bias in one's decisions due to financial or non-financial conflicts of interest; one cannot prove a negative and any attempt to do so sounds defensive and lacks credibility. Finally, both Penn and I owned stock in Genovo and it is possible that a success in the OTCD gene therapy trial could enhance the value of Genovo (and other gene therapy companies) through encouraging proof-of-concept clinical results. For example, any clinical success would likely bolster investor support for the commercial development of gene therapy that could enhance the value of most existing gene therapy companies including Genovo even if they were competitors of Genovo.

In further evaluating the role this conflict may have played in the conduct of the OTCD trial, I have reflected on the professional motivations of academic scientists such as myself and how these factors may influence decisions of the kind that have been questioned during the investigations. My primary motivation in pursuing the OTCD trial was to help children with lethal inherited diseases. If our study was successful, the same approach could potentially be applied broadly across a wide array of rare disorders. It should be recognized, however, that academic medicine is a competitive profession with the primary measure of success being recognition by your colleagues of your research accomplishments. This recognition is critical to sustaining one's research agenda through the successful competition for grants and the awarding of academic promotions and tenure. The quest for this recognition influences work plans, priorities and decisions, and is a requisite means to the ultimate goal of furthering science. Incorporating the incentive for personal financial gain into this complex dynamic is problematic specifically as it relates to the conduct of clinical trials. I learned it is very hard to convincingly uncouple drivers for academic success from the incentives derived from potential financial gain. My conclusion is that the influence of financial conflicts of interest on the conduct of clinical research can be insidious and very difficult to rule out, as I have decided was the case in the OTCD trial.

Genovo was founded before I moved to Penn as a virtual company that had acquired some of my intellectual property from the University of Michigan. Soon after my arrival to Penn, Genovo was provided the opportunity to secure substantial financial investment with a significant portion coming to my laboratory as sponsored research. Continuation of my relationship with Genovo required review and approval by Penn which undertook a thoughtful and diligent analysis of the potential conflicts of interest and put in place management plans including multiple restrictions on my activities, oversight specifically designed to manage my relationship with Genovo in the form of two committees, and a written disclosure to any subject enrolled in an Institute for Human Gene Therapy clinical trial describing a potential financial conflict of interest that Penn and I had.[2] The restrictions, aggressive in comparison to standards of the time but more standard now, included, but were not limited to: (1) waiving my rights to royalty proceeds from commercial products developed and sold by Genovo that I otherwise would have been entitled to per the inventor's distribution policy of Penn, (2) no formal employment position with Genovo and no membership on Genovo's Scientific Advisory Board, and (3) stock that was limited to less than 30% and was non-voting. The fact is that these management tools proved inadequate to assuage the concerns of financial conflicts of interest influencing my behavior in the context of the OTCD trial when reviewed following the death of Mr. Gelsinger. I conclude that it is impossible to manage perceptions of conflicts of interest in the context of highly scrutinized clinical trials, particularly where there is a tragic outcome. Disclosure of the conflict is not enough as has been suggested by others; some have suggested disclosure may actually exacerbate bias [18]. Allegations of this nature in the setting of clinical trials can erode the public's confidence in biomedical research and have far reaching negative effects and should be avoided.

My suggestion is to take a conservative approach in addressing real or perceived financial conflicts of interest in clinical trials until the community of stakeholders establishes clear and generally accepted guidelines. This conservative approach would limit direct participation in clinical trials, as defined by those responsible for the actual conduct and audit of the trial, to individuals that have no real or perceived financial conflicts of interest. This policy would not rule out participation of individuals with conflicts of interest in the preclinical work and design of the clinical trial and interpretation of clinical data; this is important since individuals with potential financial conflicts of interest may be the ones with the most knowledge of the science and the most experienced with the patient populations who are under study. However, the ultimate authority and responsibility for all aspects of the clinical trial should reside with those directly affiliated with the trial and without financial conflicts.

It must be realized, however, that a zero tolerance for real or perceived financial conflicts of interest in clinical trials (i.e., preclude the direct involvement in the clinical trial of anyone with a real or perceived financial conflict of interest) can limit the contribution of the physician-scientist to the process of bench-to-bedside or what we now call translational research. Under a zero tolerance policy, any scientist that contributes to a basic discovery that leads to a licensed patent would be precluded from direct participation in clinical trials that utilize the associated technology, independent of whether s/he has an affiliation with a company. The investigator would receive a portion of any revenue provided

---

[2] On page 11 of the OTCD gene therapy trial consent document under the header of "Sponsor Information" just above the signature space, the following statement was included: "Please be aware that the University of Pennsylvania, Dr. James M. Wilson (the Director of the Institute for Human Gene Therapy), and Genovo, Inc. (a gene therapy company in which Dr. Wilson holds an interest) have a financial interest in a successful outcome from the research involved in this study.

156   *J.M. Wilson / Molecular Genetics and Metabolism 96 (2009) 151–157*

from the licensee to the institution as part of the license which is standard practice in most institutions. Such restrictions could have the unintended consequence of impeding scientific progress. Balancing and formulation of these rules is extremely challenging but needs to be addressed.

Lesson #4: Informed consent may require objective third party participation. The OTCD gene therapy protocol and the associated consent document underwent extensive review including IRBs at three institutions, the Recombinant DNA Advisory Committee, the Oversight Committee of the General Clinical Research Center of the University of Pennsylvania, and the FDA. The subsequent investigations criticized the original consent documents for not adequately articulating the risks and for not disclosing the fact that monkeys died after being administered high dose vector. In formulating the original consent documents, the team incorporated input from the multiple constituencies noted above. Concerns were also raised that consent documents were not adequately revised during the study to incorporate disclosure of the toxicities, particularly while verbal references were made regarding encouraging results in previous subjects. Clearly, we could have done a better job in these important areas.

Adequately informing the subjects about the risks and benefits of the trial was indeed a challenge due to the complex nature of the study and the fact that this was one of the first applications of *in vivo* gene transfer in subjects with a genetic disease. This is further complicated by the requirement to prepare the consent document in a way that would be understandable to the subject; however, there are no explicit guidelines from FDA or OHRP indicating an appropriate age or grade level for readability/comprehension. Rather, the current guidance from OHRP focuses on informed consent as a process (http://www.hhs.gov/ohrp/informconsfaq.html). Many IRBs have adopted a 6th – 8th grade readability threshold for informed consent documents based on literacy rates and other factors [19]. An example of this challenge relates to a summary of the animal studies that included multiple strains of mice and two types of monkeys (macaques and baboons) injected via different routes with three different generations of vectors.

Consent was divided into two stages: the initial evaluation which was done when the subject was an outpatient, weeks to months ahead of the trial, and at the time of vector infusion, which occurred during the subject's admission to the hospital. The clinical team headed by Steve Raper took the lead in explaining the protocol and obtaining consent.

The intense scrutiny this issue received following Mr. Gelsinger's death served to illustrate some of the challenges we face in translating cutting edge discoveries into clinical evaluation, especially as it relates to informed consent. My reflections have focused on two areas. The first of which relates to non-financial conflicts of interest when the individuals involved in informed consent are also scientists behind the research or clinicians involved in the care of the patient. The scientists behind the technology believe in the potential of the technology and pursue its development with zeal in order to overcome significant uncertainties and road blocks that inevitably come up in the laboratory. This "belief" in the technology may make it difficult to objectively represent its potential limitations to the research subject in the context of informed consent. Concerns have also been raised when the Principal Investigator of the trial (i.e., the individual responsible for the well-being and consenting of the research subject) is also a physician who has or may provide medical care for the subject/patient. This dual role/relationship may confuse research with clinical care and puts the investigator in a position to heavily influence the patient's/subject's decisions.

We tried to manage these issues by precluding me from interacting with the subjects or participating in their management

based on the concern that I discovered some of the technology and therefore was invested in its success. We decided to recuse Mark Batshaw from the actual consent process since he is a metabolic disease clinician who was or may become a physician for the subjects/patients. Steve Raper was viewed as the most objective in serving in the role as clinical Principal Investigator and had the requisite qualifications based on his previous experience in clinical gene therapy and his clinical practice as a general surgeon who does procedures involving the liver.

The challenge is that the most qualified individuals to participate directly in the clinical trial are those who developed the technology and those with knowledge of the disease which unfortunately are also those with potential non-financial conflicts of interest. The crux of the problem is to assure that the subject receives a balanced and unbiased view of the risks and benefits of his/her participation in the trial and that s/he can make decisions without influence or concern over negative consequences.

One approach that has been proposed to address these non-financial conflicts of interest is to involve a third party "patient advocate" in the consent process. While this may not be feasible or even necessary in all clinical trials, it would seem prudent to consider in some cases, such as relatively novel and untested technologies in sick research subjects and/or rare diseases. An example of the apparent successful use of a patient advocate has been in the evaluation and use of the implantable artificial heart [20].

My second concern relates to the assessment of risk for a new technology that has not been tested in humans, such as was the case of adenovirus vectors for liver-directed gene therapy of subjects with a genetic disease. The onus is on the scientific team to develop as much preclinical data as they can to assess the potential utility of the technology and the types of toxicity that may be seen in humans. The fact is, however, that one must concede some level of uncertainty regarding the relevance of the preclinical models until they can be reconciled with human data. This uncertainty must be reflected clearly in the consent process.

In summary, I have highlighted some of the key lessons I learned from the OTCD investigations. This event had far reaching effects on the trajectory of gene therapy research and oversight of all clinical trials. My deepest regret is that a courageous young man who agreed to participate in this clinical trial with the hope of making life better for others with this disease lost his life in the process. The immunologic response that precipitated the lethal syndrome of systemic inflammation was unanticipated and not predicted based on the preclinical and clinical data available at the time. However, some of the problems in the design and conduct of the clinical trial that surfaced in the subsequent investigations were real and absolutely unacceptable and ultimately were my responsibility. The fact is that Mr. Gelsinger and his family, and all individuals who so selflessly volunteer to participate in clinical trials, deserve better. They deserve a clear explanation of the risks and benefits of the clinical experiment that is objective and not influenced by the biases of the professional and clinical interests of the participating investigators. They deserve a clinical trial that is conducted in strict compliance with all regulations and not tainted by the perception of financial gain by individuals and institutions. And finally, they deserve our commitment to address these complex problems so that the promise of new therapeutic strategies can realize their potential in treating their diseases.

Acknowledgments/Conflict of Interest Disclosure

The concept of writing this article emerged during discussions with the government regarding a settlement agreement. The goal was for me to openly discuss the lessons I learned from this experience to educate other investigators and minimize similar problems

J.M. Wilson/Molecular Genetics and Metabolism 96 (2009) 151–157
157

in the future. All investigations and litigation about this case have been completed and resolved. Furthermore, there are no agreements that restrict me in expressing my views openly on this topic. My thanks to the many colleagues who reviewed earlier drafts of this manuscript and provided excellent and often poignant feedback.

I am an inventor on gene therapy patents that have been licensed to multiple biopharmaceutical companies and in the past five years had served as a consultant and received grants from various companies.

References

[1] J.E. Wraith, Ornithine carbamoyltransferase deficiency, Arch. Dis. Child. 84 (2001) 84–88.

[2] A.A. Busuttil, J.A. Goss, P. Seu, T.S. Dulkanchainun, G.S. Yanni, S.V. McDiarmid, R.W. Busuttil, The role of orthotopic liver transplantation in the treatment of ornithine transcarbamylase deficiency, Liver Transpl. Surg. 4 (1998) 350–354.

[3] S. Brusilow, J. Tinker, M.L. Batshaw, Amino acid acylation: a mechanism of nitrogen excretion in inborn errors of urea synthesis, Science 207 (1980) 659–661.

[4] X. Ye, M.B. Robinson, M.L. Batshaw, E.E. Furth, I. Smith, J.M. Wilson, Prolonged metabolic correction in adult ornithine transcarbamylase-deficient mice with adenoviral vectors, J. Biol. Chem. 271 (1996) 3639–3646.

[5] X. Ye, M.B. Robinson, C. Pabin, T. Quinn, A. Jawad, J.M. Wilson, M.L. Batshaw, Adenovirus-mediated in vivo gene transfer rapidly protects ornithine transcarbamylase-deficient mice from an ammonium challenge, Pediatr. Res. 41 (1997) 527–534.

[6] F.A. Nunes, E.E. Furth, J.M. Wilson, S.E. Raper, Gene transfer into the liver of nonhuman primates with E1-deleted recombinant adenoviral vectors: safety of readministration, Hum. Gene Ther. 10 (1999) 2515–2526.

[7] Y. Yang, H.C. Ertl, J.M. Wilson, MHC class I-restricted cytotoxic T lymphocytes to viral antigens destroy hepatocytes in mice infected with E1-deleted recombinant adenoviruses, Immunity 1 (1994) 433–442.

[8] G.P. Gao, Y. Yang, J.M. Wilson, Biology of adenovirus vectors with E1 and E4 deletions for liver-directed gene therapy, J. Virol. 70 (1996) 8934–8943.

[9] S.E. Raper, Z.J. Haskal, X. Ye, C. Pugh, E.E. Furth, G.P. Gao, J.M. Wilson, Selective gene transfer into the liver of non-human primates with E1-deleted, E2A-defective, or E1–E4 deleted recombinant adenoviruses, Hum. Gene Ther. 9 (1998) 671–679.

[10] S.E. Raper, M. Yudkoff, N. Chirmule, G.P. Gao, F. Nunes, Z.J. Haskal, E.E. Furth, K.J. Propert, M.B. Robinson, S. Magosin, H. Simoes, L. Speicher, J. Hughes, J. Tazelaar, N.A. Wivel, J.M. Wilson, M.L. Batshaw, A pilot study of in vivo liver-directed gene transfer with an adenoviral vector in partial ornithine transcarbamylase deficiency, Hum. Gene Ther. 13 (2002) 163–175.

[11] N.M. King, O. Cohen-Haguenauer, En route to ethical recommendations for gene transfer clinical trials, Mol. Ther. 16 (2008) 432–438.

[12] S.E. Raper, N. Chirmule, F.S. Lee, N.A. Wivel, A. Bagg, G.P. Gao, J.M. Wilson, M.L. Batshaw, Fatal systemic inflammatory response syndrome in a ornithine transcarbamylase deficient patient following adenoviral gene transfer, Mol. Genet. Metab. 80 (2003) 148–158.

[13] M.A. Schnell, Y. Zhang, J. Tazelaar, G.P. Gao, Q.C. Yu, R. Qian, S.J. Chen, A.N. Varnavski, C. LeClair, S.E. Raper, J.M. Wilson, Activation of innate immunity in nonhuman primates following intraportal administration of adenoviral vectors, Mol. Ther. 3 (2001) 708–722.

[14] Y. Zhang, N. Chirmule, G.P. Gao, R. Qian, M. Croyle, B. Joshi, J. Tazelaar, J.M. Wilson, Acute cytokine response to systemic adenoviral vectors in mice is mediated by dendritic cells and macrophages, Mol. Ther. 3 (2001) 697–707.

[15] A.N. Varnavski, R. Calcedo, M. Bove, G. Gao, J.M. Wilson, Evaluation of toxicity from high-dose systemic administration of recombinant adenovirus vector in vector-naive and pre-immunized mice, Gene Ther. 12 (2005) 427–436.

[16] A.N. Varnavski, Y. Zhang, M. Schnell, J. Tazelaar, J.P. Louboutin, Q.C. Yu, A. Bagg, G.P. Gao, J.M. Wilson, Preexisting immunity to adenovirus in rhesus monkeys fails to prevent vector-induced toxicity, J. Virol. 76 (2002) 5711–5719.

[17] D. Shalala, Protecting research subjects–what must be done, N. Engl. J. Med. 343 (2000) 808–810.

[18] D.M. Cain, A.S. Detsky, Everyone's a little bit biased (even physicians), JAMA 299 (2008) 2893–2895.

[19] M.K. Paasche-Orlow, H.A. Taylor, F.L. Brancati, Readability standards for informed-consent forms as compared with actual readability, N. Engl. J. Med. 348 (2003) 721–726.

[20] E.H. Morreim, End-stage heart disease, high-risk research, and competence to consent: the case of the AbioCor artificial heart, Perspect. Biol. Med. 49 (2006) 19–34.

11.3 Patient Perspectives on Physician Conflict of Interest in Industry-Sponsored Clinical Trials for Multiple Sclerosis Therapeutics

Andrew J. Solomon

Solomon, AJ, et al. Patient perspectives on physician conflict of interest in industry-sponsored clinical trials for multiple sclerosis therapeutics. *Multiple Sclerosis Journal* 21(12), 1593–1599 (2015). © The Author(s), 2015.

Reprinted with permission from Sage Publications.

MULTIPLE
SCLEROSIS | MSJ
JOURNAL

Original Research Paper

Patient perspectives on physician conflict of interest in industry-sponsored clinical trials for multiple sclerosis therapeutics

Multiple Sclerosis Journal

2015, Vol. 21(12) 1593–1599

DOI: 10.1177/
1352458515569101

© The Author(s), 2015.
Reprints and permissions:
http://www.sagepub.co.uk/
journalsPermissions.nav

Andrew J Solomon, Eran P Klein, John R Corboy and James L Bernat

Abstract

Background: Pharmaceutical industry financial support of physicians, physician practices, and academic departments involved in multicenter industry-sponsored clinical trials of novel therapeutic agents is a relatively new and infrequently acknowledged source of potential physician conflict of interest. Detailed disclosure of these relationships to study participants is not uniformly a part of informed consent and documentation practices.

Objective: To understand attitudes of patients with multiple sclerosis concerning disclosure of potential physician–industry conflicts of interest created by clinical trials and how such disclosures may influence study participation

Methods: An anonymous online instrument was developed.

Results: 597 people with multiple sclerosis participated in the study. The study found that detailed disclosure of conflicts of interest is important to potential participants in industry-sponsored clinical trials for multiple sclerosis therapies and that the presence of these conflicts of interest may influence patients' decisions to participate in these studies.

Conclusions: Findings from this study support a call for uniform guidelines regarding disclosure of physician–industry relationships to prospective research participants for industry-sponsored clinical trials.

Keywords: Multiple sclerosis, clinical trials, conflict of interest, professional conduct and ethics, industry-sponsored clinical trials

Date received: 28 November 2014; accepted: 2 January 2015

Introduction

Disclosure of physician–industry financial relationships – such as physician stock ownership or compensation for consultative activities – has become a standard tool for addressing potential physician conflict of interest (COI).[1–4] Direct industry financial support of physicians, physician practices, and academic departments involved in multicenter industry-sponsored clinical trials (ISCT) of novel therapeutic agents is a relatively new and infrequently acknowledged source of potential physician COI. Detailed disclosure of these relationships to potential study participants is not uniformly included as part of informed consent and documentation practices in ISCT. We conducted a survey of multiple sclerosis (MS) patients to understand patient perspectives on the disclosure of physician compensation for participation in ISCT. MS is a

particularly fertile field for the investigation of patient attitudes toward ISCT COI management and disclosure given the rapid development and FDA approval of new therapeutics[5] and a global market value for these therapies estimated at up to US$16bn by 2016.[6]

Methods

An anonymous survey instrument of patient attitudes toward physician–industry relationships created by ISCT for MS was developed by the contributing authors and distributed through SurveyMonkey.com to people self-identifying as having MS. The survey directed respondents to questions based on specific responses, and captured an IP address to prevent multiple submissions by a single individual. The survey instrument was not previously validated. The instrument was reviewed by the University of Vermont

Correspondence to:
Andrew J Solomon
University of Vermont
College of Medicine, 1
South Prospect St., Arnold 2,
Burlington Vermont, 05401,
USA.
andrew.solomon@uvm.edu

Andrew J Solomon
University of Vermont
College of Medicine, USA

Eran P Klein
Oregon Health and Sciences
University and Portland
VA Medical Center, USA;
Department of Philosophy,
University of Washington,
USA

John R Corboy
University of Colorado
School of Medicine, USA;
Denver Veterans Affairs
Medical Center, USA

James L Bernat
Neurology Department,
Dartmouth-Hitchcock
Medical Center, USA

Table 1. Demographic Data For Survey Participants.

Gender	Female 82% (453)
	Male 18% (100)
Age	49.7 +/- 11.9
Home State	Oregon 41% (240)
	Non-Oregon 52% (308)
Years since MS diagnosis	12.8 +/- 9.8
Had participated in ISCT	Yes 13% (76)
	No 76% (454)
	Unsure 11%(65)
MS phenotype	RRMS 75% (397)
	SPMS 15% (85)
	PPMS 5% (29)
	PRMS 3% (15)
	Unknown 5% (26)

MS: multiple sclerosis, ISCT: industry sponsored clinical trial, RRMS: relapsing remitting multiple sclerosis, SPMS: secondary progressive multiple sclerosis, PPMS: primary progressive multiple sclerosis, PRMS: progressive relapsing multiple sclerosis.

Institutional Review Board prior to use and determined to be exempt from further formal committee review and approval. Recruitment was conducted through posting of an internet link to the survey in the research section of the National Multiple Sclerosis Society (NMSS) website, and regional NMSS chapters publicized the study on their own local websites, through paper or email newsletters, social media, or individual emails to members. Information about the study was also given to patients during routine clinical visits with one of the authors (AJS) at the University of Vermont Medical Center. Study information was given to patients at the Rocky Mountain Multiple Sclerosis Center at Anschutz Medical Campus in Aurora, Colorado, during routine clinical visits and was also described in a newsletter. The survey was available for completion online exclusively for three months from February 2014 through May 2014. The survey instrument is available as a supplemental file and, because the survey was navigated on the internet and subjects were automatically routed to certain questions, this pdf version of the instrument necessarily contains notation demonstrating the questions displayed to each subject based on their responses.

Results

Demographic data

Table 1 contains demographic data of survey participants. A total of 597 people with MS participated in the study and 552 completed the entire survey.

Responses from partially completed surveys were included in the results, and questions not answered were coded as missing.

The Oregon chapter of the NMSS emailed each member individually about this study while other participating state chapters relied on newsletters and social media. Of the respondents, 41% (240) identified Oregon as their home state, 52% (308) identified one of 36 additional US states as home, and 4 identified regions outside of the US. Given the large number of participants from Oregon, their responses were compared to responses from other states. Statistically significant differences were found in response to demographic questions but in no questions regarding ISCT COI. The mean age for Oregon participants was older (52 vs. 48, $p < 0.0001$) and their reported mean duration of diagnosis of MS was longer (14.4 years vs. 11.5 years, $p = 0.0007$). Fewer Oregon respondents identified as having RRMS compared to all other phenotypes of MS (67% vs. 76%, $p = 0.0170$). Oregon respondents were less likely to have participated in an ISCT (10% vs. 16%, $p = 0.02$).

Responses from subjects who had not participated in an ISCT in the past

Of the respondents 76% (454) had not participated in an ISCT for a MS medication in the past and 11% (65) were unsure if they had. For the purpose of analysis, these two groups ("non-ISCT respondents") were combined.

Non-ISCT respondents were given a hypothetical scenario which "offered the opportunity to participate in a pharmaceutical company sponsored research study of a new MS medication at your neurologist's office." Among these respondents, 87% (452) thought "a doctor involved in a research study should disclose that they or their office is paid for your participation in the study." Also, 67% (342) thought "a doctor involved in a research study should disclose how they or their office use money they are paid for your participation in the study." These results are represented in Table 2 and compared to the cohort of respondents who had participated in an ISCT in the past.

When respondents who had not participated in an ISCT in the past were offered participation in a hypothetical ISCT, disclosure of a number of additional COI relationships was also important to their decision whether to participate in the study (Table 3). Of the respondents, 79% (405) thought it was either somewhat important or extremely important "to know if

AJ Solomon, EP Klein *et al.*

Table 2. MS patients' opinions regarding disclosure of potential COI for ISCT.

	Had not participated in ISCT	Had participated in ISCT
"A doctor involved in a research study should disclose that they or their office is paid for your participation in the study"	87% (452)	75% (44)
"A doctor involved in a research study should disclose how they or their office use money they are paid for your participation in the study"	67% (342)	66% (39)
MS: multiple sclerosis, COI: conflicts of interest, ISCT: industry sponsored clinical trial.		

Table 3. Importance of disclosure of COI relationships to subjects with MS when considering participation in an ISCT.

Potential COI	Disclosure is important
Compensation toward PI salary	79% (405)
Previous payments for speaking engagements	61% (302)
Previous payments for consulting	69% (345)
Current payments for speaking engagements	70% (346)
Current payments for consulting	76% (375)
COI: conflicts of interest, MS: multiple sclerosis, ISCT: industry sponsored clinical trial, PI: primary investigator.	

the sponsoring pharmaceutical company will because of your participation pay your neurologist money that is used toward their salary" before deciding whether to participate in a study.

Of the non-ISCT respondents, 61% (302) responded that it was either "somewhat important" or "extremely important" to know if a pharmaceutical company "sometime in the past paid your neurologist to give talks about MS to doctors or patients" before deciding whether to participate in a clinical trial. Of the non-ISCT respondents, 69% (345) responded that it was either "somewhat important" or "extremely important" to know if a pharmaceutical company "sometime in the past paid your neurologist to provide advice (consulting) for the drug company." Of the non-ISCT respondents, 70% (346) responded that it was either "somewhat important" or "extremely important" to know if a pharmaceutical company "currently pays your neurologist to give talks about MS to doctors or patients," and 76% (375) responded it was either "somewhat important" or "extremely important" to know if a pharmaceutical company "currently pays your neurologist to provide advice (consulting) for the drug company."

Respondents who had *participated in an ISCT in the past*
Of the survey respondents, 13% (76) had "participated in a pharmaceutical company-sponsored research study of a MS medication" sometime in the

past. Of these respondents, 47% (35) participated in the study at a "university," 23% (17) at a "private practice office," 15% (11) at a "private research center," and 16% (12) were "not sure."

Of these respondents who had participated in an ISCT, 75% (44) indicated that "a doctor involved in a research study should disclose that they or their office is paid for your participation in the study" and 66% (39) thought "a doctor involved in a research study should disclose *how* they or their office use the money they are paid for your participation in the study." These results are displayed in Table 2 and compared to respondents who had not participated in a clinical trial in the past.

Respondents who identified their own neurologist as running the study they enrolled in were asked "Did your neurologist ever discuss whether the pharmaceutical company would provide money to run the study or pay researchers?" Of the respondents, 67% (18) responded "No" and 7% (2) "Not sure." Among respondents who were enrolled in a study with a neurologist other than their routine care provider, 50% (24) said "No" and 31% (15) did not recall such a discussion. Of those who recalled such a discussion regarding compensation for the ISCT, 53% (10) affirmed that "having this discussion before I enrolled in the study was: important to me/my decision." Respondents who recalled having a discussion with the primary investigator (PI) about compensation were asked if it was their "understanding that because of your participation money paid to the neurologist running the study would be used: only for 'overhead' (such as clinic time and space, staff salaries and supplies) associated with your participation." Of the respondents, 53% (8) of subjects who had engaged in this conversation thought that compensation would *only* pay for "overhead."

When asked "Would knowing that the neurologist running the study received money toward their salary from the pharmaceutical company because of your participation have influenced your decision to participate in the study?" 5 (7%) "would probably not have participated" or "would definitely not have participated," and 13 (18%) chose "not sure,". When asked "Would it have changed your decision to participate in the study if the pharmaceutical company also had paid the neurologist running the study to give talks about MS to doctors or patients sometime before the study started," 7 (9%) would "probably not have participated" or "definitely not have participated" and 4 (5%) responded that they "would probably not have participated" or "would definitely not have participated" if the PI was paid to give talks "while you were in the study." When asked "Would it have changed your decision to participate in the study if the pharmaceutical company also had paid the neurologist running the study to provide advice (consulting) sometime before the study started," 9 (12%) responded they either "would probably not have participated" or "would definitely not have participated" and 7 (9%) responded they "would probably not have participated" or "would definitely not have participated" if the PI was paid for such "while you were in the study."

Associations
Respondents who had not participated in an ISCT in the past were more likely to indicate that they thought "a doctor involved in a research study should disclose that they or their office is paid for your participation in the study," 87% (452) vs. 75% (44), $p = 0.0079$. However, respondents who stated they had not participated in an ISCT were just as likely as those who had participated in such a trial to indicate they thought "a doctor involved in a research study should disclose *how* they or their office use the money they are paid for your participation in the study: 66% (39) vs. 67% (342). Responses to duration of MS diagnosis and type of MS were not significantly associated with responses to any questions surrounding disclosure. In the group that had participated in an ISCT in the past, associations between responses were not assessed given the small number in this group.

For respondents who had not participated in an ISCT, women were more likely to respond that it was impor-

tant "to know if the sponsoring pharmaceutical company will because of your participation pay your neurologist money that is used toward their salary": 81.5% (322) vs. 70.0% (60), $p = 0.0146$. Women were also more likely to say it was either "somewhat important' or "very important" "to know that sometime in the past the pharmaceutical company paid your neurologist to give talks about MS to doctors or patients": 63.3% (250) vs. 47.7% (41), $p = 0.0073$. Women were also more likely to respond that it was either "somewhat important" or "very important" "to know that sometime in the past the pharmaceutical company paid your neurologist to provide advice (consulting) for the drug company" running the study: 71.14% (281) vs. 60.47% (52), $p= 0.0519$, when considering an ISCT. Demographic differences noted above between the group of respondents who lived in Oregon compared to non-Oregon respondents did not have a statistically significant influence on the above associations.

Discussion
ISCT for MS therapeutics involve financial relationships between physicians and industry that lead to improvements in the care of MS patients but that also generate potential COIs. Our study demonstrates the importance of disclosure of information concerning physician COIs in MS ISCT to potential participants, such as who receives compensation, how funds are allocated, and current and prior financial relationships with industry. This perceived importance of COI disclosure is consistent with data from other patient populations.[7–13] Our data suggest that the presence of these COIs may influence participation in MS ISCT. Findings from this study support a call for uniform guidelines regarding disclosure of physician–industry relationships to prospective research participants for ISCT.

A conflict of interest is "a set of conditions in which professional judgment concerning a primary interest (i.e., a patient's welfare, validity of research) tends to be unduly influenced by a secondary interest (such as financial gain)."[4] Contract research organizations are gradually supplanting academia's traditional role in drug development, providing new sources of funding for both academic and non-academic physicians.[14,15] Budgets for ISCTs are negotiated between sponsors and research institutions or sponsors and individual physician researchers, and can be structured to potentially generate financial surpluses on top of compensation for the time and effort of participating physicians, research staff, and payment of "overhead" expenses.[14] In academic centers, such revenue might subsidize various aspects of the research infrastructure, but some benefits may rebound to individual researchers either directly or indirectly and may support productivity or a base salary of a PI, substitute for revenue-generating clinical care, allow for additional protected academic time for other pursuits, or contribute to salaries of the support staff and research coordinators who contribute clinical and academic efforts beyond a particular ISCT. In non-academic settings, the connection between ISCT payment and physician compensation is perhaps more direct.[16] The extent to which ISCT as a source of revenue, particularly for private practice physicians, leads to the compromising of ethical standards remains a pressing but open question.[16–18]

Data on the disclosure of financial relationships to subjects participating in ISCT is limited. The patient populations studied and the specific types of COIs disclosed vary.[7–13] Respondents in the present survey overwhelmingly favored disclosure of physician financial relationships. This finding adds to emerging data across diverse disease populations indicating that patients considering participation in clinical trials favor disclosure of physician–industry relationships that may represent a COI.[7–13] Potential physician conflicts can be an important piece of information for patients as they weigh the pros and cons of volunteering for a research study and can enhance or preserve trust between a subject and investigator,[9,19] and ensure that patients make well-informed decisions that preserve their autonomy.

Compensation for ISCT for multiple sclerosis in both academic and nonacademic settings may provide incentives to expand recruitment, but this study suggests that the recruitment benefit may come at a cost. Respondents with MS who had never participated in an ISCT indicated that the presence of a potential COI might influence their decision whether to volunteer for an ISCT. Presented with a hypothetical ISCT, a majority felt it important to know about potential COIs, including a PI's salary contribution from study involvement as well as whether a PI had current or prior industry financial relationships. Our findings are in agreement with a large study of 5478 potential research participants where a sizeable minority (up to 20%) of respondents indicated they might not participate in a clinical trial if certain financial COIs, particularly individual investigators' COIs, were present.[13] While some studies have suggested that perceived COIs may not impact willingness to participate in research,[9–11,19–21] these studies also suggest that disease severity and lack of alternative treatment options, particularly in patients with advanced cancer or who were seriously ill, may

exert a stronger influence on decisions surrounding clinical trial participation.[10,11,21] The findings of the current study add to the literature indicating that potential physician COIs in ISCTs may not only increase risk for participants and jeopardize scientific integrity,[8,14,19,22] but may also have an adverse effect on recruitment.

Our study has several limitations. Our survey instrument was not validated. The authors designed questions to cover many possible forms of potential COIs that might result from financial relationships created by an ISCT. This inclusive and general language may have precluded a more nuanced understanding of the importance of those types of financial arrangements that result in COIs compared to those that do not. We also acknowledge that certain ISCT relationships can result in a net revenue loss for academic departments or practices. As with all surveys there is potential for selection and recall bias, and studies that present hypothetical decisions for respondents are categorically limited. Although participants heard about the study through their neurologist or the National MS Society web site and were presumably diagnosed accurately, there was also no direct ascertainment of diagnostic validity. Responses may have also been influenced by severity of disability and this was not assessed. We carefully worded survey questions in an attempt to use "neutral" language to eliminate bias. This ideal may not always have been met and alternative phrasing of our questions may have led to different results. Moreover, patients carry biases toward the pharmaceutical industry or physician–pharma relationships that may not have been adequately surveyed. Lastly, the subgroup in our study that had participated in an ISCT in the past and completed the survey was small, and more data are needed from those who are currently participating or have participated in ISCT for MS therapies.

Collaborations between physicians and industry have resulted in the advancement of scientific knowledge and have improved the care of patients with MS. However, changes in how COIs are disclosed and managed in clinical trials for the development of MS therapeutics are needed. Language in typical consent forms such as "the investigator is being paid by the sponsor to conduct the research study" or "the sponsor will pay the clinic or institution where the study is conducted for the costs of running the study" may not be adequate. Lack of detailed COI disclosure during the consent process risks leaving the impression that compensation will cover only research infrastructure costs, while many of these arrangements allow for a variety of potential secondary gains. Recent attempts to create more detailed disclosure guidelines of COIs for clinical research studies have been published,[23,24] but the extent of their implementation is unknown.

While many authors have recommended comprehensive and standardized disclosure of investigator relationships with industry, questions about where in the consent process such information is most effectively presented and whether potential subjects are able to understand the implications of these disclosures also need further study.[12,19]

Avoidance or minimization of potential COIs is the ultimate goal. An important step toward this goal is standardizing and making transparent current physician-industry relationships in ISCTs.[1,25,26] Development of disclosure practices for physicians in MS research may provide a model for COI disclosure in ISCT more broadly.

Conflict of interest

This study was not industry sponsored.

Andrew J Solomon received a research grant from the National Multiple Sclerosis Society and was a primary investigator in a multicenter clinical trial for a medication sponsored by Biogen Idec.

Eran P Klein has received honoraria for speaking at academic conferences and receives royalty payments for *The Birth of Bioethics* (Georgetown University Press, 2003).

John R Corboy reports that within the last year he was a primary investigator in a multicenter clinical trial for a medication sponsored by Novartis, Sun Pharma, Celgene Therapeutics, the National Multiple Sclerosis Society, and the National Institutes of Health. He has received research grants from the Juvenile Diabetes Research Foundation, the National Multiple Sclerosis Society, and Diogenix. He has served as a consultant for Novartis, Celgene Therapeutics, Teva Neurosciences, and Biogen Idec. He has received honoraria for speaking engagements from Pro CE, Rocky Mountain MS Center, via Genzyme, and for Grand Rounds at multiple academic institutions. He has been compensated for medical-legal work, as an Editor for *Neurology: Clinical Practice*, and is an uncompensated board member, NMSS Colorado-Wyoming Chapter.

James L Bernat serves on the editorial boards of *Neurocritical Care, Neurology Today*, and *Multiple Sclerosis and Related Disorders* (all unpaid) and the *Physician's Index for Ethics in Medicine* (paid). He receives royalty payments for *Ethical and Legal Issues in Neurology* (Elsevier, 2013), *Ethical Issues in*

Neurology 3rd ed (Lippincott Williams & Wilkins, 2008), and *Palliative Care in Neurology* (Oxford University Press, 2004).

Funding

This research received no specific grant from any funding agency in the public, commercial, or not-for-profit sectors.

References

1. Ross JS, Gross CP and Krumholz HM. Promoting transparency in pharmaceutical industry-sponsored research. *Am J Public Health* 2012; 102: 72–80.

2. Norris SL, Holmer HK, Ogden LA, et al. Conflict of interest disclosures for clinical practice guidelines in the national guideline clearinghouse. *PloS one* 2012; 7: e47343.

3. Holloway RG, Mooney CJ, Getchius TS, et al. Invited article: Conflicts of interest for authors of American Academy of Neurology clinical practice guidelines. *Neurology* 2008; 71: 57–63.

4. Thompson DF. Understanding financial conflicts of interest. *New Engl J Med* 1993; 329: 573–576.

5. GBI Research. *Multiple Sclerosis Therapeutics to 2019 – Treatment Diversification, Increasing Efficacy, and Pipeline Innovation Combine to Drive Growth.* July 2013. Bolton, UK: GBI. Available at: www.gbiresearch.com

6. IMS Institute for Health Informatics. *The Global Use of Medicines: Outlook Through 2016.* July 2012. NJ: IMS Inc. Available at: www.imshealth.com

7. Angelos P, Murphy TF, Sampson H, et al. Informed consent, capitation, and conflicts of interest in clinical trials: Views from the field. *Surgery* 2006; 140: 740–748.

8. Raftery J, Bryant J, Powell J, et al. Payment to healthcare professionals for patient recruitment to trials: Systematic review and qualitative study. *Health Technol Assess* 2008; 12: 1–128, iii.

9. Tosounidis TI and Kontakis GM. Clinical research: The patients' perspectives. *Injury* 2008; 39: 631–635.

10. Gray SW, Hlubocky FJ, Ratain MJ, et al. Attitudes toward research participation and investigator conflicts of interest among advanced cancer patients participating in early phase clinical trials. *J Clin Oncol* 2007; 25: 3488–3494.

11. Grady C, Horstmann E, Sussman JS, et al. The limits of disclosure: What research subjects want to know about investigator financial interests. *J Law Med Ethics* 2006; 34: 592–599, 481.

12. Weinfurt KP, Friedman JY, Allsbrook JS, et al. Views of potential research participants on financial conflicts

of interest: Barriers and opportunities for effective disclosure. *J Gen Intern Med* 2006; 21: 901–906.

13. Kim SY, Millard RW, Nisbet P, et al. Potential research participants' views regarding researcher and institutional financial conflicts of interest. *J Med Ethics* 2004; 30: 73–79.

14. Hall MA, Friedman JY, King NM, et al. Commentary: Per capita payments in clinical trials: reasonable costs versus bounty hunting. *Acad Med* 2010; 85: 1554–1556.

15. Shuchman M. Commercializing clinical trials — Risks and benefits of the CRO boom. *New Engl J Med* 2007; 357: 1365–1368.

16. Fisher JA and Kalbaugh CA. United States private-sector physicians and pharmaceutical contract research: a qualitative study. *PLoS medicine* 2012; 9: e1001271.

17. Weinfurt KP, Hall MA, Hardy NC, et al. Oversight of financial conflicts of interest in commercially sponsored research in academic and nonacademic settings. *J Gen Intern Med* 2010; 25: 460–464.

18. Fisher JA. Practicing research ethics: private-sector physicians & pharmaceutical clinical trials. *Soc Sci Med* 2008; 66: 2495–2505.

19. Licurse A, Barber E, Joffe S, et al. The impact of disclosing financial ties in research and clinical care: a systematic review. *Arch Intern Med* 2010; 170: 675–682.

20. Weinfurt KP, Hall MA, Dinan MA, et al. Effects of disclosing financial interests on attitudes toward clinical research. *J Gen Intern Med* 2008; 23: 860–866.

21. Hampson LA, Agrawal M, Joffe S, et al. Patients' views on financial conflicts of interest in cancer research trials. *New Engl J Med* 2006; 355: 2330–2337.

22. Raftery J, Kerr C, Hawker S, et al. Paying clinicians to join clinical trials: a review of guidelines and interview study of trialists. *Trials* 2009; 10: 15.

23. Rochon PA, Hoey J, Chan AW, et al. Financial conflicts of interest checklist 2010 for clinical research studies. *Open Med* 2010; 4: e69–91.

24. Weinfurt KP, Hall MA, King NM, et al. Disclosure of financial relationships to participants in clinical research. *New Engl J Med* 2009; 361: 916–921.

25. Ferris LE and Naylor CD. Physician remuneration in industry-sponsored clinical trials: the case for standardized clinical trial budgets. *Can Med Assoc J* 2004; 171: 883–886.

26. Morin K, Rakatansky H, Riddick FA, Jr, et al. Managing conflicts of interest in the conduct of clinical trials. *JAMA* 2002; 287: 78–84.

11.4 Industry Support of Medical Research: Important Opportunity or Treacherous Pitfall?

William M. Tierney, Eric M. Meslin, and Kurt Kroenke

Tierney, W, Meslin, E, Kroenke, K. Industry support of medical research: Important opportunity or treacherous pitfall? *Journal of General Internal Medicine* 31(2), 228–233 (2015). © Society of General Internal Medicine 2015.

Figure 1 reproduced from The Anatomy of Medical Research: US and International Comparisons. *Journal of the American Medical Association.* 313 (2), 2015. With permission from the American Medical Association.

JGIM

PERSPECTIVE

Industry Support of Medical Research: Important Opportunity or Treacherous Pitfall?

William M. Tierney, MD[1,2], Eric M. Meslin, PhD[2,3], and Kurt Kroenke, MD[1,2,4]

[1]Regenstrief Institute, Inc., Indianapolis, IN, USA; [2]Indiana University School of Medicine, Indianapolis, IN, USA; [3]Indiana University Center for Bioethics, Indianapolis, IN, USA; [4]Roudebush VA Center for Health Information and Communication, Indianapolis, IN, USA.

Pharmaceutical and device manufacturers fund more than half of the medical research in the U.S. Research funding by for-profit companies has increased over the past 20 years, while federal funding has declined. Research funding from for-profit medical companies is seen as tainted by many academicians because of potential biases and prior misbehavior by both investigators and companies. Yet NIH is encouraging partnerships between the public and private sectors to enhance scientific discovery. There are instances, such as methods for improving drug adherence and post-marketing drug surveillance, where the interests of academician researchers and industry could be aligned. We provide examples of ethically performed industry-funded research and a set of principles and benchmarks for ethically credible academic–industry partnerships that could allow academic researchers, for-profit companies, and the public to benefit.

KEY WORDS: ethics, research; conflict of interest; public–private partnerships; research support.

J Gen Intern Med 31(2):228–33
DOI: 10.1007/s11606-015-3495-z
© Society of General Internal Medicine 2015

Federal funding of research has decreased over the past decade.[1] At the same time, NIH has called for more collaboration between industry and academic investigators. For example, NIH's *Discovering New Therapeutic Uses for Existing Molecules* initiative will test more than 20 compounds from industry partners for their effectiveness against a variety of diseases and conditions.[2] *Accelerating Medicine Partnerships* is a collaboration among NIH, ten pharmaceutical companies, and non-profit patient advocacy organizations to identify and validate the most promising biological targets of disease for new diagnostic and drug development.[3] "Clearly, we need to speed the pace at which we are turning discoveries into better health outcomes," said NIH Director Collins. "NIH looks forward to working with our partners in industry and academia to tackle an urgent need that is beyond the scope of any one organization or sector".[4] Additionally, since passage of the Patent and Trademark Law Amendments

("Bayh–Dole") Act of 1980,[5] many academic institutions encourage faculty to patent and commercialize their discoveries, leading to mutually—scientifically and financially—beneficial partnerships between universities, their individual scientists, and private sector companies. In the wake of this engagement between academia and industry, and the enhanced scrutiny of industry payments to physicians prompted by passage of the Physician Payment Sunshine Act,[6] universities nationwide are revising their guidelines for conducting research and managing conflicts of interest.

Industry and government together have consistently funded most medical research in the U.S. (Fig. 1). Notably, industry dominates: research funding by industry in 2012 was $68 billion compared to $38 billion from federal agencies. Moreover, between 1994 and 2012, industry funding of medical research grew by 147 %, compared with 48 % for federal agencies, which was less than the 57 % inflation during those years.[7] The goal of federal research funding is to generate new knowledge that will enhance health and health care. The goal of research funding by for-profit companies is maximizing income to their shareholders. Increased knowledge and enhanced care, if they happen at all, are byproducts of the profit motive.

Can academicians' interest and industry's needs be aligned? For example, a company developing a new drug that may have fewer side effects might be interested in funding research into the incidence of adverse effects from currently marketed drugs. An academic researcher might have a strong interest in elucidating the adverse effect profile of that class of drugs when used in everyday settings among patients who are usually, if not always, excluded from pre-marketing studies.[8] Studies of how drugs and devices are used in everyday practice and the outcomes of treatment should be of mutual interest and benefit to both academic researchers and industry. For example, Bristol-Myers Squibb was about to launch a new antipsychotic drug and contracted with one of us (WMT) to conduct a study of the incidence of weight gain and diabetes among patients taking any of the currently available antipsychotics; the results were published in *JGIM*.[9]

Both academia and industry have interests in post-marketing drug surveillance.[10] The FDA requires companies to conduct post-marketing surveillance (phase IV studies) of new drugs and certain devices. Whereas academic

Received July 2, 2015
Revised July 16, 2015
Accepted July 23, 2015
Published online August 26, 2015

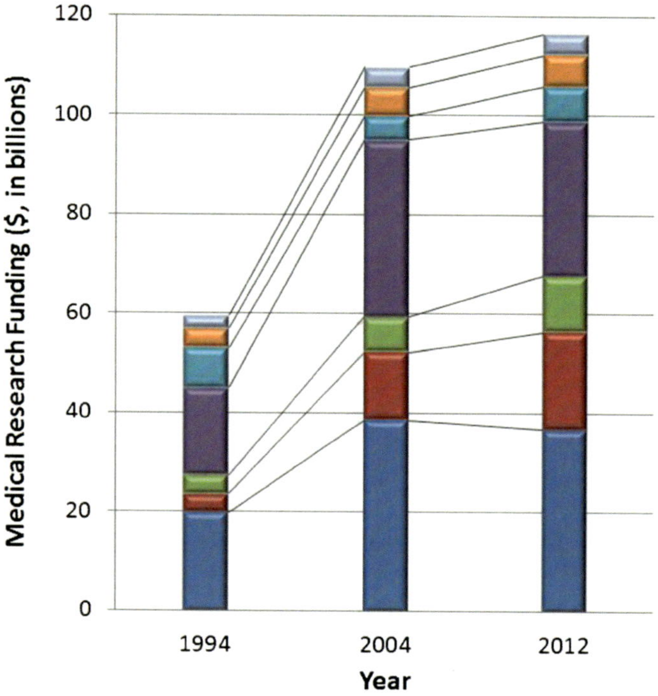

	1994	2004	2012
Foundations, Charities, Other Private	2.6	3.9	4.2
State and Local Government	3.9	5.9	6.3
Other Federal	8.0	4.8	7.1
NIH	17.6	35.6	30.9
Medical Device Firms	3.8	7.1	11.5
Biotechnology Firms	3.7	13.7	19.6
Pharmaceutical Firms	20.0	38.6	36.8

Fig. 1 Growth in medical research funding by source from 1994 to 2012 ($, in billions)[1]

investigators are interested in true estimates of benefits and risks of new treatments, for-profit drug and device companies would want to report great benefits and low risks. We believe that academic researchers are more likely to perform unbiased post-marketing studies than either researchers employed by the company marketing the drug in question or for-profit research companies whose livelihood depends on satisfying their customers.

Academic researchers and industry scientists can also share interests in generating knowledge relevant to patient care. For example, clinicians hope and expect patients to take the medications they prescribe, and pharmaceutical companies benefit when patients take them. Thus both clinician-investigators and pharmaceutical companies have obvious interests in drug adherence and in developing and validating methods for assessing and improving adherence. Industry and academic investigators can also have mutual interests in improving our ability to identify, assess, and manage important patient outcomes. For example, the Regenstrief Institute has a five-year contract with Merck Sharp & Dohme to develop and conduct mutually interesting and beneficial research projects.[11] Researchers from the Regenstrief Institute and Indiana University and scientists from Merck propose collaborative one-year projects. A review committee comprising three senior investigators from both IU/Regenstrief and Merck reviews the proposals, eliminates some, and ranks the rest. Merck decides on its allocation to the collaboration each year, and then the review committee begins at the top of the rank list and funds projects until all allocated funds are expended.

Publication of study results in peer-reviewed journals is a required deliverable of each project. Table 1 shows projects funded in the first four years of this collaboration. Importantly, like federally funded projects, the grants reimburse the salaries of IU/Regenstrief investigators and professional staff. No bonuses or extra payments are made.

Industry-funded research has a risk of bias and misconduct that can mislead readers,[12–14] consequently causing pain, suffering, and sometimes death.[15] Neither academia nor the private sector is immune from ethical scrutiny or responsibility, though public perception rarely gives high marks to the pharmaceutical industry's ethical behavior.[16] The key is minimizing bias through rigorous studies devised, conducted, and reported by academic investigators whose income is not tied to the drug being evaluated. Each of these—research methods, how they are applied, and how results are reported—is a source of bias, regardless of funding source, that rigor and vigilance can minimize in order to generate new knowledge and patient benefit.

For example, Kroenke and his colleagues received funding from Pfizer to develop screening instruments for depression (the PHQ-9) and anxiety (the GAD-7).[17] Both have become standard screening tools. The *JGIM* original article validating the PHQ-9[18] has been cited more than 3500 times, according to Web of Science[19]; it is *JGIM's* most highly cited article ever. Whereas both the PHQ-9 and GAD-7 are open-source and free to use, some survey instruments developed with federal funding require license fees,[20] an unfortunate trend where

Table 1 Funding of Projects in the First Four Years of the Regenstrief-Merck Collaboration

Project title	Brief description of project goals
Project 1: Leveraging Regenstrief's electronic medical record (EMR) and capabilities to enhance subject recruiting	Test the ability of a new identification system for EMR-enabled identification and recruitment of patients into clinical trials.
Project 2: Regenstrief-Merck Scholar's Award in Pharmacoepidemiology and Informatics	Create two annual visiting scholar positions whose focus will be primarily on the link between pharmacoepidemiology and biomedical informatics, leveraging big data analytics to: (1) improve patient care, (2) obtain better patient outcomes, and (3) lower costs.
Project 3: Building a phenotype library using Regenstrief's EMR	Define and validate a set of three algorithms for defining phenotypes of interest, validating them against human interpretation of medical charts.
Project 4a: Medication adherence in type 2 diabetes	Determine the patterns of use for medications prescribed to patients with type 2 diabetes mellitus, targeting medications for diabetes and associated metabolic disorders. Determine what patient-centered interview data might be collected, evaluate the merits of electronic monitoring of medications, and plan an intervention to improve adherence to medications. (This project was terminated due to feasibility issues.)
Project 4b: Medication adherence in respiratory disorders	Test whether monitoring asthma medication adherence using prescription records and providing feedback to patients can improve drug adherence and asthma control among patients non-adherent to their inhaled controller medications.
Project 5: Computerized reminders to promote medication adherence and utilization	Support more consistent and effective use of prescribed medications by identifying optimal physician and patient-directed strategies to improve appropriate medication adherence and utilization.
Project 6a: Usage, Benefits, and Adverse Effects of Loop Diuretics in Patients with Heart Failure or Hypertension	Identify and describe the characteristics of patients with diagnosed hypertension and heart failure using EMR data, and use prescription records to assess adherence for heart failure and hypertension medications, and relate clinical outcomes to medications prescribed and adherence.
Project 6b: Longitudinal Modeling of Heart Failure Progression	Utilize longitudinal EMR data to characterize the changes in ejection fraction and/or New York Heart Association chronic heart failure classification. Examine the impact of patient-specific covariates (drug treatment, intensity, age, weight, sex, etc.) on the rate of heart failure progression.
Project 7: Sensitivity analysis of Mini-Sentinel's protocol of active surveillance of acute myocardial infarction in association with antidiabetic agents	Better understand the sensitivity of risk estimates with respect to a set of parameters associated with design decisions. To accomplish this, the project evaluated a protocol from the Mini-Sentinel for the Active Surveillance of Acute Myocardial Infarction in Association with Use of Anti-Diabetic Agents.
Project 8: OpenMRS–Merck Strategic Collaboration	Integrate a Merck business analyst and developer into the OpenMRS community who can comprehend and assist with open-source EMR development.
Project 9: Calibrating evidence of drug risk by estimating clinical database bias	Develop methods to adjust results for more accurate answers to drug outcome research questions within the Indiana Network for Patient Care (INPC). Develop "database fingerprinting" methods that can be applied to any database in the Observational Medical Outcomes Partnership (OMOP) common data model format.
Project 10: Predictive modeling of drug–outcome associations	Develop and compare optimal predictive modeling techniques for identifying patients at risk of known drug outcomes.
Project 11: Chronic kidney disease and resistant hypertension	Define the rates of resistant hypertension in populations with and without chronic kidney disease.
Project 12: Collecting and incorporating patient-reported data into a medication adherence decision support system	Determine whether non-interruptive claims-based adherence alerts enhanced with patient-reported data and tailored recommendations can increase the number of conversations clinicians and patients have about their adherence to oral medications for diabetes. (Due to delays encountered during development and deployment, this project was discontinued.)
Project 13: Development and feasibility of a medication adherence protocol for older adults with mild cognitive impairment	Identify and quantify barriers to medication adherence in older adults with mild cognitive impairment.
Project 14: Investigation of physician reminders and recommendation scripts for HPV vaccination	Evaluate the effect of automated physician-targeted reminders and recommended scripts on first dose uptake of HPV vaccine and rates of return for second dose.
Project 15: EMR-based detection and display of hypoglycemic risk in diabetic patients	Develop a predictive model of hypoglycemia risk in patients taking insulin or sulfonylureas. Design an alert that will be delivered to providers accessing high-risk patients' EMRs.
Project 16: Melanoma algorithm development and validation	Determine the sensitivity and positive predictive value of defining melanoma in the INPC database using EMR data and data derived from natural language processing (NLP).
Project 17: Medication adherence in order adults with cognitive impairment (continuation of Project 13)	Identify and quantify barriers to adherence in older adults with mild cognitive impairment.
Osteoporosis Center of Excellence (OCOE)-1: Sub-Optimal Outcomes of Bisphosphonates Treatment in the Real World	Examine the prevalence and healthcare burden of osteoporosis patients who sustain fractures, lose bone mineral density, or remain osteoporotic despite being adherent to bisphosphonates treatment.
OCOE-2: Renal Impairment in Osteoporosis	Quantify the unmet medical need in the area of comorbid osteoporosis and chronic kidney disease, as current osteoporosis therapies are not recommended in patients with moderate to severe chronic kidney disease.
OCOE-3: Finding fractures and other phenotypes of high interest using EMR data and NLP	Develop and validate coding algorithms for fractures and other phenotypes to enhance observational studies.
OCOE-4: Broadening osteoporosis-related data in the INPC	Enhance researchers' ability to use the INPC for osteoporosis-related studies by creating the nation's largest repository of structured bone mineral density scans linked to EMR data.

(continued on next page)

Table 1. (continued)

Project title	Brief description of project goals
OCOE-5: High-volume osteoporosis and patient access registry project	Establish a large consenting cohort of patients (with links to their EMRs) for rapid recruitment for future osteoporosis-related studies.
OCOE-6: Disparities in osteoporosis treatment	Use patient and provider characteristics in multivariate models to predict which patients with osteoporosis, low bone mineral density, or fractures receive treatment with bisphosphonates or other osteoporosis drugs.
OCOE-7: Improving the capture, interpretation and use of DXA data	Upload DXA data from selected health systems' radiology departments and local clinics into INPC and assess the variability of longitudinal bone mineral density measurements in the clinical setting.
OCOE-8: Diagnosis of atypical subtrochanteric fractures in the clinical setting	Estimate the proportion of atypical femur shaft fractures in women with non-traumatic femur fractures, and identify clinical factors predicting atypical femur shaft fractures.
Cross-Collaboration Initiative (CCI) -1: Regenstrief-Merck Scholar's Award in Pharmacoepidemiology and Informatics	Create the first-ever combined pharmacoepidemiology-medical informatics fellowship to develop and train world-class leaders at the intersection of big data, pharmaceutical research, and health information technology.
CCI-2: Regenstrief Boot Camp	Hold an intensive two-day training seminar that will provide Merck and local non-Regenstrief investigators knowledge of the wide-ranging resources and capabilities available at the Regenstrief Institute.
CCI-3: EMR Summit	Hold a summit of commercial EHR and health IT developers to promote awareness and adoption of innovations in evidence-based care, patient safety, and user experience design.
CCI-4: Natural Language Processing Core	Expand Regenstrief's and Merck's capabilities to glean information from text data in support of current and future projects.
CCI-t: Electronic patient reported outcomes (ePRO) capture platform	Create a flexible, scalable, and generalizable electronic platform for generating and storing patient-reported outcomes on an unlimited variety of topics.

Total Projects = 32
Manuscripts: 14 submitted, 5 published or accepted for publication to date
29 Presentations at scientific meetings and conferences to date

patient-reported measures are frequently proprietary rather than in the public domain.[21]

Certainly there are well-documented cases where industry-funded research has been biased. For example, two systematic reviews found that studies sponsored by industry reported significantly greater benefits and less harm than studies with other sources of funding.[22,23] Similarly, there are well-known examples where industry has squelched (or attempted to squelch) study results that were unfavorable to their products.[24,25] Pharmaceutical companies have also paid ghost-writers to draft reviews of drug treatment favorable to their products, and then sought academicians to "author" the articles, with the goal of biasing the medical literature.[26] But does such obviously unethical behavior by some investigators and companies mean that industry-funded research can never be conducted by academic scientists without the results being questioned? We argue that academic–industry relationships can be "ethically credible," meaning that specific ethical principles are followed that minimize the risk that industry funding will bias the planning, conduct, or reporting of studies. Indeed, academic–industry relationships are not only possible, they are desirable as a means to maximize discoveries and patient benefits as federal research dollars are dwindling.

An example of an ethically credible partnership was the ARTIST study that was funded by Eli Lilly to assess the effects of different selective serotonin reuptake inhibitors (SSRIs) on depression and other outcomes in primary care.[27] The sponsor had postulated that its SSRI (fluoxetine) would be more effective than two competing SSRIs (sertraline and paroxetine). However, the study found no differences among the three

SSRIs as reported in a high-impact journal (*JAMA*), despite not favoring the sponsor's drug. Indeed, the evidence supporting "funding bias" has recently been questioned by social scientists as well as the Cochrane collaboration.[28,29]

To counter potential bias due to industry funding of research, the Regenstrief Institute commissioned one of us (EMM) and his colleagues at the Indiana University Center for Bioethics (IUCB) to review Regenstrief's collaboration with Merck.[11] Reviews of this kind are rare, but have been reported elsewhere.[30] During the second year of the five-year collaboration, IUCB faculty and staff reviewed the contract between Regenstrief and Merck, assessed the bioethics literature concerning industry-funded research, surveyed Indiana University/Regenstrief investigators and staff engaged in one or more Merck-funded activities, and developed a set of principles and benchmarks for ethically credible academic–industry partnerships (Table 2). IUCB reviewers found the Regenstrief-Merck collaboration to be ethically conducted overall, but that it could be improved, especially in communicating the collaboration's policies and operating principles to all faculty and staff participants.[31] The policies and procedures governing the Regenstrief-Merck collaboration were deemed to address the key ethical issues. Several benchmarks were not fully met, and the report made specific recommendations that the collaboration's leaders followed. In subsequent years, the collaboration has met all benchmarks. Specific recommendations followed were to 1) increase transparency and enhance trust by more fully educating all investigators and staff on the collaboration's policies and procedures; 2) broadcast the processes for ranking projects and selecting those to be funded; 3)

Tierney et al.: Industry Support of Medical Research   JGIM

Table 2 Principles and Benchmarks for Ethically Credible Academic–Industry Partnerships

Principle	Benchmark
Academic freedom	1. Promote investigator-initiated science and protect the ability to attract and maintain federal research support 2. Permit investigators to initiate or continue collaboration with any other qualified group, person or entity 3. Ensure that all investigators involved in the partnership are given equal opportunity to submit proposals for funding 4. Avoid obligating faculty to work outside their own self-defined scientific area
Conflict of interest policy and management	5. Protect students, fellows and post-doctoral fellows involved in collaborative projects from exploitation 6. Ensure that effective mechanisms exist to eliminate, control or manage conflicts of interest in the partnership
Intellectual property	7. Ensure that all investigators and both partners retain their proprietary and intellectual property rights throughout and after the partnership
Data-sharing, access	8. Ensure that data-sharing arrangements are explicit and that all rights to access data are fairly negotiated at the outset of the partnership
Effective governance	9. Establish parameters for what type of projects will and will not be funded (e.g., add-on projects, training, pilot studies) 10. Create ways to protect each party from an unexpected end to the partnership 11. Formally assess the efficiency, effectiveness and achievements of the partnership on an annual basis 12. Ensure that clear, comprehensive and efficient procedures exist for all governance entities of the partnership and are known to all investigators
Protection of human subjects	13. Ensure that all investigators, staff and other participants in the partnership have adequate training in the responsible conduct of research and related ethical issues 14. Ensure that all projects in the partnership aim to satisfy the highest ethical standards
Publication	15. Ensure the right of all researchers associated with the partnership to publish 16. Disseminate all research results at the conclusion of collaborative studies in a timely fashion 17. Ensure that authorship follows ICMJE guidelines
Social, scientific and industrial value	18. Maintain competitive advantage in the specified research domains 19. Structure the research to maximize potential benefit for communities and society 20. Structure the partnership to have the best chance of benefiting both partners and harming neither
Transparency	21. Widely publicize the partnership agreement and collaborative opportunities to the public and employees 22. Establish procedures for frequent and effective communication between partners 23. Ensure that both partners are aware of other partnerships each may be involved in

include a wider range of Institute and university investigators in the invitation to propose studies; 4) publicize the collaboration's distinctive conflict of interest policies; and 5) proactively assess investigators' concerns about the collaboration and provide investigators with more opportunities to learn about the collaboration and provide input.

As a result of the IUBC evaluation and the more than two decades of research collaboration with industry, the Regenstrief Institute has launched an Industry Research Office (IndRO) that facilitates conversations with prospective industry funders, identifies Regenstrief and other university principle investigators and co-investigators, helps design protocols and write proposals, manages communication and contracts, and follows the principles and benchmarks for a wider range of investigators, funders, and studies. The overriding goal of the IndRO is to provide academic researchers with alternative sources of funding their research as federal sources become increasingly constrained. In addition to faculty and staff salaries for performing research, funds from industry-sponsored studies support IndRO's management infrastructure, local clinical data repositories, and other research resources. To maintain the studies' intellectual independence and scholarly focus, all industry contracts contain a clause giving the investigators the right to publish any and all study results, and an article submitted to a peer-reviewed journal is the final required deliverable of all contracts.

The moral outrage engendered by past misbehavior on the part of the drug and device industry and academic researchers can affect all financial relationships between medical schools and industry.[32,33] If stringent ethical guidelines are followed, private sector companies can be an important source of funding for ethical, high-quality, important academic research. Universities must develop and implement policies and procedures to maximize the effectiveness and ethical conduct of all research, regardless of funding source. We are confident that this is possible and that industry, academic medical scientists, and the patients and communities they serve can all benefit.

Conflict of Interest: Dr. Tierney has received research funding from Merck Sharp & Dohme, Eli Lilly, Bristol-Myers Squibb, GlaxoSmithKline, Caremark, and Integrated Disease Management, Inc. He has never owned stock in individual medically related companies and has never received honoraria, speaking fees, or personal income from any medically related company. He is the President and CEO of the Regenstrief Institute, Inc., which has an Industry Research Office that facilitates research contracting between academic investigators and the private sector. All residual funds realized by this research support Regenstrief's local research infrastructure. No funds result in bonuses or additional income to investigators or staff.
Dr. Meslin does not now but has previously received consulting fees from Eli Lilly. He sits on the Science and Industry Advisory Committee of Genome Canada, for which he receives an annual honorarium.
Dr. Kroenke has received research funding from Eli Lilly, Pfizer, and Wyeth. He does not now but has previously received consulting fees and/or honoraria from Eli Lilly, Wyeth, Forest Laboratories, and Bristol-Myers Squibb. He has no investments in individual for-profit companies.

Corresponding Author: *William M. Tierney, MD; Regenstrief Institute, Inc., 410 West Tenth Street Suite HS2000, Indianapolis, IN 46202, USA (e-mail: wtierney@regenstrief.org).*

REFERENCES

1. **Moses H III, Matheson DHM, Cairns-Smith S, George BP, Palisch C, Dorsey R.** The anatomy of medical research: US and international comparisons. JAMA. 2015;313:174–89.

2. National Center for Advancing Translational Sciences. Discovering new therapeutic uses for existing molecules. Available at: http://www.ncats.nih.gov/research/reengineering/rescue-repurpose/therapeutic-uses/therapeutic-uses.html. Accessed April 25, 2015.

3. National Institutes of Health. Accelerating medicines partnerships. Available at: http://www.nih.gov/science/amp/index.htm. Accessed April 25, 2015.

4. National Institutes of Health. NIH launches collaborative program with industry and researchers to spur therapeutic development. Available at: http://www.nih.gov/news/health/may2012/od-03.htm. Accessed April 25, 2015.

5. Patent and Trademark Law Amendments Act of 1980, Pub. L. No. 96–517, 94 Stat. 3015, 69331 (1980) (codified as amended at 35 U.S.C. ch. 30 (2011)).

6. Patient Protection and Affordable Care Act, Pub. L. No. 111–148, 124 Stat. 119 (2010); Sec. 6002: Transparency Reports and Reporting of Physician Ownership or Investment Interests (codified as 42 U.S.C.A. § 1320a-7h).

7. USInflation.org. US inflation rate calculator. Available at: http://usinflation.org/us-inflation-rate-calculator/. Accessed July 7, 2015.

8. **Singh S, Loke YK.** Drug safety assessment in clinical trials: methodological challenges and opportunities. Trials. 2012;13:138.

9. **Farwell WR, Stump TE, Wang J, Tafesse E, L'Italien G, Tierney WM.** Weight gain and new onset diabetes associated with olanzapine and risperidone. J Gen Intern Med. 2004;19:1200–5.

10. **Psaty BM, Meslin EM, Breckenridge A.** A lifecycle approach to the evaluation of FDA approval methods and actions: opportunities provided by a new IOM report. JAMA. 2012;307(23):2491–2.

11. **Jain SH, Rosenblatt M, Duke J.** Is big data the new frontier for academic-industry collaboration? JAMA. 2014;311:2171–2.

12. **Melander H, Ahlqvist-Rastad J, Meijer G, Beermann B.** Evidence b(i)ased medicine–selective reporting from studies sponsored by pharmaceutical industry: review of studies in new drug applications. BMJ. 2003;326:1171–3.

13. **Godlee F, Smith J, Marcovitch H.** Wakefield's article linking MR vaccine and autism was fraudulent. BMJ. 2011;342:c7452.

14. **Cyranoski D.** Research integrity: cell-induced stress. Nature. 2014;511(7508):140–3.

15. **Hollon T.** Researchers and regulators reflect on first gene therapy death. Nat Med. 2000;6:6.

16. **Olsen AK, Whalen MD.** Public perceptions of the pharmaceutical industry and drug safety: implications for the pharmacovigilance professional and the culture of safety. Drug Saf. 2009;32:805–10.

17. **Kroenke K, Spitzer RL, Williams JBW, Löwe B.** The Patient Health Questionnaire somatic, anxiety, and depressive symptom scales: a systematic review. Gen Hosp Psychiatry. 2010;32:345–59.

18. **Kroenke K, Spitzer RL, Williams JBW.** The PHQ-9: validity of a brief depression severity measure. J Gen Intern Med. 2001;16:606–13.

19. Web of Science. Available at: www.isiknowledge.com. Accessed April 25, 2015.

20. **McHorney CA, Ware JE Jr, Raczek AE.** The MOS 36-Item Short-Form Health Survey (SF-36): II. Psychometric and clinical tests of validity in measuring physical and mental health constructs. Med Care. 1993;31:247–63.

21. **Newman JC, Feldman R.** Copyright and open access at the bedside. N Engl J Med. 2011;365(26):2447–9.

22. **Song F, Parekh S, Hooper L, et al.** Dissemination and publication of research findings: an updated review of related biases. Health Technol Assess 2010;14:iii. ix-xi, 1–193.

23. **Bero L.** Industry sponsorship and research outcome: a Cochrane review. JAMA Intern Med. 2013;173:580–1.

24. **Rennie D.** Thyroid storm. JAMA. 1997;277:1238–43.

25. **Blumenthal D, Campbell EG, Anderson MS, Causino N, Louis KS.** Withholding research results by academic life scientists: evidence from a national survey of faculty. JAMA. 1997;277:1224–8.

26. **Tierney WM, Gerrity MS.** Scientific discourse, corporate ghostwriting, journal policy, and public trust. J Gen Intern Med. 2005;20:550–1.

27. **Kroenke K, West SL, Swindle R, et al.** Similar effectiveness of paroxetine, fluoxetine, and sertraline in primary care: a randomized trial. JAMA. 2001;286:2947–55.

28. **Krimsky S.** Do financial conflicts of interest bias research? An inquiry into the "funding effect" hypothesis. Sci Technol Hum Values. 2013;38:566–87.

29. **Sterne JA.** Why the Cochrane risk of bias tool should not include funding source as a standard item. Cochrane Database Syst Rev. 2013;12:ED000076.

30. **Carpenter WT Jr, Koenig JI, Bilbe G, Bischoff S.** At issue: a model for academic/industry collaboration. Schizophr Bull. 2004;30:997–1004.

31. **Meslin EM, Gaffney MM, Quaid KA, Schwartz PH, Pitt AR, Rager JB.** Final summary report: Review of the Merck-Regenstrief partnership. Available at: http://hdl.handle.net/1805/6044. Accessed July 7, 2015.

32. **Rosenbaum L.** Beyond moral outrage – Weighing trade-offs of COI regulation. N Engl J Med. 2015;372:2064–8.

33. **Steinbrook R, Kassirer JP, Angell M.** Justifying conflicts of interest in medical journals: a very bad idea. BMJ. 2015;350:h2942.

References

Campbell E, Bogeli C, Rao S, Abraham M, Pierson R, Applebaum S. Industry relationships among academic institutional review board members; changes from 2005 through 2014. JAMA Intern Med. 2015;175(9):1500–6.

Dunn A, Colera E, Mandl K, Bourgeois F. Conflict of interest disclosure in biomedical research: a review of current practices, biases, and the role of public registries in improving transparency. Res Integr Peer Rev. 2016;1:1.

Elliott C. Institutional pathology and the death of Dan Markingson. Account Res. 2016. Epub ahead of print.

Kearns C, Glantz S, Schmidt L. Sugar industry influence on the scientific agenda of the National Institute of Dental Research's 1971 National Caries Program: a historical analysis of internal documents. PLoS Med. 2015;12(3):e1001798.

Resnik D. Institutional conflicts of interest policies at U.S. academic research institutions. Acad Med. 2016;91(2):242–6.

Wilson J. Lessons learned from the gene therapy trial for ornithine transcarbamylase deficiency. Mol Genet Metab. 2009;96:151–7.

Additional Suggested Reading

Dunn A, Colera E, Mandl K, Bourgeois F. Conflict of interest disclosure in biomedical research: a review of current practices, biases, and the role of public registries in improving transparency. Res Integr Peer Rev. 2016;1:1. (*A public registry of competing interests is needed in order to have a comprehensive view of COI.*)

Elliott C. Institutional pathology and the death of Dan Markingson. Account Res. 2016. Epub ahead of print. (*Apparent institutional regulatory oversight failure by a major public university is described.* 2017 24(2):65–79)

Resnik D. Institutional conflicts of interest policies at U.S. academic research institutions. Acad Med. 2016;91(2):242–246. (*Policy development for institutional conflicts of interest are incomplete.*)

Yanagawa H. Current regulatory systems for clinical trials in Japan: Still room for improvement. Clin Res Regul Aff. 2014;31(2–4):23–28. (*Describes how a country develops its research regulatory system including management of COI.*)

Data Acquisition, Management and Transparency

12

Arthur L. Caplan and Barbara K. Redman

Scientific practice and patient needs are rapidly accelerating the need for the interconnectivity of data and records. Fields especially active in this endeavor include genomic science, health outcomes research, developmental psychology, and neuroimaging studies, which generate and utilize large amounts of data housed on both public and private sites. Challenges in current efforts to build a more comprehensive data infrastructure include data stored in unconnected silos that are more or less accessible, data incompatibility, coding heterogeneity, and data storage and management too large for current infrastructures, especially as longitudinal data is added or links made to electronic health records or social media sites (Siu et al. 2016). Biobank policies and practices, data use and sharing, harmonization of definitions and policies to ease aggregation and comparison, and privacy regulations are under continuing development.

Biobanking of biological specimens including blood, urine, saliva, tissue, and cellular samples requires policies and procedures for their collection, processing, storage, and distribution (Vaught 2016). Such policies vary across national borders. They are often managed by data transfer/data use agreements. Legacy biobanks or patient data registries, collected when the individual subject was a minor, is now deceased, or cannot be located may generate unclear patient/subject consent issues for researchers, especially when data or algorithms are developed partially for commercial purposes (Mascalzoni et al. 2016). Description of types of consent may be found in Box 3 in Siu et al. (2016). Blanket consent means that donor data will be used for any research authorized by the biobank, which may ignore evidence that some donors have moral, religious, or cultural objections to particular uses of their data.

Dispute over the ethics of data use is generating new dilemmas. For example, biobanks of dried blood spots left over from mandatory newborn 'heel-stick' screening were maintained by states for long-term storage and secondary research applications and sometimes linked to public health data. Even though deidentified and subject to individual or parental requests to remove their data, scientific review and IRB approval for new public health studies subject backlash over consent in Texas and Minnesota resulted in use restrictions and in all samples being destroyed. Marginalized populations are often very skeptical about use of their data and want to be asked specifically for each use (Thiel et al. 2014). And countries like Sweden, which have built a comprehensive national infrastructure for health data are concerned about data being taken out of the reach of Swedish law (Cool 2015).

Although some funders require data sharing, it is not uniformly accepted by scientists, who see incursion on their ownership and authorship prerogatives (Zinner et al. 2016). They are concerned about the expense of resolving different format issues; cleaning, collating, annotating, and providing meta-data and disclosure of computational methods to make the data usable by others. Successful models of sharing protect data from unauthorized access, protect subjects privacy, and negotiate authorship expectations (Toga and Dinov 2015). Data practices must be especially sensitive to views of

A. L. Caplan · B. K. Redman (✉)
New York University Langone Medical Center,
New York, NY, USA
e-mail: Arthur.Caplan@nyumc.org

© Springer International Publishing AG, part of Springer Nature 2018
A. L. Caplan, B. K. Redman (eds.), *Getting to Good*, https://doi.org/10.1007/978-3-319-51358-4_12

indigenous peoples, who may want governance over their data to assure benefit to their community, assure it will not be used in a discriminatory way, and that sample disposal will be culturally acceptable (Haring et al. 2016).

Common data elements including definitions, measurement tools and standards promise to make full use of the data by being able to sum over trials. Such standards may be required by regulators such as FDA or national governmental agencies and are encouraged by the NIH (Biering-Sorensen et al. 2015) and other funders. The National Institute of Neurological Disorders and Stroke (NINDS) has developed such standards for spinal cord injury, traumatic brain injury, stroke, epilepsy, and other areas. They are important to develop a body of research as opposed to just conducting isolated studies (Cohen et al. 2015).

Commercially owned data, as that in drug development studies, has been considered protected by both state and federal law. Following serious evidence of selective reporting and methodological flaws from some of these trials, the OpenTrials movement has pressed for more disclosure. The European Medicines Agency is making study reports, both positive and negative trials, details of adverse events, with individual data available but with some commercially confidential information redacted (Abbott 2016). Trial repositories such as ClinicalTrials.gov and others across the world have been established to create a comprehensive record of clinical trials of their results and increasingly of their methods. The goal is to avoid trial duplication, understand trial quality, be able to accurately identify the state of the science in multiple areas of research investment, and make trials available for providers and patients to identify trials in which they might want to enroll or seek expanded access while remaining sensitive to subject confidentiality.

Evolving practices in data acquisition, management, and transparency provide multiple opportunities for supporting research integrity. Freely available blinded data allows study replication by independent scientists. Aggregation across multiple data sources can provide sufficient statistical power to adequately test hypotheses and make use of every subject's contribution to research.

Advice: Fields vary considerably in expectation that data will be shared. For some, such as genomics, sharing is a condition of funding.

Be alert to how the open data movement in progressing in your field and to whether resources are available to support it. If you work with vulnerable or indigenous populations, know the requirements governing confidentiality imposed by law and by the groups themselves before undertaking any inquiry. In working with commercial entities, make sure they have obtained consent for the use of both identifiable and non-identifiable data from those from whom it was obtained.

12.1   Opentrials: Towards a Collaborative Open Database of All Available Information on All Clinical Trials

Ben Goldacre and Jonathan Gray

Goldacre, B, Gray, J. OpenTrials: towards a collaborative open database of all available information on all clinical trials. *Trials* 17, 164 (2016). © 2016 Goldacre and Gray. http://creativecommons.org/licenses/by/4.0/

Goldacre and Gray *Trials* (2016) 17:164
DOI 10.1186/s13063-016-1290-8

Trials

COMMENTARY   Open Access

OpenTrials: towards a collaborative open database of all available information on all clinical trials

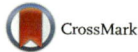 CrossMark

Ben Goldacre[1,2]* iD and Jonathan Gray[3,4]

Abstract

OpenTrials is a collaborative and open database for all available structured data and documents on all clinical trials, threaded together by individual trial. With a versatile and expandable data schema, it is initially designed to host and match the following documents and data for each trial: registry entries; links, abstracts, or texts of academic journal papers; portions of regulatory documents describing individual trials; structured data on methods and results extracted by systematic reviewers or other researchers; clinical study reports; and additional documents such as blank consent forms, blank case report forms, and protocols. The intention is to create an open, freely re-usable index of all such information and to increase discoverability, facilitate research, identify inconsistent data, enable audits on the availability and completeness of this information, support advocacy for better data and drive up standards around open data in evidence-based medicine. The project has phase I funding. This will allow us to create a practical data schema and populate the database initially through web-scraping, basic record linkage techniques, crowd-sourced curation around selected drug areas, and import of existing sources of structured and documents. It will also allow us to create user-friendly web interfaces onto the data and conduct user engagement workshops to optimise the database and interface designs. Where other projects have set out to manually and perfectly curate a narrow range of information on a smaller number of trials, we aim to use a broader range of techniques and attempt to match a very large quantity of information on all trials. We are currently seeking feedback and additional sources of structured data.

Background

Trials are used to inform decision making, but there are several ongoing problems with information management on clinical trials, including publication bias, selective outcome reporting, lack of information on methodological flaws, and duplication of effort for search and extraction of data, which have a negative impact on patient care. Randomised trials are used to detect differences between treatments because they are less vulnerable to confounding, and because biases can be minimised within the trial itself. The broader structural problems external to each individual trial result in additional biases, which can exaggerate or attenuate the apparent benefits of treatments.

To take the example of publication bias, the results of trials are commonly and legally withheld from doctors, researchers and patients, more so when they have unwelcome results [1, 2], and there are no clear data on how much is missing for each treatment, sponsor, research site, or investigator [3], which undermines efforts at audit and accountability. Information that is publicly available in strict legal terms can still be difficult to identify and access if, for example, it is contained in a poorly indexed regulatory document or a results portal that is not commonly accessed [4, 5]. In addition to this, different reports on the same trial can often describe inconsistent results because of, for example, diverse analytic approaches to the same data in different reports or undisclosed primary outcome switching and other forms of misreporting [4, 6]. There is also considerable

* Correspondence: ben.goldacre@phc.ox.ac.uk
[1]Centre for Evidence Based Medicine, Department of Primary Care Health Sciences, University of Oxford, Oxford OX2 6GG, UK
[2]Department of Non-Communicable Disease Epidemiology, London School of Hygiene and Tropical Medicine, Keppel Street, London WC1E 7HT, UK
Full list of author information is available at the end of the article

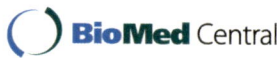

inefficiency and duplication of effort around extracting structured data from trial reports to conduct systematic reviews, for example, and around indexing these data to make it more discoverable and more used. Lastly, although large collections of structured "open data" on clinical trials would be valuable for research and clinical activity, including linkage to datasets other than those on trials, there is little available and it can be hard to search or access.

In 1999, Altman and Chalmers described a concept of "threaded publications" [7], whereby all publications related to a trial could be matched together: the published protocol, the results paper, secondary commentaries, and so forth. This suggestion has been taken up by the Linked Reports of Clinical Trials project, a collaboration of academic publishers which was launched in 2011 with the aim of using the existing CrossMark system for storing metadata on academic publications as a place where publishers can store a unique identifier (ID) on each trial to create a thread of published academic journal articles [8].

We have obtained funding for phase I of a project that expands this vision, going further than linking all academic papers on each trial: an open database of all structured data and documents on all clinical trials, cross-referenced and indexed by trial. The intention is to create a freely re-usable index of all such information to increase discoverability, facilitate audit on accessibility of information, increase demand for structured data, facilitate annotation, facilitate research, drive up standards around open data in evidence-based medicine, and help address inefficiencies and unnecessary duplication in search, research, and data extraction. Presenting such information coherently will also make different sources more readily comparable and auditable. The project will be built as structured "open data", a well-recognised concept in information policy work described as "data that can be freely used, modified, and shared by anyone for any purpose" [9].

This article describes our specific plans, the types of documents and data we will be including, our methods for populating the database, and our proposed presentations of the data to various different types of users. We do not have funding to manually populate the entire database for all data and documents on all trials, and such a task would likely be unmanageably large in any case. In the first phase, we aim to create an empty database with a sensible data schema, or structure, and then populate this through a combination of donations of existing sets of data on clinical trials, scraping and then matching existing data on clinical trials, with the option for users of the site to upload missing documents or links, and manual curation for a subset of trials. We will also create user-friendly windows onto this data. Our project start date was April 2015; our first user engagement workshop was in April 2015; and, after consultation on features and design, our first major coding phase will start in September 2015. We are keen to hear from anyone with suggestions, feature requests, or criticisms, as well as from anybody able to donate structured data on clinical trials, as described below.

Data schema

A description of the main classes of documents and data included is presented below and in Fig. 1. In overview, where possible, we will be collecting and matching registry entries; links, abstracts, or texts of academic journal papers; portions of regulatory documents describing trials; structured data extracted by systematic reviewers or other researchers; clinical study reports; additional documents such as blank consent forms; and protocols.

Types of documents and data included

Registers are a valuable source of structured data on ongoing and completed trials. There are two main categories of register: industry registers, containing information on some or all trials conducted by one company, and national registers, containing information on some or all trials conducted in one territory or covered by one regulator. National registers generally consist of structured data on 20 standard data fields set out by the World Health Organisation (WHO) [10]; industry and specialty registers are more variable [11]. The WHO International Clinical Trials Registry Platform is a "registry of registers" combining the contents of a large number of registers in one place [12]. The simple act of aggregating, deduplicating, and then comparing registers can in itself be valuable. For example, in preliminary coding and matching work, we have found that trials listed in one register as "completed" may be listed as "ongoing" in another; thus, anyone looking only in the register where the trial was "ongoing" would not have known that results were, in fact, overdue. Similarly, where the text field for primary outcome has been changed during a trial, this can be identified in serial data on one registry and flagged up on the page for that trial. Registers presenting structured data have consistent and clearly denoted fields containing information on features such as the number of participants, the interventions (ideally using standard dictionaries and data schemas for consistency with other structured data), inclusion and exclusion criteria, primary and secondary outcomes, location of trial sites, and so forth. This information is ready to be extracted, processed, or presented. As a very simple example, after extracting this information, one can calculate the total number of trial participants on an intervention globally, restrict a search to include only large trials, or facilitate search of ongoing trials within

Goldacre and Gray *Trials* (2016) 17:164

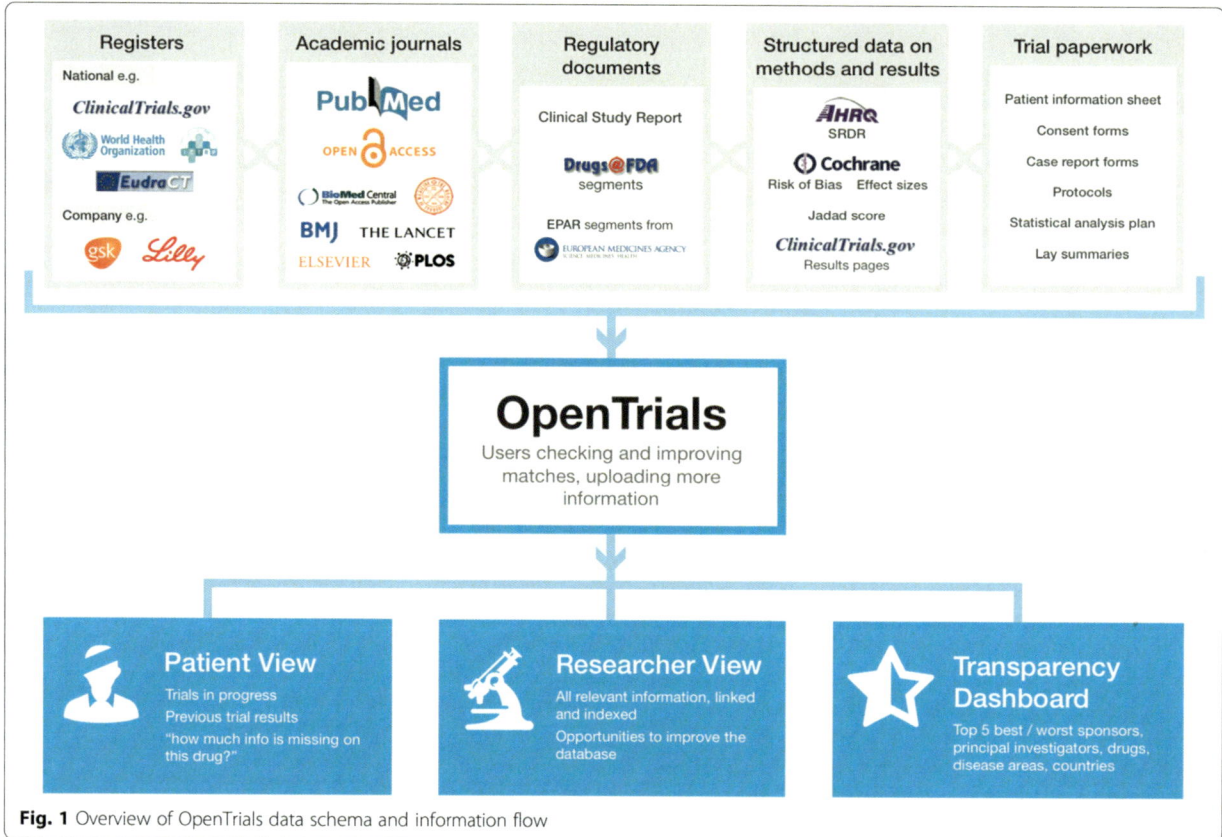

Fig. 1 Overview of OpenTrials data schema and information flow

50 miles of a location, on a specific condition, where data quality permits [13].

Academic journals are one source of information on clinical trials, in the form of semi-structured free text, although they have increasingly been found to be flawed vehicles for such data. For example, they are less complete than clinical study reports [14], inconsistent with mandated structured data on registers [15], and permissive on undisclosed switching of primary outcomes [6] and other forms of misreporting [16]. Journal articles on trials include other document types, such as commentaries and protocols. Academic journal articles reporting trial results can be matched against registry entries through various imperfect techniques, such as searching for trial ID numbers in metadata on PubMed (for very recent publications only) while applying standard search filters for trials, or using record linkage techniques on other features such as intervention or population.

Regulatory documents are an important and often neglected source of information on trials. Clinical study reports are extremely lengthy documents produced for industry-sponsored trials. They have a closely defined structure, which academic researchers have recently begun to access more frequently [14, 17]. At the other

end of the spectrum for length, there will often be free text descriptions of the methods and results of clinical trials mixed in with other information in bundles of regulatory documents released by the U.S. Food and Drug Administration and indexed on the Drugs@FDA website [18] or as part of the European public assessment report published by the European Medicines Agency for approved uses of approved drugs [19]. These documents are generally neglected by clinicians and researchers [5], poorly indexed, and hard to access and navigate. For example, the description of one trial may be buried in a few paragraphs in the middle of a long and poorly structured file, containing multiple documents, each covering multiple different issues around the approval of a product [4].

Structured data on the results of clinical trials is available from two main sources: registers that accept results reporting, such as ClinicalTrials.gov and ISRCTN (International Standard Randomised Controlled Trial Number), and structured data that has been manually extracted from free text reports on trials by researchers conducting systematic reviews or other research. This can include structured data on the characteristics of the trial (such as number of participants or a description of the interventions using standard dictionaries) or the

Goldacre and Gray *Trials* (2016) 17:164

Page 4 of 12

results of a trial (to populate fields in meta-analysis software), as well as data on the conduct of a trial or its methodological shortcomings; for example, many trials have had their risk of bias graded on various aspects of trial design using standard tools such as the Cochrane Risk of Bias Assessment Tool. There is also a Systematic Review Data Repository (SRDR) archiving structured data that has been extracted manually in the course of producing systematic reviews. SRDR is managed by the Agency for Healthcare Research and Quality (AHRQ), which has already begun to pool such data [20].

Trial paperwork includes protocols, lay summaries, and statistical analysis plans, as well as documents often currently regarded as "internal", such as blank case report forms, blank consent forms, ethical approval documents, and patient information sheets. These are generally poorly accessible and rarely indexed, but they can contain salient information. For example, it was only by examination of case report forms that the team conducting the Cochrane review on oseltamivir and complications of influenza were able to establish that the diagnostic criterion for pneumonia was "patient self-report" rather than more conventional methods such as chest x-ray, sputum, and/or medical examination [21]. As another example, when presented with a trial in which the control group received a treatment which seems to be lower than the usual standard of care, a researcher or other interested party may wish to see the consent form to establish whether the benefits and risks of participation were clearly explained to patients. Lastly, ethics committee or institutional review board paperwork may contain information on how any potential risks were discussed or mitigated or may act as an additional source of information to identify undisclosed switching of primary and secondary endpoints. By placing all of this information side by side, identifying such inconsistencies becomes more straightforward and therefore may reasonably be expected to become more commonplace.

Populating the database

Manually populating the database for all documents and data on all trials would be desirable, but it would be a major information curation project requiring very significant financial support. We initially aim to populate the database in sections, with breadth and depth in different areas, through a range of approaches, including web-scraping, basic record linkage techniques, curated crowd-sourcing, and imports or donations of existing structured and linked data.

Importing publicly accessible structured data is a straightforward way to initially seed a database of information on clinical trials. For example, the entire database of structured data on ClinicalTrials.gov can be

downloaded and re-used. This database contains structured data on features such as title, number of participants, inclusion and exclusion criteria, interventions, outcomes, and so forth [22]. There are several other sources of structured data that can be downloaded and re-used under standard Creative Commons licenses for non-commercial re-use with attribution, such as the SRDR archive hosted by AHRQ [20]. Where structured data or documents on trials are publicly accessible but not available for download as a single coherent dataset, *web-scraping* can be used. This is a well-established technique whereby large quantities of structured data can be downloaded from websites automatically using scripts to visit large numbers of web pages sequentially and to download data from tables in pages.

Once data about trials are obtained, the issue then becomes matching data on each individual trial from the various different sources, such as matching a ClinicalTrials.gov registry entry against a row of manually extracted data on results that has been downloaded from SRDR. This is a *record linkage* issue, and there is a long and established literature and code base on the subject in other domains, such as patient records. Where two records share a common ID, such as a clinical trial ID number, they can simply be merged. If there is no common unique identifier, then standard probabilistic record linkage techniques can be used on various features of the trial.

An extension of this technique can be used for targeted web-scraping. For example, all academic papers in PubMed published since 2007 that refer to a registered trial should contain the trial registry ID in the XML data of the PubMed entry (although compliance with this feature was poor initially and has improved over time). International Committee of Medical Journal Editors guidelines have stated since 2005 that all trial results reported in journals should include the trial registry ID in the abstract. Therefore, we can automate a search of PubMed to identify academic publications with a given trial ID and import or generate metadata on these documents to our thread for that trial, including the type of publication (such as protocol, results, or commentary), year of publication, author names, and journal title. Linkage of PubMed and ClinicalTrials.gov has already been successfully conducted elsewhere [23], and the use of record linkage and targeted scraping techniques can be extended to other data sources.

We will also facilitate *curated and targeted crowdsourcing*. On the main page for a trial, in our current design, there is a list of documents and data we would like to have for each trial and an icon denoting whether it is present. If it is not present, there is an "upload arrow". As an illustration, where we have a trial thread that contains a registry entry and an academic publication on results, but nothing more, then visitors can click to upload something such as a file containing structured data on results, a link to a clinical study report that they have located online, or a copy of a blank consent form. Each upload requires metadata, checking, and credit where necessary, with the option for users to flag where things have been incorrectly associated with a trial. While participatory data curation brings challenges, there is a large and growing knowledge base on this approach, both from Open Knowledge directly [24] and more broadly in the open data community.

We have also initiated collaborations around *donations of structured data*. There are many large datasets around the world where some form of record linkage has been done manually, or where structured data has been extracted from free text, to conduct a single piece of research. For example, large samples of registry entries on completed trials have been matched to academic publications and other sources of results on a specific search date to create cohorts to investigate publication bias. We have already arranged donations from researchers of three datasets of varying sizes covering varying types of data in various fields. Where disparate records pertaining to a single trial have been matched manually in this fashion, that matched data can be used in turn to validate automated record linkage techniques. It is important that the contribution and investment by those who have created such datasets be recognised and rewarded [25] while also ensuring that maximum patient benefit is derived from their work, minimising duplication of effort. By maintaining metadata on provenance, we are able to proactively give credit for all donated, imported, and externally linked data, wherever data are presented or downloadable. We are working with initial data donors on ways to do this most effectively, such as by giving credit to sources on the page for a specific trial and automatically generating a bespoke list of required acknowledgements and references for secondary users when a batch of data is downloaded and re-used. Notably, all researchers who have so far shared data in the preliminary stage of OpenTrials have expressed enthusiasm for greater public benefit from the effort which went into creating their dataset, especially as in some cases the only previous output from the creation of a large threaded dataset was a portion in a table in a published academic paper. One researcher group has expressed concern about their data being downloadable for re-use by other researchers before they have extracted adequate value from it, which is a common and legitimate concern in sharing raw data on all academic work [25]; researchers are sharing, but with a time delay.

Lastly, we are keen to populate the database manually, as perfectly as possible, and for a small number of trials

to demonstrate the value of such a resource. There are only limited resources for this in phase I funding, but we will be guided in our choice of area by sources of funding and collaborations.

We currently intend to populate the database solely for randomised trials in humans; however, because this is principally a technical service rather than a manually curated library, any increase in volume is unlikely to materially affect the feasibility of the project. We are therefore open to expanding this remit to include other types of trials. For the same reason, there is no time limit on the era of trials that can be added or on the geographical territory covered.

Presenting the data

We have developed prototype presentations of the data for different audiences and are currently running a series of user engagement workshops to improve these. Initial views are focused on search; researchers' needs for individual trials; patients' needs for individual trials; and overviews of performance metrics, which include transparency metrics on how much information is available for various classes of trial by sponsor, site, and so forth.

The webpage for researchers on a single trial is presented in Fig. 1. Across the top is the title and some basic information about the trial, extracted from a registry entry or a hierarchy of alternative sources. Below is a series of icons showing the headline documents and bundles of structured data that we would like to have on all trials. These icons are green if the relevant data or documents are present, and visitors can click through to view them; they are amber if the documents have been submitted or matched but not validated; and they are red if they are outstanding. Upload arrows are available for all missing documents so that they can be uploaded, as documents or links, by anyone who wishes to contribute.

Below that, we have various different proposed methods of presenting structured data. For example, where a trial's risk of bias has been manually assessed somewhere and that data has been imported, we can display this in free text or icons to the visitor, showing them at a glance whether the trial has significant methodological shortcomings and what those shortcomings were. We can also predict whether individual patient data (IPD) should be available for the trial on request and guide the visitor to the relevant portal (of which there are currently at least 12), using simple algorithms running on the structured data. For example, if a trial is conducted after 2007, for a currently marketed product, and sponsored by GlaxoSmithKline, the IPD should be available on request through ClinicalStudyDataRequest. com, and contextual explanatory notes for this service are also provided. This may help to increase the use

Goldacre and Gray *Trials* (2016) 17:164

of such data, which is only requested infrequently at present.

The presentation for patients (Fig. 2) is limited by the quality of the data currently available for this audience, but it has significant potential with greater user engagement. For example, we can present search options for ongoing trials for a given condition or a given drug, covering a given geographical area, filtered if necessary for an individual's eligibility by comparing their entered demographic information against structured data on the inclusion and exclusion criteria of each trial, where data quality permits. Previous efforts to do this have been hindered by the variably poor quality of information on registries for non-specialist users. Here there are many opportunities. The first is from record linkage. For example, all trials must pass through an ethics committee,

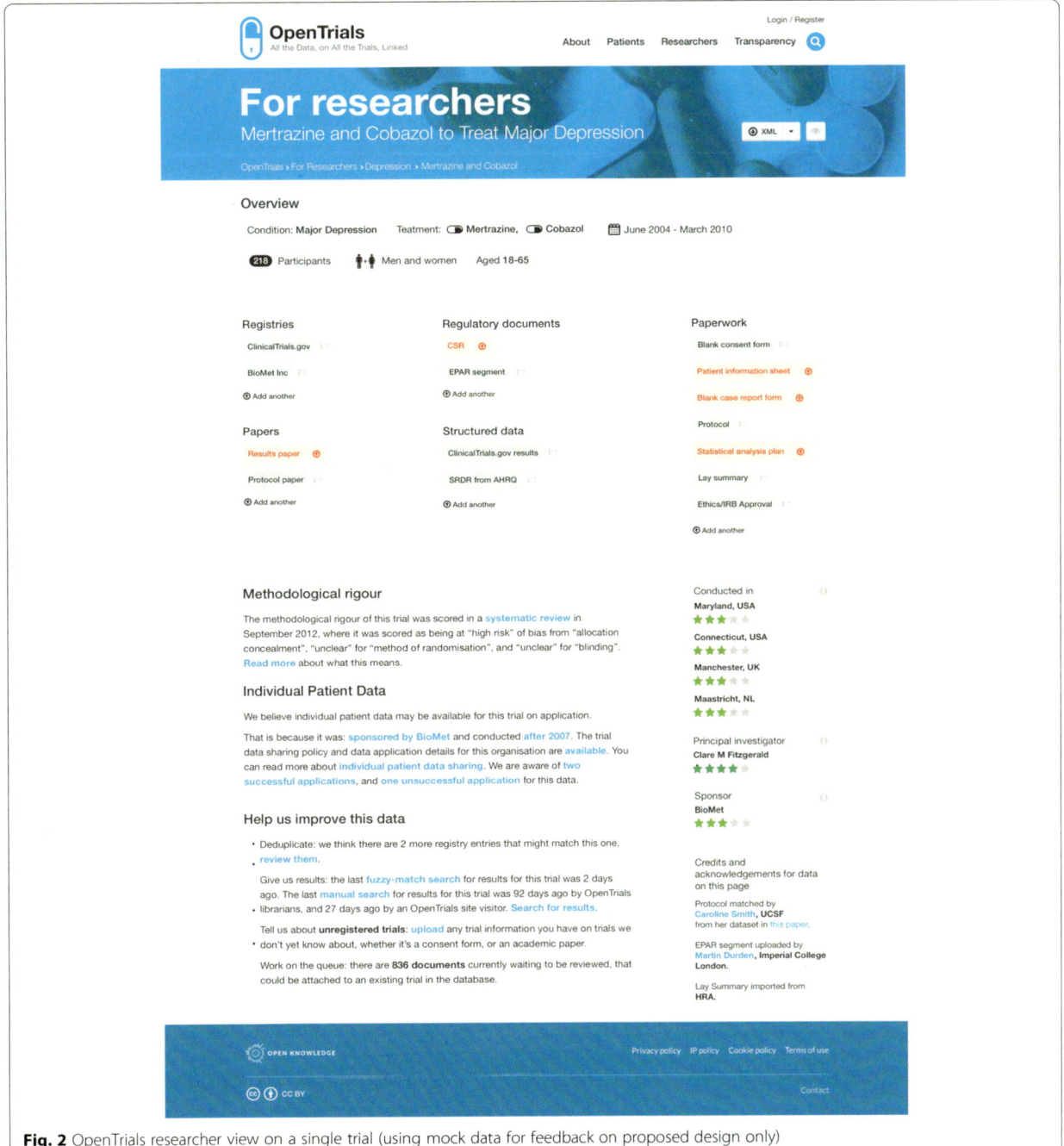

Fig. 2 OpenTrials researcher view on a single trial (using mock data for feedback on proposed design only)

Goldacre and Gray *Trials* (2016) 17:164

and all ethics committees require a lay summary. Where we can match the lay summary from ethics committee paperwork, we can present it on the patient-facing page. The second opportunity comes from using the option of crowd-sourcing and annotation, as we can also permit others to upload their own lay summaries. To this end, we have begun negotiating with science communication course leaders to work with them on using this as an exercise for their students, and are also keen that methodological shortcomings in ongoing and completed trials be communicated clearly to patients, with a view to developing a good trials guide. Here, as with other additional features to the core service, our efforts will be driven by opportunities for collaboration.

The overview of performance metrics (Fig. 3) demonstrates the value of having a large quantity of structured data in one place. For example, we can trivially produce dashboards reporting numbers of ongoing and completed trials but also, for areas or drugs where the data is reasonably complete, present metrics on transparency, such as showing how much information is currently missing for a given drug, sponsor, institution, investigator, and so forth. Such leader boards may be instrumental in driving up standards on transparency [3].

Some use cases

We envisage a wide range of users exploring a wide range of questions and are keen to hear from potential users with specific feature requests early in the development process to ensure that we can meet their needs. Some examples of use cases are presented here for illustration.

A *researcher* or *clinician* may wish to find out more about a range of trials on a drug, searching by various different features such as inclusion and exclusion criteria to match a specific population. For each individual trial, where it has already been manually graded for methodological rigour, the researcher is provided with this information immediately. Where the trial has been included in a systematic review, a link to the review is prominently displayed. If IPD is available on request, the researcher can see this immediately. Where the results on a trial have been reported in multiple different places, a researcher can rapidly review these side by side; if there are discrepancies, these may be informative. For example, there may be a more conservative analytic strategy used in the regulatory filing than in the academic paper, resulting in conflicting effect sizes or participant counts; the primary outcomes may be switched or conflict between different presentations of the results; or the names of authors and investigators may vary widely between registration and various presentations of results. Each of these elements may raise concerns for further investigation.

A *patient* interested in participating in a trial may visit the site looking for trials in progress, in their local area,

and on their medical condition. A science communication or clinical trials master of science *student* may visit the site to identify a trial that is lacking a lay summary or expert review and then write one as a learning experience and for the benefit of the wider community. An *expert patient* or *policy officer* working for a *patient group* may research a range of trials on the medicines taken by patients with their condition and find that there are many trials completed for which apparently no results have been posted. They can conduct a brief search for missing results and post any results they are able to find. Should this search yield no results, or if a professional search has already been conducted on a recent date and confirmed no results, then the patient or patient group can contact the sponsor, principal investigator (PI), or company, explaining that they represent patients using this treatment and asking them to make the results of the trial publicly accessible.

A *healthcare worker in a developing country* setting may be told of an ongoing trial by a patient and be shown a consent form or patient information sheet. Such a person can upload a copy of that document, and it will be entered into the queue of unresolved submitted documents. Here it can be seen and checked whether it matches an ongoing registered trial. If it appears to be for an unregistered trial, a new holding ID can be assigned and a new thread commenced for that trial. In this way, the OpenTrials database can facilitate field surveillance for ongoing unregistered and therefore poorly regulated or unethical research.

Trial sponsors or *university research staff* may visit the site to ensure that all their trials have results publicly available, that all other data are available, and that registry entries are not conflicting. A *journalist* or *policy officer* interested in publication bias may visit the site and explore the treatments, PIs, sites, or sponsors with the highest rates of apparently unreported results on completed trials.

A *systematic reviewer* seeking to conduct a rapid review may visit the site to search for trials and to aggregate existing extracted structured data from the site to avoid duplication of effort, before generating structured data themselves on uncoded trials and then sharing this data in turn. A researcher working on *automating systematic reviews* may use manually extracted structured data on the site, matched to free text documents, to calibrate their automated data extraction algorithms and request bespoke fields to share their extracted data back to a hidden part of the site for shared comparisons among automated review researchers.

Technical issues with data curation from multiple sources

Hosting a broad range of data and documents presents some challenges around curation, especially because

Goldacre and Gray *Trials* (2016) 17:164

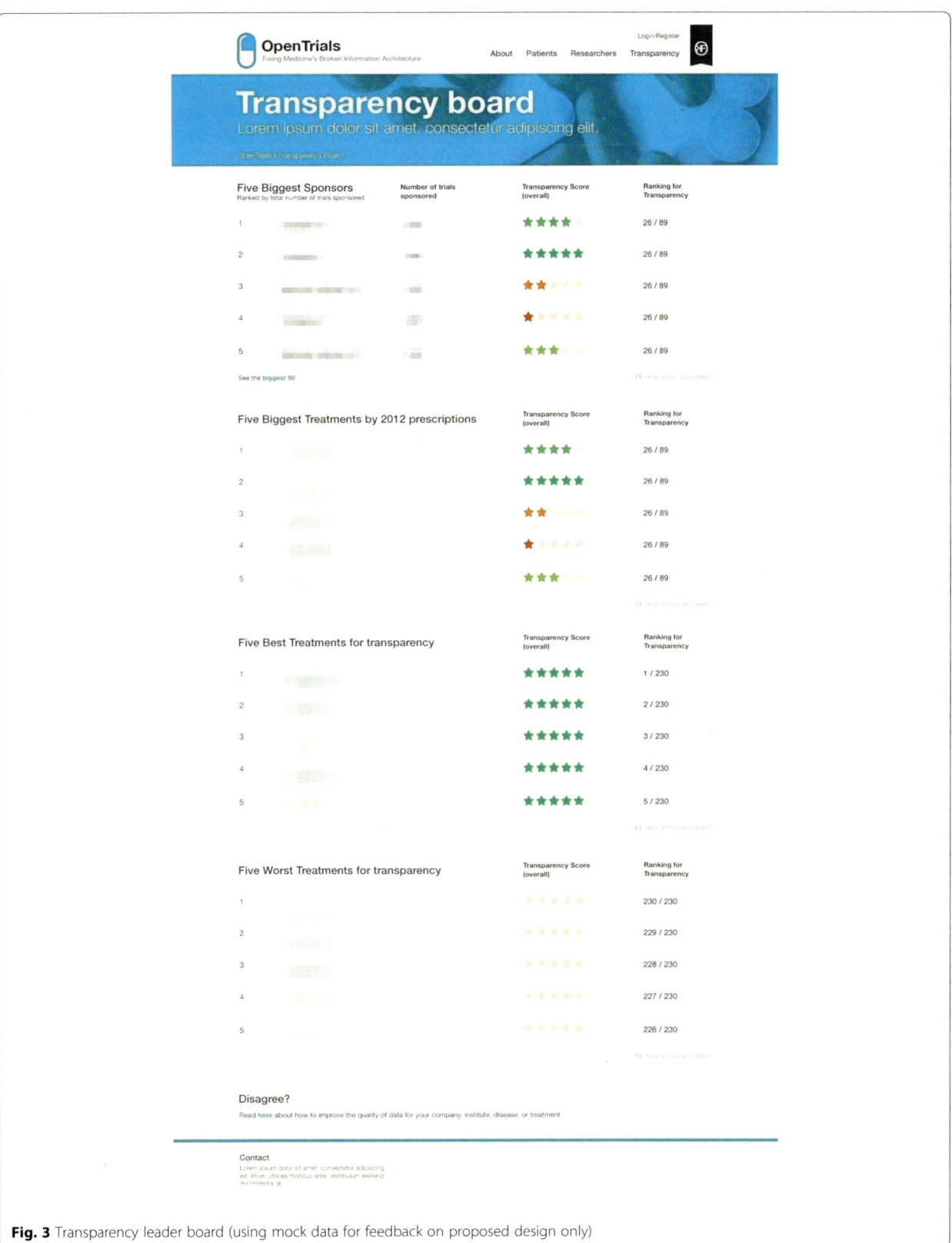

Fig. 3 Transparency leader board (using mock data for feedback on proposed design only)

different sources of structured data will use different formats and different dictionaries. Although we will exploit available mapping between different data schemas and dictionaries, we do not expect to necessarily make all sources of all structured data on all trials commensurable and presentable side by side. For example, intervention may be described in free text or as structured data using various different dictionaries, and even sample size may be labelled in different ways in different available datasets, not all of which can necessarily be parsed and merged. For simplicity, we are imposing a series of broad categories as our top-level data schema, following the list given above. This is best thought of as a thread of documents on a given trial, where a "document" means either an actual physical document (such as a consent form or a trial report) or a bundle of structured data for a trial (such as the structured results page from a ClinicalTrials.gov entry in XML format or a row of extracted data with accompanying variable names for a systematic review). This is for ease of managing multiple data sources, providing multiple bundles of structured data about each trial in multiple formats, each of which may be commonly or rarely used.

Parsers for such bundles of structured data, and mechanisms to present it in a user-friendly fashion, will be built according to need as expressed in our user groups. For example, we will parse ClinicalTrials.gov results pages in some detail and extract data on important features, such as sample size or primary and secondary outcomes, to present these on the page, because these data are consistently structured, well-curated, and available for a large number of trials. For more uncommon formats of structured data provided by systematic reviewers, we will extract some data or give options to present it on the page attractively (for example, listing "variable name" and "value"), but we will not present it on the main page for that trial. For more obscure structured data, such as the extracted data on a relational database used by a team of systematic reviewers internally (many of which may never have been included in a systematic review or a registry), we will extract some data from some fields and present these cleanly on the page but leave the rest available for download. Where anyone can provide us with a key to accompany their data schema, explaining what each variable name denotes, we will present that alongside their data. Overall, this approach represents a balance between what is achievable and perfect data curation, reflecting the fact that many users of complex structured data will be capable of using that structured data in its more raw forms.

Inconsistent structured data presents a further challenge, but also an opportunity. For example, "number of participants" may be slightly different in different data sources. This presents a challenge in terms of record

linkage validating a match between data sources to ensure that both records do pertain to the same trial. It also presents a challenge in terms of data presentation, as a choice must be made regarding which to present in a user-friendly front page for a trial. This is an example of the issues covered in our user engagement workshops. However, it also presents an opportunity to identify and flag inconsistencies in data on the same feature of the same trial in different places, to facilitate research on the reasons for this, and to establish whether such inconsistencies have resulted in bias.

By comparison, indexing and threading free text documents present far fewer challenges. For each uploaded document, we expect to have some metadata covering provenance, date of upload, type, any available structured data from the source (subject to the issues above), and some optional additional extracted data.

Open data in medicine

Open data is a widely recognised concept outside medicine, but to date there has been relatively little activity around open data in healthcare, and in particular almost none on clinical trials. The concept of "open data" arose in the open source software movement and in public sector information policy work. It now refers to a rapidly growing set of ideals, norms, and practises for publishing information from government, academia, civil society, and the private sector. Open data principles and standards stipulate how information should be disclosed: in machine-readable formats, for example, and with open licenses that remove restrictions on re-use [9]. The removal of legal and technical restrictions on re-use is intended to facilitate new forms of collaboration, innovation and re-use of data, such as through analysis, new applications and services, or collaborative databases and data "ecosystems" which combine and curate data from multiple sources.

Existing notable examples of open data include the OpenStreetMap project, a collaborative open data project to create a free map of the world, integrating geospatial data from many different sources, including the public sector, private sector, researchers, individuals, and civil society organisations. To date, this project has over 2 million registered and contributing users, with their data widely used as an alternative to proprietary geospatial information providers [26]. The Wikidata project, a sister project to Wikipedia, curates statistical data from a variety of different sources and currently has had over 230 million edits from 15,000 active users [27]. Both of these projects have been relatively successful in aligning the activities of different users to facilitate the collaborative development of a shared resource which can be re-used and developed in a wide variety of different contexts. The integration of these projects into different applications, services and workflows has also contributed in turn to their further development, population, and sustainability.

We hope that the OpenTrials project can become a similar collaborative open database project for medicine, and that it can help to catalyse a better data infrastructure for information about clinical trials. While many existing databases are limited to specific use cases (such as for compliance with regulation or for particular research communities), there is an opportunity to create a shared data infrastructure for medicine through a combination of flexible and extensible schemas and data structures, user interfaces catering to different users and use cases, proactively seeking collaboration with organisations and researchers who operate in this area, and being responsive to their needs. This will entail not just the technical work of collation, cleaning and presentation of data from multiple sources but also the social and political work of aligning the interests and activities of different organisations, researchers and users around collaborative activity. Elsewhere, Open Knowledge (the organisation leading the technical aspects of building the OpenTrials database) has used the phrase *participatory data infrastructures* to describe flexible information systems—with their various technical, legal, administrative and social components—that are responsive to the needs and interests of multiple different users and groups [28]. By being responsive, the data infrastructure can be extended to include fields and indicators which are not currently captured in existing information systems, which can make it more useful as a research resource, a tool for driving policy change and improvement in data quality, or for other as yet unforeseen purposes. In addition to this, the very act of requesting shares of bulk data can itself be a positive forward push.

As a minimum, we hope that OpenTrials and related projects will contribute to advancing norms and practices around access to data and documents in medicine, including the expectation that such information will be shared as structured open data that can be more readily matched, analysed and collaboratively improved.

Intellectual property and privacy

There are various intellectual property (IP) issues presented by such a database, such as regarding third-party IP in articles, documentary materials or datasets. There are various approaches to managing these issues. For example, if a copy of a consent form is made available to us by a trial participant, then we believe there is a clear public interest in its being publicly accessible and available for download (with personal information redacted where needed). However, such forms can be lengthy written documents published without explicit permission to republish or re-use. While it seems unlikely that

anyone would have a sincere commercial IP reason to withhold such documents from public access, it is possible to have other reasons to prefer that they be kept inaccessible or to have a blanket policy on restricting third-party use of all documents or a preference to host it on their own service; therefore, they may use IP law to prevent it from being either hosted or shared with doctors, researchers, and patients.

Here we believe the most sensible option is to pursue a simple three-stage policy: (1) link out to such documents, wherever possible, if they are publicly accessible in any form, but take a copy for archive in case the publicly accessible version disappears; (2) host the text if such documents are not accessible, assuming good faith and public interest, but provide a service for "take down" requests; and (3) treat each request for withdrawal on a case-by-case basis, seeking funding for legal expenses to defend public interest as and where this seems appropriate.

With respect to privacy, we propose to avoid hosting IPD to protect patient privacy. Instead, we will link to sources where IPD is available upon request and monitor the availability of these sources.

Practical issues

The project has received phase I funding from the Laura and John Arnold Foundation, given to Open Knowledge and the Centre for Open Science, with BG as principal investigator. User engagement, database design, front-end design and coding will be carried out by Open Knowledge, and the back-end database is provided by the Centre for Open Science. We have a small steering committee meeting regularly for the daily running of the project and a larger advisory group with a wide range of users and stakeholders for intermittent guidance on build, strategic direction and sustainability. In terms of outcome measures, we have targets for the quantity of data imported and the number of active users, as well as policy impacts, such as raised expectations of access to documents and around structured open data on clinical trials.

Our objective for phase I is to create a functioning database with a practical schema; populate it through scraping, record linkage, data donations, crowd-sourcing, and a small amount of pilot curation; and create user-friendly web interfaces onto the data. We believe that this will provide a clear working demonstration of the value of a matched and indexed database of all structured data and documents on all clinical trials, and that it will enable us to work towards obtaining further funding to populate the database—the key financial challenge—and develop new features to meet demand from researchers, clinicians, policy makers, patients and other users. We are also considering alternative options for sustainability, such as offering a paid service whereby OpenTrials librarians can curate and enter data as perfectly as possible for a given set of trials in exchange for a fee, enabling research sites or sponsors to facilitate access to information on their trials and demonstrate compliance and transparency, although this raises potential conflicts of interest that would need to be managed. If, after producing a functioning service, it proves impossible to make the project financially sustainable, then we have a no-cost wind-down plan in place, sharing all code and data to appropriate platforms (e.g., GitHub and Figshare). Where further features and infrastructure have been developed using functions on the site, we will aim to reserve a fund to permit a static archive with functioning APIs so that any other projects dependent on OpenTrials features or data can continue to operate.

There are several clear shortcomings and challenges to the OpenTrials plan which we have attempted to mitigate within the confines of limited funding as described above. These challenges include limitations on financial and person-time resources that prevent us from creating a comprehensive, manually curated library of all information on all trials; the challenges around ensuring integrity of material submitted openly online; the challenges of maintaining information infrastructure over a term that exceeds stand-alone academic project grants; and the challenges around engaging a community to solicit wider sharing of documents and structured data. We are keen to hear feedback on additional strategies to meet these challenges.

Conclusions
We are building an open free database and web service to identify, aggregate, store, match, index and share all available documents and data on all clinical trials. We are keen to receive feedback on the current methods, design, and data schema; feature requests; offers or suggestions of further data sources; and collaborations or methods to expand or improve the specification. Progress can be viewed at www.OpenTrials.net where the service will be hosted.

Abbreviations
AHRQ: Agency for Healthcare Research and Quality; ID: identifier; IP: intellectual property; IPD: individual patient data; ISRCTN: International Standard Randomised Controlled Trial Number; PI: principal investigator; SRDR: Systematic Review Data Repository; WHO: World Health Organisation.

Competing interests
OpenTrials is funded by the Laura and John Arnold Foundation. BG has received funding from the Laura and John Arnold Foundation, the Wellcome Trust, the World Health Organisation and the West of England Academic Health Science Network. BG receives income from speaking and writing for lay audiences on problems in science, including publication bias and better access to documents. Open Knowledge is a non-profit organisation which receives funding from a variety of philanthropic and research sources.

Authors' contributions
BG developed the initial concept for OpenTrials. BG and JG further developed the concept and design of OpenTrials. BG wrote the first draft of the manuscript. Both authors contributed extensively to subsequent drafts, and both read and approved the final manuscript.

Acknowledgements
OpenTrials is funded by the Laura and John Arnold Foundation. The design and structure of this project has been developed through the course of several years of discussion and practical prototyping with various collaborators and coders, including Louise Crow, Anna Powell-Smith, Tobias Sargent, Sam Smith, Emma Beer, Iain Chalmers, Liam Smeeth and Rufus Pollock.

Author details
[1]Centre for Evidence Based Medicine, Department of Primary Care Health Sciences, University of Oxford, Oxford OX2 6GG, UK. [2]Department of Non-Communicable Disease Epidemiology, London School of Hygiene and Tropical Medicine, Keppel Street, London WC1E 7HT, UK. [3]Policy and Research, Open Knowledge, St John's Innovation Centre, Cowley Road, Cambridge CB4 0WS, UK. [4]University of Amsterdam, Amsterdam, Netherlands.

Received: 8 September 2015 Accepted: 28 February 2016
Published online: 08 April 2016

References
1. Schmucker C et al. Extent of non-publication in cohorts of studies approved by research ethics committees or included in trial registries. PLoS One. 2014; 9:e114023.
2. Song F. et al. Dissemination and publication of research findings: an updated review of related biases. Health Technol Assess. 2010;14(8).
3. Goldacre B. How to get all trials reported: audit, better data, and individual accountability. PLoS Med. 2015;12:e1001821.
4. O'Connor AB. The need for improved access to FDA reviews. JAMA. 2009; 302:191–3.
5. Chan AW. Out of sight but not out of mind: how to search for unpublished clinical trial evidence. BMJ. 2012;344:d8013.
6. Mathieu S, Boutron I, Moher D, Altman DG, Ravaud P. Comparison of registered and published primary outcomes in randomized controlled trials. JAMA. 2009;302:977–84.
7. Chalmers I, Altman DG. How can medical journals help prevent poor medical research? Some opportunities presented by electronic publishing. Lancet. 1999;353:490–3.
8. Altman DG, Furberg CD, Grimshaw JM, Shanahan DR. Linked publications from a single trial: a thread of evidence. Trials. 2014;15:369.
9. Open Knowledge – Source Code. The Open Definition. http:// opendefinition.org/. Accessed 19 March 2016.
10. World Health Organisation (WHO). International standards for clinical trial registries. Geneva: WHO; 2012. http://apps.who.int/iris/bitstream/10665/ 76705/1/9789241504294_eng.pdf. Accessed 19 March 2016.
11. Moja LP et al. Compliance of clinical trial registries with the World Health Organization minimum data set: a survey. Trials. 2009;10:56.
12. World Health Organisation (WHO). International Clinical Trials Registry Platform. http://www.who.int/ictrp/en/. Accessed 19 March 2016.
13. Pfiffner PB, Oh J, Miller TA, Mandl KD. ClinicalTrials.gov as a data source for semi-automated point-of-care trial eligibility screening. PLoS One. 2014;9: e111055.
14. Wieseler B et al. Completeness of reporting of patient-relevant clinical trial outcomes: comparison of unpublished clinical study reports with publicly available data. PLoS Med. 2013;10:e1001526.
15. Hartung DM et al. Reporting discrepancies between the ClinicalTrials.gov results database and peer-reviewed publications. Ann Intern Med. 2014;160:477–83.
16. Boutron I, Dutton S, Ravaud P, Altman DG. Reporting and interpretation of randomized controlled trials with statistically nonsignificant results for primary outcomes. JAMA. 2010;303:2058–64.
17. Doshi P, Jefferson T, Del Mar C. The imperative to share clinical study reports: recommendations from the Tamiflu experience. PLoS Med. 2012;9:e1001201.
18. U.S. Food and Drug Administration (FDA). Drugs@FDA FDA approved drug products. http://www.accessdata.fda.gov/scripts/cder/drugsatfda/. Accessed 19 March 2016.
19. European Medicines Agency. European public assessment reports: background and context. http://www.ema.europa.eu/ema/index. jsp?curl=pages/medicines/general/general_content_000433. jsp&mid=WC0b01ac058067fa25. Accessed 19 March 2016.

Goldacre and Gray *Trials* (2016) 17:164

20. Ip S et al. A Web-based archive of systematic review data. Syst Rev. 2012;1:15.
21. Jefferson T et al. Oseltamivir for influenza in adults and children: systematic review of clinical study reports and summary of regulatory comments. BMJ. 2014;348:g2545.
22. Zarin DA, Tse T, Williams RJ, Califf RM, Ide NC. The ClinicalTrials.gov results database—update and key issues. N Engl J Med. 2011;364:852–60.
23. Huser V, Cimino JJ. Linking ClinicalTrials.gov and PubMed to track results of interventional human clinical trials. PLoS One. 2013;8:e68409.
24. Open Knowledge. Global Open Data Index. http://index.okfn.org/. Accessed 19 March 2016.
25. Fecher B, Friesike S, Hebing M. What drives academic data sharing? PLoS One. 2015;10:e0118053.
26. OpenStreetMap. Stats. https://wiki.openstreetmap.org/wiki/Stats. Accessed 19 March 2016.
27. Wikidata. Wikidata:Statistics. https://www.wikidata.org/wiki/Wikidata:Statistics. Accessed 19 March 2016.
28. Gray J, Davies TG. Fighting phantom firms in the UK: from opening up datasets to reshaping data infrastructures? Working paper presented at the Open Data Research Symposium at the 3rd International Open Government Data Conference, Ottawa, ON, Canada, 27. 2015. http://papers.ssrn.com/abstract=2610937. Accessed 19 March 2016.

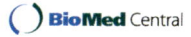

12.2 International Charter of Principles for Sharing Bio-specimens and Data

Deborah Mascalzoni, Edward S. Dove, Yaffa Rubinstein, Hugh J. S. Dawkins, Anna Kole, Pauline McCormack, Simon Woods, Olaf Riess, Franz Schaefer, Hanns Lochmüller, Bartha M. Knoppers, and Mats Hansson

Mascalzoni, D, et al. International Charter of principles for sharing bio-specimens and data. *European Journal of Human Genetics* 23(6), 721-728 (2016). 2015 Macmillan Publishers Limited All rights reserved 1018-4813/15. An imprint of SpringerNature.

*EJHG*Open
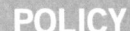

European Journal of Human Genetics (2015) 23, 721–728
© 2015 Macmillan Publishers Limited All rights reserved 1018-4813/15
www.nature.com/ejhg

International Charter of principles for sharing bio-specimens and data

Deborah Mascalzoni*[,1,2], Edward S Dove[3], Yaffa Rubinstein[4], Hugh JS Dawkins[5,6,7,8], Anna Kole[9], Pauline McCormack[10], Simon Woods[10], Olaf Riess[11], Franz Schaefer[12,13], Hanns Lochmüller[10], Bartha M Knoppers[3] and Mats Hansson[1]

There is a growing international agreement on the need to provide greater access to research data and bio-specimen collections to optimize their long-term value and exploit their potential for health discovery and validation. This is especially evident for rare disease research. Currently, the rising value of data and bio-specimen collections does not correspond with an equal increase in data/sample-sharing and data/sample access. Contradictory legal and ethical frameworks across national borders are obstacles to effective sharing: more specifically, the absence of an integrated model proves to be a major logistical obstruction. The Charter intends to amend the obstacle by providing both the ethical foundations on which data sharing should be based, as well as a general Material and Data Transfer Agreement (MTA/DTA). This Charter is the result of a careful negotiation of different stakeholders' interest and is built on earlier consensus documents and position statements, which provided the general international legal framework. Further to this, the Charter provides tools that may help accelerate sharing. The Charter has been formulated to serve as an enabling tool for effective and transparent data and bio-specimen sharing and the general MTA/DTA constitutes a mechanism to ensure uniformity of access across projects and countries, and may be regarded as a consistent basic agreement for addressing data and material sharing globally. The Charter is forward looking in terms of emerging issues from the perspective of a multi-stakeholder group, and where possible, provides strategies that may address these issues.
European Journal of Human Genetics (2015) **23**, 721–728; doi:10.1038/ejhg.2014.197; published online 24 September 2014

INTRODUCTION TO THE INTERNATIONAL CHARTER OF PRINCIPLES FOR SHARING BIO-SPECIMENS AND DATA

Sharing data and bio-specimens is essential for the discovery, new knowledge creation and translation of various biomedical research findings into improved diagnostics, biomarkers, treatment development, patient care, health service planning and general population health. The growing international agreement on the need to provide access to research data sets to optimize their use and fully exploit their long-term value has been articulated in many documents, including the OECD Principles and Guidelines for Access to Research Data from Public Funding, the Toronto Statement, and more recently the Global Alliance for Genomics and Health's White Paper.[1–3] Contemporaneously, the ambitious aims set out in the International Rare Disease (RD) Research Consortium (IRDiRC.org), which seeks to develop 200 therapies and to diagnose most RDs by 2020, and the decision of the European Commission asking all members states to develop a national plan for RDs,[4] provide further impetus. Although sharing of data and samples is thought to be beneficial for most health-related research, it is of highest importance for RD research because of the scarcity of research participants, samples, data, resources and researchers for any given RD.

Ideally, data and bio-specimens should be made widely available to the most inclusive and ethically responsible research community, but there is often resistance by institutions and individuals who fear that they will not receive recognition for their investment in building collections. Real and perceived risks of discrimination of vulnerable patients groups because of health-related data sharing also exist and must be considered in any legislation or guidelines. Collecting data and storing biological samples in accordance with ethical and scientific standards requires intellectual, institutional and economic resources and, critically, the participation of patients and the wider community including otherwise healthy volunteers.

All data and material sharing agreements should be ethically robust and mindful of the responsibilities owed to the donors to make best ethical use of the samples and data consistent with their consent.

Researchers face very different requirements for data and sample sharing. Data Transfer Agreement (DTA) and Material Transfer Agreement (MTA) are often written in legal terms, and so are not easily understood by scientists or institute administration officers who serve as a conduit for these agreements. Hence the need to provide a simplified overview of basic principles and a practical template

[1]Center for Research Ethics and Bioethics Uppsala University, Uppsala, Sweden; [2]Center for Biomedicine, EURAC Research, Bolzano, Italy; [3]Centre of Genomics and Policy, Mc Gill University, Montreal, Quebec, Canada; [4]Office for Rare Diseases Research, National Center for Advancing Translational Sciences, National Institutes of Health, Bethesda, MD, USA; [5]Office of Population Health Genomics, Department of Health, Perth, Western Australia, Australia; [6]Centre for Population Health Research, Curtin Health Innovation Research Institute, Curtin University of Technology, Bentley, Western Australia, Australia; [7]School of Pathology and Laboratory Medicine, University of Western Australia, Nedlands, Western Australia, Australia; [8]Center for Comparative Genomics, Murdoch University, Murdoch, Western Australia, Australia; [9]EURORDIS, Rare Disease Europe, Paris, France; [10]PEALS (Policy, Ethics & Life Sciences) Research Centre, Newcastle University, Newcastle upon Tyne, UK; [11]Institute of Medical Genetics and Applied Genomics, University of Tübingen, Tübingen, Germany; [12]Pediatric Nephrology Division at Heidelberg University Hospital, Heidelberg, Germany; [13]Institute of Genetic Medicine, Newcastle University International Centre for Life, Newcastle upon Tyne, UK
*Correspondence: Dr D Mascalzoni, Center for Research Ethics and Bioethics, Uppsala University, Husargatan 3, BMC, Entrance A11 Box 564, SE-751 22 Uppsala, Sweden. Tel: +46 18 471 61 97; Fax: +46 18 471 66 75; E-mail: deborah.mascalzoni@crb.uu.se
Received 13 June 2014; revised 1 August 2014; accepted 20 August 2014; published online 24 September 2014

(the MTA/DTA). The principles are equally valid and applicable for Access Agreements (AAs).

The Charter, together with the template for general MTA/DTA, constitutes an enabling tool to improve the governance and audit of sharing data and specimens across multiple international settings. It is written in simplified language to make it accessible and usable by scientists and other stakeholders, and provides a consistent set of principles that will improve interoperability nationally and internationally.

The Charter has been developed to provide a common overview and foundational framework of the practice of sharing, and to frame a minimum list of the terms needed to achieve an equitable and ethically grounded data sharing agreement through multi-stakeholder engagement and consensus, including patient representatives, clinicians, researchers, institutions and government agencies. This Charter is the result of a careful negotiation of different stakeholder's interest: that includes a stakeholders workshop held in Brussels in October 2013. During the 2-day workshop, RD patient representatives, legal experts, ethical experts, industry representatives and scientists debated the issues and produced consensus positions that informed the Charter. The model is the result of further analysis and is built on earlier consensus documents and position statements, which provided the P3G general legal framework and generic MTA.[5] The Charter has then been considered by the RD Connect Patient Ethics Council and RD Connect Patient Advisory Council, which endorsed the Draft Charter as the patient consulting bodies of RD Connect.

The MTA/DTA provides a clear and simplified template that can be applied to different research contexts. It follows the Charter's principles and incorporates them in a mutual template agreement between researchers (or institutions) that comprise best practices and values. Ideally, both the provider and recipient should not only fulfil legal requirements but also comply with ethical and quality assurance mechanism recommendations to achieve the highest ethical standards. Therefore, the suggested items constitute a best practice guideline.

The following five principles[6] for the custodianship of bio-specimen repositories and data, constitute the common premise for the Charter:

- Respect for privacy and autonomy: custodianship implies protection of participants' privacy. Privacy protection measures should be in place and informed consent must provide provisions for future as yet unspecified research using data and bio-specimens.
- Reciprocity: custodianship also implies giving back. Feedback of general results should be channelled to institutions and patients.
- Freedom of scientific enquiry: custodianship should encourage openness of scientific enquiry, and should maximize data and bio-specimen use and sharing so as to exploit their full potential to promote health.
- Attribution: the intellectual investment of investigators involved in the creation of data registries and bio-repositories is often substantial, and could be acknowledged by mutual agreement.
- Respect for intellectual property: the sharing of data and bio-specimens needs to protect proprietary information and address the requirements of institutions and third-party funders.

As described by Knoppers *et al*,[7] the sharing of personal data is a form of data processing, in accordance with the EU directive 95/46/EC on personal data protection. The processing of personal data requires authorization from a data protection authority or an ethics review board, unless directly permitted by law. Health-related personal data are classified as sensitive, implying that confidentiality laws apply and that processing requires consent from the data subject or permission

by law (on consent, see below). Different types of data are associated with different degrees of intellectual investment by the researchers, which should be reflected in sharing agreements. The sharing and integration of data across research groups and national borders implies that data (and metadata) must be sufficiently equivalent. As suggested by the DataSHaPER platform for harmonizing data collection in epidemiological research, the level of equivalence with regard to primary information collected (eg, serum cholesterol level) and qualifying factors that may affect the interpretation of data (eg, whether the subject had been fasting before measurement) is likely to be context- or consortium specific.[8] Issues about the quality of data accordingly have to be separately addressed by each party before sharing and being described in an MTA/DTA.

Wherever possible, the complete anonymization of data and bio-specimens should be avoided, based on the principle that this would make it impossible to add relevant data as science progresses, and precludes re-contacting donors and data subjects to communicate future medical discoveries that may benefit them.[9] This also reflects RD patients' views on the need to optimize data value in order to seek results for patients and for the benefit of the broader community. Similar considerations and issues concerning the anonymization of data in large cohort population databases and biobanks have been expressed more recently, and form an integral part of the consensus being developed internationally;[10,11] for a discussion, see also.[12–15] Donors of bio-specimens and data should therefore be informed that confidentiality will be taken seriously with the help of strict coding measures, as described below, but that there is no guarantee of complete anonymity because of the nature of the research and advances in technology.

At the time of the collection of data and bio-specimens, their future specific use may be difficult to anticipate or may only be described in very broad general terms, for example, for cancer research, RD research or medical research. The question about the acceptability of broad consent[16,17] has been deeply debated in the ethics and legal literature,[13–15,18–20] and there is some consensus on its acceptability[21,22] provided proper on-going ethical and legal oversight are in place (approval by ethics review boards for every single project is mandatory).

The need to re-contact and involve patients in research though, may also lead to the development of patient centric approaches to consent that provide a dynamic interaction. A number of patient centric consent strategies exploiting online technologies have been developed to help address the limits of a pure broad consent approach. Obviously longitudinal population projects are in constant contact with their participants but dynamic consent models[14,15,22] offer an alternative way to overcome the tension between broad and specific consent also in non-longitudinal research such as clinical trials, by ensuring ongoing information and participant involvement after general consent has been provided at the time of bio-specimens collection. Different research platforms and legal frameworks may require more detailed consent, but for the sharing procedures related to prospective sampling and data acquisition we propose and outline a minimal requirement strategy. Therefore, we further propose that templates for informed consent in research projects of an epidemiological character can be accepted if based on the notion of broadly described purposes for future research, provided this is subject to ethics approval and supported by a policy of regular updates to donors and a clear option to withdraw. In fact, even when the purpose is described only in general or broad terms, information regarding the process of research may be specific on the relevant issues, for example, that the research project implies the sharing of data across research groups and national borders, that complementary information may be added through linkage to different registries' medical records, that it involves genetic analyses and collaboration with both academic and commercial partners, whether or not there is any provision for return of research findings, etc. So to overcome the lack of detailed research information at the time of consent, we suggest an integrated approach entailing broad consent coupled with provision of on-going information about the general development of project, for instance by proper communication with the participants/donors through email, phone, a newsletter, patient organizations contacts and regular website updates dedicated to them.[22]

A sizeable number of samples currently exist in clinical biobanks as well as patient data registries for which there is little or no expressed consent for research, data/material sharing to other groups especially industry, or where the scope of the consent may be unclear. These samples may have been collected at a time when research ethics had not been developed to the standard they are now. In RD, there may not be an opportunity to obtain an equivalent sample or data set for research. Rules and recommendations regarding information and consent procedures need to take into account the complexity of patient perceptions as well as the different characteristics of different cohorts and collections.[23,24]

In order for researchers to be able to share samples and data of this kind, a common framework of how to manage informed consent concerns is needed. Legal frameworks may differ between countries making it possible in some countries to use archived samples and data without explicit consent, while researchers in other countries are obliged to obtain new consent. However, this does not necessarily constitute an obstacle for sharing across borders as each institution needs only to adhere to their national legal requirements on the information and consent procedures in order to satisfy the ethical requirements necessary to send samples and data abroad.[25,26] A recipient in another country can then use them either in a joint venture together with the sender or for MTA regulated projects, even if sampling and acquisition of data is differently regulated in that country, provided the objectives of the research are the same. Approval of these single projects by an ethics review board is always required.

Respect for autonomy, in the sense of having a direct say on how one's samples and data will be used in some cases may involve re-consent where according to the ethics committee the scope of the original consent may preclude the suggested research use. This is particularly relevant where the development of new techniques could not have been anticipated when the samples were first collected. Although ethics review is always requested for every single project, a general requirement to obtain new informed consent in all cases may be impractical and would also involve a potential for selection bias because of drop outs, decreasing the scientific value of the data and the sample collection.[27,28] The potential psychological impact on the research participants of re-contacting and re-consenting should be considered, although neglecting to inform patients on this basis should never be the default position and should be carefully evaluated in order to avoid paternalistic approaches.[14] RD research may be particularly vulnerable to selection bias because the number of available samples and data are intrinsically low for each condition, ultimately jeopardizing research, which is in the interests of all parties. However, careful consideration of the time, effort and other resources required to adequately re-consent patients should be given, as low numbers of patient research participants may also result in benefits of re-consent with low drop-out rates. The actual balance and trade-off between respect for autonomy and optimizing provision of new

treatment opportunities should be sensitive to and recognize the needs of the RD community and the wider public.

Where legal provisions requiring informed consent were in place at the time of sample/data collection, re-consent or notification with an opt-out option, should be pursued. A clear distinction should be made between collections in which a previous consent was obtained and where a question was not asked, and one where a patient actively declined an option or in which the information provided excluded some options (eg, 'your data will not be shared with any commercial organizations'). In these instances, re-consenting or notification with opt-out should be also pursued. For some older cohorts, the researcher may still find re-consent achievable within reasonable efforts, using this also as an opportunity to update or collect new data. Other projects may be particularly vulnerable to drop outs and one may want to use a scheme with notification and opt-out, thus still respecting the autonomy of participants.

Where it is determined that re-contacting patients is unfeasible or when inclusion of small sample numbers from across a large number of collections and registries are of outmost importance or when samples are held in older collections, an acceptable option could be a waiver on re-consent. This option is not feasible in every legal system and requires an adequate assessment of the reasons for asking for a waiver to the ethics review board. Optional re-consent as well as notification with an opt-out clause or general waiver of re-consent for specific cases may create some efficiencies and still maintain ethically responsible and practical ways to access samples an data spread across many sites globally. Where a waiver for re-consent is required, a careful explanation of the reasons that lead to this solution should be provided to the ethics review board. The permission by the ethics board to use the samples should specifically state the permission to share abroad and foresee genetic analysis where appropriate. The sharing of data and bio-specimens without consent needs to be compliant with the appropriate legal framework.

In the case of bio-specimens and data from minors or collected when the person was a minor, re-consent or notification with opt-out clause should be always pursued. Data and bio-specimens from deceased persons should be anonymized and used with ethics approval. Some legal systems may impose specific restrictions (eg, UK's Human Tissue Act 2004).

Institutions and organizations may have legitimate proprietary interests associated with data collected by researchers.[9] Biobank research infrastructures and data collections require investments and intense labour, and therefore a legitimate institutional interest based on the need to protect local investments exists. There is also another layer of institutional interest: the integrity of a research endeavour that has collected data based on original and promising hypotheses.[29–31] The effective dissemination of research results is thus associated with established criteria for acknowledging intellectual contributions and originality through rules of authorship and intellectual property rights. Custodianship implies the duty of recognizing the role of research institutions and their legal and ethical duties to participants and patients. There is agreement that general aggregated research results should be either on open access databases or at least disseminated to institutions and patients.

With regard to biobanks where the amount of samples may be limited, it is recommended that the samples are used only for studies reviewed by a competent and well-balanced data access committee so as to ensure good scientific quality. This is motivated primarily by ethical concerns for the protection of patient interests of reaping the fruits of their donated samples in terms of truly improved diagnosis and treatment opportunities. Data collections do not face scarcity but clinical quality registries are dependent on the trust of patients and therefore good communication processes are required to maintain this trust. Also, the submission of new data and reports using clinical registries that are of low scientific quality may jeopardize the trust and willingness of patients to consent and to continuously contribution data. To this end, caretakers of the clinical registry should also be granted a right to assess the quality of an application to acquire data for a study, as a parallel to an intellectual property right, because they have invested both personal intellectual and institutional resources in order to create the registry. They should be the rightful protectors of the integrity of the clinical registry in this sense. In practice, most networks of bio- and data repositories do have some kind of scientific evaluation committee to make these kinds of decisions, and we believe for good reason. The protocols of investigators who request access to clinical registries or biobanks should be vetted by a representative data access committee for scientific quality and the bona fides of applicants should also be authenticated, for example, through checking on their background and institution affiliation with the institution or university signing the MTA/DTA as co-responsible for the scientific integrity of the applicant.

The Charter briefly outlines the guiding principles for data and bio-specimen sharing together with the MTA/DTA that encloses these ethical principles in a template model. The Charter, developed within the framework of international research consortia projects, aims to provide a tool to be used for effective, ethically grounded sharing in the international context.

CHARTER OF PRINCIPLES FOR SHARING DATA AND BIO-SPECIMEN
Guiding principle
1. Sharing data and biological samples (bio-resources) is essential for accelerating biomedical research projects that will provide benefits to current and future patients.

Research conducted through biobanks and registries is more effective if access to sufficient data is granted, and the use of data is maximized through data sharing. Ensuring secure data and sample sharing ethically and legally protects bio-resources, as well as the donors and all the partners involved in research.

Sharing data and bio-specimens
2. DTA/(MTA: DTAs and MTAs should always be used to govern data/material transfer between parties.

DTAs and MTAs are legal contracts that help ensure that the parties signing the agreement will comply with a set of rules defined by the involved parties. These documents state the scope of the use of data or bio-specimens, the limits posed by the informed consent used for the original collection, special limitations, duration of sharing and use, and other special conditions including donors' expectations, etc.

Security and privacy regulations
3. Data and bio-specimens shall always be collected, stored and exchanged in a secure manner, through secure channels. Double coding and encryption are highly recommended for data handling. The type of data and bio-specimens provided to researchers should be described clearly in the DTA or MTA.

4. Data sharing should only occur when proper ethics review board approvals are in place (approval for the collection of the materials and approval for the single research projects).

5. Anonymization of data and bio-resources should generally be avoided because it will make it impossible to add individual-level data

as science progresses, and precludes re-contacting donors to communicate future medical discoveries that may benefit them.

6. Donors should be informed that the confidentiality of their information will be protected through secure technology and strict coding measures, but that there is no guarantee of complete confidentiality because of the evolving variety of techniques and technology advances in genome and gene sequencing that may lead to the potential identification of the individual.

7. Sharing occurring in international contexts should ensure that fundamental privacy interests are respected. The processing of personal data abroad requires authorization from a data inspection authority or by duly authorized institutional review board (IRB) unless directly permitted by law (general authorizations).

The European Medicines Agency has recommended a strict nomenclature, which we have adapted here with regard to both bio-specimen and data (Hansson[31]):

- Identified data and bio-specimens: data labelled or linked to the individual in a way that makes them directly identifiable (name and surname or social security numbers).
- Coded data (may be single or double coded): personally identifying information is removed from data and bio-specimens and replaced with a code. In the case of double-coding, two or more codes are assigned to the same donor's data held in different data sets, with the key connecting the codes back to the donor's direct identifiers held by a third party and not available to the researchers.
- Anonymized data and bio-specimens: data and samples that have been identified earlier or coded, but the identification, or the code and the code key have been destroyed, and thus there is no longer any link to the individual.
- Anonymous data and bio-specimens: there are no links to the individual donor, the data and bio-specimens were never associated with identifiers, and the risk of identification of individuals is very low. There may be general descriptions such as 'man, aged 50–55 years, cholesterol level 240 mg per 100 ml.'

For all above-mentioned categories, it is assumed that international and national regulations on access, informed consent, coding and data protection apply.

Health-related personal data are classified as sensitive, implying that data protection and confidentiality laws apply and that processing requires consent from the data subject or legal permission. Data sharing of personal data is a form of data 'processing', in accordance with National and International Regulation such as the EU directive 95/46/EC on personal data protection or in the US, HHS Regulations for the Protection of Human Subjects (http://www.hhs.gov/ohrp/humansubjects/guidance/45cfr46.html#46.102) and the Health Insurance Portability and Accountability Act (HIPAA) Privacy Rule, 45 CFR 164.514(b).[2]

Ensuring the scientific use of data and bio-specimens
8. Without distinction, access and use of data and samples should always be based on the scientific validity, quality and potential of the request. Those who contribute, collect, curate and annotate samples/data, however, should have first rights to publish within a given time period (usually no longer than 1 year).

9. In addition, the identity and bona fide of the requestors should be authenticated. Proper attribution and intellectual property should be accorded as appropriate, and the security of the data and samples should always be ensured.

In recognition of the contribution of the samples and data of patients, research participants and their families, the protocols of those requesting access for use should be vetted for their scientific validity and quality.

Acknowledgment of the bio-resources and data providers

10. The sharing of data and bio-specimens should follow criteria for the acknowledgement of intellectual contributions and originality through rules of authorship and intellectual property rights.

Many consider data collections and genomic databases a public good contributing to the improvement of public health, often serving as an incentive for governmental spending. This in itself will motivate the sharing of data and bio-specimens. However, it does not exclude the recognition of the interests of the researchers who have invested a great deal of intellectual effort in establishing the databases, registries and bio-specimen collections. An analogous example is the publication of scientific results, which can also be seen as instrumental to public health. However, unlike the sharing of data and bio-specimens, the dissemination of research results is associated with established criteria for the acknowledgement of intellectual contributions and originality through rules of authorship and intellectual property rights. We suggest five categories that should reflect different ladders of merit and following levels of recognition as proposed in the table below:

- Data included in official governmental administrative databases

  These sets of data should be available for research. As they are created for public interest they should not lead to authorship or special recognition.

- Data from health quality registries organized by researchers/clinicians

  These registries are normally organized within the national health-care systems and should in principle be publicly available for research. However, there is often a dedicated group of doctors/researchers who invest intellectual as well as material resources in collecting and systematizing data. This should be recognized in the acknowledgements of an article that builds on the collected data but not lead to authorship. There may be a fee-for-service for providing access to the data.

- Descriptive data directly accessible through health records or available instruments

  These data should in principle be openly available with due reference to the original source of the instrument. Some instruments are also made publicly available for a fee.

- Hypothesis-generated data and bio-specimens collection available after screening or within a specific project, or processed data

  Should in principle be available, but the principal investigator (PI) and researchers in the project should have time to explore and confirm preliminary findings. There may be a fee for service for providing access to the data. Normally, the conditions for the sharing of data should be part of the original agreement with the funder and be subject to the review process of the scientific journals. Requests for data and bio-specimens could include an offer of co-authorship to the PI when significant contribution to

the acquisition, analysis or interpretation of data is made and acknowledgements to the consortium or the biobank.

- Processed data: for example, GWAS data, omics data, whole-genome sequence data

  The processing of bio-specimens to obtain data is a considerable investment by the institution and reflects a significant contribution to the acquisition, analysis and interpretation of data. Therefore, requests for data and bio-specimens could include an offer of co-authorship to the PI or the consortium and a note in the acknowledgements.

- Acknowledgement for biobanks/data providers

  Biobanks are infrastructure created with the purpose of providing data and bio-specimens for research purposes. Authorship may not be a proper recognition mean. A recommended way to recognize the role of the data/bio-specimen provider is through the emerging bio-resource research impact factor (BRIF). As described by P3G, BRIF is 'a tool to calculate the research impact of bio-resources based on a unique digital resource identifier and on a metrics algorithm somewhat analogous to the journal impact factor.' Further information on BRIF can be found on the P3G website at http://www.p3g.org/brif-bioshare-pilot-study.

The kind of acknowledgment foreseen for the use of bio-resources and data should be clearly defined. For all categories, it is assumed that European and national regulations on access, informed consent, coding and data protection apply.

It is recommended in appropriate cases that when data from a common database is analysed, the results should be fed back to the common database. In order to recognize intellectual contributions, the researcher/research group who carried out the analyses should be entitled to a period of exclusivity of use of the results in order to explore their potential. Following the tradition of a 'grace period' in association with balancing publication interests versus investigating patentability, 6 months to 1 year of such exclusive use should be usually granted.

Quality of data and bio-specimens

11. Quality of data and bio-specimens must be ensured by the provider.

The quality of data and bio-specimens must be ensured in accordance with international standards. The integration of data across research groups and national borders implies that data must be sufficiently equivalent. As suggested by the DataSHaPER platform for harmonizing data collection in epidemiological research, the level of equivalence with regard to primary information collected (eg, serum cholesterol level) and qualifying factors that may affect the interpretation of data (eg, whether the subject had been fasting before measurement) is likely to be context- or consortium specific. Accordingly, issues concerning the quality of data have to be sorted out separately by each consortium before sharing.

Informed consent

12. Informed consent: informed consent to the general scope of the research project is mandatory. If broad consent is used, regular updates on the development and the aggregated results of the project/biobank are recommended, as they serve as reminders of on-going participation and keep the participants involved. Informed consent should also offer the clear option for the participant to

Charter of principles for international sharing
D Mascalzoni et al

726

withdraw from the research. Ongoing ethics oversight by proper review or ethics review boards is recommended.

At the time of data and sample collection, future research use may be difficult to anticipate or may only be describable in very broad general terms, for example, for 'cancer research', 'rare disease research' or 'medical research'. Therefore, broad consent with ethics approval, with the right to withdraw from the study, is acceptable if there is a continuous flow of information on project developments. We therefore suggest that templates for informed consent in research projects of an epidemiological character may be based on broad consent if they are supported by a commitment by the PI/project to provide regular updates in a timely and sufficiently comprehensive manner. Information especially relevant for data sharing should be disclosed in the information sheets.

In the information provided, it should be clearly specified whether or not:

- the research project reasonably anticipates the sharing of data across research groups and national borders.
- complementary information may be added through linkage to different data registries, medical records, etc.
- the project involves genetic analyses.
- the project involves collaboration with both academic and commercial partners.

Participants should be allowed to have some options to express choices, or at least be provided clear information on the policy for return of incidental findings, the destination of data and biospecimens after death or in the case of the termination of the project, and the involvement of relatives in research. A description of the communication of information strategy flowing from the project should be provided, and should include the general development of project timelines and newsletters or website updates dedicated to the donors.

Use of previously collected data and samples

13. For the use of previously collected data and bio-specimen where consent is absent or not fit for purpose, we recommend a case by case assessment by an ethics board. According to national legal requirements, either re-consent or a notification with opt-out schemes should be required in order to enable the institution to use and share internationally. This is especially important where minors (at the time of the collection) are involved. In some cases – where re-contact of patients is unfeasible and disproportionate to benefits (very old collections) – a waiver for re-consent can be granted by an ethics review board (please refer to national legal requirements). In this case, a clear outline of the reasons for requiring the waiver should be provided to the ethics board. A clear distinction should be made between collections in which a previous consent was obtained and where a question was not asked – and – one where a patient actively declined some options, for which re-consent is required.

Return of results to sharing partner institutions

14. Any agreement on sharing should regulate:

- Return of results significant for individuals that provided the bio-materials (the source institution remains responsible for that).
- Return of aggregated or other types of results to the source biobank/database.

Results from research may have a specific value for public health and individual health. Custodianship implies recognizing the role of research institutions and their legal and ethical duties to participants and patients. There is also agreement that aggregated research results should be disseminated to institutions and patients; regardless of the kind of policy of return of results adopted, these should be made explicit. Short reports should be provided by the research team to the data providers (institutions, biobanks) in order to ensure awareness of results relevant to their collections or to the donors. These reports may contain a publication list and relevant results important for further research developments or directly relevant to donors.

Intellectual property

15. The sharing of data and bio-resources must be done in a way that protects proprietary information and addresses the interests of institutions and third-party funders. These parties may have legitimate proprietary interests associated with data collected by researchers.

The intellectual investment of investigators involved in the creation and maintenance of data registries and bio-repositories is often substantial, and should be appropriately acknowledged.

MTA/DTA TEMPLATE
Mutual agreement between provider and recipient
Provider of data...
     Recipient of data... (This must be an institution officially registered by national/regional authorities.)
     MTA/DTA must be signed before any exchange takes place

1.   *Provider.* Provider...................................... hereby declares that:
     The (name country) .... from which the human biological material is collected has a legal and ethical framework providing a high level of quality, security and privacy protection concerning medical research involving human biological material; and that health data exchange is in accordance with local regulation (please note that some regulations, such as those from the EU, require compliance with their rules even if the research is conducted abroad).

     Data/bio-specimens provided consist of the following: .... (description including type of material and type of data: primary data and which type, genotypes, aggregate data, etc.)

     The bio-specimens provided refer to .... (no. of individuals) and are composed of ..... (no. of tubes and quantity of material referred to the scope).

     The material will be de-identified, stripped of all personally identifying information, without any direct means of identification. Bio-specimens will be double-coded (no direct identifier shall be on the tubes).

     To ensure the confidentiality and security of the associated data, transfer and processing will be handled safely and associated data will not be transported together with bio-specimens.

     To ensure traceability of the material to be de-identified, a code will be applied to the tubes. The mechanism to re-identify the data will remain with the provider.

     To ensure exchange and transport security, biosafety (packaging, labelling description of transport means and insurance for bio-specimens) will be observed.

     The project from which the data and bio-specimens were collected was approved by a local ethics committee or IRB.

     Informed consent for storage and distribution was obtained (enclose a copy of the model in use), and that:

- the informed consent contained the clause necessary for allowing bio-specimens and data sharing abroad (in case of an international project).
- the informed consent allowed the research described in the project description section.

2. *Recipient.* Recipient………………………………….. hereby declares that:

- the data will be used solely for the scope of the project described below, and no attempt will be made to sell the data/material or share it with a third party. The data/samples will be used for the following purpose: (description of the biomedical research project of the Recipient (or of the joint project): ………………………………….(aims should be clear, including the duration of the project…………………………..
- authorization from the local ethics review committee or IRB ……………………….(date and copy enclosed).
- when consented to, will ensure the return of results relevant to the health of individuals ……………….. and …………………… ……………………………………(description of the type of data that must be returned).
- will not harm the persons who provided bio-specimens by naming the provenience of the bio-specimens unless approved by the Provider.

3. *Terms and conditions (for Recipient).* Conditions of use include:

- no attempt to re-identify the participants
- adherence to use limitations stated in approved application
- no third-party data or sample sharing/selling without authorization from Provider
- primary data must not be patented
- that the use of the material has, for example, medical/public health objectives
- informing the resource of issues related to data integrity and/or the privacy of the participants as applicable
- compliance with original consents and applicable laws and institutional policies
- access granted for a limited time period (eg, 6 months or ……………), after which Recipient must reapply.

Documents to be provided by the recipient institution:

1. Authorization from a local ethics committee or a regional or local competent authority for the project for which the data are provided (by Recipient or, in the case of a joint project, by both parties).
2. Documents by the national data protection authority that reference the applicable laws that allow research using sensitive and health data, including genetic data.

4. *Receipt and handling of imported biological material.* The Recipient must document and follow the procedures for the receipt and proper storage of the type of biological material handled.

Provider has to prepare and ship the biological material in accordance with postal regulations, such as IATA (International Air Transport Association) and ADR (European Agreement on International Carriage of Dangerous Goods).

5. *Publication.* Prior review of publications before submission may be required (eg, to ensure the privacy/confidentiality of data and that the results will not cause stigmatization). Recipients should acknowledge the biobank/data provider in any publication/presentation (or other clauses).

6. *Is the material used to be returned or destroyed?* Recipient will comply with the destruction/return of unused bio-specimens and of data related to the bio-specimens at the end of the project or of the duration stated above

Description of the requirement (destruction/return)………… …………………………………..

7. *Intellectual property rights.* (Requires a specific agreement case by case. See general Introduction)……………………… ………………………………………………………………………… ………

8. *Who controls the data/bio-specimens in the resource?* Control of the bio-specimens remains with Provider, who can at any time demand the return or destruction of data and bio-specimens if a breach in the agreement occurs.

9. *Obligation to report.* Annual…………… (or other) and final reports to Provider are required. Reports should include ……………………………………………………………………… (specify required content).

10. *Responsibilities of the biobank/consortia.* Biobanks and research consortia have the right to terminate/alter this agreement with the researcher/institution, for the safety of the patients/participants or because of any infringements of the obligations stated in the present DTA/MTA. The Recipient understands and agrees that Provider does not bear any responsibility or accept any liability arising from the Recipient's use of the data or bio-specimens.

Time, place and signatures of the persons legally responsible for the institutions involved.

CONFLICT OF INTEREST
The authors declare no conflict of interest.

ACKNOWLEDGEMENTS
We thank the RD Connect Patient Ethics Council and RD Connect Patient Advisory Council (Jean Jacques Cassiman, Tracy Dudding, Muriel Gevrey, Emma Heslop, Joseph Irwin, Julian Isla, Sigurður Jóhannesson, Lydia Lemonnier, Chantal Loirat, Dorthe Lykke, Milan Macek, Caron Molster, Kay Parkinson, Odile Perrousseaux, Marita Pohlschmidt, Daniel Renault, Peter Reussner, Francoise Rouault, Balthasar Schaap, Inge Schwersenz, Chris Sotirelis, Volker Straub, Oliver Timmis, Johannes van Delden, Marieke van Meel, Elizabeth Vroom, Urban Wiesing) and all RD-connect partners for their valuable inputs. This work has been supported by the European Union Seventh Framework Programme (FP7/2007–2013) under grant agreements no. 305444 (RD-Connect), 305121 (Neuromics), and no. 305608 (EURenOmics) and RD Connect from the Australian National Health and Medical Research Council APP1055319 under the NHMRC-European Union Collaborative Research Grants scheme'. In addition, DM and MH have received funding from the Innovative Medicines Initiative project BTCure (grant agreement no. 115142-1), the BioBanking and Molecular Resource Infrastructure of Sweden project (financed by the Swedish Research Council), Euro-TEAM, BiobankCloud, BioSHaRE and Biobanking and Biomolecular Resources Research Infrastructure (BBMRI)LPC (313010). BMK and ESD wish to thank the Government of Canada through Genome Canada and the Canadian Institutes of Health Research, the Quebec Breast Cancer Foundation, and the Ministère de l'enseignement supérieur, de la recherche, de la science et de la technologie du Québec through Génome Québec. The funders had no influence on the design or the writing of the article.

1 Global Alliance White Paper. http://oicr.on.ca/oicr-programs-and-platforms/global-alliance/white-paper.
2 OECD principles and guidelines for access to research data from public funding. http://www.oecd.org/dataoecd/9/61/38500813.pdf.
3 Birney, Prepublication data sharing, Toronto International Data Release, *Nature* **461**: 168–170.
4 European Council (EC 2009/c 151/02) Council recommendation on an action in the field of rare Diseases 2009.
5 Knoppers BM, Chisholm M, Kaye J *et al*: A P3G generic access agreement for population genomic studies. *Nat Biotechnol* **31**: 384–385.
6 Ness RB. on behalf of the American College of Epidemiology Policy Committee: biospecimen "ownership": point. *Cancer Epidemiol Biomarkers Prev* 2007; **16**: 188–189.
7 Knoppers BM, Harris JR, Tassé AM, Budin-Ljøsne I, Kaye J, Deschênes M, Zawati MH: Towards a data sharing Code of Conduct for international genomic research. *Genome Med* 2011; **3**: 46.
8 Fortier I, Burton PR, Robson PJ *et al*: Quality, quantity and harmony: the DataSHaPER approach to integrating data across bioclinical studies. *Int J Epidemiol* 2010; 1–11.
9 O'Brien SJ: Stewardship of human bio-specimens, DNA, genotype, and clinical data in the GWAS era. *Annu Rev Genomics Hum Genet* 2009; **10**: 193–209.
10 McGuire A, Gibbs RA: No longer de-identified. *Science* 2006; **312**: 370–371.
11 Gymrek M *et al*: Identifying personal genomes by surname inference. *Science* 2013; **339**: 321.
12 Hansson MG, Gattorno M, Stjernschantz Forsberg J, Feltelius N, Martini A, Ruperto N: Ethics bureaucracy – a significant hurdle for collaborative follow-up of drug effectiveness in rare childhood diseases. *Arch Dis Childhood* 2012; **97**: 561–563.
13 Kaye J: Broad consent is informed consent. *BMJ* 2011; **343**.
14 Kaye J: From patients to partners: participant-centric initiatives in biomedical research. *Nat Rev Genet* 2012; **13**: 371–376.
15 Kaye J: The tension between data sharing and the protection of privacy in genomics research. *Annu Rev Genomics Hum Genet* 2012; **13**: 415–431.
16 Lunshof JE, Chadwick R, Vorhaus DB, Church GM: From genetic privacy to open consent. *Nat Rev Genet* 2008; **9**: 406–411.
17 Hansson MG, Dillner J, Bartram CR, Carlsson J, Helgesson G: Should donors be allowed to give broad consent to future biobank research? *Lancet Oncol* 2006; **7**: 266–269.
18 Caulfield T: Biobanks and blanket consent: the proper place of the public good and public perception rationales. *Kings Law J* 2007; **18**: 209–226.

19 Arnason V: Coding and consent: moral challenges of the database project in Iceland. *Bioethics* 2004; **18**: 27–49.
20 Mascalzoni D, Hicks A, Pramstaller P, Wjst M: Informed consent in the genomics era. *PLoS Med* 2008; **5**: e192.
21 Sheehan M, Martin J: Can broad consent be informed consent? *Public Health Ethics* 2011; **4**: 226–235.
22 Mascalzoni D, Paradiso A, Hansson M: Rare disease research: breaking the privacy barrier. *Appl Translational Genomics* 2014; **3**: 23–29.
23 Hoeyer K: Donors perceptions of consent to and feedback from biobank research: time to acknowledge diversity. *Public Health Genomics* 2010; **13**: 345–352.
24 Steinsbekk KS, Solberg B: Biobanks – when is re-consent necessary? *Public Health Ethics* 2011; **4**: 236–250.
25 Budin-Ljøsne I, Tassé AM, Knoppers BM, Harris JR: Bridging consent: from toll bridges to lift bridges? *BMC Med Genomics* 2011; **4**: 69.
26 Van Veen EB *et al*: TuBaFrost 3: regulatory and ethical issues on the exchange of residual tissue for research across Europe. *Eur J Cancer* 2006; **42**: 2914–2923.
27 Kaijser M: Examples from Swedish biobank research; in: Levin M, Hansson MG (eds.): *Biobanks as Resources for Health*. Uppsala: Uppsala University, 2003, pp 33–50, may be downloaded at www.crb.uu.se.
28 Helgesson G, Dillner J, Carlsson J, Bartram CR, Hansson MG: Ethical framework for previously collected biobank samples. *Nat Biotech* 2007; **25**: 973–975.
29 Shamoo AE, Resnik DB: *Responsible Conduct of Research*. 2nd edn. New York: Oxford University Press, 2009.
30 Hansson MG, Simonsson B, Feltelius N, Stjernschantz Forsberg J, Hasford J: Medical registries represent vital patient interests and should not be dismantled by stricter regulation. *Cancer Epidemiol* 2012; **36**: 575–578.
31 Hansson MG: Ethics and biobanks. *Br J Cancer* 2009; **100**: 8–12.

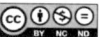

12.3 Facilitating a Culture of Responsible and Effective Sharing of Cancer Genome Data

Lillian L. Siu, Mark Lawler, David Haussler, Bartha Maria Knoppers, Jeremy Lewin, Daniel J. Vis, Rachel G. Liao, Fabrice Andre, Ian Banks, J. Carl Barrett, Carlos Caldas, Anamaria Aranha Camargo, Rebecca C. Fitzgerald, Mao Mao, John E. Mattison, William Pao, William R. Sellers, Patrick Sullivan, Bin Tean Teh, Robyn L. Ward, Jean Claude ZenKlusen, Charles L. Sawyers, and Emile E. Voest

Siu, L, et al. Facilitating a culture of responsible and effective sharing of cancer genome data. *Nature Medicine* 22(5), 464-471 (2016). An imprint of Springer Nature.

PERSPECTIVE

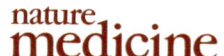

Facilitating a culture of responsible and effective sharing of cancer genome data

Lillian L Siu[1,21], Mark Lawler[2,21], David Haussler[3], Bartha Maria Knoppers[4], Jeremy Lewin[1], Daniel J Vis[5], Rachel G Liao[6], Fabrice Andre[7], Ian Banks[8], J Carl Barrett[9], Carlos Caldas[10], Anamaria Aranha Camargo[11], Rebecca C Fitzgerald[10], Mao Mao[12], John E Mattison[13], William Pao[14], William R Sellers[15], Patrick Sullivan[16], Bin Tean Teh[17], Robyn L Ward[18], Jean Claude ZenKlusen[19], Charles L Sawyers[20] & Emile E Voest[5]

Rapid and affordable tumor molecular profiling has led to an explosion of clinical and genomic data poised to enhance the diagnosis, prognostication and treatment of cancer. A critical point has now been reached at which the analysis and storage of annotated clinical and genomic information in unconnected silos will stall the advancement of precision cancer care. Information systems must be harmonized to overcome the multiple technical and logistical barriers to data sharing. Against this backdrop, the Global Alliance for Genomic Health (GA4GH) was established in 2013 to create a common framework that enables responsible, voluntary and secure sharing of clinical and genomic data. This Perspective from the GA4GH Clinical Working Group Cancer Task Team highlights the data-aggregation challenges faced by the field, suggests potential collaborative solutions and describes how GA4GH can catalyze a harmonized data-sharing culture.

There is broad consensus that the identification of aberrations in tumor DNA is key not only to achieving a better understanding of cancer but also to developing an improved process for selecting patients

[1]Princess Margaret Cancer Centre, University of Toronto, Toronto, Canada. [2]Centre for Cancer Research and Cell Biology, Queen's University, Belfast, UK. [3]UC Santa Cruz Genomics Institute, University of California, Santa Cruz, California, USA. [4]Centre of Genomics and Policy, McGill University, Montreal, Canada. [5]The Netherlands Cancer Institute, Amsterdam, the Netherlands. [6]The Global Alliance for Genomics and Health, Toronto, Canada. [7]Gustave Roussy and Université Paris Sud, Villejuif, France. [8]Patient's Advocacy Committee, European Cancer Organization, Brussels, Belgium. [9]Translational Sciences, Oncology iMED, AstraZeneca, Waltham, Massachusetts, USA. [10]Department of Oncology, University of Cambridge, Cambridge, UK. [11]Hospital Sírio-Libanês, São Paulo, Brazil. [12]Yonsei Cancer Research Institute, Yonsei University College of Medicine, Seoul, Korea. [13]Kaiser Permanente, Pasadena, California, USA. [14]Roche Innovation Center Basel, Pharma Research and Early Development, Roche, Basel, Switzerland. [15]Novartis Institutes for Biomedical Research, Cambridge, Massachusetts, USA. [16]Advocacy for Canadian Children Oncology Network, Vancouver, Canada. [17]National Cancer Centre Singapore, Singapore. [18]University of Queensland, St. Lucia, Australia. [19]The Cancer Genome Atlas, National Cancer Institute, National Institutes of Health, Bethesda, Maryland, USA. [20]Memorial Sloan Kettering Cancer Center, New York, New York, USA. [21]These authors contributed equally to this work. Correspondence should be addressed to M.L. (mark.lawler@qub.ac.uk).

Received 21 November 2015; accepted 21 March 2016; published online 5 May 2016; doi:10.1038/nm.4089

for specific treatments. The latter is embraced by patients and their oncologists for the promise it holds of improving therapeutic outcomes through precision medicine, and by payers and governments because of its potential to reduce healthcare costs. Several governments and government-sponsored initiatives have recognized that linking and sharing clinical information and genomic knowledge are key requisites for delivering twenty-first-century cancer care (https://www.whitehouse.gov/blog/2015/01/20/watch-president-obamas-2015-state-union), including the recently announced "moonshot" effort to cure cancer, endorsed by US President Obama[1]. Examples of initiatives with a clinico-genomic data-sharing aspiration include the US-based Precision Medicine Initiative and the UK's 100,000 Genomes Project, both of which have cancer as a major focus of their activities[2,3]. The goal of these and of other projects is to show how a genomically informed understanding of diseases such as cancer can transform patient care.

To this end, many institutions worldwide have developed cancer-molecular-profiling initiatives to identify relevant biological drivers and to use this information to inform biomarker-guided clinical trials. These initiatives, coupled with the increased utility of next-generation sequencing (NGS), compared to conventional sequencing approaches, and its ever-decreasing costs, have fueled an unprecedented expansion of genomic data generated from people with cancer. However, these efforts typically either occur at an institutional level or are compartmentalized within disease-specific activities[4,5]. The analysis and storage of annotated genomic data in such isolated "silos" prevents collective data curation and data sharing, which makes the analysis of phenotype–genotype relationships prone to inconsistent interpretation—especially for low-frequency variants—owing to the use of different bioinformatics algorithms. A global unified approach is required to maximize our ability to recognize biological patterns between groups of patients, whose information may reside currently in different databases or institutions, and to use this knowledge to drive preventive or therapeutic interventions. The benefits afforded by data aggregation are substantial, and they would address a number of scenarios that the cancer community encounters (**Box 1**).

The sharing of aggregated data has thus become a substantial rate-limiting step in the development of cancer-prevention and treatment strategies. This not only has implications for patient populations with uncommon histologies or rare phenotypes, but is also increasingly relevant for cancer treatment in general, given a rise in the molecular

Box 1 Hypothetical examples illustrating importance of data sharing

Hypothetical examples

1. A group from country A employed a targeted panel to assess a selected set of hot-spot mutations in 50 genes and published these results on the basis of an analysis of 1,000 patients with colorectal cancer. A group in country B, capable of performing whole-exome sequencing, has identified that one of these hot spots, in the presence of another specific mutation, may adversely affect clinical outcome in colorectal cancer. To confirm their hypothesis, the country B group would like to collaborate with the group in country A to determine whether remaining DNA samples and clinical data can be shared.
2. A research group from country A reported favorably on a variant in gene X that may predict response for drug Y. Their findings indicated that the variant is significantly associated with progression-free survival at 6 months after the initiation of treatment. A group from country B investigated the same gene variant for the same drug, but found no statistical relationship at 3 months and 24 months after treatment initiation. A research group from country C now wants to perform a meta-analysis to determine whether the findings of both trials are in agreement, but it requires the original and individualized clinical and genomic data from the groups in countries A and B.
3. Two large studies have recently been published suggesting that the use of drug Z may confer a better prognosis in breast cancer among patients who have a common somatic variant. There are many large oncology practices worldwide that capture the use of drug Z in their patients' EHRs. Can this information be collected and integrated to provide a reliable validation of this finding?
4. One of 500 patients in a clinical trial in country A responded to drug X, and this patient's tumor is known to harbor a rare germline variant. A large institution in country B is currently considering running a similar trial for the same drug. The sharing of the details of such incidental findings would have an important bearing on the new trial.

stratification of individuals with common malignancies into smaller groups to tailor their treatment, either through drug repurposing or by using innovative precision-medicine protocols.

Although the importance of open access to genomic information is clearly recognized[6–9], multiple technical and logistical barriers for effective data sharing persist, including data noncomparability, coding heterogeneity, difficulties in the storage and transfer of large data sets and nonstandardized bioinformatics analyses. Additionally, regulatory, legal and ethical processes are not designed for global data sharing and thus require urgent attention.

In the face of this fragmented landscape, the GA4GH was established in 2013 with a vision to promote the responsible and effective sharing of genomic and clinical data and to transfer the benefits of this "team science" approach directly to patients (**Box 2**). In this Perspective, we highlight the challenges that a global clinical and genomic data-sharing approach presents, suggest potential solutions and highlight key initiatives (some of which are sponsored by GA4GH) to foster these activities in the molecular-profiling landscape (**Table 1**).

Challenges in data sharing

In recognition of the urgent need to generate and maximize the value of high-throughput molecular data in cancer research, international efforts such as The Cancer Genome Atlas (TCGA)[10] and the International Cancer Genome Consortium (ICGC)[11] were established to unify genomics-driven research efforts. Although these initiatives were groundbreaking and laid the foundation for future opportunities, the utility of data sharing can only be maximized once its scope is extended beyond information derived solely from tumor samples collected at a single time point and without clinical correlates (as was the case with initiatives such as TCGA and ICGC). Ideally, attendant clinical data would include a longitudinal series of samples with detailed clinical, genomic and pathological information[12]. The analysis of a single tumor sample per patient can cause researchers to inadvertently ignore the phenomena of tumor heterogeneity and clonal evolution, and it obscures the dynamics of disease progression at both the clinical and molecular levels[13]. In most cases, longitudinal data, including clinical co-morbidities, and the effects of different medications and environmental exposures, are required for a granular assessment that enables the identification of correlates for favorable or poor clinical outcome, and of patient-specific *de novo* resistance

mechanisms under treatment pressure. However, longitudinal data with detailed clinical and pathological information are more difficult to harmonize and share between institutions.

Clinical data: challenges and potential solutions

The data in most electronic health-record (EHR) systems are not vetted for quality assurance and are not structured in a way that readily enables easy extraction. These problems are magnified when we attempt to extract and compare data across institutions, and they become substantial barriers to cross-border data-sharing initiatives.

In contrast to rare diseases, for which initiatives such as Human Phenotype Ontology[14,15], PhenoTips[16] and PhenoDB[17] have underpinned the development of a standardized human-phenotypic ontology, the cancer field lacks a universally accepted lexicon. Tools such as the PheWAS (developed from the Vanderbilt-led Phenome-Wide Association Study) were developed to facilitate unbiased interrogation of the EHR to detect associations between a specific genetic variant and a wide range of clinical outcomes and phenotypes[18]. Although the PheWAS and similar tools have been applied thus far

Box 2 Description of GA4GH

GA4GH is a not-for-profit worldwide alliance of more than 380 international stakeholders from 38 countries, with a current focus on rare diseases and cancer[30] and an emerging interest in infectious disease. GA4GH operates through a series of Working Groups (WG): Data WG, Regulatory and Ethics WG, Security WG and Clinical WG, which develop initiatives, policies, recommendations and application–program interfaces (APIs) that promote and harmonize responsible and effective data sharing. Although GA4GH produces recommendations, it does not seek to enforce data standards, but rather to persuade potential stakeholders of the added value of a collaborative data-sharing culture. The first plenary meeting of GA4GH stakeholders took place in March 2014 at the Wellcome Trust in London, UK, with subsequent conferences in San Diego, California, USA, and Leiden, the Netherlands. This Perspective was undertaken after discussions during the third GA4GH plenary meeting in Leiden, and in response to a number of international data-sharing initiatives (including the recently launched AACR's transatlantic data-sharing project GENIE[68]).

PERSPECTIVE

Table 1 Key cancer-molecular-profiling and big-data initiatives, including GA4GH-enabled initiatives

Examples of initiatives	Description[a]	How is this initiative enabling data sharing?
National and international molecular-screening platforms		
SPECTA (screening patients for efficient clinical trial access)[64]	SPECTA represents a pan-European collaboration that involves more than 40 clinical centers in 16 European countries, which had an initial focus on colorectal cancer but is now expanding to various other tumor types.	• Molecular-screening platform that matches patients' genomic profiles to potential clinical trials
Precision-medicine clinical trials		
National Cancer Institute's Molecular Analysis for Therapy Choice (NCI–MATCH)[65]	A complex basket trial evaluating a new or existing agent against a specific molecular aberration across tumor types. NCI–MATCH will be available at more than 2,400 clinical sites across the US.	• Enables sharing of clinical and genomic data to facilitate access to innovative targeted therapies
Targeted Agent and Profiling Utilization Registry (TAPUR)[66] and Drug Rediscovery Protocol (DRUP)	In these two trials, genomic analysis identifies a particular abnormality that allows patients access to a molecularly targeted agent already shown to be effective against this "actionable" mutation in at least one cancer.	• Intercontinental, parallel data-sharing approach to facilitate patient access to "approved" treatments
Big-data initiatives		
The Cancer Genome Atlas (TCGA)[10]	An NCI–NHGRI collaboration that has generated comprehensive catalogs of the key genomic changes in major types and subtypes of cancer.	• Supports open access to genomic data
International Cancer Genome Consortium (ICGC)[11] and *ICGCMed*[b]	A consortium created to coordinate large-scale, comprehensive molecular characterization of 50 different tumor types and/or subtypes. *ICGCMed* is the next generation project of ICGC, with a stated aim to link genomic data with longitudinal clinical data.	• Supports open access to data • Links genomic and clinical data/outcomes (*ICGCMed*)
Cancer Core Europe (CCE)[67]	A consortium of six European cancer centers that share a common translational genomic platform to conduct next-generation clinical trials.	• Establishes a European virtual e-cancer hospital
100,000 Genomes Project[3]	A project supported by Genomics England to sequence 100,000 whole genomes, with a focus on rare diseases, cancer and infectious diseases.	• Enables sharing of clinical and WGS data for clinical actionability
CancerLinQ[20]	An ASCO-led initiative to create a data-informatics system that will collect, analyze and learn from complete EHRs, with the primary goal of improving the quality of care provided to people with cancer.	• Enables sharing of clinical and genomic data • Addresses data security and access issues
The Cancer Genome Collaboratory	A Canadian NSERC, Genome Canada and CIHR-supported initiative to make ICGC data available for cloud computing in a community cloud infrastructure (http://www.genomecanada.ca/en/cancer-genome-collaboratory).	• Enables sharing of clinical and genomic or NGS data • Co-locates compute with big data sets
Genomics Evidence Neoplasia Information Exchange (GENIE)[68]	An AACR-enabled transatlantic initiative to integrate genomic profiles and longitudinal clinical outcomes at seven different cancer centers in the US, Canada and Europe.	• Enables sharing of clinical and genomic or NGS data • Addresses data security and access issues
GA4GH-enabled data-sharing initiatives		
BRCA challenge[b]	A global initiative to pool data on *BRCA1/2* genetic variants and corresponding clinical data (http://www.genomicsandhealth.org/work-products-demonstrati on-projects/brca-challenge-0).	• Creates a curated catalog, *BRCA* Exchange
Beacon Project[b]	A simple, online web service that allows users to query an institution's databases to determine whether they contain a genetic variant of interest (http://www.genomicsandhealth.org/work-products-demonstration-projects/beacon-project-0).	• Enables sharing of genetic data
Matchmaker Exchange[b]	A collaborative effort to facilitate the matching of cases with similar phenotypic and genotypic profiles through standardized APIs (http://www.genomicsandhealth.org/work-products-demonstration-projects/matchmaker-exchange-0).	• Establishes federated platforms through standardized APIs
Other data sharing or harmonization initiatives		
BD2K (big data to knowledge)[26,b]	A trans-NIH program to support the development of innovative approaches and tools to maximize and accelerate the integration of data science into biomedical research.	• Develops new methods and standards for sharing genomic information
Electronic Medical Records and Genomics (eMERGE)[19]	A national network that combines DNA biorepositories with EHR systems for large-scale, high-throughput genetic research.	• Finds solution to link EHR data to genomic data
Genome Data Commons (GDC)	An interactive knowledge system to store, analyze and distribute cancer-genomics data generated by NCI and other research organizations (http://www.cancer.gov/news-events/press-releases/2014/GenomicDataCommonsNewsNote).	• Enables sharing of clinical and genomic data • Finds solution to data warehousing
Helix Nebular Project	A European partnership between information-technology providers and research centers that aims to develop a science cloud to meet the growing demand for computing power (http://www.helix-nebula.eu).	• Enables sharing of clinical and genomic data through cloud computing
Health Level 7 International (HL7) and fast healthcare interoperability resources (FHIR)	An international collaboration dedicated to providing frameworks and standards for the exchange, sharing and integration of electronic health information (http://www.hl7.org/fhir/).	• Develops standards for sharing EHR data
ICGC–TCGA dialogue for reverse-engineering assessments and methods (DREAM)[28,b]	An international effort to improve standard methods for identifying cancer-associated mutations and rearrangements in WGS data.	• Standardizes WGS and bioinformatics algorithms • Identifies best pipelines for harmonizing mutation calling

[a]Description of each initiative is adapted from its related publication or website. AACR, American Association for Cancer Research; API, application programming interface; ASCO, American Society of Clinical Oncology; CIHR, Canadian Institutes of Health Research; EHR, electronic health record; EORTC, European Organisation for Research and Treatment of Cancer; GA4GH, Global Alliance for Genomics and Health; NCI, National Cancer Institute; NGS, next-generation sequencing; NHGRI, National Human Genome Research Institute; NIH, US National Institutes of Health; NSERC, Natural Sciences and Engineering Research; WG, Working Group; WGS, whole-genome sequencing. [b]Collaborations with GA4GH.

mainly to germline genetic diseases, as in initiatives conducted by the Electronic Medical Records and Genomics (eMERGE) Network[19], they could potentially support similar approaches in somatic diseases such as cancer.

The tracking of longitudinal clinical outcomes is crucial to linking clinical and molecular data for prognostic or predictive relevance; however, efficacy outcomes (such as objective responses and time to disease progression based on validated criteria, and overall survival) and toxicity information (as classified by the National Cancer Institute (NCI) common terminology criteria for adverse events (CTCAE) are not routinely captured in patient EHRs outside the context of clinical trials.

Solutions to these clinical-data challenges are at a less mature stage than are the solutions for genomic data, but they are developing. Standards are emerging for how to represent data from EHRs in a way that can be shared between institutions. Leading among these is the international fast healthcare interoperability resources effort (FHIR) (http://www.hl7.org/fhir/), which is being developed in conjunction with the Health Level 7 International (HL7) infrastructure. Technical tools are now emerging that use standards such as the FHIR to federate data from EHRs in a functional way that can perform aggregation, cleaning and parsing of data longitudinally over time and from multiple disparate sources. It is crucial that in such activities, the quality of the merged data is assured and controlled. A key example of such an effort is CancerLinQ[20], a system that the American Society of Clinical Oncology (ASCO) is custom-building to gather data through direct electronic feeds from numerous oncology practices. CancerLinQ aims to measure, monitor and learn through the analysis of pooled information to improve the quality of cancer care and to provide clinical-decision support.

The tools described above require well-developed and widely accepted ontologies or vocabularies to standardize the classification of diseases; examples of these include the International Classification of Diseases (ICD) (http://www.who.int/classifications/icd/en/) and the Systematized Nomenclature of Medicine Clinical Terms (SNOMED CT) (http://www.nlm.nih.gov/snomed/). In an effort to resolve the lack of standardized phenotypic-variation descriptors in malignancy, particularly in the genomic era, a task team of the GA4GH Clinical Working Group is developing approaches to support the alignment of and mapping across ontologies in cancer by leveraging specialist resources, such as those provided by the National Cancer Institute Thesaurus[21] and the Human Phenotype Ontology[14,15].

Genomic data: challenges and potential solutions

Genomic-data sharing in cancer research has been successful within large consortia such as TCGA and the ICGC. Databases such as the Cancer Genomics Hub (CGHub), the European Genome–Phenome Archive, and the ICGC data portal provide cancer genomics data to researchers at a rate of multiple petabytes per month—representing the largest exchange of genomic information in any area of research[22]. New databases, such as the Genome Data Commons (GDC) of the NCI (USA) (created as part of the development of a Precision Cancer Medicine knowledge system; http://www.cancer.gov/news-events/press-releases/2014/GenomicDataCommonsNewsNote) and the 100,000 Genomes Project (UK)[3], are being constructed. However, these systems are not designed to handle data generated on a scale of millions of samples, as is anticipated with widespread clinical application of NGS. This is an entirely new data-engineering challenge.

Most cancer-genomics data generated by clinical applications are held separately in silos by different medical institutions or by their

contractors. This makes aggregated data analysis more difficult. Because the data sets are large, now consisting of multiple petabytes (10^{15} bytes), a simple transmission of genome-sequencing data between geographically remote repositories is increasingly infeasible.

The aggregation problem is made more difficult by substantial heterogeneity in the procedures for data collection, storage and representation. Problems of data size can be overcome by sharing only the mutation and gene-expression information from the clinical samples, and not the raw data produced by sequencing machines. However, a lack of consensus in the mutation-calling process, in the methods for gene-expression quantification and even in the data formats used to express this information is hampering current aggregation efforts. Nonstandardized *ad hoc* functional annotation and a lack of consensus between institutions on the clinical importance of genomic variants further limit the universal applicability of NGS data for guiding improvements in patient care[8]. In particular, there are no widely accepted definitions of driver mutations in cancer and "clinically actionable" results[23,24]. This represents a serious barrier to the integration of clinical genomics into healthcare delivery.

Solutions presented by the GA4GH

In response to these diverse challenges, collaborative efforts, including GA4GH-enabled initiatives, have proposed[25] and/or are implementing multiple solutions. Recognizing the need to link diverse genomic-data repositories, the GA4GH Data Working Group, in collaboration with initiatives such as the US National Institutes of Health (NIH) Big Data to Knowledge (BD2K) Center in Translational Genomics[26], are pioneering new standards and methods for sharing genomic information. They are developing a universal application-programming interface (API) that will facilitate the creation of a global, cohesive genome-informatics ecosystem, which would maximize data sharing at scale. Specific task teams within the GA4GH Data Working Group are implementing particular functionalities in the GA4GH API to enable expressive and universal representation of genetic variation; gene and transcript expression; annotation of genomics features; and relationships between genotype and phenotype.

Furthermore, to facilitate the harmonization of mutation-calling procedures among institutions, the ICGC and TCGA invited the cancer-genomics and bioinformatics communities to work together to identify the best pipelines for the detection of mutations in DNA-sequencing reads for cancer genomes[27]. This has led to the establishment of the ICGC–TCGA dialogue for reverse-engineering assessments and methods (DREAM) somatic mutation calling challenge ('the SMC–DNA meta-pipeline challenge'), a crowd-sourced benchmark of somatic-mutation detection algorithms[28]. The Benchmarking Task Team of the GA4GH Data Working Group is working closely with the DREAM teams to identify the most effective algorithms for widespread use by the scientific and clinical community. The need to identify and share the best data-analysis pipelines has also stimulated considerable work on so-called containerized computation in genomics. In this approach, the development of code that executes different programs for data processing, analysis and interpretation facilitates easier exchange between different institutions and different computing environments than was previously possible. This would be analogous to the strategy used by the company Docker, in which shipping containers across the world's ports are standardized so that one set of machinery is sufficient at any port to handle any shipping container. In containerized computing, one type of packaging for data and programs enables analysis of the data on all computing systems. The Containers and Workflows Task Team of

PERSPECTIVE

the GA4GH Working Group is devoted to this area. Furthermore, containerized code that has been battle-tested in the DREAM challenges and by large consortium efforts is now being applied to clinical NGS analysis in cancer—a strategy proposed by groups such as the next-generation sequencing standardization of clinical testing (Nex-StoCT) II informatics work group for the analysis of germline variations in disease[29].

With regard to the lack of consensus on what constitutes an "actionable" mutation, GA4GH is driving the Actionable Cancer Genome Initiative (ACGI)[30]. The main goals of the ACGI are to identify a list of "actionable" genes in different cancers with canonical targetable mutations, as well as rare variants of uncertain importance, and to aggregate data related to these aberrations—their evidence-based curated actionability calls and phenotypic or clinical information (including longitudinal data)—in a searchable format to enhance patient care.

Data-warehousing and data-access challenges
One question that members of the GA4GH have considered in detail is whether the world's genomic and clinical information will reside in a single physical database, or whether it will be made available through a federated network that spans a series of interlinked data repositories in many countries. Although both approaches have their supporters, GA4GH is investigating how a federated model (which may involve a relatively small number of large databases) could be organized to fulfill data-warehousing requirements, while supporting improved data access for data consumers. In a federated system, some data are likely to be on commercial clouds (for example, Amazon, Google, Microsoft or one of the 30 cloud providers in the Helix Nebula Marketplace associated with Europe's Helix Nebula Project; http://www.helix-nebula. eu/) and the rest on government clouds, private clouds or other dedicated systems. The recent decision by the NIH to allow private and commercial cloud-computing solutions to be applied to the storage and analysis of the vast genomic data that is housed in its repository— the database of Genotypes and Phenotypes (dbGaP)[31]—is timely. It opens up competition between different cloud solutions in genomics. The creation of a competitive market for such cloud solutions will enable secure and organized data storage at low cost, with sufficient elasticity to provide a dynamic platform that ensures rapid and efficient analysis of large data sets[32] (http://www.genomicsandhealth. org/working-groups/our-work/cloud-security).

Optimized, interoperable technical standards are needed for the analysis of data that are distributed across multiple sites, as suggested above. Beyond the data-harmonization challenges, there are also substantial technical challenges to ensuring coordinated version control; data uniqueness and integrity; location transparency; harmony and efficiency in access procedures; privacy and security requirements; and to maintaining compliance with institutional and legal regulations at the regional, national and international levels.

Furthermore, in conjunction with the GA4GH's API-based standardization efforts (as well as its file-based standards efforts), the Containers and Workflows Task Team of the GA4GH's Data Working Group is developing mechanisms that will allow a computational procedure to be ported to different institutions, where it can be run locally with reliably consistent results and minimal customization required. This allows a single institution to perform complex analysis of large data sets at remote sites. On the other hand, when only smaller data items are needed from a remote site, these can be obtained with a simple Internet query, again by using the API. A mechanism for queries of this type is in development by the GA4GH Beacon Project (http://www.genomicsandhealth.org/

work-products-demonstration-projects/beacon-project-0) (**Table 1**). Having a range of solutions such as these to data-aggregation and analysis problems is critical to the success of a federated system.

Ethical, regulatory and security challenges
Even if technical challenges are addressed, global data sharing will require a marked shift in the conventional ethics framework, especially given diversity in countries' legal and regulatory requirements. We may have reached the limits of applying current informed-consent procedures with an increased data-sharing culture that is posing new consent-related challenges (**Box 3**). Broad consent is a practical, overarching solution, although this practice can be contentious if it is not accompanied by proper governance[33]. Because informed consent is usually conducted as a once-off task, respect for individual autonomy demands ongoing oversight to respect the trust of participants who give researchers the right to use their data and samples for "future unspecified research." To ease these concerns, new variations of consent documents have been proposed (for example, tiered or dynamic consent and open consent)[33–37], and novel governance models have been suggested[38]. It is important that the consent model chosen correspond to the nature of the study. Thus, broad consent is particularly suited for longitudinal studies (for example, UK Biobank; http://www. ukbiobank.ac.uk/), and open consent for those who wish to put their genome data in the public domain (for example, Personal Genome Project; http://www.personalgenomes.org/).

However, challenges to the development of consent procedures remain. For example, it is not possible to implement the rights of the individual to withdraw their archived data in an international study if data are anonymized[39]. In addition, it is even more challenging to protect participants' privacy, given the unique identifying

---

Box 3 Consent models for biomedical research

In all situations indicated below, the principles of respect for the individual 'data donor' and ethically responsible data sharing are implicit to the process.

Specific consent
In this situation, consent is limited to data generated from a particular research protocol, applied for a specific disease type.

Specific and "related conditions" consent
This consent process adds the possibility for the consent for use of research data to be extended to other, related disease domains.

Tiered consent
Here a series of options is provided, with the research participant being able to indicate consent for one, some or all of the options indicated.

Dynamic consent
This is a continuous consent process, with the opportunity for the participant to indicate their consent (or lack of consent) for their data to be used in an evolving series of research studies that develops over time from the original research protocol.

Broad consent
This indicates consent for future unspecified research studies, whose ethical principles are ensured through oversight from an independent research-ethics committee.

Open consent
For an open consent model, all future biomedical research is indicated, with resulting research data becoming accessible to other researchers.

PERSPECTIVE

nature of genetic information[40–43]. Germline data collection (whether preplanned or incidentally detected) increases the complexity, if researchers have promised to re-contact individuals to notify them particularly if new genetic findings come to light after original use. Further complicating matters, conventional national or institutional review boards may not have the expertise to assess the risks and compliance regulations that are associated with international data-sharing projects, and current oversight systems are, in many cases, not adequately equipped for privacy breaches[44].

The GA4GH has approached these complex issues from a fundamental human-rights perspective, by proposing and adopting a Framework for Responsible Sharing of Genomic and Health-Related Data that emphasizes both the rights of all citizens to benefit from the advances of science and the rights of scientists to be recognized for their work[45]. This approach is complementary to and bolsters conventional bioethics principles, but employing a legal human-rights perspective embeds responsible clinico-genomic data sharing within a recognized and endorsed international legal framework. The approach thus provides an environment in which the ethics principles espoused by this Framework can be recognized and adhered to by all stakeholders. This Framework can also foster responsible data sharing more strongly than a conventional bioethics approach by offering legal protection in several areas, such as privacy; anti-discrimination and fair access; and procedural fairness[44].

It will require an ethics and regulatory framework that fosters cross-border, collaborative, open data sharing to address the complex issues highlighted above. Given the substantial legal and ethical variations between different countries and/or jurisdictions, there is an urgent need for harmonization. To that end, the implementation of the GA4GH Framework[46] will enable responsible data sharing, while still respecting individual rights. The adoption of and adherence to the following GA4GH-enabled principles, policies and tools within

the Framework will provide a blueprint for addressing the complex ethical, legal and security issues outlined.

As an overarching enabler of the activities and human-rights aspirations outlined above, the GA4GH Framework underpins all aspects of its genomic and clinical data-sharing activities going forward. As part of this framework, the GA4GH Regulatory and Ethics Working Group produced a 'GA4GH Consent Policy'[47], which balances the need to respect the autonomous decision-making rights of each individual patient with the promotion of the common good of international genomic and health-related data sharing. Three consent tools[48] have been created for GA4GH by the Public Population Project in Genomics and Society–International Policy interoperability and data Access Clearinghouse (P3G–IPAC; http://www.p3g.org/ipac): (i) *Legacy Consent and International Data Sharing*: This allows researchers to address the adequacy of previously collected "legacy" consents (consents taken at the time of the study that may not have envisaged the complexity of future scientific use(s) of samples or data). (ii) *Clauses for International Data Sharing*: This provides advice and templates for researchers who wish to add clauses or addenda on international data sharing to their existing consent document(s). (iii) *Generic International Data Sharing Prospective Consent Form*: This provides an adaptable consent template for international data sharing for prospective studies.

GA4GH's Regulatory and Ethics Working Group has prepared a 'Privacy and Security Policy'[49] that requires a proportionate approach, which involves weighing the real risks and benefits, as well as a concordance of terms such as pseudonymized; de-identified; coded, etc., to address the "Babel" of nomenclature[50]. GA4GH's Regulatory and Ethics Working Group has also published a "safe harbor" mechanism for privacy protection[44] in cross-border sharing, which elucidates the criteria for mutually agreed-upon data-protection principles[25]. To specifically address privacy and security mechanisms, the GA4GH

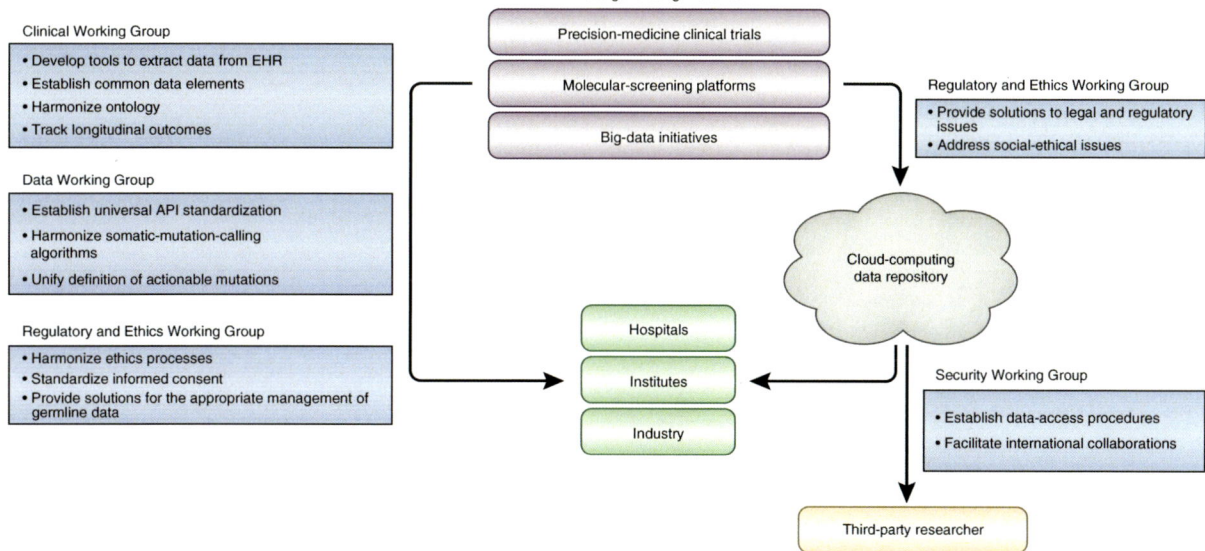

Figure 1 Data-sharing vision as facilitated by GA4GH through its working groups, each of which focuses on particular data-sharing challenges: for example, Clinical Working Group, establish common data elements; Data Working Group, establish universal API standardization; Regulatory and Ethics Working Group, harmonize ethics processes; Security Working Group, establish data-access procedures. GA4GH provides guidance to facilitate responsible, effective and secure data sharing. Groups such as hospitals, institutes and pharmaceutical companies that are conducting data-generating initiatives are encouraged to share clinical and genomic information under the framework developed by GA4GH, including collaborations with third-party researchers via robust access procedures.

PERSPECTIVE

Security Working Group has created a *Security Infrastructure Policy Paper*[51] that documents the standards and implementation practices for protecting the privacy and security of shared genomic and clinical data. For cases in which the data are highly phenotypic—that is, there are sufficient data elements that, either alone or in combination with other information, could serve to re-identify an individual—a form of a controlled-access approach may be the most appropriate, such as the one used by the Data Access Compliance Office in the ICGC[7]. GA4GH is, however, considering the potential of a registered system of access for less-sensitive data as an intermediary tier between closed and open access.

It is also extremely important to ensure ethics compliance and responsible conduct by researchers. To this end, the GA4GH's Regulatory and Ethics Working Group has developed an accountability policy[52]. Additionally, the ethical standards associated with the commercial usage and sale of aggregated, anonymized data are unclear and will require consideration. In addition, it is crucial to educate the cancer community at large to ensure the responsible use and sharing of clinical and genomic information[53].

Concluding remarks

The development of responsible and effective practices for sharing genomic and clinical data that are generated from biospecimens is increasingly important for patients (including those who have cancer), as it enables research discoveries to be applied rapidly for their benefit. Patients are actively pursuing approaches that ensure their rights to share information for the overall benefit of citizens and societies[54,55]. A European survey conducted in 2012 of 811 individuals with cancer revealed that more than 91% of patients wanted their samples to be retained for future research, and a substantial number of them also indicated that they would participate in biomarker testing to enable personalization of their treatment[56]. More recently, a survey of 100 people with breast cancer indicated that more than 75% of them would share de-identified data with researchers not involved in their care, and that 60% of patients were additionally prepared to share identified data[57]. As a follow up to these studies, the GA4GH is collaborating with a number of institutions and prominent patient-advocacy groups to develop a survey to measure the specific attitudes of individuals with cancer to the sharing of genomic and/or clinical data.

Patients with cancer are emphasizing that they no longer want to be passive recipients but are increasingly active participants in both high-quality research and its clinical adoption; these principles are enshrined in the European Cancer Patients Bill of Rights[58,59], which was launched in the European Parliament on World Cancer Day 2014. Substantial challenges in relation to the privacy of data exist, particularly in Europe, in the context of both the Clinical Trials Directive (http://www.ec.europa.eu/health/human-use/clinical-trials/directive/index_en.htm) and the recently approved General Data Protection Regulation[60]. However, patients are increasingly recognizing the value of genomics research, its clinical translation[61] and the need for responsible data sharing[62]. That said, issues such as discrimination must be addressed adequately and with clear patient education and input[62,63], not only in terms of their access to optimal-quality care (including precision cancer care) but also in relation to socio-economic factors such as employment rights and the availability of affordable insurance; without such attention, their enthusiasm for participating in genomics research and for acting as advocates for responsible data sharing may waver. Individuals with cancer generally have a positive attitude to sharing their data (http://www.free-the-data.org/);

we need to ensure that data sharing happens in a timely, responsible and effective manner, so that its value in improving health care can be realized as rapidly as possible.

The GA4GH is committed to engaging with key stakeholders, including researchers, healthcare professionals and patients with cancer, to establish a globally effective genomic and clinical data-sharing ecosystem that addresses the diverse challenges that we have articulated in this Perspective (**Fig. 1**). GA4GH's success in fostering "a coalition of the willing" within the international community, in combination with its ability to develop and implement technical informatics solutions within a harmonized and secure ethical and legal framework, can help to deliver a powerful, globally accessible clinico-genomic platform and to foster an associated philosophy that supports data-driven advances for patients and societies.

ACKNOWLEDGMENTS
This manuscript is written on behalf of the GA4GH Clinical Working Group (WG). We thank the Data WG, Regulatory and Ethics WG and Security WG for their important contributions. L.L.S. is supported by the Cancer Care Ontario Research Chair and Applied Cancer Research Units Grant; M.L., C.C. and R.C.F. are supported by Cancer Research UK; D.H. is funded by the US National Institutes of Health (award #U54HG007990). B.M.K. is supported by the Quebec Breast Cancer Foundation; C.L.S. is supported by the Howard Hughes Medical Institute and US National Cancer Institute (Grant #CA008748); E.E.V. is supported by the Barcode for Life Foundation and the Hartwig Medical Foundation.

COMPETING FINANCIAL INTERESTS
The authors declare competing financial interests: details are available in the online version of the paper.

Reprints and permissions information is available online at http://www.nature.com/reprints/index.html.

1. McCarthy, M. US president endorses "moonshot" effort to cure cancer. *Br. Med. J.* **352**, i213 (2016).
2. Collins, F.S. & Varmus, H. A new initiative on precision medicine. *N. Engl. J. Med.* **372**, 793–795 (2015).
3. Siva, N. UK gears up to decode 100,000 genomes from NHS patients. *Lancet* **385**, 103–104 (2015).
4. Meric-Bernstam, F. *et al.* Feasibility of large-scale genomic testing to facilitate enrollment onto genomically matched clinical trials. *J. Clin. Oncol.* **33**, 2753–2762 (2015).
5. André, F. *et al.* Comparative genomic hybridisation array and DNA sequencing to direct treatment of metastatic breast cancer: a multicentre, prospective trial (SAFIR01/UNICANCER). *Lancet Oncol.* **15**, 267–274 (2014).
6. Walport, M. & Brest, P. Sharing research data to improve public health. *Lancet* **377**, 537–539 (2011).
7. Joly, Y., Dove, E.S., Knoppers, B.M., Bobrow, M. & Chalmers, D. Data sharing in the post-genomic world: the experience of the International Cancer Genome Consortium (ICGC) Data Access Compliance Office (DACO). *PLoS Comput. Biol.* **8**, e1002549 (2012).
8. Rehm, H.L. *et al.* & ClinGen—the Clinical Genome Resource. *N. Engl. J. Med.* **372**, 2235–2242 (2015).
9. US National Institutes of Health. National Institutes of Health genomic data sharing policy https://gds.nih.gov/PDF/NIH_GDS_Policy.pdf (27 August 2014).
10. Cancer Genome Atlas Research Network. *et al.* The Cancer Genome Atlas Pan-Cancer analysis project. *Nat. Genet.* **45**, 1113–1120 (2013).
11. International Cancer Genome Consortium. *et al.* International network of cancer genome projects. *Nature* **464**, 993–998 (2010).
12. Aparicio, S. & Caldas, C. The implications of clonal genome evolution for cancer medicine. *N. Engl. J. Med.* **368**, 842–851 (2013).
13. Alizadeh, A.A. *et al.* Toward understanding and exploiting tumor heterogeneity. *Nat. Med.* **21**, 846–853 (2015).
14. Köhler, S. *et al.* The Human Phenotype Ontology project: linking molecular biology and disease through phenotype data. *Nucleic Acids Res.* **42**, D966–D974 (2014).
15. Groza, T. *et al.* The Human Phenotype Ontology: Semantic Unification of Common and Rare Disease. *Am. J. Hum. Genet.* **97**, 111–124 (2015).
16. Girdea, M. *et al.* PhenoTips: patient phenotyping software for clinical and research use. *Hum. Mutat.* **34**, 1057–1065 (2013).
17. Hamosh, A. *et al.* PhenoDB: a new web-based tool for the collection, storage, and analysis of phenotypic features. *Hum. Mutat.* **34**, 566–571 (2013).
18. Denny, J.C. *et al.* Systematic comparison of phenome-wide association study of electronic medical record data and genome-wide association study data. *Nat. Biotechnol.* **31**, 1102–1111 (2013).

19. McCarty, C.A. *et al.* The eMERGE Network: a consortium of biorepositories linked to electronic medical records data for conducting genomic studies. *BMC Med. Genomics* **4**, 13 (2011).

20. Schilsky, R.L., Michels, D.L., Kearbey, A.H., Yu, P.P. & Hudis, C.A. Building a rapid learning health care system for oncology: the regulatory framework of CancerLinQ. *J. Clin. Oncol.* **32**, 2373–2379 (2014).

21. Sioutos, N. *et al.* NCI Thesaurus: a semantic model integrating cancer-related clinical and molecular information. *J. Biomed. Inform.* **40**, 30–43 (2007).

22. Stein, L.D., Knoppers, B.M., Campbell, P., Getz, G. & Korbel, J.O. Data analysis: Create a cloud commons. *Nature* **523**, 149–151 (2015).

23. Van Allen, E.M. *et al.* Whole-exome sequencing and clinical interpretation of formalin-fixed, paraffin-embedded tumor samples to guide precision cancer medicine. *Nat. Med.* **20**, 682–688 (2014).

24. Andre, F. *et al.* Prioritizing targets for precision cancer medicine. *Ann. Oncol.* **25**, 2295–2303 (2014).

25. Kosseim, P. *et al.* Building a data sharing model for global genomic research. *Genome Biol.* **15**, 430 (2014).

26. Paten, B. *et al.* The NIH BD2K center for big data in translational genomics. *J. Am. Med. Inform. Assoc.* **22**, 1143–1147 (2015).

27. Boutros, P.C. *et al.* Global optimization of somatic variant identification in cancer genomes with a global community challenge. *Nat. Genet.* **46**, 318–319 (2014).

28. Ewing, A.D. *et al.* & ICGC–TCGA DREAM Somatic Mutation Calling Challenge participants. Combining tumor genome simulation with crowdsourcing to benchmark somatic single-nucleotide-variant detection. *Nat. Methods* **12**, 623–630 (2015).

29. Gargis, A.S. *et al.* Good laboratory practice for clinical next-generation sequencing informatics pipelines. *Nat. Biotechnol.* **33**, 689–693 (2015).

30. Lawler, M. *et al.* & Clinical Working Group of the Global Alliance for Genomics and Health (GA4GH). All the world's a stage: facilitating discovery science and improved cancer care through the global alliance for genomics and health. *Cancer Discov.* **5**, 1133–1136 (2015).

31. Tryka, K.A. *et al.* NCBI's Database of Genotypes and Phenotypes: dbGaP. *Nucleic Acids Res.* **42**, D975–D979 (2014).

32. Global Alliance for Genomics and Health. White Paper: creating a global alliance to enable responsible sharing of genomic and clinical data https://genomicsandhealth. org/about-the-global-alliance/key-documents/white-paper-creating-global-alliance-enable-responsible-shar (3 June 2013).

33. Kaye, J. The tension between data sharing and the protection of privacy in genomics research. in *Ethics, Law and Governance of Biobanking*, Vol. 14 (ed. Mascalzoni, D.) 101–120 (Springer, the Netherlands, 2015).

34. Haga, S.B. & Beskow, L.M. Ethical, legal, and social implications of biobanks for genetics research. *Adv. Genet.* **60**, 505–544 (2008).

35. Wolf, L.E. & Lo, B. Untapped potential: IRB guidance for the ethical research use of stored biological materials. *IRB* **26**, 1–8 (2004).

36. Lunshof, J.E., Chadwick, R., Vorhaus, D.B. & Church, G.M. From genetic privacy to open consent. *Nat. Rev. Genet.* **9**, 406–411 (2008).

37. Lolkema, M.P. *et al.* Ethical, legal, and counseling challenges surrounding the return of genetic results in oncology. *J. Clin. Oncol.* **31**, 1842–1848 (2013).

38. O'Doherty, K.C. *et al.* From consent to institutions: designing adaptive governance for genomic biobanks. *Soc. Sci. Med.* **73**, 367–374 (2011).

39. Zika, E., Schulte In den Bäumen, T., Kaye, J., Brand, A. & Ibarreta, D. Sample, data use and protection in biobanking in Europe: legal issues. *Pharmacogenomics* **9**, 773–781 (2008).

40. Homer, N. *et al.* Resolving individuals contributing trace amounts of DNA to highly complex mixtures using high-density SNP genotyping microarrays. *PLoS Genet.* **4**, e1000167 (2008).

41. Lin, Z., Owen, A.B. & Altman, R.B. Genetics. Genomic research and human subject privacy. *Science* **305**, 183 (2004).

42. Gymrek, M., McGuire, A.L., Golan, D., Halperin, E. & Erlich, Y. Identifying personal genomes by surname inference. *Science* **339**, 321–324 (2013).

43. Erlich, Y. & Narayanan, A. Routes for breaching and protecting genetic privacy. *Nat. Rev. Genet.* **15**, 409–421 (2014).

44. Knoppers, B.M. International ethics harmonization and the global alliance for genomics and health. *Genome Med.* **6**, 13 (2014).

45. Knoppers, B.M., Harris, J.R., Budin-Ljøsne, I. & Dove, E.S. A human rights approach to an international code of conduct for genomic and clinical data sharing. *Hum. Genet.* **133**, 895–903 (2014).

46. Global Alliance for Genomics and Health. Framework for responsible sharing of genomic and health-related data https://genomicsandhealth.org/node/6611 (10 September 2014).

47. Global Alliance for Genomics and Health. Consent policy https://genomicsandhealth. org/consent-policy-pdf-27-may-2015 (27 May 2015).

48. Global Alliance for Genomics and Health. GA P3G–IPAC consent tools https:// genomicsandhealth.org/ga-p3g-ipac-consent-tools (6 August 2014).

49. Global Alliance for Genomics and Health. Privacy and security policy https:// genomicsandhealth.org/privacy-and-security-policy-pdf-26-may-2015 (26 May 2015).

50. Global Alliance for Genomics and Health. Data sharing lexicon. https://genomicsandhealth. org/files/public/GA4GH_DataSharingLexicon_Mar15.pdf (15 March 2016).

51. Global Alliance for Genomics and Health. Security infrastructure: standards and implementation practices for protecting the privacy and security of shared genomic and clinical data https://genomicsandhealth.org/security-infrastructure-version-11 (12 March 2015).

52. Global Alliance for Genomics and Health. Accountability policy https:// genomicsandhealth.org/ga4gh-accountability-policy (10 February 2016).

53. Christensen, K.D. *et al.* & MedSeq Project Team. Are physicians prepared for whole genome sequencing? a qualitative analysis. *Clin. Genet.* **89**, 228–234 (2016).

54. Pillai, U. *et al.* Factors that may influence the willingness of cancer patients to consent for biobanking. *Biopreserv. Biobank.* **12**, 409–414 (2014).

55. Mancini, J. *et al.* Consent for biobanking: assessing the understanding and views of cancer patients. *J. Natl. Cancer Inst.* **103**, 154–157 (2011).

56. Tejpar, S. *et al.* Awareness and understanding of stratified/personalized medicine in patients treated for cancer: a multi-national survey (37th European Society for Medical Oncology Congress) 1382P (Oxford University Press, 2012).

57. Rogith, D. *et al.* Attitudes regarding privacy of genomic information in personalized cancer therapy. *J. Am. Med. Inform. Assoc.* **21**, e2, e320–e325 (2014).

58. Lawler, M. *et al.* & European Cancer Concord (ECC). A Bill of Rights for patients with cancer in Europe. *Lancet Oncol.* **15**, 258–260 (2014).

59. Lawler, M. *et al.* A catalyst for change: the European cancer Patient's Bill of Rights. *Oncologist* **19**, 217–224 (2014).

60. European Commission. Proposal for a regulation of the European Parliament and of the council on the protection of individuals with regard to processing of personal data and on the free movement of such data (general data protection regulation) http://ec.europa.eu/justice/data-protection/document/review2012/com_2012_11_ en.pdf, (25 January 2012).

61. Husedzinovic, A., Ose, D., Schickhardt, C., Fröhling, S. & Winkler, E.C. Stakeholders' perspectives on biobank-based genomic research: systematic review of the literature. *Eur. J. Hum. Genet.* **23**, 1607–1614 (2015).

62. McGuire, A.L. *et al.* To share or not to share: a randomized trial of consent for data sharing in genome research. *Genet. Med.* **13**, 948–955 (2011).

63. Green, R.C., Lautenbach, D. & McGuire, A.L. GINA, genetic discrimination, and genomic medicine. *N. Engl. J. Med.* **372**, 397–399 (2015).

64. Lacombe, D. *et al.* European perspective for effective cancer drug development. *Nat. Rev. Clin. Oncol.* **11**, 492–498 (2014).

65. Conley, B.A. & Doroshow, J.H. Molecular analysis for therapy choice: NCI MATCH. *Semin. Oncol.* **41**, 297–299 (2014).

66. Schilsky, R.L. Implementing personalized cancer care. *Nat. Rev. Clin. Oncol.* **11**, 432–438 (2014).

67. Eggermont, A.M. *et al.* Cancer Core Europe: a consortium to address the cancer care-cancer research continuum challenge. *Eur. J. Cancer* **50**, 2745–2746 (2014).

68. American Association for Cancer Research. Project GENIE (Genomics Evidence Neoplasia Information Exchange) http://www.aacr.org/Documents/GENIE_Info Graph.pdf.

References

Abbott A. Europe's drug regulator opens vaults of clinical-trials data. Nature. 2016;538(7626):440.

Biering-Sorensen F, et al. Common data elements for spinal cord injury clinical research: a National Institute for Neurological Disorders and Stroke project. Spinal Cord. 2015;53(4):263–77.

Cohen M, Thompson C, Yates B, Zimmerman L, Pullen C. Integrating common data elements across studies to advance research. Nurs Outlook. 2015;63(2):181–8.

Cool A. Detaching data from the state: biobanking and building Big Data in Sweden. BioSocieties. 2015; epub ahead of print:1–19.

Haring R, Henry W, Hudson M, Rodriguez E, Taualii M. Views on clinical trial recruitment, biospecimen collection, and cancer research: population science from landscapes of the Haudenosaunee (People of the Longhouse). J Cancer Educ. 2016; July 9 epub head of print.

Mascalzoni D, et al. International Charter of principles for sharing biospecimens and data. Eur J Hum Genet. 2016;23(6):721–8.

Siu L, et al. Facilitating a culture of responsible and effective sharing of cancer genome data. Nat Med. 2016;22(5):464–71.

Thiel D, Plastt T, Platt J, King S, Kardia S. Community perspectives on public health biobanking: an analysis of community meetings on the Michigan BioTrust for Health. J Community Genet. 2014;5:125–38.

Toga A, Dinov I. Sharing big biomedical data. J Big Data. 2015;2:7.

Vaught J. Biobanking comes of age: the transition to biospecimen science. Annu Rev Pharmacol Toxicol. 2016;56:211–28.

Zinner D, Pham-Kanter G, Campbell E. The changing nature of scientific sharing and withholding in academic life sciences research: Trends from national surveys I 2000 and 2013. Acad Med. 2016;91(3):433–40.

Additional Suggested Reading

Cool A. Detaching data from the state: biobanking and building Big Data in Sweden. BioSocieties. 2015; epub ahead of print:1–19. (*Describes reconsideration of data policies by Sweden in the wake of Big Data*).

Krumholz H. Big data and new knowledge in medicine: the thinking, training and tools needed for a learning health system. Health Aff. 2014;33(7):1163–1170. (*Consolidates information from research and health care into tools for a learning health care system.*)

Metcalf J, Crawford K. Where are human subjects in Big Data research? The emerging ethics divide. Big Data Soc. 2016;1–14. (*Describes growing discontinuities between data science in research and current research ethics regulation.*)

International Research Involving Resource-Constrained Countries

13

Arthur L. Caplan and Barbara K. Redman

While there has been an accelerating development of scientific capacity around the globe, in much of the world research ethics review systems are still developing and policies are variable. (Subjects protection regulations for many countries may be found on the US Office of Human Research Protection website). Policies and research ethics frameworks are not yet harmonized, and varied intellectual property and trade laws may limit data transfer.

Community engagement has become an expected part of international research with low and middle income countries (LMICs). Especially contentious is the duty to provide ancillary or continuing care to research participants. India instituted policies requiring that any subject injured in research be given care for the rest of their lives, although this policy was subsequently revised. In countries where quality health services are not available, researchers must attend to risks of exploitation when clinical trials are the only option for care or when the sponsor of a study does not intend to make the agent available, should it prove beneficial at a reasonable price, post the conclusion of a study.

For LMICs, health services research is of high importance in order to improve delivery of proven therapeutics. Populations larger than those available in a single country are important for research in rare diseases and for common diseases in which prevention or treatment offer moderate success. This situation necessitates enrollment of thousands of research participants in multiple countries (Yusuf and Wittes 2016). This means identifying a central IRB that can insure comprehension and consent to research in many nations and settings. Determining what is reasonable compensation for recruiting in populations of different economic backgrounds and protecting against stigma for participating in certain types of research such as mental health, HPV, HIV, or sex work are challenges that must be anticipated and managed.

Trials of surgical interventions offer another example. Less than 1% of surgical patients are enrolled in clinical trials, largely not in international collaborations. Yet, 80% of deaths from surgically correctible disorders occur in LMICs, offering opportunity for public health gains if surgical trials were undertaken in those countries (Søreide et al. 2013).

The International Society for Stem Cell Research, an independent non-profit organization established in 2002 as a forum for education in stem cell research, has developed global standards (Daley et al. 2016). This is a prominent example of an attempt at scientific self-regulation in a contentious area of science that spans the globe. But there are still many doctors and clinics in many nations offering bogus stem cell 'therapies' for untested and unproven indications.

Science is increasingly accomplished by international teams. Much effort is being put into developing research and research ethics capacity in LMIC, a necessary condition for research integrity so that health problems of those countries can be studied by partnerships among developed country researchers, native scientists and local communities.

Advice: Having experience in a multi-national research team is a plus. It will teach you how to navigate research regulatory systems across nations and in LMICs which is the future of human research in many fields. Thinking early about how to achieve community involvement, what policies can minimize any suggestion of exploitation, what the circumstances are under which studies can be terminated prematurely and how recruitment can be respectful of local values while honoring international standards is crucial to doing ethical research in LMICs.

13

A. L. Caplan · B. K. Redman (✉)
New York University Langone Medical Center,
New York, NY, USA
e-mail: Arthur.Caplan@nyumc.org

© Springer International Publishing AG, part of Springer Nature 2018
A. L. Caplan, B. K. Redman (eds.), *Getting to Good*, https://doi.org/10.1007/978-3-319-51358-4_13

13.1   The H3Africa Policy Framework: Negotiating Fairness in Genomics

Jantina de Vries, Paulina Tindana, Katherine Littler, Michè
le Ramsay, Charles Rotimi, Akin Abayomi, Nicola Mulder,
and Bongani M. Mayosi

deVries, J, et al. The H3Africa policy framework: negotiating airness in genomics, *Trends in Genetics* 31(3), 117–119
(2015). © 2015 The Authors. Published by Elsevier Ltd.

Scientific Life

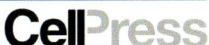

The H3Africa policy framework: negotiating fairness in genomics

Jantina de Vries[1], Paulina Tindana[2], Katherine Littler[3], Michèle Ramsay[4], Charles Rotimi[5], Akin Abayomi[6], Nicola Mulder[7], and Bongani M. Mayosi[8]

[1] Department of Medicine, University of Cape Town, UCT Centre for Clinical Research, Old Main Building, Groote Schuur Hospital, Observatory, Cape Town 7925, South Africa
[2] Navrongo Health Research Centre, Ghana Health Service, PO Box 114, Navrongo, Ghana
[3] Wellcome Trust, Gibbs Building, London, NW1 2BE, UK
[4] Division of Human Genetics, School of Pathology, Faculty of Health Sciences, University of the Witwatersrand and National Health Laboratory Service, PO Box 1038, Johannesburg 2000, South Africa
[5] Sydney Brenner Institute for Molecular Bioscience, University of the Witwatersrand, Johannesburg, Parktown 2193, South Africa
[6] Center for Research on Genomics and Global Health, MSC 5635, Bethesda, MD 20892-5635, USA
[7] NSB-H3A Biobank, National Health Laboratory Services of South Africa, Faculty of Medicine and Health Sciences, Stellenbosch University, Tygerberg Hospital, Cape Town 7505, South Africa
[8] Institute of Infectious Disease and Molecular Medicine, UCT Faculty of Health Sciences, Observatory 7925, South Africa

Human Heredity and Health in Africa (H3Africa) research seeks to promote fair collaboration between scientists in Africa and those from elsewhere. Here, we outline how concerns over inequality and exploitation led to a policy framework that places a firm focus on African leadership and capacity building as guiding principles for African genomics research.

Introduction

The historical underrepresentation of people of African ancestry in genomics research [1,2], with only a few studies focusing on or including people of African ancestry, has the potential of widening the health gap between Africa and the rest of the world by generating knowledge and interventions that may help in understanding or treating disease in Africa [3]. The H3Africa Consortium seeks to harness genomics technologies to investigate diseases pertinent to African patients [2]. Central to this aim is fostering collaboration between scientists in Africa and elsewhere. Of ethical importance is that H3Africa builds equitable partnerships between researchers and other key stakeholders. Equitable, or fair, partnerships can help build strong research systems [4]. They are also a means to counter exploitation and promote mutual respect and trust [5], and offer an opportunity to ensure that research is responsive to local health needs and that data interpretation is contextualised.

H3Africa builds on a growing body of work seeking to define what constitutes fair partnerships [6–10]. Here, we outline four key components of that policy framework that together seek to establish more 'fair' ways of working together, most notably by advocating preferential access to funding, samples, and data for African researchers. We hope that these examples can set a new standard for international collaborative health research that involves samples and data from African patients.

African leadership

An important aspect of H3Africa research is that it is under the leadership of scientists on the African continent, with grants awarded to, and managed by, African institutions. The expectation is that such research will be more successful in capitalising on the insight and experience of African clinicians and researchers, help in data interpretation and translation of results to the clinical setting, and build research capacity [2,6,7]. In the case of H3Africa, funding was allocated exclusively to researchers with a primary institutional affiliation in Africa, and the majority of co-applicants also had to be based in Africa. In addition, the majority of funds have to be spent in Africa. The H3Africa Steering Committee comprises H3Africa lead investigators (currently 23) and two representatives of the two funding bodies that support it. Additional representatives of the funding bodies join the meetings but do not have voting rights. The effect is that African scientists are developing the policies governing the genomic research taking place, and that H3Africa is establishing a South-to-South network (i.e., a collaboration network between scientists based in the Global South) of genomic scientists, with the academic discourse now occurring in Africa and between African scientists [11,12]. This is one recognised element of fair partnerships [7,8].

The H3Africa policy framework

H3Africa has developed policies for sample and data sharing, as well as the terms of reference for the committee deciding on sample and data access [2]. The various policies were developed by several H3Africa Working Groups, comprising representatives of each of the currently funded 21 research projects. These policies took about 12 months to develop in an iterative process involving the working

Corresponding author: de Vries, J. (Jantina.devries@uct.ac.za).
Keywords: Africa; genomics; ethics; fairness; H3Africa.

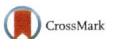
CrossMark

Scientific Life

Trends in Genetics March 2015, Vol. 31, No. 3

groups, the H3Africa members, and contact sessions at the H3Africa meetings. Policy proposals are pending ratification by the H3Africa Steering Committee. The policy framework offers three further examples of how notions of fairness were incorporated in the work of the Consortium.

The data-sharing policy

In line with international standards, H3Africa researchers are required to make genomic data available for secondary research. H3Africa researchers are granted a minimum of 11 months before genomic and phenotype data are publicly released, after which the data are under publication embargo for a further 12 months or until the first publication. Therefore, the total timeframe for the public release of data is 23 months. This is significantly longer than for other projects funded by the same agencies*. The reason for this extended period of exclusive access is to enable African scientists to analyse and publish their data before others can, and is similar to a previous large genomics research project that occurred in Africa [13]. Training is currently under way through H3A-BioNet, a continental bioinformatics network that offers courses, mentorship, and infrastructural support for the analysis of genomic data. In addition to these extended timelines, applicants wishing access to data need to describe how their proposed use will contribute to capacity building and health improvement in Africa. The hope is that, by prompting secondary users to consider this, there will be greater awareness of the need to establish a more fair way of working with researchers in Africa.

The sample-sharing policy

A prominent ethical concern in research in Africa relates to ownership over samples and, to a lesser extent, data. Samples and their movement across borders seem to have become symbolic of concerns over exploitation and fairness and, therefore, have become stringently regulated in many African countries [14]. Examples of regulatory approaches are strict export criteria, and requirements for export permits and material transfer agreements.

The proposal that samples collected in H3Africa need to be shared for secondary use through one of the H3Africa biorepositories in development, has created considerable controversy. This proposal generated suspicions that H3Africa research is just a way of making available African samples to researchers elsewhere. To address such concerns, careful thought has gone into developing a policy framework that would not only allay such fears, but also promote African-led research on African samples. The current policy proposal is that external researchers can apply for samples but, for a period of 3 years, they will only be made available either to researchers based in Africa, or to researchers outside of Africa who both work with researchers in Africa and develop a clear plan for capacity building. In other words, for 3 years, samples can

only be used for research that strengthens African research capacity. Unlike data, biospecimens are a limited resource that can be depleted, so careful consideration is required when providing access to these. Integrated into the policy is a requirement for new data generated from these samples to be submitted to the same public repository as H3Africa data.

The data and biospecimen access committee

A final component of the policy framework where considerations of fairness have been discussed is the composition of the committee that will decide on access requests: the Data and Biospecimen Access Committee (DBAC). Given that the DBAC will control access to African samples, H3Africa researchers felt that it was necessary for this committee to comprise primarily individuals based in Africa, but that it could also include researchers outside of Africa with experience working in Africa, to allow relevant expertise from across the world to be brought to bear. Ideally, the DBAC should have representation from across relevant scientific disciplines, such as genomics, bioinformatics, and ethics, as well as nonscience stakeholders, such as a patient advocate.

The future of genomic research in Africa

The focus on Africa seeks to ensure that African researchers have a fair chance to develop the capacity for genomic research and investigate diseases that they believe are pertinent to Africa. It also seeks to ensure that data will be interpreted in the context where they were collected. We hope that H3Africa will set a new gold standard for collaborative genomic research in Africa, and possibly for broader collaborative health research.

The exclusive focus on the 'Africanness' of researchers in their various roles (as primary applicants, secondary data and sample users, or members of the DBAC) of course raises important questions, both about what 'Africanness' really means, and about the ethical implications of restricting the utility of samples and data in this way. What should matter is that research that is conducted is of the highest ethical and scientific standard and leads to maximum patient benefit in the shortest period of time, regardless of where the research is conducted. This should be based on principles of fairness and inclusivity. The question is whether H3Africa policies will successfully and sustainably foster African-led genomic research, and build a generation of African scientists that are internationally competitive.

Acknowledgements

This work reports on the policy framework for H3Africa that was developed with the input from a large number of people. We express thanks to all those that continue to contribute to the success of H3Africa projects. J.D.V. and B.M. are supported by a Wellcome Trust H3Africa grant (RHD Gen, WT099313MA); M.R. is supported by a NIH H3Africa grant (AWI-Gen, 1U54HG006938); C.R. is supported by a NIH H3Africa grant (ACCME, U54HG006947); A.A. is supported by a NIH H3Africa grant (1UH2HG007092); and N.M. is supported by an H3Africa grant (H3A BioNet, U41HG006941).

---

*See the Draft NIH Data Sharing Policy available from http://grants.nih.gov/grants/guide/notice-files/NOT-OD-13-119.html. For information about the Wellcome Trust position, see http://www.wellcome.ac.uk/About-us/Policy/Spotlight-issues/Data-sharing/Guidance-for-researchers/index.htm (both accessed 3 December 2014)

References

1 Rosenberg, N.A. *et al.* (2010) Genome-wide association studies in diverse populations. *Nat. Rev. Genet.* 11, 356–366

Scientific Life

Trends in Genetics   March 2015, Vol. 31, No. 3

2 H3Africa Consortium (2014) Research capacity. Enabling the genomic revolution in Africa. *Science* 344, 1346–1348

3 Need, A.C. and Goldstein, D.B. (2009) Next generation disparities in human genomics: concerns and remedies. *Trends Genet.* 25, 489–494

4 Edwards, D. *et al.* (2014) *Negotiating research contracts. Creating opportunities for stronger research and innovation systems*, Council on Health Research for Development, Geneva

5 Emanuel, E.J. *et al.* (2004) What makes clinical research in developing countries ethical? The benchmarks of ethical research. *J. Infect. Dis.* 189, 930–937

6 Chu, K.M. *et al.* (2014) Building research capacity in Africa: equity and global health collaborations. *PLoS Med.* 11, e1001612

7 Whitworth, J.A.G. *et al.* (2008) Strengthening capacity for health research in Africa. *Lancet* 372, 1590–1593

8 Binka, F. (2005) Editorial: North–South research co-llaborations: a move towards a true partnership? *Trop. Med. Int. Health* 10, 207–209

9 Costello, A. and Zumla, A. (2000) Moving to research partnerships in developing countries. *BMJ* 321, 827–829

10 Tucker, T.J. and Makgoba, M.W. (2008) Public health. Public–private partnerships and scientific imperialism. *Science* 320, 1016–1017

11 Wonkam, A. and Mayosi, B.M. (2014) Genomic medicine in Africa: promise, problems and prospects. *Genome Med.* 6, 11

12 Ramsay, M. *et al.* (2011) Africa: the next frontier for human disease gene discovery? *Hum. Mol. Genet.* 20, R214–R220

13 Parker, M. *et al.* (2009) Ethical data release in genome-wide association studies in developing countries. *PLoS Med.* 6, e1000143

14 De Vries, J. *et al.* (2011) Ethical issues in human genomics research in developing countries. *BMC Med. Ethics* 12, 5

13.2 Sponsorship in Non-commercial Clinical Trials: Definitions, Challenges and the Role of Good Clinical Practices Guidelines

Raffaella Ravinetto, Katelijne De Nys, Marleen Boelaert, Ermias Diro, Graeme Meintjes, Yeka Adoke, Harry Tagbor, and Minne Casteels

Ravinetto, R, et al. Sponsorship in non-commercial clinical trials: definitions, challenges and the role of Good Clinical Practices guidelines. *BMC International Health and Human Rights* 15, 34 (2015). © 2015 Ravinetto et al. http://creativecommons.org/licenses/by/4.0/

Ravinetto *et al. BMC International Health and Human Rights* (2015) 15:34
DOI 10.1186/s12914-015-0073-8

BMC International Health and
Human Rights

DEBATE

Open Access

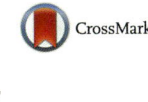

Sponsorship in non-commercial clinical trials: definitions, challenges and the role of Good Clinical Practices guidelines

Raffaella Ravinetto[1,2*], Katelijne De Nys[2,3], Marleen Boelaert[4], Ermias Diro[5], Graeme Meintjes[6], Yeka Adoke[7], Harry Tagbor[8] and Minne Casteels[2]

Abstract

Background: Non-commercial clinical research plays an increasingly essential role for global health. Multiple partners join in international consortia that operate under the limited timeframe of a specific funding period. One organisation (the sponsor) designs and carries out the trial in collaboration with research partners, and is ultimately responsible for the trial's scientific, ethical, regulatory and legal aspects, while another organization, generally in the North (the funder), provides the external funding and sets funding conditions. Even if external funding mechanisms are key for most non-commercial research, the dependence on an external funder's policies may heavily influence the choices of a sponsor. In addition, the competition for accessing the available external funds is great, and non-commercial sponsors may not be in a position to discuss or refuse standard conditions set by a funder. To see whether the current definitions adequately address the intricacies of sponsorship in externally-funded trials, we looked at how a "sponsor" of clinical trials is defined in selected international guidelines, with particular focus on international Good Clinical Practices codes, and in selected European and African regulations/legislations.

Discussion: Our limited analysis suggests that the sponsors definition from the 1995 WHO Good Clinical Practices code has been integrated as such into many legislations, guidelines and regulations, and that it is not adequate to cover today's reality of funding arrangements in global health, where the legal responsibility and the funding source are de facto split. In agreement with other groups, we suggest that the international Good Clinical Practices codes should be updated to reflect the reality of non-commercial clinical research. In particular, they should explicitly include the distinction between commercial and non-commercial sponsors, and provide guidance to non-commercial sponsors for negotiating with external funding agencies and other research counterparts.

Summary: Non-commercial sponsors of clinical trials should surely invest in the development of adequate legal, administrative and management skills. By acknowledging their role and specificities, and by providing them with adapted guidance, the international Good Clinical Practices codes would provide valuable guidance and support to non-commercial clinical research, whose relevance for global health is increasingly evident.

Background

The North–south divide in access to health is very large. Clinical research & development (R&D) follows a similar pattern, and this despite rapid evolution in the field of clinical trials in the South. There is a clear tendency to relocate trials to resource-poor settings [1, 2], either for

reasons of *external validity*, i.e. to challenge findings obtained in the North on new drugs and devices in a variety of epidemiological settings and populations; or for *convenience* reasons, represented by lower costs, less stringent review, and potentially higher recruitment rates; or for *global health* reasons, when the choice for a location in the South is driven by the need to address the specific health needs of the local population.

In recent years, there has been a significant increase in clinical research carried out under non-commercial North–south collaborations, prompted by *global health*

* Correspondence: rravinetto@itg.be
[1]Clinical Sciences Department, Institute of Tropical Medicine Antwerp, Antwerp, Belgium
[2]Clinical Pharmacology and Pharmacotherapy, KU Leuven, Leuven, Belgium
Full list of author information is available at the end of the article

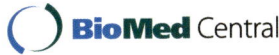

556   A. L. Caplan and B. K. Redman

Ravinetto *et al. BMC International Health and Human Rights* (2015) 15:34   Page 2 of 7

reasons. Non-commercial clinical research as well as public-private partnerships are essential for R&D of medical products of no direct commercial interest, for assessing the effectiveness and feasibility of medical products and health interventions in specific contexts/ groups, and for providing independent evaluation of such products and interventions [3, 4]. The increased availability of funds and technological investment for global health [5, 6], by philanthropic charities, foundations, public-private partnerships, bilateral/multilateral aid, and sometimes pharmaceutical companies, provide opportunities for non-commercial research groups to design, carry out and sponsor scientifically sound clinical research in traditionally neglected areas, e.g. infectious neglected diseases and tuberculosis.

In commercial research, the same organization (usually, a pharmaceutical company) funds, designs and carries out a trial. But the new context of North–South collaborations often leads to complex arrangements, with multiple partners joining in international consortia that often have an ad hoc structure and operate under the limited timeframe of a specific funding period.

Only in few cases will academic sponsors be able to conduct trials without external funding. Generally, one agency in the North (usually a foundation or a public authority) provides the funding and sets conditions for such funding, and another organization (henceforward called the sponsor), usually but not always located in the North, designs and conducts the trial, in collaboration with research partners. The financial arrangements between the funding agency and the research partners are formalized in contracts defining respective roles and responsibilities, and they may be quite complex. The main contract is usually signed between the funder and the non-commercial research consortium, and it defines the conditions under which the agreed funding will be disbursed. The liability issues generated by the testing of new medicines, devices or protocols should be carefully considered in contractual agreements. The set-up of a complex multi-institutional partnership may sometimes be at odds with the concept of "single sponsorship", which was developed for ensuring the protection of participants in the context of commercial trials. Single sponsorship is rooted in the need to clearly identify the legal responsibility, and does not hinge upon the "funding" aspect. Noteworthy, most funding agencies are unwillingly to take on the role of sponsor and often they may not be suitable for this.

Non-commercial international research is not immune from any risks for exploitation, depending on how it is designed and conducted and on how findings are implemented and disseminated. Exploitation can arise when the ambitions of the academic sponsors or the strategical plans of the funders prevail on the interests of the

communities. Hence the importance to strengthen the regulatory framework for non-commercial research, starting with the key question on the legal responsibility.

The concept of sponsorship merits closer scrutiny in this context. To enlighten the debate we examined how a "sponsor" of clinical trials is defined in selected international or national guidelines and legislation, and discuss whether current definitions adequately address the intricacies of sponsorship in externally (i.e. "outside of the sponsor")-funded trials.

Discussion

Among international guidelines, we considered those that most often inspire national legislations: the Declaration of Helsinki, the International Ethical Guidelines for Biomedical Research Involving Human Subjects (CIOMS), and the Good Clinical Practices (GCP) code of the World Health Organization (WHO) and of the International Conference for Harmonization (ICH). However, the Helsinki Declaration [7] and the CIOMS Guidelines [8] do not give a specific definition of what a "sponsor" is nor of its duties, even if both mention "sponsors" among the actors of medical research, and the CIOMS Guidelines also talk of "externally sponsored research" in relation to trials carried out in a different host country. Therefore, the Helsinki Declaration and the CIOMS Guidelines were excluded from the comparative analysis.

The selection of the international regulations and national guidelines/legislations included in the analysis was guided by our experience in North–South collaborative trials that bring together African and European institutions. Thus, we focused on the European and African regulatory environment. Among international regulations, we considered the European Union (EU) Directive, which is the main reference for European Member States and funding agencies. Among national guidelines/legislation, we considered the UK Clinical Trials Regulation, which is the main reference for some Commonwealth countries and for UK funding agencies, and the regulations/legislation of host countries of our research projects, i.e. Belgium, South Africa, Ethiopia, Uganda and Ghana.

Sponsor's definitions

Table 1 gives an overview of the definition of sponsor in the selected documents. The WHO/GCP Guidelines, issued in 1995 [9], define the sponsor as "an individual, a company, an institution or an organization which takes responsibility for the initiation, management *and/or financing* of a clinical trial". The ICH/GCP Guidelines, issued in 1996 [10], use exactly the same definition, which leaves some degree of ambiguity about whether the sponsor should be primarily responsible for the "initiation and management" of a trial, or for its "financing",

Ravinetto *et al. BMC International Health and Human Rights* (2015) 15:34

Table 1 Overview of the definition of sponsor

Guideline/regulation	Year	Sponsor's definition
WHO GCP	1995	An individual, a company, an institution or an organization which takes responsibility for the initiation, management and/or financing of a clinical trial.
ICH GCP	1996	An individual, a company, an institution or an organization which takes responsibility for the initiation, management and/or financing of a clinical trial.
EU Directive	2002	An individual, company, institution or organization which takes responsibility for the initiation, management and/or financing of a clinical trial
Belgian Law	2004	An individual, company, institution or organization which takes responsibility for the initiation, management and/or financing of a clinical trial
UK Regulation	2004	Takes responsibility for the initiation, management and financing (or arranging the financing) of that trial.
South Africa GCP	2006	An individual, company, institution, or organisation which takes responsibility for the initiation, management, and/or financing of a clinical trial
Uganda Guidelines	2007	The sponsor is responsible for providing all the necessary financial support for initiation and completion of the research project
Uganda Guidelines	2014	The sponsor as such is not defined
Ghana GCP	2013	An individual, company, institution or organization which takes responsibility for the initiation, management and/or financing of a trial. This excludes an individual company, institution or organization which has been requested to provide money for a trial and does not benefit in any way from the results of the trial
EU Regulation	2014	An individual, company, institution or organisation which takes responsibility for the initiation, the management and for setting up the financing of the clinical trial
Ethiopia GCP	Not dated	An individual, a company, an institution or an organization which takes responsibility for the initiation, management and/or financing of a clinical trial.

or for both. This definition reflects the situation of the '90s, when clinical trials were mainly conducted in Western contexts by commercial sponsors assuming both roles. Both GCP codes accept the notion of "sponsor-investigator", which only refers to an individual, thus is not applicable to non-commercial sponsors in global clinical research.

The same definition was found in the South African [11] and Ethiopian [12] GCP guidelines (where the "funder" is mentioned but not defined), and in the 2001/20/EC/EU Directive [13]. The definition of the EU Directive was incorporated into national legislations, such as the Belgian Law of 2004 [14]. Noteworthy, the Belgian Law distinguishes between commercial and non-commercial sponsors and is explicit about the fact that the same responsibilities hold for both, although it assures some rights (such as data ownership) for non-commercial sponsors.

However, the recent European Regulation on Clinical Trials on Medicinal Products for Human Use [15] introduced an important clarification in the definition of a sponsor: "an individual, company, institution or organisation which takes responsibility for the initiation, the management *and for setting up the financing* of the clinical trial". This definition clarifies that the sponsor is equally scientifically, legally and financially responsible but, by replacing the wording "financing" with the

wording "setting up the financing", it acknowledges that the budget can either come from the sponsor itself or from sources external to the research group. The UK regulators had already incorporated this nuance in their definition of sponsor, which is the one taking responsibility for the initiation, management *and financing (or arranging the financing)* of a trial [16].

The shift in the European legislation is in line with the growing attention paid to non-commercial research. Previously there was a description of the features of non-commercial clinical trials (i.e. those conducted without the participation of the pharmaceutical industry) and of non-commercial sponsors (i.e. universities, hospitals, public scientific organisations, non-profit institutions, patient organisations or individual researchers) [17]. The new regulation is much more explicit in acknowledging the importance of clinical trials conducted by non-commercial sponsors, which often rely on external funding from funds or charities.

Also in Africa, we find definitions which depart from the WHO/GCP guidelines, to be better rooted in the current reality. The previous (2007) Uganda National Guidelines for Research Involving Humans as Research Participants stated that the sponsor is responsible for *providing all the necessary financial support* for initiation and completion of the research project, while the detailed description of the sponsor's responsibilities

Ravinetto *et al. BMC International Health and Human Rights* (2015) 15:34

covered the different aspects of trial initiation and management [18]. The recent new Guidelines, issued in July 2014 [19], do not include anymore a formal definition of sponsor; however, the sponsor is still held responsible for providing all the necessary for implementation of the trial, including post-research obligations, while the detailed description of its responsibilities still covers the different aspects of trial initiation and management. In the Ghana GCP code [20], a clarification was added to the WHO/GCP definition, to clarify that an individual, company, institution or organization that provides money for a trial without benefiting from its results, is excluded from the definition of sponsor. Thus, for externally funded trials, the sponsor's legal responsibility remains with the organization that initiates and manages the trial.

Sponsor versus funder

This analysis suggests that the WHO/GCP definition of sponsor has been integrated as such into many international and national legislations, guidelines and regulations, and is not entirely adequate to cover the reality of funding arrangements in global health today (even if the difference between commercial and non-commercial sponsors is sometimes acknowledged). Some guidelines (South Africa, Ethiopia) mention the "funder" in addition to the sponsor, and some others (UK, Ghana, EU) reflect the fact that two or more different entities may respectively initiate/conduct a trial, and (co-)finance it. The former entity is the legal sponsor, while the latter is the external funder. But some ambiguity remains between "sponsor" and "funding agency". This was further confirmed by the unsatisfactorily results of a complementary literature search: the wording "sponsor" was often inaccurately referred to as the organization that funds a research, i.e. in a "lay" meaning (like for the "sponsor" of an event), rather than in the GCP meaning. This ambiguity may contribute to the poor awareness of some inexperienced sponsors, especially in the non-commercial sector, of the scope of their own responsibilities.

The legal sponsor is ultimately responsible for the scientific, ethical, regulatory and legal aspects of the trial, and also for financial aspects (i.e., if an external funder withdraws, the sponsor will be responsible to look for funds to complete the trial). It is therefore its primary role and responsibility to ensure that sufficient resources are planned for full compliance with ethical and GCP requirements. Sponsors' poor awareness of such requirements, which are described more in details in Table 2, may lead to underestimation of the overall study budget. In the specific case of externally-funded research, this will lead them to requesting insufficient financial resources from the funding agency.

Non-commercial sponsors often face budgetary problems because of the poor flexibility of the external funding [21, 22]. Some funding bodies will not accept a miscellaneous budget line for contingency/incidentals and are unwilling to review or supplement the budget once agreements have been finalized (which often happens before detailed protocols have been developed, and even before the clinical sites' needs are thoroughly assessed). The lack of flexibility is problematic also in other situations [23], e.g. when recruitment is slower than anticipated because of reasons beyond control of investigators, or when exchange rate with the local currency fluctuates over time: for instance, depreciation will make it more difficult to buy equipments abroad, while appreciation will decrease the local value of foreign funds.

As mentioned above, the poor awareness of GCP requirements may lead sponsors to requesting insufficient financial resources from the funding agency. But in other cases the budget awarded by the funding agency is much lower than the initially requested one, and may be insufficient to meet all costs required for full GCP-compliance, e.g. adequate external monitoring or data management set-up, costs that are unfortunately often the first to be cut in such situation.

Negotiations between non-commercial sponsors and funders

One could argue that it is the sponsor's responsibility to ensure that adequate funding and funding's conditions are negotiated for carrying out a trial according to appropriate standards, and to reject unsatisfactory conditions. Even though some sponsors underestimate the budget, in reality many cost items may be impossible to foresee in advance [22]. Awareness of GCP-requirements and good negotiation skills are both essential to ensure that the positions of the funding agency and the research consortium are sufficiently reflected in the final contract, but in practice, contracts are often based on the standard templates of the funding agency. Many non-commercial sponsors lack a legal department with enough human resources to conduct such negotiations. According to an analysis of the Council in Health Research for Development (COHRED), for instance, various research institutions in Africa and Asia have weak contracting capacity [24]. In addition, non-commercial sponsors often find themselves in a position of power unbalance *vis-à-vis* the funding agency. The competition for accessing the external funds available for health research is great, and most North- or South-based non-commercial sponsors may not be in a position to negotiate the rules set by the funding agencies. They have to balance the risk of a contract that does not reflect particular quality requirements ("contractual risk") versus the risk of being unable to conduct research relevant for a given population ("ethical risk").

Ravinetto *et al. BMC International Health and Human Rights* (2015) 15:34   Page 5 of 7

Table 2 Overview of sponsor's specific responsibilities in the international GCP codes

WHO GCP 1995	ICH GCP 1996
5.1 Selection of the Investigator(s)	5.1 Quality Assurance and Quality Control
5.2 Delegation of responsibilities	5.2 Contract Research Organization
5.3 Compliance with the protocol and procedures	5.3 Medical Expertise
5.4 Product information	5.4 Trial Design
5.5 Safety information	5.5 Trial Management, Data Handling, and Record Keeping
5.6 Investigational product	5.6 Investigator Selection
5.7 Trial management and handling of data	5.7 Allocation of Responsibilities
5.8 Standard operating procedures	5.8 Compensation to Subjects and Investigators
5.9 Compensation for subjects and investigators	5.9 Financing
5.10 Monitoring	5.10 Notification/Submission to Regulatory Authority(ies)
5.11 Quality assurance	5.11 Confirmation of Review by IRB/IEC
5.12 Study reports	5.12 Information on Investigational Product(s) (IPs)
5.13 Handling of adverse events	5.13 Manufacturing, Packaging, Labelling, and Coding IP(s)
5.14 Termination of the trial	5.14 Supplying and Handling IP(s)
	5.15 Record Access
	5.16 Safety Information
	5.17 Adverse Drug Reaction Reporting
	5.18 Monitoring
	5.19 Audit
	5.20 Noncompliance
	5.21 Premature Termination or Suspension of a Trial
	5.22 Clinical Trial/Study Reports
	5.23 Multicenter Trials

The way forward?

In externally-funded clinical research, the legal responsibility and the funding source are often de facto split. The liability risks of sponsors, as well as those of researchers and other research actors have been described [25]. However, to our knowledge the responsibilities of the funding agencies have not been described so far, even if in non-commercial research many choices may be positively or negatively influenced/determined by their policy.

Some guidelines are subject to periodical update, which allows taking new challenges into account. An example of this dynamic is given by the revision of the Helsinki Declaration, preceded by a public debate. Conversely, the WHO/ and ICH/GCP Guidelines, which orient most national legislators, were issued respectively in 1995 and 1996 and never updated. A revision is urgently needed, to better reflect the current reality of clinical trials including the perspective of non-commercial research [23, 26]. More in particular, we are not aware of any processes for the update of the WHO/GCP. Concerning the ICH/GCP, an "Integrated addendum" was published on 11th June 2015, with the objective to "modernize the ICH E6 Guideline by supplementing with additional recommendations which will facilitate broad and consistent international implementation of new methodologies". This draft text, now transmitted to the National Regulatory Authorities of the ICH region for internal and external consultation (accessed on 27th August 2015 at http://www.ich.org/products/guidelines/efficacy/efficacy-single/article/addendum-good-clinical-practice.html), does not address the definition of sponsor.

We suggest in the first place that the international GCP codes should include the distinction between commercial and non-commercial sponsors.

Non-commercial sponsors should pay special attention to the research legal framework and try to improve the contractual agreements with the funding agency, so that responsibilities and liability issues are fairly shared, and other important aspects are duly clarified. To be able to do so, non-commercial organisations that wish to act as sponsor in clinical trials should invest in the development of adequate legal, administrative and management skills, just as they do for scientific skills. This would also enable them to negotiate fair and meaningful contracts for other key-activities in clinical research, such as the supply of investigational products, the transfer and

560

A. L. Caplan and B. K. Redman

Ravinetto *et al. BMC International Health and Human Rights* (2015) 15:34

Page 6 of 7

sharing of trials' data and samples, and the policy insurance contract(s) [24]. To help cope with this, we suggest that the WHO/ and ICH/GCP Guidelines include as annexes some adapted model contract templates or standard checklists, with clauses for "reasonable flexibility", to guide the negotiation with external funding agencies. The same applies to templates and guidance for negotiation with other research counterparts, e.g. insurance policies, data and material transfer agreements etc.

Limitations of this analysis

Our analysis is meant to launch a debate aiming at better legislation on non-commercial sponsorships, based on the analysis of a sample of guidelines, laws and regulations. The international regulations and national guidelines/legislations included in this analysis were selected with focus on the European and (English-speaking) African regulatory environment. This led to exclusion of other influential guidelines and legislations, such as the ones from the United States, India, and Brazil, so more research is needed to investigate this issue in more regulatory environments.

While focusing on the sponsor's definition and role, we did not look at the complex dynamics that may exist within North–South research consortia, or at the possible power unbalance between Northern and Southern partners. As noted by Hoekman and colleagues, despite the increasing globalization of clinical trials, the scientific leadership of research tends to remain rooted in the North [27], which may be translated into unfair benefit sharing with local researchers, institutions and communities in the South. This phenomenon should be investigated more in-depth in its own right.

Conclusion

The current definitions of "sponsor" in clinical research do not reflect the challenges met by non-commercial sponsors in externally-funded research, especially but not only in the South, and in particular they do not adequately cover the reality of funding arrangements in clinical research in a global health context today. A revision of the WHO/ and ICH/GCP Guidelines is needed, to better reflect the current reality of independent clinical research.

By acknowledging the role and specificities of non-commercial sponsors, and by providing adapted guidance on standard research contracts, the international GCP codes would provide valuable guidance and support to non-commercial clinical research, whose relevance for global health is increasingly evident. This will only succeed if representatives of institutions involved in non-commercial clinical trials in the North and in the South (researchers, sponsors, administrators, legal experts etc.) are actively involved in the

next, and increasingly urgent, GCP revision. It is of crucial importance that this review process is as inclusive, representative and transparent as possible.

Abbreviations
CIOMS: Council for International Organizations of Medical Sciences; COHRED: Council in Health Research for Development; EU: European Union; GCP: Good Clinical Practices; ICH: International Conference for Harmonization; R&D: Research & Development; UK: United Kingdom; WHO: World Health Organization.

Competing interests
We declare that we do not have competing interests.

Authors' contributions
RR wrote the draft paper, with the support of KDN, ED, GM, YA, HT, MB and MC. All the co-authors equally critically read the initial draft, contributed to the developments of the final version, and approved the final manuscript.

Authors' information
RR is the Head of the Clinical Trials Unit at the Institute of Tropical Medicine Antwerp (ITM CTU), and she carried out a doctoral research at KU Leuven, under the guidance of MC, KDN and MB. This paper is part of her PhD project. ED, GM, YA and HT are academic researchers conducting non-commercial clinical trials in sub-Saharan Africa, some in collaboration with the ITM CTU.

Acknowledgments
There was no specific funding for this paper. The Clinical Trials Unit of the Institute of Tropical Medicine is supported by the Department of Economy, Science and Innovation of the Flemish Government.

Author details
¹Clinical Sciences Department, Institute of Tropical Medicine Antwerp, Antwerp, Belgium. ²Clinical Pharmacology and Pharmacotherapy, KU Leuven, Leuven, Belgium. ³Clinical Trial Center, University Hospitals Leuven, Leuven, Belgium. ⁴Public Health Department, Institute of Tropical Medicine Antwerp, Antwerp, Belgium. ⁵Department of Internal Medicine, University of Gondar, Gondar, Ethiopia. ⁶Institute of Infectious Disease and Molecular Medicine and Department of Medicine, University of Cape Town, Cape Town, South Africa. ⁷College of Health Sciences, Makerere University School of Public Health, Kampala, Uganda. ⁸School of Public Health, Kwame Nkrumah University of Science and Technology, Kumasi, Ghana.

Received: 11 January 2015 Accepted: 15 December 2015
Published online: 30 December 2015

References
1. Levinson DR. US Department of Health and Human Services, Office of Inspector General. Challenges to FDA's ability to monitor and inspect foreign clinical trials, 2001. OEI-01-08-00510. Accessed 19th November 2014 from http://oig.hhs.gov/oei/reports/oei-01-08-00510.pdf
2. European Medicines Agency. Reflection paper on ethical and GCP aspects of clinical trials of medicinal products for human use conducted outside of the EU/EEA and submitted in marketing authorisation applications to the EU Regulatory Authorities, 2012. EMA/121340/2011. Accessed 19th November 2014 from http://www.ema.europa.eu/docs/en_GB/document_library/Regulatory_and_procedural_guideline/2012/04/WC500125437.pdf
3. Burrows JN, Elliott RL, Kaneko T, Mowbray CE, Waterson D. The role of modern drug discovery in the fight against neglected and tropical diseases. Med Chem Commun. 2014;5:688–700.
4. G-Finder. Neglected diseases research and development: the public divide. Policy Cures 2013, Sydney, Australia. Accessed 19th November 2014 from http://www.policycures.org/downloads/GF_report13_all_web.pdf
5. Kilama WL, Chilengi R, Wanga CL. Towards an African-Driven Malaria Vaccine Development Program: History and Activities of the African Malaria Network Trust (AMANET). Am J Trop Med Hyg. 2007;77 Suppl 6:282–8.
6. Druml C, Singer EA, Woltz M. Report of the first meeting of the Vienna initiative to save European Academic Research. The Middle Eur J of Med. 2006;118/5-6 Suppl 1:1–12.
7. World Medical Association. Declaration of Helsinki: Ethical Principles for Medical Research Involving Human Subjects. Adopted by the 18th General

Ravinetto *et al. BMC International Health and Human Rights* (2015) 15:34

Page 7 of 7

Assembly, Helsinki, 1964, last amended by 60th General Assembly. Fortaleza, Brazil: World Medical Association; 2013.

8.   Council for International Organizations of Medical Sciences (CIOMS) in collaboration with the WHO. International Ethical Guidelines for Biomedical Research Involving Human Subjects. Geneva, Switzerland: CIOMS; 2002.

9.   World Health Organization. Technical report series No. 850, annex 3, guidelines for good clinical practices for trials on pharmaceutical products. Geneva, Switzerland: WHO; 1995.

10. International Conference of Harmonization. ICH Tripartite Guideline for Good Clinical Practices E6 (R1). Geneva, Switzerland: ICH Secretariat; 1996.

11. Department of Health. Guidelines for Good Practice in the Conduct of Clinical Trials with Human Participants in South Africa 2006. Accessed on 19th November 2014 from http://www.kznhealth.gov.za/research/guideline2.pdf

12. Ethiopia Food, Medicine and Health Care Administration and Control Agency (FMHACA). Narrated GCP. Not dated. Accessed 23 December 2014 from http://www.fmhaca.gov.et/documents/GCP_narreted.pdf

13. Directive 2001/20/EC of the European Parliament and of the Council of 4 April 2001 on the approximation of the laws, regulations and administrative provisions of the Member States relating to the implementation of good clinical practice in the conduct of clinical trials on medicinal products for human use. Last accessed on 19/9/2015 at http://ec.europa.eu/health/files/eudralex/vol-1/dir_2001_20/dir_2001_20_en.pdf

14. Belgian Law concerning experiments on the human person. 2004. Accessed 23 December 2014 from http://www.ejustice.just.fgov.be/cgi_loi/change_lg.pl?language=fr&la=F&cn=2004050732&table_name=loi

15. Regulation (EU) No 536/2014 of the European parliament and of the Council of 16 April 2014 on clinical trials on medicinal products for human use, and repealing Directive 2001/20/EC (2014). Official Journal of the European Union. Accessed 23 December 2014 from http://eur-lex.europa.eu/legal-content/EN/TXT/?uri=uriserv:OJ.L_.2014.158.01.0001.01.ENG

16. MEDICINES – UK The Medicines for Human Use (Clinical Trials) Regulations, 2004. No. 1031. Accessed 23 December 2014 from http://www.legislation.gov.uk/uksi/2004/1031/pdfs/uksi_20041031_en.pdf

17. European Commission. Entreprise and Industry Directorate General. Draft guidance on 'specific modalities' for non-commercial clinical trials referred to in Commission Directive 2005/28/EC. 2006. Accessed 23 December 2014 from http://ec.europa.eu/health/files/pharmacos/docs/doc2006/07_2006/guide_noncommercial_2006_07_27_en.pdf

18. Uganda National Council for Sciences and Technology. Uganda National Guidelines for Research Involving Humans as Research Participants 2007. Accessed 19th November 2014 from http://www.uncst.go.ug/dmdocuments/Guideline,%20Human%20Subjects%20Guidelines%20Marc.pdf

19. Uganda National Council for Sciences and Technology. Uganda National Guidelines for Research Involving Humans as Research Participants. 2014. Accessed 19th November 2014 from http://www.uncst.go.ug/dmdocuments/Human%20Subjects%20Protection%20Guidelines%20July%202014.pdf

20. Food and Drugs Authority. Guidelines for Good Clinical Practice in Ghana 2013. Accessed 19th November 2014 from http://www.fdaghana.gov.gh/images/stories/pdfs/downloads/drugs%20guidelines/GUIDELINES%20FOR%20GOOD%20CLINICAL%20PRACTICE%20IN%20GHANA.pdf

21. Ravinetto RM, Talisuna A, De Crop M, van Loen H, Menten J, Van Overmeir C, et al. Challenges of non-commercial multicentre North-South collaborative clinical trials. TMIH. 2012;18(2):237–41. doi:10.1111/tmi.12036.

22. Idoko OT, Kochhar S, Agbenyega TE, Ogutu B, Ota MO. Review: impact, challenges, and future projections of vaccine trials in Africa. Am J Trop Med Hyg. 2013;88(3):414–9.

23. McMahon AD, Conway DI, MacDonald TM, McInnes GT. The unintended consequences of clinical trials regulations. PLoS Med. 2009;3(11):e1000131. doi:10.1371/journal.pmed.1000131.

24. Marais D, Toohey J, Edwards D and IJsselmuiden C. Where there is no lawyer: Guidance for fairer contract negotiation in collaborative research partnerships. Council in Health Research for Development (COHRED) 2013. Geneva & Pietermaritzburg. Last accessed on 19/9/15 at http://www.cohred.org/wp-content/uploads/2012/04/Fair-Research-Contracting-Guidance-Booklet-e-version.pdf

25. Singh JA. Research and legal liability. Acta Trop. 2009;112 Suppl 1:S71–5.

26. Lang T, Cheah PY, White NJ. Clinical research: time for sensible global guidelines. Lancet. 2011;377:1553–5.

27. Hoekman J, Frenken K, Zeeuw D, Heerspink HL. The geographical distribution of leadership in globalized clinical trials. PLoS One. 2012;7(10):e45984.

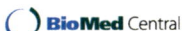

13.3   Improving the Informed Consent Process in International Collaborative Rare Disease Research: Effective Consent for Effective Research

Sabina Gainott, Cathy Turner, Simon Woods, Anna Kole, Pauline McCormack, Hanns Lochmüller, Olaf Riess, Volker Straub, Manuel Posada, Domenica Taruscio, and Deborah Mascalzoni

Gainotti, S, Turner, C, Woods, S, Kole, A, McCormack, P, et al. Improving the informed consent process in international collaborative rare disease research: effective consent for effective research. *European Journal of Human Genetics* 24, 1248–1254 (2016). © 2016 Macmillan Publishers Limited, part of Springer Nature. All rights reserved 1018–4813/16.

European Journal of Human Genetics (2016) 24, 1248–1254
© 2016 Macmillan Publishers Limited, part of Springer Nature. All rights reserved 1018-4813/16
www.nature.com/ejhg

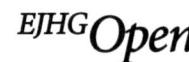

ARTICLE

Improving the informed consent process in international collaborative rare disease research: effective consent for effective research

Sabina Gainotti[*,1,9], Cathy Turner[2], Simon Woods[3,9], Anna Kole[4,9], Pauline McCormack[3,9],
Hanns Lochmüller[2,9], Olaf Riess[5], Volker Straub[2], Manuel Posada[6,9], Domenica Taruscio[1,9] and
Deborah Mascalzoni[7,8,9]

The increased international sharing of data in research consortia and the introduction of new technologies for sequencing challenge the informed consent (IC) process, adding complexities that require coordination between research centres worldwide. Rare disease consortia present special challenges since available data and samples may be very limited. Thus, it is especially relevant to ensure the best use of available resources but at the same time protect patients' right to integrity. To achieve this aim, there is an ethical duty to plan in advance the best possible consent procedure in order to address possible ethical and legal hurdles that could hamper research in the future. Therefore, it is especially important to identify key core elements (CEs) to be addressed in the IC documents for international collaborative research in two different situations: (1) new research collections (biobanks and registries) for which information documents can be created according to current guidelines and (2) established collections obtained without IC or with a previous consent that does not cover all CEs. We propose here a strategy to deal with consent in these situations. The principles have been applied and are in current practice within the RD-Connect consortia – a global research infrastructure funded by the European Commission Seventh Framework program but forward looking in terms of issues addressed. However, the principles established, the lessons learned and the implications for future research are of direct relevance to all internationally collaborative rare-disease projects.
European Journal of Human Genetics (2016) 24, 1248–1254; doi:10.1038/ejhg.2016.2; published online 10 February 2016

INFORMED CONSENT FOR RARE DISEASE RESEARCH IN THE ERA OF GLOBAL DATA SHARING AND NEXT-GENERATION SEQUENCING

Fostering global data sharing that allows collaborative work on scarce and disparate resources is essential for research into rare diseases (RDs).[1]

The challenges posed by new sequencing technologies and the world-wide dimension of data sharing require research consortia to adapt existing informed consent (IC) procedures to a new reality and ensure that consent processes are relevant and useful for ongoing and new collections.

For RD patients, research is often the only hope for future treatments and in some cases the only possibility for getting a diagnosis. This creates a status of special vulnerability in RD patients that could lead them to accept conditions which they might not in other circumstances. Therefore, it is especially important to identify guidance that will foster the right to enjoy the benefits of scientific progress for RD patients and at the same time respect patients' rights and values:[2-7] we regard it as an ethical duty to plan ahead the best possible consent procedures in order to anticipate and avoid ethical and legal hurdles that could hamper research in the future.

RD-Connect is a global research infrastructure[8] aimed at developing an integrated platform in which omics data will be combined with clinical phenotype information and biomaterial from multiple RD projects including EURenOmics[9] and NeurOmics.[10]

We suggest that RD-Connect poses relevant ethical challenges, which are common to other international research projects focused on omics research and can therefore be used to learn common lessons. There are sensitive topics that need special consideration in the consent process such as return of incidental findings to participants; the ties to family members and possible obligations arising from research results; the future use of samples; the limits or the foreseen sharing of data derived from next-generation sequencing (NGS);[11] as well as the difficulty to explain and enforce the right to withdraw from research in the light of global sharing. The very nature of genomic research promotes a widespread dissemination and ongoing reuse of data and participants should be made aware that different actors and bodies (ie, research ethics committees (RECs), internal governing boards and external reviewers) will be responsible to decide on their behalf for future uses and for reviewing and evaluating access requests from external researchers.[12-14] This means that the protection of their integrity is delegated to a system that should be explained and disclosed.[12-14]

[1]National Centre for Rare Diseases, Istituto Superiore di Sanità, Rome, Italy; [2]Institute of Genetic Medicine, Newcastle University International Centre for Life, Newcastle upon Tyne, UK; [3]PEALS (Policy, Ethics and Life Sciences) Research Centre, Newcastle University, Newcastle upon Tyne, UK; [4]EURORDIS, Rare Disease Europe, Paris, France; [5]Institute of Human Genetics and Applied Genomics, University of Tubingen, Tubingen, Germany; [6]Institute of Rare Diseases Research, SpainRDR & CIBERER, ISCIII, Madrid, Spain; [7]Center for Research Ethics and Bioethics, Uppsala University, Uppsala, Sweden; [8]Center for Biomedicine, EURAC Research, Bolzano, Italy
*Correspondence: Dr S Gainotti, National Centre for Rare Diseases, Istituto Superiore di Sanità, v.le Regina Elena 299, 00162 Rome, Italy. Tel. +39 0649904095, Fax: +39 0649904370; E-mail: sabina.gainotti@iss.it
[9]These authors are partners in RD-Connect.
Received 7 August 2015; revised 23 November 2015; accepted 8 December 2015; published online 10 February 2016

In fact specific features of omics research, and in this case of the global RD-Connect platform, raise particular challenges for the IC process as they add new ethical and legal complexities and require coordination and harmonisation between different research centres worldwide.[15–17]

IC is traditionally discussed in terms of its function as a means to ensuring respect for personal autonomy, integrity, self determination and the right to privacy.[18]

In RD research respecting privacy can be especially challenging since, in certain cases, it would suffice to link basic information like the name of the disease and the name of the treating physician or the specific ultra-rare sequence change and the place of origin to trace back individual patients.[19–22] In 'undiagnosed cases' clinical and genetic data (and occasionally also patient images) are often entered into databases expressly conceived to facilitate the matching of cases with similar phenotypic and genotypic profiles (eg, the Matchmaker Exchange project http://www.matchmakerexchange.org/).

Family contact and therefore re-identification is common practice to build a full data set, and it is often necessary to be able to re-contact and re-identify patients. This is usually accepted by patients and relatives because it is only through the promotion of research that they will progress towards a diagnosis or a cure,[23] but requires that participants are carefully informed of the risk as codification cannot ensure a zero risk of re-identification.[22]

To address those special concerns we tried to determine the kind of information that should be required for this type of research in international consortia in the form of core elements (CEs) required for informing patients in research.

The CEs recommended in our guidelines are in response to particular legal and ethical requirements identified through an extensive literature analysis and on the values identified through stakeholder involvement.

Key values identified by stakeholders at a workshop held in Rome in April 2014 with patients, scientists, industry and ethicists include:

1. Respect for patients' and patients' families' integrity;
2. The right to enjoy the benefits of scientific advancement;
3. Altruism and solidarity.[24]

All such values are assumed to hold within an environment where trust is well-placed.[25] RD research is often conducted in a context in which the research is closely tied to patient care and is merged in the route to diagnosis. The current request made by key funders for research to be conducted in the international context of data sharing, possibly with unspecified partners, may not always be clear enough to patients. The link between research and this close, clinical relationship should be made transparent and explicit so respecting the special trust granted by participants.[26]

Also, participants should be offered the possibility to decide the level of accessibility of their data, especially in matchmaking databases where researchers must decide to make a case 'private' (visible and accessible only by themselves), 'matchable' (visible by all users and accessible upon request) and 'public' (visible and accessible by all users).

The discussed sharing practice can get really problematic if it does not also include an explicit sharing of responsibilities, which could be facilitated through the adoption of a 'Code of Conduct' and a system of unique identifiers for researchers.[27] Researchers not directly involved in a caring relationship with the RD patient might perceive that they are not bound by the same medical or deontological framework as are treating clinicians.

INFORMED CONSENT FOR NEW RESEARCH COLLECTIONS

In the last decade, there has been a shift from a specific IC paradigm to a paradigm that tries to take into account the values of beneficence, solidarity, justice, reciprocity, mutuality, citizenship and universality.[28–33]

Different models such as broad consent and dynamic consent have been proposed as possible solutions to some of the ethical challenges described above, like future uses and international sharing of samples and data derived from NGS, return of incidental findings to participants and family members and difficulty to enforce the right to withdraw from research.[34–37]

Focus groups carried out with RD patient representatives (http://rd-connect.eu/platform/ethics/rd-pec/)[38] highlighted that RD patients generally find acceptable broadly described purposes for the use of biomaterials and data for biobanks. However, many would prefer to see access to their data more strictly controlled. Also, RD patients foresaw a number of possible risks for themselves, their children and/or other family members; most notably discrimination in such areas as employment, health-care access and financial matters.

Therefore, we propose that if broadly descriptive consent is to be adopted, then this should be supplemented by providing participants with additional safeguards and opportunities for being updated.[39] Patients may accept data sharing and find broadly described purposes of a research acceptable, provided there is clarity about governance of data and samples, re-contact policies, privacy measures, ethical oversight, clear withdrawal policy and a commitment to keep participants informed if major changes in these areas occur.

For RD patients, research is often the only hope for future treatments and in some cases the only possibility for getting a diagnosis, and RD patients and their families are usually highly motivated to participate and have a significant role in the research process. The need to re-contact and involve patients in research takes advantage of patient-centric approaches to consent that provide dynamic interaction exploiting online technologies to help address new challenges. Online tools can assist with ongoing information and participant involvement regarding new studies.[40,41]

During the IC process, new research participants as well as participants who are re-consenting are entitled to understand to what extent they are involved in research and the kind of control that is granted to them on the use of their data and samples.

The challenges of this procedure are on many levels and include the need to explain genomic research in simple language as well as to provide information about the potential foreseeable uses of data and samples.[11,42,43]

It is therefore important that:

- Researchers make a sincere attempt to provide clear information in patient friendly form and include the CEs (as defined below);
- Information is provided to patients at least when major changes occur and by sharing general results (brochures, colloquium, internet pages, mass media);
- The formal decision (consent) should take place after the information process, allowing participants appropriate time to think, reflect and ask questions;
- A description of the communication of information strategy for the future (after the collection) is provided to the participant;
- Wherever possible patient/participant representatives are consulted on the quality, detail and clarity of the information provided before a study starts.

1250

CORE INFORMATION ELEMENTS

There are some essential requirements for a valid IC,[17,44,45] including age and legal capacity of the participant, freedom of choice and voluntariness – implying the right to withdraw from research at any moment without prejudice. IC in human research must clearly describe research objectives, procedures, risks involved and expected benefits to potential participants. As voluntariness is a precondition of participation in research and IC aims to support a free informed decision, the elements that mostly impact the risk/benefit ratio of the project should always be disclosed.

A broad description of the kind of research expected at the time of the collection is acceptable, provided transparent information about the CEs is provided.

CEs should be included in the IC material for ongoing and future collections occurring in global consortia[46,47] (Box 1):

1. *Study procedure:* descriptions should address how and for how long the storage and conservation of samples and data is planned; access policies; security measures; the use and sharing of the data for research; and information on options for future uses.
2. *Reasonably anticipated benefits:* participants are made aware that there will probably be no direct personal benefits, though it might be reasonable to describe potential secondary benefits, for example, in the case of registries, participants may be kept up-to-date about ongoing clinical trials for their RD. Also, participants without a clear diagnosis may benefit in terms of advancing knowledge on the causes of their condition and possibly find the causative gene.
3. *Foreseeable informational risks:* these include the potential loss of confidentiality caused by misuse of data, misconduct, hacking, the chance of information about a family member being divulged in one's country and abroad, also in jurisdictions that may have different data protection provisions in place. The current evidence does not allow us to draw conclusions about the efficacy of de-identification methods;[48] therefore, participants should be aware that their data will be accessed, shared and linked to other sets of information, that there exist different data protection regulations in different countries and that, while all reasonable efforts will be made to protect confidentiality, the purpose and extent of further usage cannot be foreseen. Participants should be made aware specifically if their medical records will be accessed and how these may be used alongside data from research studies.
4. *International data sharing:* in a research scenario where the data are shared widely and frequently, the sharing process must be clearly described. Several studies show that research participants across a range of populations and disease groups wish to be informed whether wide data-sharing procedures are implemented.[49,50] Participants should be informed that their coded data will be placed in international archives such as the European Genome-phenome Archive (EGA), where access to data will be overseen and decided by a data access committee according to established principles and criteria. Information on the use of interoperable identifiers allowing matching between different databases also needs to be provided. Interoperable identifiers, created by using the same data elements in different databases with different algorithms will enable researchers to follow patients over time and across diseases, registries, studies and countries and avoid duplicating efforts by matching data collected at different times and by different entities, including linking patients' clinical information recorded in registries to biological samples available in one or more biobanks.
5. *Use of NGS techniques:* participants must be informed that their samples are likely to be analysed using large-scale genome

---

Box 1 Essential elements of IC documents for International Consortia on RD

Information elements that are relevant in IC documents for biobank and observational studies in RD Research

- General (name of the PI, Institution, funding, duration, over-sight, contact persons)
- Aims, research uses of data (eg, cancer research and RD research)
- Voluntariness of participation and possibility to withdraw
- Procedures involved in participation, including interviews and blood taking
- Kinds of samples and data that will be collected
- Potential physical, psychological and social risks (informational risks)
- Potential benefits of participation
- Protections in place locally to ensure the confidentiality of samples and data
- Access to data/samples for research purposes: who will have access, who should control and what the procedures in place (data access committee)
- Access to data/samples for purposes such as validation and quality control
- Study oversight
- Compensation/reimbursement
- Custodianship of samples
- Study dissemination plans (professional journals/lay versions/codified or aggregated results only/specific results/patient pictures and occasionally short professional video sequences).

CEs for the IC of studies participating to international RD research

- Possibility of data sharing across research groups and national borders
- Possibility of large-scale genome sequencing techniques
- Return of secondary findings
- Hosting of the data in open access database (eg, in RD-Connect the European Genome-Phenome Archive)
- Use of interoperable identifiers for the de-identification of participants
- Access by industry if foreseen and prospects for third-party commercialisation and intellectual property
- Possible linkage to different data (registries, medical records, etc.)
- Withdrawal procedures, such as sample retrieval and/or destruction and difficulties in ensuring the right to withdraw for the data already shared
- Permission to re-contact

---

sequencing techniques that carry potential for clinically relevant discoveries for individuals and families. A brief description of the techniques used should be given and the aim of the analysis explained, including the possibility of discovering previously unknown mutations relating to their condition as well as 'disease modifier' genes which do not directly cause the condition but might affect its severity and its course.

6. *Return of secondary findings and access to sequences:* this is a very sensitive issue that needs to be addressed.[51] As there are no shared guidelines on this matter the IC should at least state if return is

planned or not. If not, when sequencing is performed, it should be clear whether individuals may ask permission to access their sequencing in order to seek advice elsewhere. If return is planned, then it should be detailed how the re-contact will occur; if the health-care system will be involved, then what are the researchers' options if results have implications for family members. Return of secondary findings should always be optional and not forced. As it is unclear to what extent or how secondary findings may impact individuals in future discoveries, this is a strong argument for asking the participants if they want to be re-contacted or not.

7. *Procedures for data access:* Core elements should also include details of the procedures for data access[52] and the persons entitled to access the data, *including industry access* with prospects for third-party commercialisation and intellectual property procedures.[53]

8. *Right to withdraw:* a research participant holds a right to withdraw from research at any time,[18] but wide sharing and an open research programme create a problem for the execution of the right to withdraw. It must be acknowledged therefore that there may be some practical limitations in respecting the right to withdraw, in particular that while it is always possible to withdraw and deny access for future research projects, it may be impossible to withdraw from a specific research project for which one's data may have already been accessed.[12] The name of the person legally responsible for data as well as specimen custodianship must be available.

9. *Permission to re-contact:* permission to re-contact should always be pursued in order to allow unexpected events to be addressed in the future. If the project does not ask permission then this may lead to the impossibility of re-contact in the future.

10. *The information strategy on a general level should be described:* the strategy may vary greatly from project to project but it should be clear whether the plan foresees individual information being returned or whether the study is planning to publish newsletters, or information on a webpage dedicated to patients.

We suggest the inclusion of the following items in the IC, as it seems reasonable and will provide greater flexibility to researchers and participants:

11. Destination of data and biospecimens after death or in the case of the termination of the project;

12. Access to research results by family members if foreseen, or after death.

Participants should preferably be allowed to express choices with regard to the CEs. CEs are moving targets and the need to re-contact patients in the future is foreseeable. Therefore, we strongly recommend that permission is sought to be able to re-contact participants and ask them for contact details. Of course they may freely refuse this option.

USE OF EXISTING BIOSPECIMENS COLLECTION

The use of biological samples and data outside the purpose originally described in the consent form is usually considered as 'secondary use'.[54] The original consent, usually describing the aims of the 'primary use' of donation and/or data collection may not contemplate one or more CEs previously defined.[17]

Given the scarcity of biospecimens in RDs, existing collections are extremely precious. As such, every effort should be made to use existing data and samples by looking at feasible ways for preserving and maximising their use in the future.[55,56]

In some jurisdictions, institutional review boards/research ethics committees (IRBs/RECs) can determine whether sharing a participant's data for research purposes is consistent with the IC of study participants from whom the data were originally obtained. However, IRBs/REC can differ in their decisions even in countries where there is guidance or legislation.[15]

In international consortia using RD data and samples we suggest that, whenever possible, the original IC document used in existing collections be revised by the local investigator subject to IRB/REC approval to ensure that IC is compliant. If CEs are missing and re-contact is feasible (as in the case of regular follow-up visits with the researcher), then a re-consent is required. This may be done by actively asking participants' permission (opt-in) or by sending participants a notification and a description of the research project and presuming his/her consent unless s/he declines participation (opt-out).

Although the 'opt-in' option is always preferable, there may be instances in which the request may not be highly sensitive (few CEs missing in the original IC document), the costs of re-consent may be considered as too high for researchers in terms of possible drop outs, the re-contact may involve very old cohorts or the number of people to be re-consented may be very high. However, this is not likely to be the case in RD research.

For some cohorts, the researcher may still find re-consent achievable within reasonable efforts, using this also as an opportunity to update or collect new data. Other projects may be particularly vulnerable to drop outs and here one may want to use a scheme with notification and opt-out.

A clear distinction should be made between collections in which a previous consent was obtained and a question was not asked, and one where a patient actively declined an option or in which the information provided excluded some options (eg, 'your data will not be shared with any commercial organisations'). In the last instances, opt-in re-consenting should always be pursued in order to verify whether these options are now acceptable to the participant.

OPT-IN RE-CONSENT

Opt-in procedures require the participant/donor to actively give permission. Rare disease research may be particularly vulnerable to selection bias because the number of available samples and data is intrinsically low for each condition. However, careful consideration of the time, effort and other resources required to adequately re-consent patients should be given, as re-consent may also result in the benefits of better patient engagement, reducing drop-out rates and increasing donors' motivation to participate in research projects. Also, re-consent would be the occasion to effectively broaden the scope of participants' consent, thus ensuring its broad validity in future research projects.

An analysis of the costs associated with consent should also include an examination of the costs of 'no consent' or badly designed consent for the use of samples and information. If research participants feel that relevant information has been withheld from them, then this may result in a loss of public trust in research; and therefore, a reduction in participation in future studies, loss of opportunity for follow-up and loss of patient organisation support in research projects.[57] Some studies indicate that patients are more willing to share their data when procedures are in place that give them more control over the way their data are used.[58] Establishing a better dialogue about research with a patient cohort may lead to a more motivated, informed and proactive patient community.[59] Trust and transparency

1252

may be increased and drop-out rates may reduce, as the NeurOmics experience illustrates below.

OPT-OUT STRATEGIES

In an opt-out procedure, the participant/donor receives a notification and a description of the research project and consent is presumed unless he/she declines participation. Opt-out methods are designed to minimise the burdens of eliciting IC from a large number of patients while providing those who do not wish to contribute the opportunity to exercise that preference[60] although studies show that donors/participants are not always favourable to opt-out schemes.[61-63] Therefore, this option may only be justified when re-contact is not achievable with reasonable efforts.

The fact that opt-out options do not affect research in terms of drop outs is supported by the report of a Swedish study.[64] Recent legislation in Finland also supports this view, and foresees the implementation of opt-out options for registries and biobanks.[65]

WAIVER OF CONSENT

Although having a valid consent in place is the most ethical option, there are instances in which a waiver may be requested to ethical boards, especially where it is determined that re-contacting patients requires disproportionate effort or is impossible (perhaps because of lack of contact details or patients lost to follow-up). This waiver should contain an explanation why participants should or could not be re-contacted. New consent procedures may ensure that this occurrence will be minimised in the future by asking specific permission to look up contact information for re-contacting patients.

This option is not feasible in every legal system and requires an adequate assessment of the reasons for asking for a waiver from the ethics review board.

The 'moral endorsement' of patient organisations could be sought in order to ensure that the patient community is aware of, and agrees with, certain uses of data and samples related to their diseases.[66]

Indeed patient associations often have an educational role, and patient representatives dedicate a lot of time and efforts to explain to other RD patients the kind of research that is conducted and highlighting the importance of participating in clinical and observational research.

Even if re-consent is perceived as burdensome and detrimental to research by many researchers, positive outcomes can come by its practice.

THE NEUROMICS EXPERIENCE

The NeurOmics project is facing many of these consent and re-contact issues now. As a partner project of RD-Connect,[10] NeurOmics is undertaking whole-exome sequencing and deep phenotyping of 1100 genetically-undiagnosed rare neuromuscular and neurodegenerative disease patients.

NeurOmics has therefore worked closely with RD-Connect in order to recommend CEs to be included in any consent forms used by partners contributing samples. Templates were circulated to all partners collecting samples and data in January 2013. This template included permission to have samples included in genetic research, specified how data would be accessed – including by international and commercial partners, made clear that unrelated findings would not be returned, asked for permission to re-contact and made clear the right to withdraw from the research. Partners were asked to check existing consent forms against this template.

NeurOmics investigators are requested to confirm that the consent necessary to share data is in place when entering phenotype data into the project's clinical database, PhenoTips.[67] Where this consent is not yet obtained, it is expected that patients will be re-contacted and re-consented following the guidelines proposed here (Figure 1) and drawn up by RD-Connect, NeurOmics and patient groups.

This has now resulted in the confirmed consent and therefore possible sharing of data for 976 of 1065 patients entered into the PhenoTips system. In the meantime, those remaining 89 patients are being re-contacted according to the proposed guidelines. In spite

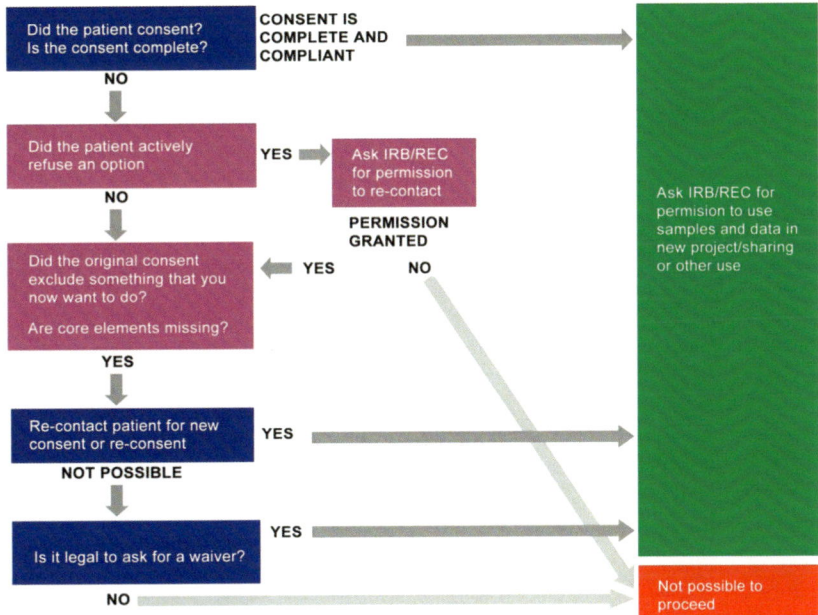

Figure 1 Procedures for using already collected samples.

of time and resource implications, which have understandably been a concern for partners, this re-contact has worked well and has had benefits beyond the obtaining of consent.

At the University of Newcastle, patients for whom consent was incomplete were contacted by telephone and/or letter in order to explain the changing research needs, data-sharing intentions and to request consent. This resulted in only one patient declining the request, around 80% returning new consents and 20% with no response so far – (still ongoing). Clinicians involved reported added benefits – up-to-date clinical and family information could be obtained, patients and their families were generally motivated to be involved in research, hear more about it and give further samples if required. Several patients reported that it was good to know that their (historic) sample was still being used and that they had not been forgotten. The clinicians were also able to use the contact to answer questions or concerns and manage patient expectations where required. The team at Newcastle University feel that this has resulted in a more engaged patient cohort and have reported this as a very positive outcome of investing the resources needed to undertake this updating of consent.

CONCLUDING REMARKS

In the era of genomic research and global data sharing, participants must deal with an unprecedented mass of information and complexity. Moreover, the information given today may be obsolete in the near future. The risks and the aims of research and the benefits of participation are not always completely foreseeable at the time the data and/or samples are collected.

In this current work we propose that, for the IC of prospective cases, broadly described research purposes with ongoing updates for participants is the best current solution. This allows for the requirement of research to have a flexible tool as well as the need for transparency and good ethical standards. Achieving a good balance between the level of understanding that is required for meaningful IC,[11,68] especially for data sharing in genomics, and the need for practical solutions, is burdensome without a system in place to engage participants. Therefore, dynamic options may be the future of research, especially in projects where a share of funding is devoted to the development of IT platforms.

If this option is not yet implementable, then we propose that at least:

- Regular updates on development and aggregated results of the project/biobank are given to participants;
- Patient participation is promoted at a more institutional level by involving patient organisations in governance, developing policies, practices and documentation.

Regarding established collections, the decision to ask for re-consent through active opt-in or opt-out procedures, or to ask for a waiver of consent from the IRB/REC, should be guided by a careful evaluation of the following elements:

- Possibility of re-contact and re-consent of patients within a reasonable effort (also dependent on researchers' resources, eg, availability of contact details and possibility to meet the patient during follow-up visits);
- Specificity of the original IC and number of CEs missing;
- Rarity of the collection and the disease under study;
- Endorsement by patient associations directly involved with the research and collections at stake.

The process of IC that we propose here is intended to enhance the involvement of participants, but we are aware that there are instances for which the applicability is not certain, for example, in very old collections.

The effort to create a good ethical framework for prospective use, including clear governance and good IC procedures, is an ethical obligation in the light of good, sound, well-thought procedures that allow scientific research to happen. Although our emphasis is on good ethical guidance, we understand that different legal jurisdictions may require different standards, even though the ethical principles are broadly applicable across different contexts. But, without doubt, it is necessary to plan ahead for better consent and ethical practices in future collections.

CONFLICT OF INTEREST

The authors declare no conflict of interest.

ACKNOWLEDGEMENTS

This work has been supported by the European Union Seventh Framework Programme (FP7/2007–2013) under grant agreements no. 305444 (RD-Connect), 305121 (Neuromics), and no. 305608 (EURenOmics) and RD-Connect from the Australian National Health and Medical Research Council APP1055319 under the NHMRC-European Union Collaborative Research Grants scheme' as well as the IMI project BTCure (grant agreement number 115142-1), the BioBanking and Molecular Resource Infrastructure of Sweden project, Biobanking and Biomolecular Resources Research Infrastructure (BBMRI)LPC. We thank the RD-Connect Patient Ethics Council and RD-Connect Patient Advisory Council (Jean Jacques Cassiman, Tracy Dudding, Muriel Gevrey, Emma Heslop, Joseph Irwin, Julian Isla, Sigurður Jóhannesson, Lydia Lemonnier, Chantal Loirat, Dorthe Lykke, Milan Macek, Caron Molster, Kay Parkinson, Odile Perrousseaux, Marita Pohlschmidt, Daniel Renault, Peter Reussner, Françoise Roualt, Balthasar Schaap, Inge Schwersenz, Chris Sotirelis, Oliver Timmis, Johannes van Delden, Marieke van Meel, Elizabeth Vroom and Urban Wiesing) and all RD-connect partners for their valuable inputs. We also thank RD researchers and patient representatives who participated to the workshop on informed consent held in Rome in 23–24 April 2014: Marco Crimi, Erica Daina, Fabrizio Farnetani, Vera Frankova, Elisabeth Hulier Ammar, Javier Judez, Daniel Renault, Françoise Roualt, Chris Sotileris, Virgilia Toccaceli and Paola Torreri.

1 International Rare Diseases Research Consortium (IRDIRC). Available at http://www.irdirc.org/ (accessed 29 September 2015).
2 EURORDIS Position Paper "WHY Research on Rare Diseases" Paris, October 2010. Available at http://www.eurordis.org/sites/default/files/publications/why_rare_disease_research.pdf (accessed 29 September 2015).
3 Regulation (EC) No 141/2000 of the European Parliament and the Council of 16 December 1999 on Orphan Medicinal Products; Official Journal of the European Communities, 22.1.2000: L 18/1-18/5.
4 Communication from the Commission to the European Parliament, the Council, the European Economic and Social Committee and the Committee of the Regions on Rare Diseases - Europe's challenges {SEC(2008)2713} {SEC(2008)2712} /* COM/ 2008/0679 final */.
5 Council Recommendation of 8 June 2009 on an action in the field of rare diseases (2009/C 151/02); Official Journal of the European Union, 3.7.2009: C 151/7 -151/10.
6 UNESCO. Venice statement on the right to enjoy the benefits of scientific progress and its applications, 2009. Available at http://unesdoc.unesco.org/images/0018/001855/185558e.pdf (accessed 29 September 2015).
7 Knoppers BM, Harris JR, Budin-Ljøsne I, Dove ES: A human rights approach to an international code of conduct for genomic and clinical data sharing. *Hum Genet* 2014; **133**: 895–903.
8 Thompson R, Johnston L, Taruscio D *et al*: RD-Connect: an integrated platform connecting databases, registries, biobanks and clinical bioinformatics for rare disease research. *J Gen Intern Med* 2014; **29** (Suppl 3): S780–S787.
9 EURenOmics: Cutting edge technologies for rare kidney diseases. Available at www.eurenomics.eu (accessed 29 September 2015).
10 NeurOmics: Integrated European Project on Omics Research of Rare Neuromuscular and Neurodegenerative Diseases. Available at www. http://rd-neuromics.eu/project-welcome/. (accessed 29 September 2015).
11 McGuire AL, Caulfield T, Cho MK: Research ethics and the challenge of whole-genome sequencing. *Nat Rev Genet* 2008; **9**: 152–156.

12 Melham K, Briceno Moraia L, Mitchell C, Morrison M, Teare H, Kaye J: The evolution of withdrawal: negotiating research relationships in biobanking. *Life Sci Soc Policy* 2014; **10**: 16.
13 Kosseim P, Dove ES, Baggaley C *et al*: Building a data sharing model for global genomic research. *Genome Biol* 2014; **15**: 430.
14 Tabor HK, Berkman BE, Hull SC *et al*: Genomics really gets personal: how exome and whole genome sequencing challenge the ethical framework of human genetics research. *Am J Med Genet A* 2011; **155**: 2916–2924.
15 Wallace SE, Knoppers BM: Harmonised consent in international research consortia: an impossible dream? Genomics. *Soc Policy* 2011; **7**: 35–46.
16 Budin-Ljøsne I, Isaeva J, Maria KB *et al*: Data sharing in large research consortia: experiences and recommendations from EnGaGe. *Eur J Hum Genet* 2014; **22**: 317–321.
17 Budin-Ljøsne I, Tassé AM, Knoppers BM *et al*: Bridging consent: from toll bridges to lift bridges? *BMC Med Genomics* 2011; **4**: 69.
18 World Medical Association Declaration of Helsinki - Ethical Principles for Medical Research Involving Human Subjects. Adopted by the 18th WMA General Assembly, Helsinki, Finland, June 1964. Last amended by the 64th WMA General Assembly, Fortaleza, Brazil, October 2013.
19 McGuire AL, Gibbs RA: Genetics. No longer de-identified. *Science* 2006; **312**: 370–371.
20 Lowrance WW, Collins FS: Ethics. Identifiability in genomic research. *Science* 2007; **317**: 600–602.
21 Malin B, Sweeney L: How (not) to protect genomic data privacy in a distributed network: using trail re-identification to evaluate and design anonymity protection systems. *J Biomed Inform* 2004; **37**: 179–192.
22 El Emam K, Rodgers S, Malin B: Anonymising and sharing individual patient data. *Br Med J* 2015; **350**: h1139.
23 Kent A: Consent and confidentiality: whose information is it anyway? *J Med Ethics* 2003; **29**: 16–18.
24 Woods S, McCormack P: Disputing the ethics of research: the challenge from bioethics and patient activism to the interpretation of the Declaration of Helsinki in clinical trials. *Bioethics* 2013; **27**: 243–250.
25 O'Neill O. *Autonomy and Trust in Bioethics*. Cambridge University Press: Cambridge, 2002
26 Berkman BE, Hull SC, Eckstein L: The unintended implications of blurring the line between research and clinical care in a genomic age. *Per Med* 2014; **11**: 285–295.
27 Knoppers BM, Harris JR, Tassé AM *et al*: Towards a data sharing Code of Conduct for international genomic research. *Genome Med* 2011; **3**: 46.
28 Chadwick R, Berg K: Solidarity and equity: new ethical frameworks for genetic databases. *Nat Rev Genet* 2001; **2**: 318–321.
29 Graeme L: Genetic databases: assessing the benefits and the impact on human and patient rights—A World Health Organisation Report. *Eur J Health Law* 2004; **11**: 79–84.
30 Knoppers BM, Chadwick R: Human genetic research: emerging trends in ethics. *Nat Rev Genet* 2005; **6**: 75–79.
31 Hoedemaekers R, Gordijn B, Pijnenburg M: Solidarity and justice as guiding principles in genomic research. *Bioethics* 2007; **21**: 342–350.
32 Gottweis H, Gaskell G, Starkbaum J: Connecting the public with biobank research: reciprocity matters. *Nat Rev Genet* 2001; **12**: 738–739.
33 Praisnack B, Buyx A: A solidarity-based approach to the governance of research biobanks. *Med Law Rev* 2013; **21**: 71–91.
34 Hansson MG, Dillner J, Bartram CR, Carlson JA, Helgesson G: Should donors be allowed to give broad consent to future biobank research? *Lancet Oncol* 2006; **7**: 266–269.
35 Mascalzoni D, Hicks A, Pramstaller P, Wjst M: IC in the genomics era. *PLoS Med* 2008; **5**: e192.
36 Kaye J: Broad consent is informed consent. *Br Med J* 2011; **343**: d6900.
37 Sheehan M, Martin J: Can broad consent be IC? *Public Health Ethics* 2011; **4**: 226–235.
38 McCormack P, Kole A, Turner C, Woods S: Consent, collaboration and cures: the views of rare disease patients on systems for sharing data and biospecimens. *Figshare* 2015; https://dx.doi.org/10.6084/m9.figshare.1318777.v1.
39 Mascalzoni D, Dove E, Rubinstein Y *et al*: International Charter of principles for sharing bio-specimens and data. *Eur J Hum Genet* 2014; **23**: 721–728.
40 Kaye J, Whitley EA, Lund D, Morrison M, Teare H, Melham K: Dynamic consent: a patient interface for twenty-first century research networks. *Eur J Hum Genet* 2015; **23**: 141–146.
41 Kaye J, Curren L, Anderson N *et al*: From patients to partners: participant-centric initiatives in biomedical research. *Nat Rev Genet* 2012; **13**: 371–376.
42 Ponder M, Statham H, Hallowell N *et al*: Genetic research on rare familial disorders: consent and the blurred boundaries between clinical service and research. *J Med Ethics* 2008; **34**: 690–694.

43 Kaye J, Heeney C, Hawkins N, de Vries J, Boddington P: Data sharing in genomics: re-shaping scientific practice. *Nat Rev Genet* 2009; **10**: 331–335.
44 Council for International Organizations of Medical Sciences. International Ethical Guidelines for Biomedical Research Involving Human Subjects, 2002. Available at http://www.cioms.ch/publications/guidelines/guidelines_nov_2002_blurb.htm (accessed 29 September 2015).
45 Organisation for Economic Co-operation and Development. Guidelines for Human Biobanks and Genetic Research Databases (HBGRDs). Available at http://www.oecd.org/dataoecd/41/47/44054609.pdf (accessed 29 September 2015).
46 Rubinstein YR, Groft SC, Hull S *et al*: IC process for patient participation in rare disease registries linked to biorepositories. *Contemp Clin Trials* 2011; **33**: 5–11.
47 Mallette A, Tassé AM: P3G generic Information Pamphlet and Consent Form (2014). Available at http://www.p3g.org/system/files/biobank_toolkit_documents/P3G%20Generic%20Info%20Pamphlet%20and%20Consent%20Form%20for%20Biobanks.pdf (accessed 29 September 2015).
48 El Emam K, Jonker E, Arbuckle L *et al*: A systematic review of re-identification attacks on health data. *PLoS One* 2011; **6**: e28071.
49 Oliver JM, Slashinski MJ, Wang T *et al*: Balancing the risks and benefits of genomic data sharing: genome research participants' perspectives. *Public Health Genomics* 2012; **2**: 106–114.
50 Ludman EJ, Fullerton SM, Spangler L *et al*: Glad you asked: participants' opinions of re-consent for dbGaP data submission. *J Empir Res Hum Res Ethics* 2010; **5**: 9–16.
51 Appelbaum PS, Parens E, Waldman CR *et al*: Models of consent to return of incidental findings in genomic research. *Hastings Cent Rep* 2014; **44**: 22–32.
52 Shabani M, Knoppers BM, Borry P: From the principles of genomic data sharing to the practices of data access committees. *EMBO Mol Med* 2015; **7**: 507–509.
53 Nicol D: The impact of commercialisation and genetic data sharing arrangements on public trust and the intention to participate in biobank research. *Public Health Genomics* 2015; **18**: 160–172.
54 P3G Observatory, Lexicon, online. Available at http://www.p3gobservatory.org/lexicon/list.htms (accessed 29 September 2015).
55 Høyer K: Donors perceptions of consent to and feedback from biobank research: time to acknowledge diversity? *Public Health Genomics* 2009; **13**: 345–352.
56 Steinsbekk KS, Solberg B: Biobanks—when is re-consent necessary? *Public Health Ethics* 2011; **4**: 236–250.
57 Resnik DB: Re-consenting human subjects: ethical, legal and practical issues. *J Med Ethics* 2009; **35**: 656–657.
58 Damschrodera LJ, Prittsc JL, Neblod MA *et al*: Patients, privacy and trust: patients' willingness to allow researchers to access their medical records. *Soc Sci Med* 2007; **64**: 223–235.
59 Levy D, Splansky GL, Strand NK *et al*: Consent for genetic research in the Framingham Heart Study. *Am J Med Genet A* 2010; **152A**: 1250–1256.
60 Brothers KB, Westbrook MJ, Wright MF *et al*: Patient awareness and approval for an opt-out genomic biorepository. *Per Med* 2013; **10**: 349–359.
61 Kaufman D, Bollinger J, Dvoskin R, Scott J: Preferences for opt-in and opt-out enrollment and consent models in biobank research: a national survey of Veterans Administration patients. *Genet Med* 2012; **14**: 787–794.
62 McCartney M: Care.data doesn't care enough about consent. *BMJ* 2014; **348**: g2831.
63 Moberly T: Care.data must become an opt-in system, say doctors. *BMJ* 2014; **348**: g4284.
64 Johnsson L, Hansson MG, Eriksson S *et al*: Patients' refusal to consent to storage and use of samples in Swedish biobanks: cross sectional study. *BMJ* 2008; **337**: a345.
65 Forsberg JS, Soini S: A big step for Finnish biobanking. *Nat Rev Genet* 2014; **15**: 6.
66 Renault D: Patients perspective in EURenOmics on consent and re-consent. Presentation made at the Workshop on informed consent, Rome, 23–24 April 2014.
67 Girdea M, Dumitriu S, Fiume M *et al*: PhenoTips: Patient phenotyping software for clinical and research use. *Hum Mutat* 2013; **34**: 1057–1065.
68 Lunshof JE, Chadwick R, Vorhaus DB, Church GM: From genetic privacy to open consent. *Nat Rev Genet* 2008; **9**: 406–411.

Supplementary Information accompanies this paper on European Journal of Human Genetics website (http://www.nature.com/ejhg)

13.4 The Standard of Care Debate: Can Research in Developing Countries Be Both Ethical and Responsive To Those Countries' Health Needs?

David Wendler, Ezekiel J. Emanuel, and Reidar K. Lie

Wendler, D, Emanuel, E, Lie, R. The standard of care debate: Can research in developing countries be both ethical and responsive to those countries' health needs? *American Journal of Public Health* 94(6), 923–928 (2004).

| HEALTH POLICY AND ETHICS FORUM |

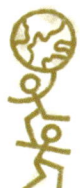

The Standard of Care Debate: Can Research in Developing Countries Be Both Ethical and Responsive to Those Countries' Health Needs?

| David Wendler, PhD, Ezekiel J. Emanuel, MD, PhD, and Reidar K. Lie, MD, PhD

To avoid exploitaiton of host communities, many commentators argue that subjects must receive the best methods available worldwide. Others worry that this requirement may block important research intended to improve health care, especially in developing countries.

To resolve this dilemma, we propose a framework for the conditions under which it is acceptable to provide subjects with less than the best methods. Specifically, institutional review boards should assume a default of requiring the "worldwide best" methods, meaning the best methods available anywhere in the world, in all cases.

However, institutional review boards should be willing to grant exceptions to this default for research studies that satisfy the following 4 conditions: (1) scientific necessity, (2) relevance for the host community, (3) sufficient host community benefit, and (4) subject and host community nonmaleficence. (*Am J Public Health.* 2004;94:923–928)

THE DISTRIBUTION OF HEALTH care around the world is marked by dramatic inequalities. Individuals in developed countries typically have access to safe water, new vaccines, and effective medications; individuals in developing countries often have access to little or no health care at all. These inequalities in health care have contributed to significant inequalities in health, with individuals who happen to live in the developing world experiencing far greater disease burdens and far shorter lives than individuals in the developed world. These inequalities have also led to a debate over what clinical investigators can do to improve health care in developing countries and thereby reduce health disparities between rich and poor.[1–6]

To protect host communities from exploitation, most commentators argue that efforts to improve health care in the developing world should never involve research that uses less than the "worldwide best"[7] methods, meaning the best methods available anywhere in the world.[8–15] Most notably, paragraph 29 of the Declaration of Helsinki states: "The benefits, risks, burdens, and effectiveness of a new method should be tested against those of the best current prophylactic, diagnostic, and therapeutic methods."[7] Similarly, Shapiro and Meslin, chairman and executive director of the US National Bioethics Advisory Commission write: "In our view, an experimental intervention should normally be compared with an established, effective treatment . . . whether or not that treatment is available in the host [developing] country."[16(p140)]

A ban on research using less than the worldwide best methods would definitively address the potential for such research to exploit host communities. Yet, such a ban may also block important research designed to improve health care for the world's poor. Is it possible to address the potential for exploitation while allowing research that has the potential to benefit the host communities?

The debate over what standard of care should be required for individuals participating in research trials typically focuses on research conducted in developing countries by investigators from developed countries. This focus makes sense. Most clinical research is conducted by investigators from developed countries, and most communities lacking access to good health care are located in developing countries. Nonetheless, researchers from developing countries may also exploit host communities. And communities in developed countries sometimes lack access to the best methods available worldwide, increasing the potential that they may be exploited. A complete analysis, then, should address the potential for exploitation independent of the nationality of the investigators,

or the geographic location of the study.

SCIENTIFIC NECESSITY

Some critics argue that research using less than the best methods available worldwide—medications, procedures, interventions, vaccines—is never scientifically necessary.[9,10,15] They conclude that requiring the best methods in all cases would allow investigators to obtain the same scientific information while providing greater benefits to subjects. This argument has focused on the controversial HIV vertical transmission trials.

So-called long-course treatment, also known as the 076 regimen, was—and remains—the best method for preventing transmission of HIV infection from mother to child. Unfortunately, the "early prenatal visits, intravenous infusion during labor, and cost" associated with long-course treatment make it neither affordable nor feasible in developing countries, where the burden of HIV disease is greatest.[17(p786)] To identify a method to help individuals in developing countries, investigators compared a less expensive, more easily administered "short course" of zidovudine (AZT) to what these individuals typically receive to prevent vertical trans-

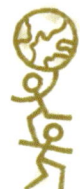

mission—namely, no treatment at all. Criticism of these trials was widespread, with commentators arguing that the control arms could have used long-course AZT rather than no treatment, thus reducing the number of HIV-infected babies in the trials without undermining the scientific importance of the resulting data.[8–10,13]

Before the start of the short-course trials, data from South Africa showed wide variation in the HIV vertical transmission rate in untreated individuals over time, even at the same location.[18] These data provided compelling evidence, *ex ante*, that any assessment of short-course AZT needed an untreated control arm to determine whether the intervention was better than no treatment at all. This need for a no-treatment control arm was confirmed by the results of the trials themselves.

The transmission rates found in the trials—18.9% to 27.5% in the placebo arm[19–23] and 9.9% to 18% in the short-course arm—confirm that an equivalence trial

could well have shown a long-course transmission rate of 8%, and a short-course transmission rate of 17% (Table 1). Comparing this short-course transmission rate to the 076 placebo transmission rate of 25% would suggest that short-course treatment is better than placebo and possibly worth pursuing. Yet, the variability in the placebo transmission rate reveals that the placebo rate in an equivalence trial might have been 19%, suggesting that short-course treatment was not worth pursuing. The important point is that this result was a realistic possibility *at the outset,* implying that the trials needed a no-treatment arm to determine whether the short course was better than no treatment at all.

The literature, perhaps shaped by the debate over the HIV vertical transmission trials, has focused on what investigators may use as *controls* in clinical trials. Yet, a total ban on research using less than the best methods would also prevent investigators from assessing active agents that are

expected to be less effective than the worldwide best methods. This frequently overlooked implication of a total ban on less than the best methods is illustrated by the landmark nevirapine trials.

Approximately 75% of HIV vertical transmission occurs during or after delivery.[24] Thus, a treatment administered during delivery might offer a feasible, economical way to reduce HIV vertical transmission in developing countries, despite the fact that it would not affect the 25% of transmission that occurs during gestation.[25] This line of reasoning led investigators to nevirapine, a well-tolerated, low-cost, potent antiviral. A single 200-mg oral dose of nevirapine given during labor passes quickly through the placenta and has a long serum half-life.[26] Hence, a single dose of nevirapine given to the mother during labor, and to the infant within 72 hours of birth, might offer a feasible and affordable treatment for vertical HIV transmission in developing countries.

Because nevirapine does not offer protection against the approximately 25% of vertical transmission that occurs in utero, it was recognized at the time that it would be less effective than long-course AZT therapy. Hence, the requirement that trial participants receive the worldwide best methods implies that participants may not receive nevirapine alone, precluding assessment of nevirapine as a single agent. The human costs of this requirement are highlighted by the fact that trials conducted on nevirapine as a single agent have revolution-

ized perinatal HIV treatment in developing countries, potentially saving millions of lives.[27]

Determining whether a trial using less than the best methods is scientifically necessary requires clinical judgment based on the relevant probabilities: What are the chances the trial will answer an important question? What are the chances the same question can be answered by a trial using only the best methods? Because there is no infallible algorithm to answer these questions, institutional review boards will have to decide whether to allow less than the best methods on a case-by-case basis. To maximize subject benefit, institutional review boards should assume a default of requiring the best methods in all cases. From there, institutional review boards should allow research using less than the best methods only when scientifically necessary to answer an important question.

HOST COMMUNITY RELEVANCE

Provision of the best methods to everyone in the world would render incremental improvements in health care for developing countries otiose. To take just 1 example, approximately 10 million children die each year from diseases that could be prevented by aid amounting to less than 1% of the gross national product of developed countries.[28,29] Provision of such aid would save millions of lives and render unnecessary any research to assess whether less than the

TABLE 1—Outcomes of Short-Course AZT Vertical Transmission Trials: 1999–2000

Trial, Country, Year	Placebo Transmission Rate, %	Short-Course Transmission Rate, %	Long-Course Transmission Rate, %
076 Regimen, United States, 1999	25.5	NA	8.3
Placebo trial, Thailand, 1999	18.9	9.9	NA
Ivory Coast, 1999	24.9	15.7	NA
Ivory Coast, Burkina Faso, 1999	27.5	18.0	NA
Equivalence, Thailand, 2000	NA	10.5	6.5
Nevirapine, Uganda, 1999	25.1	13.1	NA

Note. AZT = zidovudine; NA = not available.

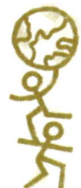

best methods may be partially effective in combating these diseases. Tragically, this aid has not been provided. In this context, research using less than the best methods sometimes represents the best hope for communities in developing countries to address their most significant health needs. When it does, when these trials address an important health need of communities in developing countries, the moral importance of helping the poor provides a strong argument in their favor.

SUFFICIENT HOST COMMUNITY BENEFIT

Even when scientifically necessary, and relevant to an important health concern of the host community, research using less than the best methods retains the potential to exploit host communities by failing to provide them with a fair level of benefits. The fairness of the benefits to the host community depends on the burdens and risks it bears and the extent to which others benefit from its participation in the trial.[30] In particular, as the host community assumes greater burdens, or others enjoy greater benefits from its participation, the institutional review board should insist that the host community receive correspondingly greater benefits to ensure a fair trial.

Beforehand, it may be unclear whether the tested method, even if proved effective, will be implemented in the host community. In such cases, the fact that the trial addresses an important

health concern may not in itself offer a fair level of benefits. Similarly, trials may produce so much benefit for others that the information provided to the host community does not represent a fair proportion of the overall benefits.[11] In these cases, the host community should receive additional benefits, such as development of clinics or training of nurses, to ensure that the overall benefits it receives are fair given the burdens it experiences and the benefits others receive from its participation.[30]

The need for a fair level of benefits highlights the fact that a ban on research using less than the worldwide best methods, although intended to *minimize* the potential for exploitation, may *increase* it in practice. To ensure that the host community receives sufficient benefits, investigators might focus their research on methods that the host communities can implement, if proved successful. Insisting that investigators use the worldwide best methods may force them to abandon these attempts to assess methods that can be implemented in the host communities, thereby increasing the chances for exploitation.

SUBJECT AND HOST COMMUNITY NONMALEFICENCE

The principle of nonmaleficence implies that research using less than the best methods should be allowed only when it will not make research subjects or the host community prospectively worse off.[31] To satisfy this

requirement, such research should not harm the existing health care system. For instance, research should not rely on nurses or laboratories that are needed to care for patients in the host community. Second, it is important to ensure that research using less than the worldwide best methods does not make subjects prospectively worse off than they would be in the absence of the trial. Provided there is clinical equipoise between the proposed new treatment and the local methods of care, individuals who enroll will receive either the methods they would have received otherwise, if any, or a method not known to be inferior to it.[32] When this condition is met, research participation can offer subjects an important benefit by providing access to medical interventions not otherwise available to them.

Satisfaction of these 4 conditions—scientific necessity, host country relevance, sufficient benefit, nonmaleficence—ensures that research using less than the worldwide best methods addresses an important health concern of the host community and offers the host community sufficient benefit without making subjects worse off. This potential to help the world's poor provides an important ethical argument in favor of allowing such research.

POSSIBLE OBJECTIONS

1. *These trials violate investigators' clinical obligations.* The US National Bioethics Advisory Commission and others argue that researchers gain moral obli-

gations to provide the best care possible when they enter into clinical relationships with research subjects.[31,33–35] This view implies that investigators should not conduct research using less than the best methods even when it satisfies the 4 conditions outlined: a potential for future benefit, no matter how great, cannot justify the violation of researchers' obligations to provide present subjects with the best methods. Although this argument seems compelling, it is not clear that it accurately reflects clinicians' obligations.

Clearly, investigators have clinical obligations that go beyond the scientific needs of particular research trials. Investigators cannot justify trials using less than the best methods simply by arguing that in the absence of the trial, subjects would receive nothing. For instance, an investigator working in the developing world cannot decide against providing her subjects with cardiopulmonary resuscitation at little or no cost simply on the grounds that, in her absence, they would not receive it. At the same time, investigators' clinical obligations do not seem to imply they must provide the worldwide best methods in all cases. It is widely agreed that investigators assessing whether aspirin reduces mortality from heart attacks in a developing country would not be required to provide subjects with coronary artery bypass surgery,[36] much less coronary intensive care in case of a myocardial infarction.[37] What implications does the fact that clinicians need not provide these worldwide best

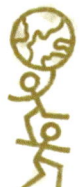

methods have for the standard of care debate?

One's moral obligations depend in part on the costs associated with the available alternatives.[38–40] Whether I have a moral obligation to save a drowning child depends upon what is required, and what I must forgo. If I can save the child at little or no cost to myself or others, then I am obligated to do so. If saving the child would put me at great risk of death, or prevent me from saving several other children, I am not obligated to do so.

Physicians' obligations to their patients are similarly shaped by the relevant costs. This is obvious, although often implicit, in the context of standard medical care. To take an example relevant to developing countries, the Elizabeth Glaser Pediatric AIDS Foundation devoted a $100 million grant from the US Agency for International Development to blocking vertical transmission of HIV from mother to child in the developing world.[41] Long-course AZT therapy (the 076 regimen) is the worldwide best method for blocking vertical transmission of HIV from mother to child. Hence, the claim that clinicians are obligated to provide those for whom they care with the best methods implies that the clinicians working on this project are obligated to provide long-course AZT to block vertical transmission of HIV.

Assuming a cost of $250 per mother–child pair treated, provision of long-course AZT would translate into approximately 65 000 fewer HIV-infected children compared with the back-

ground infection rate without treatment. Conversely, devoting the same money to single-dose nevirapine, at $4 per mother–child pair, translates into approximately 270 000 fewer HIV-infected children compared with the background infection rate without treatment. That is, providing nevirapine rather than long-course AZT has the potential to save an additional 200 000 lives.

This difference supports the claim that the foundation made the ethically appropriate choice—supply nevirapine—even though its decision entails that the foundation's clinicians will fail to provide the worldwide best methods to block vertical transmission when they could have done so. This conclusion suggests that the provision of less than the best methods can be consistent with physicians' clinical obligations when providing the best methods would entail unacceptably high costs. Determining exactly how high the associated costs must be to justify providing less than the best methods will be difficult, and institutional review boards will have to use their judgment. Under the proposed 4 conditions, researchers may use less than the best methods only when their use is scientifically necessary to address an important health concern of the host community. Insisting that researchers provide all subjects with the best methods in such cases would entail a high cost, represented by the importance of the health concern that thereby goes unaddressed.

2. *These trials rely on a double standard.* Some commentators

argue that it is unethical to conduct research in the *developed* world using less than the best methods. Hence, allowing such trials in the *developing* world relies on a double standard: "Acceptance of a standard of care that does not conform to the standard in the sponsoring country results in a double standard in research. Such a double standard . . . permits research designs that are unacceptable in the sponsoring country."[8(p854)]

The fact that a particular trial design is allowed in one place but not another does not in itself constitute a double standard.[42] For there may be relevant differences—environmental, genetic, social, cultural differences—that render the same design acceptable in one place, but not the other. To take a straightforward example, no one would argue that approving research using bovine-derived drugs in the United States but not in India constitutes an ethical double standard.

Because patients in developed countries typically have access to the worldwide best methods, research using less than the best methods typically does not have sufficient social value to justify its risks. In contrast, such research may have sufficient social value in developing countries, where the existing standard of care is something less than the worldwide best. This suggests that research using less than the worldwide best methods can be ethically acceptable in developing countries, even though the very same research would be unethical in a developed country.

Furthermore, when a developed country makes a reasonable decision not to provide a worldwide best treatment on grounds of cost-effectiveness, it may be acceptable to conduct research in that country on less effective methods.[43] For instance, a new type of erythropoietin has been developed that is expected to be as effective as existing versions for postchemotherapy supportive care, and more easily administered. During the time this newer drug is on patent, it is likely to be very expensive, and a developed country may decide on cost-effectiveness grounds to provide its citizens with the older, less-convenient version. Assuming this decision is a reasonable one, it seems ethically acceptable to conduct trials in that country that compare proposed new treatments to the older version, rather than the worldwide best version.

3. *These trials are counterproductive.* Some critics argue that research using less than the best methods may be counterproductive, reducing pressure on host governments to reform, or pharmaceutical companies to provide treatments at an affordable price. "The issue of the affordability of drugs should be tackled by getting governments, pharmaceutical companies, donors, and other international agencies to cooperate in making drugs cheaper rather than by looking for other, probably inferior, regimens for people in less-developed countries."[44(p842)]

This possibility highlights the importance of assessing the ethical acceptability of research

HEALTH POLICY AND ETHICS FORUM

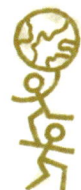

using less than the best methods in light of *all* feasible alternatives. If an individual study, or even series of studies using less than the worldwide best methods would impair a realistic chance that the host country will receive state-of-the-art health care for the condition under study, such studies should be prohibited. However, when there are no realistic alternatives for the foreseeable future to address the health concern in question, use of less than the worldwide best methods may represent the best hope for the host communities. Here too, institutional review boards must use their judgment. What are the chances that the research use of less than the best methods will lead to the development of a feasible and economical treatment? What are the chances, in the absence of these trials, that the best methods will be provided for the condition in question?

SUMMARY

Critics rightly point out that research using less than the worldwide best methods has the potential to be scientifically unnecessary, counterproductive, exploitive, inconsistent with investigators' clinical obligations, and based on an ethical double standard. Fortunately, these possibilities, although important, are not inevitable. Investigators should be allowed to use less than the worldwide best methods only when doing so is ethically appropriate and has the potential to provide sufficient benefit for the host communities.

Specifically, institutional review boards should assume a default of requiring the best methods in all cases and approve research using less than the worldwide best methods only when it satisfies the following 4 conditions: (1) scientific necessity: investigators must use less than the worldwide best methods to answer the scientific question posed by the trial; (2) relevance for the host community: answering the scientific question posed by the trial will help address an important health need of the host community; (3) sufficient host community benefit: the trial will produce a fair level of benefit for the host community; and (4) subject and host community nonmaleficence: subjects and the host community will not be made prospectively worse off than they would be in the absence of the trial. ■

About the Authors

The authors are with the Department of Clinical Bioethics at the National Institutes of Health, Bethesda, Md. Reidar K. Lie is also with the Department of Public Health and Primary Health Care, University of Bergen, Norway.

Requests for reprints should be sent to David Wendler, PhD, Department of Clinical Bioethics, National Institutes of Health, Building 10, Room 1C118, Bethesda, MD 20892 (e-mail: dwendler@nih.gov).

This article was accepted October 2, 2003.

Note. *The opinions expressed are the authors' own and do not reflect any position or policy of the National Institutes of Health, Public Health Service, or Department of Health and Human Services.*

Contributors

D. Wendler conceived the project and wrote the first draft of the article. All the authors helped revise the article.

Acknowledgments

The work for this project was completed as part of the authors' responsibilities as employees of the National Institutes of Health.

References

1. Macklin R. After Helsinki: unresolved issues in international research. *Kennedy Inst Ethics J.* 2001;11:17–36.

2. Levine RJ. The "best proven therapeutic method" standard in clinical trials in technologically developing countries. *IRB: Rev Human Subjects Res.* 1998;20:5–9.

3. Lie RK. Ethics of placebo-controlled trials in developing countries. *Bioethics.* 1998;12:307–311.

4. Varmus H, Satcher D. Ethical complexities of conducting research in developing countries. *N Engl J Med.* 1997; 337:1003–1005.

5. Resnik DB. The ethics of HIV research in developing nations. *Bioethics.* 1998;12:286–306.

6. Killen J, Grady C, Folkers GK, Fauci AS. Ethics of clinical research in the developing world. *Nature Rev.* 2002;2:210–215.

7. Declaration of Helsinki, paragraph 29, revised October 2000. Available at: http://www.wma.net/e/home/html. Accessed January 10, 2004.

8. Lurie P, Wolf SM. Unethical trials of methods to reduce perinatal transmission of the human immunodeficiency virus in developing countries. *N Engl J Med.* 1997;337:853–856.

9. Angell M. The ethics of clinical research in the third world. *N Engl J Med.* 1997;337:847–849.

10. Angell M. Ethical imperialism? Ethics in international collaborative clinical research. *N Engl J Med.* 1988;319: 1081–1083.

11. Angell M. Investigators' responsibilities for human subjects in developing countries. *N Engl J Med.* 2000;342: 967–969.

12. Rothman KJ, Michels KB. The continuing unethical use of placebos. *N Engl J Med.* 1994;331:394.

13. Rothman D. The shame of medical research. *The New York Review of Books.* Available at: http://www.nybooks.com/articles/13907. Accessed January 10, 2004.

14. Annas G. Prominent opinion: the ethics of international research trials in the developing world. *J Med Ethics.* 2001;2:7010.

15. Brennan TA. Proposed revisions to the Declaration of Helsinki—will they weaken the ethical principles underlying human research? *N Engl J Med.* 1999; 341:527–531.

16. Shapiro HT, Meslin EM. Ethical issues in the design and conduct of clinical trials in developing countries. *N Engl J Med.* 2001;345:139–142.

17. Dabis F, Msellati P, Meda N, et al. 6-month efficacy, tolerance, and acceptability of a short regimen of oral zidovudine to reduce vertical transmission of HIV in breastfed children in Cote d'Ivoire and Burkina Faso: a double-blind placebo-controlled multicentre trial. *Lancet.* 1999;353:786–792.

18. Karim SSA. Placebo controls in HIV perinatal transmission trials: a South African's viewpoint. *Am J Public Health.* 1998;88:564–566.

19. Conner EM, Sperling RJ, Gelber R, et al. Reduction of maternal–infant transmission of human immunodeficiency virus type 1 with zidovudine treatment. *N Engl J Med.* 1994;331: 1173–1180.

20. Shaffer N, Chuachoowong R, Mock PA, et al. Short-course zidovudine for perinatal HIV-1 transmission in Bangkok, Thailand: a randomized controlled trial. *Lancet.* 1999;353: 773–780.

21. Wiktor SZ, Ekpini E, Karon JM, et al. Short-course oral zidovudine for prevention of mother-to-child transmission of HIV-1 in Abidjan, Cote d'Ivoire: a randomized trial. *Lancet.* 1999; 353: 781–785.

22. Lallemont M, Jourdain G, Le Coeur S, et al. A trial of shortened zidovudine regimens to prevent mother-to-child transmission of human immunodeficiency virus type 1. *N Engl J Med.* 2000;343:982–991.

23. Guay LA, Musoke P, Fleming T, et al. Intrapartum and neonatal single-dose nevirapine compared to zidovudine for prevention of mother-to-child transmission of HIV-1 in Kampala, Uganda: HIVNET 012 randomised trial. *Lancet.* 1999;354:795–802.

24. Rouzioux C, Costagliola D, Burgard M, et al. Estimated timing of mother-to-child human immunodeficiency virus type 1 transmission by use of a Markov model: the HIV infection in newborns

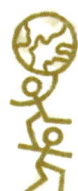

French collaborative study group. *Am J Epidemiol.* 1995;142:1330–1337.

25. Consensus statement. Science, ethics, and the future of research into maternal infant transmission of HIV-1. *Lancet.* 1999;353:832–835.

26. Mirochnick M, Fenton T, Gagnier P, et al. Pharmacokinetics of nevirapine in human immunodeficiency virus type 1–infected pregnant women and their neonates. *J Infect Dis.* 1998;178:368–374.

27. Marseille E, Kahn JG, Mmiro F, et al. Cost effectiveness of a single-dose nevirapine regimen for mothers and babies to decrease vertical HIV-1 transmission in sub-Saharan Africa. *Lancet.* 1999;354:803–809.

28. Jha P, Mills A, Hanson K, et al. Improving the health of the global poor. *Science.* 2002;295:2036–2039.

29. Attaran A, Sachs J. Defining and refining international donor support for combating the AIDS pandemic. *Lancet.* 2002;357:57–61.

30. Participants in the 2001 Conference on Ethical Aspects of Research in Developing Countries. Fair benefits for research in developing countries. *Science.* 2002;298:2133–2134.

31. National Bioethics Advisory Commission. Ethical and policy issues in international research: clinical trials in developing countries. Available at: http://www.georgetown.edu/research/nrcbl/nbac/pubs.html. Accessed January 10, 2004.

32. Freedman B. Equipoise and the ethics of clinical research. *N Engl J Med.* 1987;317:141–145.

33. Lurie P, Wolfe SM. HIVNET nevirapine trials [letter]. *Lancet.* 1999;354:1816.

34. Lurie P, Wolfe SM. Science, ethics, and the future of research into maternal infant transmission of HIV-1 [letter]. *Lancet.* 1999;353:1878–1879.

35. Omene JA. Science, ethics, and the future of research into maternal infant transmission of HIV-1 [letter]. *Lancet.* 1999;353:1878.

36. Bloom BR. The highest attainable standard: ethical issues in AIDS vaccines. *Science.* 1998;279:186–188.

37. Kass N, Faden R. HIV research, ethics, and the developing world. *Am J Public Health.* 1998;88:548–550.

38. Kagan S. *The Limits of Morality.* Oxford, England: Oxford University Press; 1989:64–70.

39. Raz J. *Practical Reason and Norms.* Oxford, England: Oxford University Press; 1975:15–32.

40. Beauchamp T, Childress J. *The Principle of Biomedical Ethics.* 5th ed.

Oxford, England: Oxford University Press; 2001:14–21.

41. Brown D, Faler B. US to give AIDS foundation $100 Million Grant. *Washington Post.* August 1, 2002:A8.

42. Orentlicher D. Universality and its limits: when research ethics can reflect local circumstances. *J Law Med Ethics.* 2002;30:403–410.

43. Freedman B. Placebo-controlled trials and the logic of clinical purpose. *IRB.* 1990;12:1–6.

44. Msamanga G. Letter to the editor. *N Engl J Med.* 1998;338:842.

References

Daley G, Hyun I, Apperley J, Barker R, Benvenisty N, et al. Setting global standards for stem cell research and clinical translation: the 2016 ISSCR Guidelines. Stem Cell Rep. 2016;6:787–97.

Søreide K, Alderson D, Bergenfelz A, Beynon J, Connor S, et al. Strategies to improve clinical research in surgery through international collaboration. Lancet. 2013;382:1140–51.

Yusuf S, Wittes J. Interpreting geographic variations in results of randomized, controlled trials. N Engl J Med. 2016;375(23):2263–71.

Additional Suggested Reading

Benatar S, Daibes I, Tomsons S. Inter-philosophies dialogue: creating a paradigm for global health ethics. Kennedy Inst Ethics J. 2016;26(3):323–346. (*Philosophical look at global health ethics is provided.*)

Daley G, Hyun I, Apperley J, Barker R, Benvenisty N, et al. Setting global standards for stem cell research and clinical translation: the 2016 ISSCR Guidelines. Stem Cell Rep. 2016;6:787–797. (*Stem cell research is an example of self-regulation by an emerging area of science.*)

Folayan M, Peterson K, Haire B, Brown B, Audu K, et al. Debating ethics in HIV research: Gaps between policy and practice in Nigeria. Dev World Bioeth. 2015;15(3):214–225. (*One developing country addresses gaps between policy and practice in an area of research important to the health of their people.*)

Pratt B, Lwin K, Zion D, Nosten F, Loff B, Cheah P Exploitation and community engagement: Can community advisory boards successfully assume a role minimizing exploitation in international research? Dev World Bioeth. 2013;15(1):18–26. (*Community advisory boards to research projects are expected to provide strong recommendations to make international research fair.*)

Appendix: Montreal Statement on Research Integrity in Cross-Boundary Research Collaborations, 2013

3rd World Conference on Research Integrity

Montreal Statement on Research Integrity in Cross-Boundary Research Collaborations, 2013.

Reprinted with permission from the International Council for Science.

© Springer International Publishing AG, part of Springer Nature 2018
A. L. Caplan, B. K. Redman (eds.), *Getting to Good*, https://doi.org/10.1007/978-3-319-51358-4

Montreal Statement on Research Integrity in Cross-Boundary Research Collaborations

Preamble. Research collaborations that cross national, institutional, disciplinary and sector boundaries are important to the advancement of knowledge worldwide. Such collaborations present special challenges for the responsible conduct of research, because they may involve substantial differences in regulatory and legal systems, organizational and funding structures, research cultures, and approaches to training. It is critically important, therefore, that researchers be aware of and able to address such differences, as well as issues related to integrity that might arise in cross-boundary research collaborations. Researchers should adhere to the professional responsibilities set forth in the *Singapore Statement on Research Integrity*. In addition, the following responsibilities are particularly relevant to collaborating partners at the individual and institutional levels and fundamental to the integrity of collaborative research. Fostering the integrity of collaborative research is the responsibility of all individual and institutional partners.

Responsibilities of Individual and Institutional Partners in Cross-Boundary Research Collaborations

General Collaborative Responsibilities

1. Integrity. Collaborating partners should take collective responsibility for the trustworthiness of the overall collaborative research and individual responsibility for the trustworthiness of their own contributions.

2. Trust. The behavior of each collaborating partner should be worthy of the trust of all other partners. Responsibility for establishing and maintaining this level of trust lies with all collaborating partners.

3. Purpose. Collaborative research should be initiated and conducted for purposes that advance knowledge to the benefit of humankind.

4. Goals. Collaborating partners should agree at the outset on the goals of the research. Changes in goals should be negotiated and agreed to by all partners.

Responsibilities in Managing the Collaboration

5. Communication. Collaborating partners should communicate with each other as frequently and openly as necessary to foster full, mutual understanding of the research.

6. Agreements. Agreements that govern collaborative research should be understood and ratified by all collaborating partners. Agreements that unduly or unnecessarily restrict dissemination of data, findings or other research products should be avoided.

7. Compliance with Laws, Policies and Regulations. The collaboration as a whole should be in compliance with all laws, policies and regulations to which it is subject. Collaborating partners should promptly determine how to address conflicting laws, policies or regulations that apply to the research.

8. Costs and Rewards. The costs and rewards of collaborative research should be distributed fairly among collaborating partners.

9. Transparency. Collaborative research should be conducted and its results disseminated transparently and honestly, with as much openness as possible under existing agreements. Sources of funding should be fully and openly declared.

10. Resource Management. Collaborating partners should use human, animal, financial and other resources responsibly.

11. Monitoring. Collaborating partners should monitor the progress of research projects to foster the integrity and the timely completion and dissemination of the work.

Responsibilities in Collaborative Relationships

12. Roles and Responsibilities. Collaborating partners should come to mutual understandings about their roles and responsibilities in the planning, conduct and dissemination of research. Such understandings should be renegotiated when roles or responsibilities change.

13. Customary Practices and Assumptions. Collaborating partners should openly discuss their customary practices and assumptions related to the research. Diversity of perspectives, expertise and methods, and differences in customary practices, standards and assumptions that could compromise the integrity of the research should be addressed openly.

14. Conflict. Collaborating partners should seek prompt resolution of conflicts, disagreements and misunderstandings at the individual or institutional level.

15. Authority of Representation. Collaborating partners should come to agreement on who has authority to speak on behalf of the collaboration.

Responsibilities for Outcomes of Research

16. Data, Intellectual Property and Research Records. Collaborating partners should come to agreement, at the outset and later as needed, on the use, management, sharing and ownership of data, intellectual property, and research records.

17. Publication. Collaborating partners should come to agreement, at the outset and later as needed, on how publication and other dissemination decisions will be made.

18. Authorship and Acknowledgement. Collaborating partners should come to agreement, at the outset and later as needed, on standards for authorship and acknowledgement of joint research products. The contributions of all partners, especially junior partners, should receive full and appropriate recognition. Publications and other products should state the contributions of all contributing parties.

19. Responding to Irresponsible Research Practices. The collaboration as a whole should have procedures in place for responding to allegations of misconduct or other irresponsible research practice by any of its members. Collaborating partners should promptly take appropriate action when misconduct or other irresponsible research practice by any partner is suspected or confirmed.

20. Accountability. Collaborating partners should be accountable to each other, to funders and to other stakeholders in the accomplishment of the research.

The Montreal Statement on Research Integrity in Cross-Boundary Research Collaborations was developed as part of the 3rd World Conference on Research Integrity, 5-8 May 2013, in Montréal, as a global guide to the responsible conduct of research. It is not a regulatory document and does not represent the official policies of the countries or organizations that funded or participated in the Conference.

Index

A
Accumulation of evidence, 1
Authorship
    article retraction, 173
    correction/retraction, 173
    ethical responsibilities, 173
    ghost, 173
    honorary, 173
    ICMJE criteria, 173
    inclusion/exclusion, 173
    inflation, 216–219
    integrity, 173
    order and inclusion/exclusion, 173
    pre-study, 173
    publications, 173
    third party sign-off, 173
Avoiding plagiarism, 289–351

B
Barn door, 224–232
Belmont report, 162–169
Biobanking
    biological specimens, 515
    heel-stick screening, 515
    policies and procedures, 515
Bio-specimens, 530–538
Biomedical sciences, 224–232
Biomedical workforce, 249–250
Bogus stem cell therapies, 549
Bone morphogenetic proteins
    in spine, 9–20

C
Campbell, E., 465
Cancer genome data, 539–546
Care debate, 570–575
Caplan, A.L., 1, 51, 95, 113, 173, 223, 261, 371, 385,
    435, 465, 515, 549
Common data elements, 516

Conflict of interest (COI), 435
    advices, 466
    description, 465
    IRB members, 465, 466
    MA, 465
    potentiality, 465
    situations, 465
Council for International Organizations of Medical
    Sciences (CIOMS), 113

D
Data acquisition, 516
Data infrastructure, 515
Data monitoring committees, 142–148
Data safety monitoring boards (DSMBs), 113
Data sharing, 515, 516
Detrimental research practices, 177–183

E
Elliott, C., 465
The Endless Frontier, 52–54
Ethical modernization, 394–417
Ethical review
    in South Asia, 133–140
Ethics reforms in Korea, 394–417
European Medicines Agency, 516

F
Fabrication, 385
Falsification, 385
Financial incentives, 74–76
Flint water crisis, 78–93
Format issues, 515

G
Gene therapy, 490–497
Ghost authorship, 173

© Springer International Publishing AG, part of Springer Nature 2018
A. L. Caplan, B. K. Redman (eds.), *Getting to Good*, https://doi.org/10.1007/978-3-319-51358-4

Global research, 549
Grinnell, F., 1
Guatemala STD experiments, 59–69

H
H3Africa policy framework, 550–552
Heterogeneity of disease, 1
Honorary authorship, 173
Human subjects' protection, 435
    Belmont report, 113
    CIOMS, 113
    Food and Drug Administration, 113
    IRB review, 113
    scientific review committees, 113
    virtuous investigator, 113
    vulnerable groups, 113

I
Industry support of medical research, 506–512
Infuse trials, 41–47
Institutional conflicts of interest, 465
Institutional review board (IRB)
    animal care and use committees, 113
    goal, 113
    institutions/trials, 113
    OHRP, 113
International Council of Medical Journal Editors (ICMJE), 173
International Society for Stem Cell Research, 549
Irreproducibility
    biological systems, 95
    outcome assessment, 95
    reagents and antibodies, 95
    systematic reviews, 95

L
Low and middle income countries (LMICs)
    central IRB, 549
    clinical trials, 549
    community engagement, 549
    health services research, 549
    multi-national research, 549
    research capacity, 549
    surgical trials, 549

M
Mentee, mentor-relationship, 223
    Mentor projectsmentee relationship, 223
    in research, 223
    quality of experience, 223
Mentorship, 256–258
Meta-analyses (MA), 465
Multiple sclerosis therapeutics, 498–504

N
National Caries Program (NCP), 467–489
National Institute of Dental Research (NIDR), 467–489
National Institute of Neurological Disorders and Stroke (NINDS), 516
National Institute of Health (NIH) research, 59–69
Non-commercial clinical trials, 554–560

O
Office of Human Research Protections (OHRP), 113
Office of Research Integrity (ORI), 173, 234–248, 385
OpenTrials movement, 516–528
Ornithine transcarbamylase deficiency, 490–497

P
Peer review, 372–375
    date editorial, 371
    double-blind, 371
    erroneous rejection, 371
    mentors, 371
    post-publication review, 371
    quality control, 371
    quality of scientific work, 371
    research integrity, 371
    reviewer comments, 371
    single-blind, 371
    studies, 371
Pharmaceutical marketing, 208–214
Pharmaceuticalisation
    in South Asia, 133–140
Physician conflict of interest, 498–504
Plagiarism, 262–272, 385
    acquisition, 261
    "Dear Plagiarist", 261
    electronic tools, 261
    frequency, 261
    language development, 261
    literature, 261
    research integrity, 261
    screening, 261
Policies and research ethics frameworks, 549
Post-publication culture, 376–378
Post-publication peer review, 380–383
Practice of science, 23–39
Predatory journals, 173
Pregnant women, 150–160
Professional responsibility, 251–255
Publication-pollution denialism, 174–176
Published research findings, 2–8

Q
Quality time, 107–110

R
Randomized placebo-controlled
        trial (RCT), 1
    Reproducibility, 96–101, 103–106
    independent investigators, 95
    integrity, 95
    and irreproducibility, 95
    reaffirming scientific standards, 95
    reliability, 95
    replication, 95
    reviewer, 95
    scientific practices, 95
Research agenda capture, 465
Research ethics, 114–129
Research integrity, 23–39, 429–432
Research integrity officers (RIOs), 435

Research methods
    accumulating evidence, 1
    allied discipline, 1
    clinical trial, 1
    multiple therapies, 1
    scientific memoir, 1
    scientific practice, 1
    trial recruitment, 1
Research misconduct, 177–183, 435
    and data fraud, 421–427
    developing policies, 385
    ethics reforms in Korea, 394–417
    FFP, 386
    finding of, 385
    Japan, 385
    integrity, 436–452
    in medical research, 387–393
    mentoring, 234–248
    PHS agencies, 385
    scandalous cases, 385
    statistical anomalies, 385
    trainees, 224–232
    the United Kingdom, 385
Resnik, D., 465
Responsible conduct of research (RCR), 223

S
Self-plagiarism, 289–351
Science policy
    contract flows notion, 51
    evolving form, 51
    political discourse, 51
    public audience, 51
    public resources, 51
    science self-governance yielded regulations, 51
Science self-governance yielded regulations
    human and animal subjects protection, 51
    public accountability, 51

Second-language writing, 261
Self-plagiarism, 261
Self-regulation, 435
Siu, L., 515
South Asia
    pharmaceuticalisation and ethical review, 133–140
Spine
    bone morphogenetic proteins, 9–20
Stigma, 549
Systematic review, 190–205

T
Text-based plagiarism, 274–286
Trial repositories, 516

U
US Office of Human Research Protection website, 549

W
Whistleblower, 453–455
    Commission on Research Integrity, 435
    competitor's program, 435
    description, 435
    ethical integrity, 435
    FFP, 435
    institution/organization and society, 435
    regulatory area, 435
    research integrity, 435
    Woo Suk Hwang case, 435
Woo Suk Hwang case, 435

Z
Zika vaccines, 150–160